Informatik aktuell

Herausgeber: W. Brauer
im Auftrag der Gesellschaft für Informatik (GI)

Hans-Peter Meinzer Thomas M. Deserno
Heinz Handels Thomas Tolxdorff (Hrsg.)

Bildverarbeitung für die Medizin 2009

Algorithmen – Systeme – Anwendungen

Proceedings des Workshops
vom 22. bis 25. März 2009 in Heidelberg

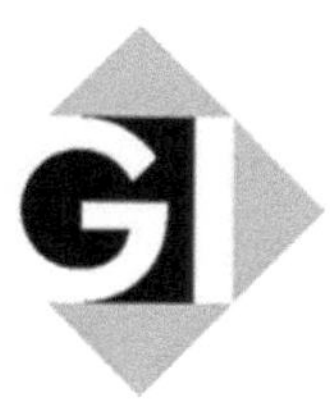

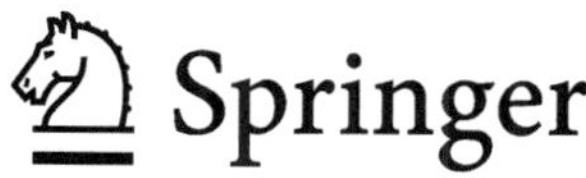

Herausgeber

Hans-Peter Meinzer
Deutsches Krebsforschungszentrum
Abteilung für Medizinische und Biologische Informatik / H0100
Im Neuenheimer Feld 280, 69120 Heidelberg

Thomas Martin Deserno, geb. Lehmann
Rheinisch-Westfälische Technische Hochschule Aachen
Universitätsklinikum Aachen
Institut für Medizinische Informatik
Pauwelsstraße 30, 52074 Aachen

Heinz Handels
Universität Hamburg
Universitätsklinikum Hamburg-Eppendorf
Institut für Medizinische Informatik
Martinistraße 52, 20246 Hamburg

Thomas Tolxdorff
Charité – Universitätsmedizin Berlin
Institut für Medizinische Informatik
Hindenburgdamm 30, 12200 Berlin

Bibliographische Information der Deutschen Bibliothek
Die Deutsche Bibliothek verzeichnet diese Publikation in der Deutschen Nationalbibliografie; detaillierte bibliografische Daten sind im Internet über http://dnb.ddb.de abrufbar.

CR Subject Classification (1998): A.0, H.3, I.4, I.5, J.3, H.3.1, I.2.10, I.3.3, I.3.5, I.3.7, I.3.8, I.6.3

ISSN 1431-472-X
ISBN 978-3-540-93859-0 Springer Berlin Heidelberg New York

Springer Berlin Heidelberg New York
Springer ist ein Unternehmen von Springer Science+Business Media

springer.de

Printed in Germany

Satz: Reproduktionsfertige Vorlage vom Autor/Herausgeber
Gedruckt auf säurefreiem Papier SPIN: 12603060 33/3142-543210

Bildverarbeitung für die Medizin 2009

Veranstalter

DKFZ	Abteilung Medizinische und Biologische Informatik Deutsches Krebsforschungszentrum (DKFZ), Heidelberg
BVMI	Berufsverband Medizinischer Informatiker
DAGM	Deutsche Arbeitsgemeinschaft für Mustererkennung
DGBMT	Fachgruppe Medizinische Informatik der Deutschen Gesellschaft für Biomedizinische Technik im VDE
GI	Fachgruppe Imaging und Visualisierungstechniken der Gesellschaft für Informatik
GMDS	Arbeitsgruppe Medizinische Bild- und Signalverarbeitung der Gesellschaft für Medizinische Informatik, Biometrie und Epidemiologie
IEEE	Joint Chapter Engineering in Medicine and Biology, German Section
DGaO	Deutsche Gesellschaft für angewandte Optik

Tagungsvorsitz

Prof. Dr. Hans-Peter Meinzer

Abteilung Medizinische und Biologische Informatik
Deutsches Krebsforschungszentrum (DKFZ), Heidelberg

Lokale Organisation

Ingmar Wegner
Stefanie Hauser
Alexander Seitel
Uwe Engelmann
u.v.m.

Abteilung Medizinische und Biologische Informatik
Deutsches Krebsforschungszentrum (DKFZ), Heidelberg

Verteilte BVM-Organisation

Prof. Dr. Thomas M. Deserno, Jens Hoffmann
Rheinisch-Westfälische Technische Hochschule Aachen (Tagungsband)

Prof. Dr. Heinz Handels, Dipl.-Ing. Martin Riemer
Universitätsklinkum Hamburg-Eppendorf (Begutachtung)

Prof. Dr. Hans-Peter Meinzer, Dipl. Inform. Alexander Seitel
Deutsches Krebsforschungszentrum Heidelberg (Anmeldung)

Prof. Dr. Thomas Tolxdorff, Dagmar Stiller
Charité – Universitätsmedizin Berlin (Internetpräsenz)

Programmkomitee

Prof. Dr. Til Aach, Rheinisch-Westfälische Technische Hochschule Aachen
Prof. Dr. Reto Bale, Medizinische Universität Innsbruck
Prof. Dr. Dirk Bartz, Universität Leipzig
Prof. Dr. Dr. Johannes Bernarding, Universität Magdeburg
Priv.-Doz. Dr. Jürgen Braun, Charité – Universitätsmedizin Berlin
Prof. Dr. Thorsten M. Buzug, Universität zu Lübeck
Prof. Dr. Florian Dammann, Klinikum Göppingen
Prof. Dr. Thomas M. Deserno, Rheinisch-Westfälische Technische Hochschule Aachen
Prof. Dr. Hartmut Dickhaus, Universität Heidelberg
Dr. Jan Ehrhardt, Universitätsklinikum Hamburg-Eppendorf
Prof. Dr. Dr. Karl-Hans Englmeier, GSF Forschungszentrum München
Prof. Dr. Rudolf Fahlbusch, International Neuroscience Institute Hannover
Prof. Dr. Bernd Fischer, Universität zu Lübeck
Prof. Dr. Heinz Handels, Universitätsklinkum Hamburg-Eppendorf
Priv.-Doz. Dr. Peter Hastreiter, Universität Erlangen-Nürnberg
Prof. Dr. Jürgen Hoffmann, Universität Tübingen
Prof. Dr. Alexander Horsch, Technische Universität München & Universität Tromsø, Norwegen
Dr. Stephan Jacobs, Universität Leipzig
Prof. Dr. Dr. Hans-Gerd Lipinski, Fachhochschule Dortmund
Dr. Omid Majdani, Medizinische Hochschule Hannover
Prof. Dr. Jürgen Meixensberger, Universität Leipzig
Prof. Dr. Hans-Peter Meinzer, Deutsches Krebsforschungszentrum Heidelberg
Prof. Dr. Heinrich Müller, Universität Dortmund
Priv.-Doz. Dr. Arya Nabavi, Universität Kiel
Prof. Dr. Nassir Navab, Technische Universität München
Prof. em. Dr. Heinrich Niemann, Universität Erlangen-Nürnberg
Prof. Dr. Dietrich Paulus, Universität Koblenz-Landau
Prof. Dr. Heinz-Otto Peitgen, Universität Bremen
Prof. Dr. Dr. Siegfried J. Pöppl, Universität zu Lübeck
Prof. Dr. Bernhard Preim, Universität Magdeburg
Prof. Dr. Karl Rohr, Universität & Dt. Krebsforschungszentrum Heidelberg
Prof. Dr. Georgios Sakas, Fraunhofer Institut Darmstadt
Prof. Dr. Dietmar Saupe, Universität Konstanz
Prof. Dr. Jörg Schipper, Universität Düsseldorf
Prof. Dr. Rainer Schubert, Private Universität für Gesundheitswissenschaften, Medizinische Informatik und Technik Innsbruck
Prof. Dr. Uwe Spetzger, Universität Leipzig
Prof. Dr. Thomas Tolxdorff, Charité – Universitätsmedizin Berlin
Prof. Dr. Axel Wismüller, University of Rochester, New York, USA
Prof. Dr. Herbert Witte, Universität Jena
Dr. Thomas Wittenberg, Fraunhofer Institut Erlangen
Prof. Dr. Ivo Wolf, Hochschule Mannheim

Preisträger des BVM-Workshops 2008 in Berlin

Erstmalig wurde auf der BVM 2008 der mit 1.000 € dotierte BVM-Award an eine herausragende Diplom-, Bachelor-, Master- oder Doktorarbeit aus dem Bereich der Medizinischen Bildverarbeitung vergeben. Die je mit einem Preisgeld von 250 € dotierten BVM-Preise zeichnen besonders hervorragende Arbeiten aus, die auf dem Workshop präsentiert wurden.

BVM-Award 2008 für seine herausragende Diplomarbeit

Alexander Schmidt-Richberg (Universitätsklinikum Hamburg-Eppendorf)
Variationeller Ansatz für eine integrierte Segmentierung und nicht-lineare Registrierung

BVM-Preis 2008 für die beste wissenschaftliche Arbeit

Stefan Wörz mit *Winz ML, Rohr K* (Universität & DKFZ Heidelberg)
Geometric alignment of 2D gel electrophoresis images

BVM-Preis 2008 für den besten Vortrag

Lena Maier-Hein mit *Tekbas A, Seitel A, Pianka F, Müller SA, Schawo S, Radeleff B, Tetzlaff R, Franz AM, Rau AM, Wolf I, Kauczor HU, Schmied BM, Meinzer HP* (DKFZ & Universität Heidelberg)
In-vivo targeting of liver lesions with a navigation system based on fiducial needles

BVM-Preis 2008 für die beste Posterpräsentation

Nils Papenberg mit *Modersitzki J, Fischer B* (Universität zu Lübeck)
Registrierung im Fokus

Danksagung

Die Herausgeber dieser Proceedings verzichten auf das sonst übliche Vorwort, um mehr Platz für Beiträge zu haben. Dennoch möchten wir allen herzlich danken, die zum Gelingen des BVM-Workshops 2009 beigetragen haben: den Mitarbeitern des DKFZ Heidelberg für die Organization vor Ort, Frau Dagmar Stiller für die Pflege der Internetpräsentation, Herrn Alexander Seitel für die Pflege des BVM-Emailverteilers und der webgestützten Workshopanmeldung, Herrn Martin Riemer für die web-basierte Durchführung des Reviewingprozesses und Herrn Jens Hoffmann für die Überarbeitung der LaTeX-Styles sowie für die Entwicklung der web-basierten Beitragseinreichung. Dem Springer-Verlag, der nun schon zum zwölften Mal die BVM-Proceedings herausbringt, wollen wir für die gute Kooperation ebenfalls unseren Dank aussprechen; insb. Frau Dorothea Glaunsinger. Für die finanzielle Unterstützung bedanken wir uns herzlich bei unseren Sponsoren, insbesondere der Firma CHILI, die den BVM-Award gestiftet hat.

Inhaltsverzeichnis

Die fortlaufende Nummer am linken Seitenrand entspricht den Beitragsnummern, wie sie im endgültigen Programm des Workshops zu finden sind. Dabei steht V für Vortrag, P für Poster und S für Softwaredemonstration.

Visualisierung

Bildanalyse 1

Segmentierung 1

Bildanalyse 2

Navigation

Registrierung 1

Registrierung 2

Algorithmen 1

Segmentierung 2

Algorithmen 2

Anwendungen 1

Bildanalyse 3

Segmentierung 3

Anwendungen 2

Poster

Softwarepräsentationen

Adapted Transfer Function Design for Coronary Artery Evaluation

Sylvia Glaßer[1], Steffen Oeltze[1], Anja Hennemuth[2], Skadi Wilhelmsen[3], Bernhard Preim[1]

[1]Department of Simulation and Graphics, University of Magdeburg
[2]MeVis Research GmbH, Bremen
[3]Centre of Radiology, University Hospital, Magdeburg
glasser@isg.cs.uni-magdeburg.de

Abstract. We present an approach for adapted transfer function (TF) specification to highlight pathologic changes of the coronary artery vessel wall based on contrast medium-enhanced computed tomography (CT) datasets. The TFs are combined with common visualization techniques for the evaluation of coronary arteries in CT image data. The presented mapping of CT values in Hounsfield Units (HU) to optical properties such as color and opacity leads to a different color coding for different plaque types.

1 Introduction

Coronary artery disease (CAD) is the leading cause of death in western nations [1]. Recent developments in multislice spiral computed tomography (MSCT) allow for a high spatial resolution with short acquisition times and thus for noninvasive evaluation of the coronary arteries. In contrast to conventional angiograms, MSCT image data also enable an assessment of the vessel wall's cross-sectional area. Furthermore, MSCT image data have a great potential for noninvasive identification, characterization, and quantification of atherosclerotic CAD [2].

Atherosclerotic CAD is the result of accumulatations in the artery wall, so-called plaques. They can be classified into soft, fibrous and hard plaques. Soft plaques are prone to rupture and thus very dangerous for the patient, whereas fibrous plaques and hard plaques consist of more dense accumulations and are assumed to be more stable. Hard plaques are characterized by calcium deposits. The quantification of coronary calcium is important in assessing the patient's whole plaque burden. A plaque does not necessarily lead to a significant stenosis. Especially the early states of atherosclerotic CAD can be compensated by a positive remodelling of the vessel wall.

Common strategies for the visualization of the coronary artery tree based on MSCT image data are maximum intensity projection (MIP), multiplanar reformation (MPR), curved multiplanar reformation (CPR) for 2D views and direct volume rendering techniques (DVR) for a 3D view [2, 3, 4]. The mapping from CT values in Houndsfield Units (HU) to optical properties such as color and opacity is described by a transfer function (TF). The windowing function, which is a special instance of a TF, maps an interval of HU values to gray values. The user can manipulate the interval's width and center and thus influence brightness and contrast.

We will present visualization techniques that facilitate a visual separation of hard plaques and highlight the coronary artery wall including soft and fibrous plaques. In contrast to the method presented by Wesarg et. al [5] we also account for non-stenotic plaque deposits. Due to varying HU values of the bloodpool caused by the contrast medium, the TFs have to be adapted to each dataset.

2 Materials and Methods

We developed our techniques based on 12 contrast medium-enhanced MSCT coronary angiograms from a 64-slice scanner (Siemens Sensation 64). For each dataset the segmentation of the coronary artery lumen [6] and the skeleton of the segmentation result were available. For the TF specification the mean density and standard derivation of the bloodpool (μ_{blood}, σ_{blood}) and the vessel wall (μ_{wall}, σ_{wall}) have to be approximated.

2.1 Approximation of blood density values

The segmentation result primarily consists of voxels representing the contrast medium-enhanced blood and is used for the approximation of the blood density distribution. Because of other densities originating from surrounding tissue or interpolation issues, μ_{blood} and σ_{blood} could not be directly derived from the segmentation. The approximation therefore is carried out by means of an iterative reduction of a cost function. Costs are defined as differences between the approximated normal distribution and the distribution of all segmented voxels. Results for μ_{blood} and σ_{blood} indicate that the mean density of the blood strongly differs for each dataset. Thus, a static threshold for a separation of hard plaques from blood is not applicable. We use a threshold s, similar to the threshold of the Agatston score [7]. To avoid overestimation, which may arise due to artifacts or contrast medium accumulation in small branches, we define s as $s = \mu_{\text{blood}} + 3\sigma_{\text{blood}}$.

2.2 Approximation of vessel wall density values

The approximation of the vessel wall density values is based on the evaluation of a coronary artery segment and its skeleton. The vessel wall of this segment is analyzed by means of intensity profile volumes (IPV). The IPV calculation is carried out in 4 steps (Fig. 1):

1. Selection of a long, non-branching segment of the coronary artery tree. The selection is carried out by traversing the skeleton of the segmentation.

2. The real vessel centerline is approximated by the segment skeleton.
3. For each skeleton voxel, n rays perpendicular to the skeleton are casted.
4. The rays are sampled and the sampled intensities are saved in the IPV.

After the IPV extraction, the vessel wall densities can be approximated. For each skeleton voxel, the sampled intensities representing the vessel wall will appear as vertical structures in a slice of the IPV (Fig. 1(b)). The IPV is slicewise convoluted with a Gaussian and a Sobel filter. The convolutions are followed by a search for vertical structures to obtain a sample of vessel wall intensities. Based on this sample, μ_{wall} and σ_{wall} is calculated.

2.3 TF specification

We developed two TFs, the TF_{2D} and the TF_{3D}, for 2D and 3D visualizations. They differ only in the interval size of the vessel wall densities. We use $\mu_{\text{wall}} \pm \sigma_{\text{wall}}$ for the TF_{3D} and $\mu_{\text{wall}} \pm 2\sigma_{\text{wall}}$ for the TF_{2D}. This is motivated by a possible occlusion of inner structures of the vessel wall in 3D visualizations. Therefore, we also use smaller opacity values for the vessel wall for the TF_{3D} than for the TF_{2D}. In comparison, the vessel wall and hard plaques are mapped to higher opacity values, whereas absolute transparency is assigned to the surrounding tissue and the contrast medium-enhanced blood.

We intuitively use colors from beige to white for hard plaques, since these structures usually appear white or light gray in conventional CT-displays. For the vessel wall, we employ a color scale from blue over red to green to provide high contrasts for the visualization of different plaque deposits and thus different densities in the vessel wall.

For a more intuitive view, the TF_{2D} is combined with the windowing TF. The user can now choose interesting HU value intervals by manipulating the parameters of the windowing TF. The CPR and MPR view as well as the 3D spatial variation of the coronary artery tree are linked with each other. On the one

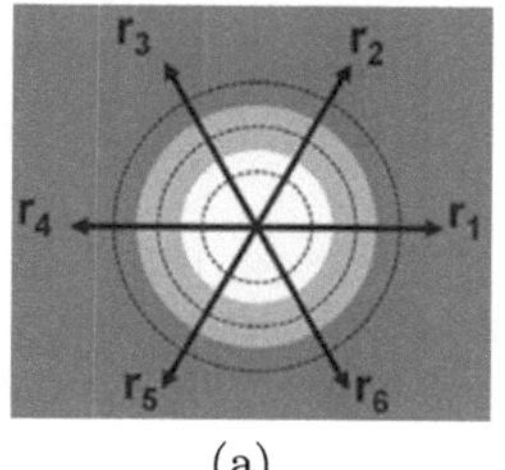

(a)

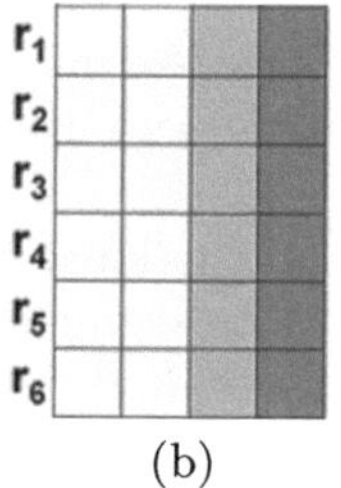

(b)

Fig. 1. Extraction of a slice of the intensity profile volume (IPV). For each voxel v of the skeleton of a vessel segment, n (e.g. 6) rays perpendicular to the centerline are casted (a). Along the rays, intensities are sampled and saved in a slice of the IPV (b). A cross-section of an ideal vessel (white) and the vessel wall (light gray) with surrounding tissue (dark gray) leads to vertical structures in the IPV slice for v. The IPV has as many slices as the number of centerline voxels.

hand, the user can traverse the CPR view with the correspondending MPR view being updated. On the other hand, it is possible to pick an interesting vessel part in the 3D view with the other views being updated accordingly. The presented techniques have been integrated in the MeVisLab platform (www.mevislab.de).

3 Results

For each of the 12 datasets, we created adapted TFs based on the specific parameters μ_{blood}, σ_{blood}, μ_{wall} and σ_{wall}. We combined the adapted TFs with common 2D and 3D visualizations (Fig. 2). Our method highlights not only stenotic plaque deposits, but also displays smaller plaques without a significant stenosis.

3D visualizations show the spatial variation of the coronary artery tree and indicate the patient's whole plaque burden by highlighting all hard plaques (Fig. 2a). In the combined CPR-MPR view, the plaques are highlighted with different colors depending on the plaque type (Fig. 2b).

The methods and visualizations were discussed with an experienced radiologist. First comparisons between conventional views and the TF_{2D} and TF_{3D} color coded visualizations indicate, that hard plaques, especially smaller ones, can be better detected in the colored view. Furthermore, the color coding of the vessel wall with different colors for fibrous and soft plaque deposits gives indications about the plaque type. An absolute identification is impossible due to overlapping density intervalls of these types [8].

4 Discussion

We presented a method for the visualization of the coronary artery wall and atherosclerotic plaque based on adapted TFs. Our method highlights hard plaques and soft and fibrous plaques by color coding of the vessel wall. Also early stages of the CAD consisting of non-stenotic plaque deposits can be visualized. The adapted TFs were combined with common visualization techniques of CT coronary angiograms. An informal evaluation with one radiologist revealed that our method is a useful extension for conventional CT coronary angiogram evaluation.

Problems arise due to the local vessel wall density approximation. Falsifications in MPR views of other segments could be observed in 2 datasets. Potential improvements are the individual creation of a local TF for each vessel segment or a global approximation of the vessel wall density. The highlighting of dense structures such as hard plaques leads to the highlighting of coronary stents as well. A further improvement of the visualization could be the segmentation of stents in a preprocessing step.

Acknowledgement. We thank Dr. Stephan Achenbach (University of Erlangen-Nürnberg, Germany) for providing the image data and MeVis Research for providing advanced MeVisLab features.

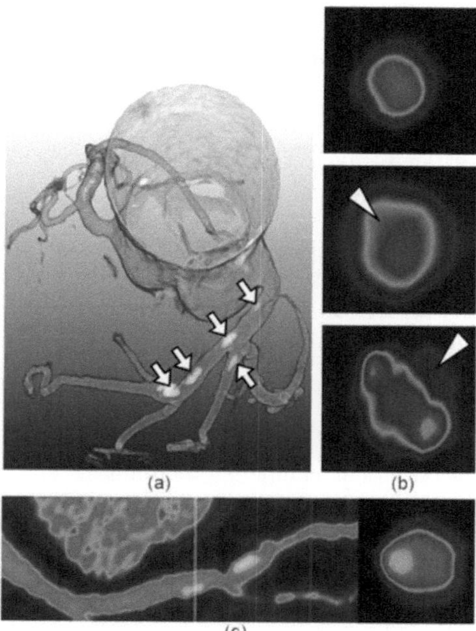

Fig. 2. Visualizations of coronary arteries with adapted TFs. (a) DVR visualization provides an overview about the spatial variation and of hard plaques (arrows). (b) MRP views provide cross-sectional views of the coronary artery walls. The type of the plaque (arrowheads) may be inferred from the color coding: MPR view without plaques (top), greenish colors indicate fibrous plaques (middle) and pinkish colors indicate soft plaques, which are prone to rupture (bottom). (c) shows the combined CPR-MPR view. The transparent white bar indicates the current position in the CPR view (left) of the cross-sectional MPR view (right).

References

1. American Heart Association. Heart disease and stroke statistics - 2007 update. Circulation. 2007;115:e69–e171.
2. Schoepf UJ, Becker CR, Ohnesorge BM, et al. CT of coronary artery disease. Radiology. 2004;232(1):18–37.
3. Kanitsar A, Fleischmann D, Wegenkittl R, et al. CPR - curved planar reformation. Proc IEEE Vis. 2002; p. 37–44.
4. Straka M, Cervenansky M, Cruz AL, et al. The VesselGlyph: Focus & context visualization in CT-angiography. Proc IEEE Vis. 2004; p. 385–392.
5. Wesarg S, Fawad Khan M, Firle EA. Localizing calcifications in cardiac CT data sets using a new vessel segmentation approach. J Digit Imaging. 2006;19(3):249–257.
6. Hennemuth A, Boskamp T, Fritz D, et al. One-click coronary tree segmentation in CT angiographic images. LNCS. 2005;1281:317–21.
7. Agatston AS, Janowitz WR, Hildner FJ, et al. Quantification of coronary artery calcium using ultrafast computed tomography. J Am Coll Cardiol. 1990;15(4):827–832.
8. Pohle K, Achenbach S, MacNeill B, et al. Characterization of non-calcified coronary atherosclerotic plaque by multi-detector row CT: Comparison to IVUS. Atherosclerosis. 2007;190:174–180.

Multimodal Visualization of DTI and fMRI Data Using Illustrative Methods

Silvia Born[1], Werner Jainek[1], Mario Hlawitschka[2], Gerik Scheuermann[3], Christos Trantakis[4], Jürgen Meixensberger[4], Dirk Bartz[1]

[1]ICCAS / VCM, Universität Leipzig
[2]Institute for Data Analysis and Visualization, University of California, Davis, USA
[3]Institut für Informatik, Universität Leipzig
[4]Klinik für Neurochirurgie, Universitätsklinikum Leipzig
silvia.born@iccas.de

Abstract. Designing multimodal visualizations combining anatomical and functional brain data is a demanding task. Jainek et al. [1] applied illustrative rendering techniques to obtain a high-quality representation of the location and characteristic of brain activation areas (derived from MRI and fMRI). Here, we present the integration of DTI data into this system. Reconstructed nerve fibers connecting functional areas with each other and lower brain areas are embedded into the complex rendering pipeline. Further, we enhanced perception of depth and shape by applying silhouettes and dithered halftoning.

1 Introduction

Exploring the brain's anatomy and function with advanced imaging modalities is common practice in medicine and the neurosciences. Multimodal visualizations of these imaging data constitute supportive tools for clinicians and researchers, because they contain all relevant information, are easy to grasp and provide new insight into the known data (concerning, e.g., spatial relationships). However, deriving these visualizations of high quality is a challenging task and an issue of ongoing research. Numerous such multimodal brain visualizations exist (such as [2, 3]) , but (to our knowledge) no illustrative approaches have been employed so far. However, they appear to be quite suitable for this task, since the goal of these methods is to mimic hand-drawn sketches (as, e.g., in anatomy atlases) and discern important from unimportant information by emphasizing major features and neglecting irrelevant details. In this paper, we, therefore, present our illustrative approach of multimodal brain visualization. Our goal is to represent the location of brain functionalities (MRI and fMRI data) and the course of connecting fiber tracts (reconstructed from DTI data), while avoiding visual clutter. Further, we aim at conveying information about the connectivity of different brain areas. The latter is especially important for understanding brain anatomy and function but also for the planning of surgical interventions in the clinical context since an injury of these structures can lead to severe neurological deficits beyond the injury of the functional areas itself.

2 Material and methods

The work presented here is based on a system adopting advanced illustrative rendering techniques to obtain high-quality visualizations of anatomical and functional brain data [1]. Interactive frame rates, which are achieved by an efficient GPU implementation, facilitate user interaction and the usage of additional exploration tools such as clipping, distance measurements, and annotations. The presented data is based on a clinical dataset consisting of a T_1-weighted MRI scan, an fMRI sequence (finger tapping), and a DTI dataset (baseline and six gradients). For preprocessing the brain surface, different cortical areas and the border between white and gray matter were segmented in the MRI dataset using Freesurfer [4, 5]. The fMRI dataset was analyzed and the activity map was created.

2.1 Improvement of shape perception

We use illustrative mesh rendering to display brain anatomy. For visualizing brain activity areas, however, direct volume rendering is applied because surface meshes depict only one activation threshold and prevent further insight into the characteristic of the activation itself. A clipping plane divides the brain into an opaque and a transparent part to improve the visibility of the activation areas (see Figure 1). Nevertheless, the exact location of these areas with respect to the cortical surface is still difficult to perceive. For the human visual system,

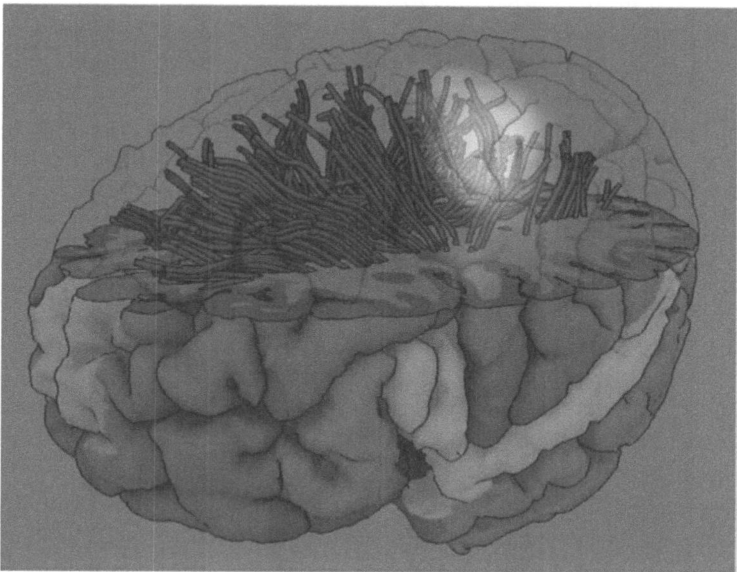

Fig. 1. Combined visualization of cortical anatomy, brain activity (light spot), and nervous pathways.

occlusion and motion parallax are essential cues for depth perception [6]. We enhance these depth cues by emphasizing the shape of the cortical gyri and sulci using silhouettes (detected by depth gradients and normal similarities [7]) and gentle surface shading. For surface shading, a diffuse light source and ambient occlusion shading is used. Langer and Bülthoff revealed that this kind of lighting condition is most appropriate for representing shape from shading and more suitable than, e.g., using a direct light source [8]. Because the cortex surface is rendered transparently, common diffuse shading is hardly visible, and we apply dithered halftoning according to [7]. This illustrative method is capable of conveying diffuse lighting and ambient occlusion shading [9] on transparent surfaces without introducing clutter.

2.2 Integration of nerve fibers

The exploration of diffusion tensor data allows insight into the path of nerve fibers and thus the connectivity of brain areas. Diffusion information can be visualized either directly, e.g., by glyphs [10] or by reconstructed fiber tracts using streamlines or streamtubes [11]. We use streamtubes because they are easier to interprete and provide better depth perception.

For the streamtubes, a second-order tensor field was reconstructed from the six diffusion-weighted DTI scans by a linear least-squares fit [12] using the Stejskal-Tanner formula [13]. Then, fourth-order Runge-Kutta integration is applied to construct the fiber tracts by trilinear interpolation on the tensor field [14]. A lower limit on the fractional anisotropy is used to ensure that fibers are only propagated in areas with anisotropic diffusion characteristic.

The obtained geometrical models are integrated into the scene, which is divided into several layers depending on position of camera, clipping plane, and surface meshes. All layers are rendered into textures for intermediate storage, which are then combined for the final render output. During these steps, the rendering of illustrative elements, such as silhouette detection and shading, is carried out. For further details about the general rendering pipeline, please refer to [1].

3 Results

The final visualization (see Figure 1) gives the user detailed insight into the structure of the brain (e.g., shape of gyri and sulci, position of different cortical areas, the border between white and gray matter, and cortical thickness) and location and characteristic of the fMRI activation areas. Nervous pathways connecting functional areas of interest or leading from functional to lower brain areas, can also be detected rather easily in this visualization. However, fiber tracking is only possible in the white matter, whereas the activation areas are located in the gray matter. Therefore, the visualized connection between nerve fibers and functional areas is no precise but an approximated contact or infiltration.

Fig. 2. Enhancement of shape and depth perception with silhouettes (b) and additional dithered halftoning (c). Applying only slight surface shading on a transparent surface provides hardly any depth cues (a).

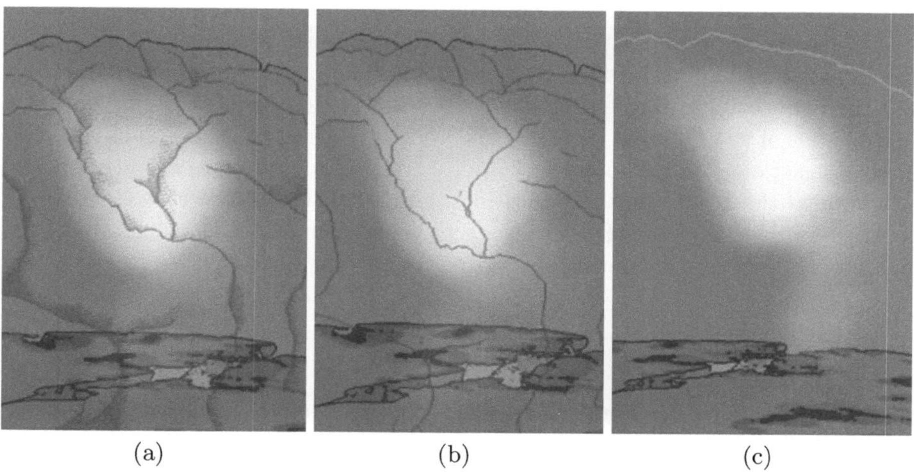

(a) (b) (c)

The enhancements concerning shape and depth perception are displayed in Figure 2. The activation areas are partly occluded by the silhouettes and shaded areas (dithered halftoning) depicting the brain surface. Due to these two effects and motion parallax, which arises during user interaction, the ability to locate these brain functions is improved considerably.

The preprocessing time is rather high, since the segmentation of the MRI data requires several hours of runtime. The fMRI analysis is carried out in the department for neuroradiology. Concerning the DTI data, the creation of the tensor field takes less than one second and the fiber tracking can be computed in about 10 seconds. Per frame a total of about 3.7 million triangles and 180 volume slices are rendered. On a Windows machine (Intel Core 2 Duo Processor T8300 (2.4GHz), 4GB RAM, Nvidia GeForce 8600M GS graphics card) a frame rate of 2.8 is achieved for the visualization as illustrated in Figure 1 (output resolution of 700x700 pixels).

4 Discussion

We have presented an illustrative approach for a combined display of MRI, fMRI, and DTI data. Several methods have been used to include a great amount of information into the visualization, while keeping it uncluttered and easy to understand. Effort has been put into obtaining a good shape perception of the cortical surface and the visualization of the location of brain function. Therefore, the shape of the transparently rendered brain surface has been accentuated by stronger silhouettes and shading effects (dithered halftoning). Furthermore, streamtubes representing nerve fibers have been reconstructed from DTI data and integrated into the visualization system.

Suitable applications are high-quality visualizations of research results in the area of the neurosciences where brain anatomy, function, and especially connectivity play an important role. The integration of further DTI visualization techniques (e.g., illuminated streamlines) conveying brain connectivity are planned.

Moreover, this visualization approach can be applied as a digital and interactive brain atlas helping medical students explore and understand brain anatomy and the connectivity of different areas. In addition to the already implemented annotations of the different cortex areas, adding further structures such as blood vessels, ventricles, or pathologies (tumors) would provide more orientation and insight into the brain anatomy and interconnectivity. In any case, a trade-off between a higher number of structures and visual clutter needs to be found, e.g., by focus-and-context renderings according to specific user queries.

References

1. Jainek W, Born S, Bartz D, et al. Illustrative hybrid visualization and exploration of anatomical and functional brain data. Computer Graphics Forum. 2008;27(3):855–862.
2. Köhn A, Weiler F, Klein J, et al. State-of-the-art computer graphics in neurosurgical planning and risk assessment. Proc Eurographics Short Papers. 2007; p. 117–120.
3. Beyer J, Hadwiger M, Wolfsberger S, et al. High-quality multimodal volume rendering for preoperative planning of neurosurgical interventions. Proc IEEE Visualization. 2007; p. 1696–1703.
4. Fischl B, Liu A, Dale A. Automated manifold surgery: Constructing geometrically accurate and topologically correct models of the human cerebral cortex. IEEE Trans Med Imaging. 2001;20(1):70–80.
5. Fischl B, van der Kouwe A, Destrieux C, et al. Automatically parcellating the human cerebral cortex. Cerebral Cortex. 2004;14:11–22.
6. Goldstein E. Sensation and perception. Belmont: Wadsworth Publishing; 2006.
7. Strothotte T, Schlechtweg S. Non-photorealistic computer graphics. San Francisco: Morgan Kaufman; 2002.
8. Langer M, Bülthoff H. Perception of shape from shading on a cloudy day: Technical report No.73. Tübingen: Max-Planck-Institut für Biologische Kybernetik; 1991.
9. Jainek W. Illustrative Visualization of Brain Structure and Functional MRI Data. Tübingen: Eberhard-Karls-Universität; 2007.
10. Kindlmann G, Westin C. Diffusion tensor visualization with glyph packing. Proc IEEE Visualization. 2006; p. 1329–1335.
11. Zhang S, Demiralp C, Laidlaw D. Visualizing diffusion tensor MR images using streamtubes and streamsurfaces. IEEE Trans Vis Comput Graph. 2003;9(4):454–462.
12. Basser P, LeBihan D. Fiber orientation mapping in an anisotropic medium with NMR diffusion spectroscopy. Proc Ann Meet Soc Magn Reson Med. 1992; p. 1221.
13. Stejskal E, Tanner J. Spin diffusion measurements: Spin echoes in the presence of a time-dependent field gradient. J Chem Phys. 1965;42:288–292.
14. Weickert J, Hagen H. Visualization and Processing of Tensor Fields. Berlin: Springer; 2005.

Automatische Annotation medizinischer 2D- und 3D-Visualisierungen

Konrad Mühler[1], Bernhard Preim[1]

[1]Institut für Simulation und Graphik, Otto-von-Guericke-Universität Magdeburg
muehler@isg.cs.uni-magdeburg.de

Kurzfassung. Wir stellen ein Framework vor, mit dem medizinische 2D- und 3D-Visualisierungen automatisch annotiert werden können. Annotationstexte wie St beirukturbenennungen oder Kurzbefunde werden so in der Darstellung platziert, dass sie gut lesbar sind und keine anderen Texte oder Strukturen verdecken. Weiterhin führen wir Techniken ein, mit denen sich eine Überfrachtung von Schichtbildern mit Annotationen vermeiden lassen. Unser System kommt sowohl in der chirurgischen OP-Planung wie auch in medizinischen Ausbildungssystemen zum Einsatz.

1 Einleitung

Annotationen spielen bei der Gestaltung von verständlichen Visualisierungen eine wichtige Rolle. Sie bereichern diese sowohl um Informationen wie auch um Hinweise zur Lenkung der Aufmerksamkeit. In chirurgischen Planungssystemen können durch Annotationen Informationen zu einzelnen Strukturen direkt in der Visualisierung eingeblendet werden und müssen nicht umständlich aus anderen Quellen entnommen werden. Solche Informationen können beispielsweise Volumina oder Abmaße von Strukturen sowie Kommentare und Kurzbefunde sein. In Trainings- und Lernsystemen sind automatische Annotationen hilfreich, um Lernenden das Auffinden von Strukturen in den noch ungewohnten 3D-Darstellungen zu erleichtern. Neben automatisch in eine Visualisierung eingefügten Annotationen sind auch zusätzliche, durch den Nutzer eingebrachte, Annotationen relevant, z.B. Bemerkungen eines Radiologen für den planenden Chirurgen.

Annotationen sollten bestimmte Voraussetzungen erfüllen: Die zu annotierenden Regionen werden mit einem Ankerpunkt versehen, der über eine Annotationslinie die Verbindung zum Annotationstext (Label) herstellt. Der Label sollte dabei keine anderen Regionen oder Label verdecken. Die verschiedenen Annotationslinien sollten sich nicht schneiden, um die Zuordnung der Label nicht unnötig zu erschweren. Außerdem sollten die Label so nah wie möglich an den annotierten Regionen platziert werden.

Das Problem der automatischen Annotation von Darstellungen wird seit längerem erforscht. Im Bereich von 2D-Darstellungen liegt der Fokus dabei auf der Annotation von geografischen Karten [1]. [2] platzieren sämtliche Annotationen außerhalb an den Rändern einer Darstellung, was allerdings aufgrund der großen

Objekt-Text-Distanz sowie der starken Häufung von Labeln zu einer erschwerten Zuordnung von Annotationen führt. Trotz vieler Verfeinerungen und Optimierungen der Algorithmen ist kein Verfahren bekannt, welches die Besonderheiten von 2D-Schichtbildern mit segmentierten Regionen und die Problematik der schichtbasierten Kohärenz behandelt.

Für 3D-Darstellungen wurden verschiedene Verfahren vorgestellt. [3] und [4] platzieren die Label innerhalb der Objekte und verformen die einzeiligen Label, um sie der Form der Objektes anzupassen. Hier stellt die schwere Lesbarkeit der Label sowohl durch die Verformung als auch die schlechten Kontraste mit den Oberflächen ein großes Problem dar. Verfahren zur externen Annotation polygonaler Modelle stellten [5] und [6] vor. [5] fixierten dabei die Annotationen in festen Regionen links und rechts neben der Visualisierung. Bei [6] werden die sichtbaren Objekte in einem ColorIDBuffer gerendert, um auf dem resultierenden Bild mit Hilfe einer Distanztransformation mögliche Ankerpunkte innerhalb der Objekte zu identifizieren. Der Text wird nach verschiedenen Layoutparadigmen (kreisförmig, links-rechts verteilt) um die Szene angeordnet, wobei Überschneidungen der Verbindungslinien vermieden werden. Das Verfahren ist allerdings auf einzeilige Label und eine kompakte Szene beschränkt.

Als Annotationssysteme für medizinische Bilddaten sind [7], [8] und [9] zu nennen. Bei [7] und [8] können 2D-Schichtbilddaten manuell mit Annotationen versehen werden. Der Nutzer ist dabei selbst für die Platzierung verantwortlich. Auch müssen die Annotationen für jedes Schichtbild einzeln neu ausgeführt werden. [9] stellen ein Annotationssystem für den AnatomyBrowser vor, bei dem die Annotationen für 3D-Darstellungen aus einer bestimmten Sicht neben die Darstellung gestellt werden. Überschneidungen von Verbindungslinien werden nicht berücksichtigt.

2 Methoden

2.1 Automatische Annotation in 2D

Wir haben ein Verfahren entwickelt, mit dem sich segmentierte Strukturen in 2D-Schichtbildern automatisch annotieren lassen. Die Datengrundlage der Regionen bilden dabei die MultiCodedSegmentationMasks [10]. Das Verfahren durchläuft zur Annotation eines Schichtbildes 5 Schritte: (I) Zunächst werden die Zusammenhangskomponenten analysiert, um so die zu annotierenden Regionen und freien Bereiche für die Label zu ermitteln. (II) Mit Hilfe einer Distanztransformation wird für jede Region ein Ankerpunkt bestimmt (der Punkt mit der größten Entfernung zum Rand der Region). (III) Mit Hilfe der Distanztransformation werden anschließend für jeden Label anhand seiner Größe alle möglichen Positionen für eine Platzierung in den freien Bereichen ermittelt. (IV) Die Label werden initial an die Position mit der geringsten Distanz zum jeweiligen Ankerpunkt platziert, um abschließend in mehreren Iterationsschritten mögliche Konflikte wie Überschneidungen zu lösen (V). Dabei wirken sich die im 3. Schritt einmalig ermittelten Platzierungspositionen geschwingikeitssteigernd aus, so dass das gesamte Verfahren in Echtzeit ablaufen kann.

Abb. 1. Annotationen in 2D-Schichtbildern: (a) Annotation wichtiger Strukturen des Halses zur OP-Planung. (b) Annotation von Gefäßen der Leber. Dabei wurden benachbarte Regionen der gleichen Struktur gruppiert und kleine Strukturen eingekreist.

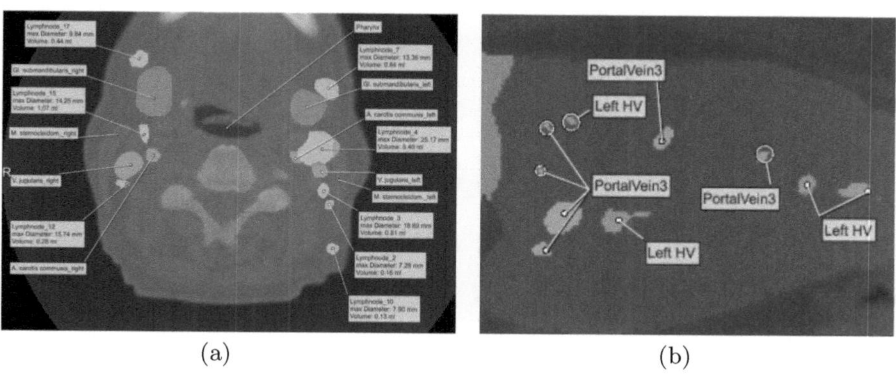

(a) (b)

Gruppierung: Gerade bei vaskulären Strukturen ist es typisch, dass diese in vielen einzelnen, kleineren Regionen in einem Schichtbild auftreten. Aus diesem Grund können Annotationen der gleichen Struktur in unserem Verfahren gruppiert werden, wenn die verschiedenen Ankerpunkte nahe genug beieinander liegen (Abb. 2(b)).

Kleine Strukturen: Sehr kleine, nur wenige Voxel große Regionen würden durch Annotationspunkte und -linien meist vollständig verdeckt werden. Daher werden sehr kleine Regionen mit einem Kreis umschlossen (Abb. 2(b)).

Innere Annotationen: Werden große Teile eines Schichtbildes von einer einzelnen Struktur verdeckt, z.B. dem Leberparenchym, so würden alle Label der innen liegenden Strukturen weit weg von diesen am Rand des Schichtbildes platziert werden müssen, um die große Struktur nicht zu verdecken. Daher berücksichtigt unser Verfahren verschiedene Stufen von Wichtigkeiten einzelner Strukturen. So ist es möglich, dass Label wichtiger Strukturen (z.B. Gefäße) auch Regionen unwichtiger Strukturen überdecken dürfen (z.B. das Leberparenchym).

Kohärenz zwischen Schichtbildern: Wenn die optimalen Positionen der Label für jedes Schichtbild neu berechnet werden, springen die Label beim Durchgehen der Schichtbilder, was störend wirkt und ein Lesen der Label unmöglich macht. Aus diesem Grund berücksichtigt unser Verfahren die im vorherigen Schichtbild durch einen Text belegte Position bei der Neuberechnung. Es wird versucht, den Text solange an dieser Position zu platzieren, wie keine Konflikte oder Überlappungen auftreten und eine Maximaldistanz zum jeweiligen Ankerpunkt nicht überschritten wird.

2.2 Automatische Annotation in 3D

Ein großer Nachteil des Ansatzes von [6] ist die ausschließliche Annotation von sichtbaren Objekten, da eine vollständige Opazität aller Objekte angenommen

Abb. 2. Annotationen in 3D-Visualisierungen: (a) Annotation von Leberterritorien mit ihren Volumina. Der Tumor wurde als sichtbar klassifiziert und daher mit einer normalen Linie annotiert. (b) Annotation der vergrößerten Lymphknoten eines Halses. Für nicht sichtbare Lymphknoten wird per Pfeil die Richtung und Lage angezeigt.

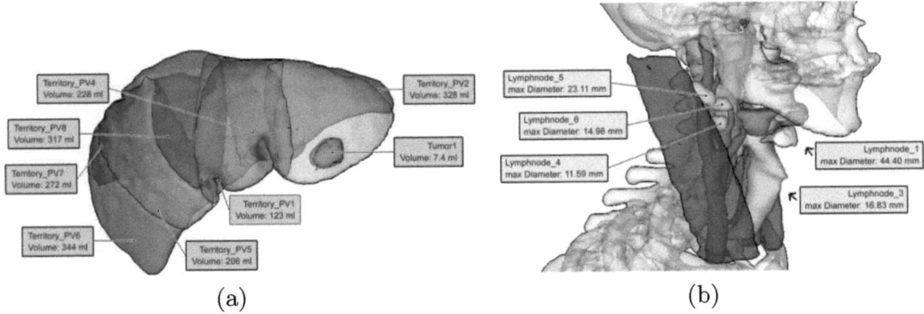

(a) (b)

wird. Dies macht die Annotation von Strukturen unmöglich, die durch stark transparente Strukturen verdeckt werden. Wir haben daher das Verfahren um die Möglichkeit erweitert, Strukturen jeglicher Art zu annotieren. Dazu wird für den Fall, dass kein unverdeckter Bereich der Struktur sichtbar ist, ein Hilfsankerpunkt anstelle des sonst aus der Distanztransformation errechneten Ankerpunktes bestimmt. Dabei hat sich das Zentrum der projizierten Bounding Box der jeweiligen Struktur als gute Annäherung erwiesen. Damit ist zwar nicht in jedem Fall die Lage des Ankerpunktes innerhalb der Struktur gewährleistet – z.B. bei extrem konkaven Strukturen. Jedoch tritt dieser Fall in der praktischen Nutzung kaum auf. Je nach dem Grad der Verdeckung wird ein anderer Annotationsstil genutzt. Um den Grad der Verdeckung zu ermitteln, wird an der Stelle des Hilfsankerpunktes ein Strahl in die Szene geschickt und ermittelt, in welchem Maße die zu annotierende Struktur noch sichtbar ist. Gilt die Struktur dabei als sichtbar, so wird sie mit einer normalen Annotationslinie annotiert. Ist die Struktur nicht mehr sichtbar, soll sie aber dennoch annotiert werden (z.B. um auf ihre Bedeutung hinzuweisen), so weist ein Pfeil anstelle einer Annotationslinie in die Richtung der Struktur (Abb. 2). Der Betrachter bekommt so zum Einen die Existenz einer aktuell verdeckten Struktur vermittelt. Zum Anderen kann er durch Anklicken des Labels eine automatische Kameraneupositionierung erreichen [11], so dass die Struktur sichtbar wird.

3 Ergebnisse

Mit Hilfe unseres Annotationsframeworks ist es möglich, medizinische 2D- und 3D-Visualisierungen automatisch mit unterschiedlichen Texten zu annotieren. Bisher aufwändig manuell erstellte Annotationen für Planungsergebnisse bspw. in der Leber- oder HNO-Chirurgie (Abb. 2) können nun automatisch erzeugt werden. Annotationen in 2D unterstützen das Auffinden von Strukturen in Schichtbildern (Abb. 2(a)) und fördern im Zusammenspiel mit 3D-Darstellungen die

Übertragung von 2D-Informationen auf die 3D-Szene. Techniken, wie die Zusammenfassung von Annotationen, verhindern die Überfrachtung von Darstellungen mit Annotationen (Abb. 2(b)). Zusätzlich zu den automatisch erzeugten Annotationen kann der Nutzer eigene Annotationen hinzufügen (z.B. durch Aufziehen von Kugeln in der Darstellung) bzw. bestehende erweitern. Dies können Kommentare eines Experten für einen Lernenden oder Kurzbefunde eines planenden Chirurgen sein. Die dazu erfassten Texte fließen in die automatische Annotationsvisualisierung ein, so dass es auch hier zu keinen Überlappungen kommt.

4 Diskussion

Auch wenn das vorgestellte Framework wesentliche Anforderungen an ein automatisches Annotationssystem für medizinische Visualisierungen erfüllt, wünschen sich unsere medizinischen Partner weitere Interaktionen mit den Labeln selbst. So ist ein erweitertes Ausklappen der Label denkbar, um ausführlichere Informationen. Auch müssen die verschiedenen Darstellungsstile und Interaktionsformen einer genaueren Evaluierung durch ein größeres Kollektiv medizinischer Experten unterzogen werden.

Danksagung. Dieses Projekt wurde im Zusammenhang mit dem SOMIT-FUSION-Projekt durch das BMBF gefördert (FKZ 01-BE03B). Wir danken MeVis-Research für die Bereitstellung von MeVisLab.

Literaturverzeichnis

1. Christensen J, Marks J, Shieber S. An empirical study of algorithms for point-feature label placement. ACM Trans Graph. 1995;14:203–232.
2. Bekos MA, Kaufmann M, et al. Mutli-stack boundary labeling problems. In: Conf. on Fd. of Software Techn. and Theoretical Comp. Science; 2006. p. 81–92.
3. Götzelmann T, Ali K, et al. Form follows function: Aesthetic interactive labels. In: Computational Aesthetics; 2005. p. 193–200.
4. Ropinski T, Praßni JS, et al. Internal labels as shape cues for medical illustration. In: Vision, Modeling, and Visualization; 2007. p. 203–212.
5. Preim B, Raab A. Annotation von topographisch komplizierten 3D-Modellen. In: SimVis; 1998. p. 128–140.
6. Ali K, Hartmann K, Strothotte T. Label layout for interactive 3D illustrations. J WSCG. 2005;13(1):1–8.
7. Chronaki C, Zabulis X, Orphanoudakis SC. I2Cnet medical image annotation service. Med Inform. 1997;22(4):337–347.
8. Goede PA, Lauman JR, et al. Methodology and implementation for annotating digital images for context-appropriate use in an academic health care environment. J Am Med Inform Ass. 2004;11(1):29–41.
9. Lober WB, Trigg LJ, et al. IML: An image markup language. In: American Medical Informatics Association Fall Symposium; 2001. p. 403–407.
10. Tietjen C, Mühler K, et al. METK - The medical exploration toolkit. Proc BVM. 2008; p. 407–411.
11. Mühler K, Neugebauer M, et al. Viewpoint selection for intervention planning. In: IEEE/Eurographics Symposium on Visualization; 2007. p. 267–274.

Structure Size Enhanced Histogram
A Transfer Function for 3D Volume Visualization

Stefan Wesarg, Matthias Kirschner

Technische Universität Darmstadt, GRIS, Medical Computing
stefan.wesarg@gris.informatik.tu-darmstadt.de

Abstract. Direct volume visualization requires the definition of transfer functions (TFs) for the assignment of opacity and color. Multi-dimensional TFs are based on at least two image properties, and are specified by means of 2D histograms. In this work we propose a new type of a 2D histogram which combines gray value with information about the size of the structures. This structure size enhanced (SSE) histogram is an intuitive approach for representing anatomical features. Clinicians – the users we are focusing on – are much more familiar with selecting features by their size than by their gradient magnitude value. As a proof of concept, we employ the SSE histogram for the definition of two-dimensional TFs for the visualization of 3D MRI and CT image data.

1 Introduction

Transfer functions (TFs) are tools for assigning optical properties to scalar volume data sets [1]. For direct volume rendering of such data, e.g. opacity can be set depending on the gray value at a given voxel position. Since the location of boundaries is of high interest, early work focused on the extraction of isocontours [2] and on finding optimal threshold values that correspond to intensity transitions [3]. A better distinction between different structures can be achieved when additional parameters like gradient magnitude are used for generating multi-dimensional TFs [4]. However, the definition of those TFs is a difficult task, and several techniques for helping the user have been proposed [5, 6, 7].

Based on two image properties, a 2D histogram can be created and used for the TF generation [4, 1]. One fundamental problem with all histograms is the fact that any spatial information is lost. One possible solution for that problem is the classification of the 2D histogram entries by their mean spatial position, i.e. replacing the frequency value at each 2D bin with a class label [8, 9]. For special applications, it is also useful to use distance information as second input for the 2D histogram instead of gradient magnitude [10, 11].

In this work we present a novel type of 2D histogram that combines gray value with information about the size of structures in the image data. For computing this structure size enhanced (SSE) histogram, we estimate the size of the structures by employing a multi-scale approach. Opacity assignment is based on the location of each bin in the SSE histogram. Spatial information is added by employing a distance map for a coarse classification of the 2D bins, or as an alternative by utilizing the approach of Roettger et al. [9].

2 Materials and methods

The main reason for the usage of 2D histograms for TF generation is the fact that different tissue types often share more or less the same gray value range in the image data – e.g. soft tissue in CT images. Thus, in a 1D histogram these structures are represented within a small range around one single bin. A special benefit of 2D histograms based on gray value and gradient magnitude is the distinction between the structures' boundaries and their inner region. A rendering that emphasizes these boundaries reveals much of the interesting information contained in the image data.

Considering how humans perceive different structures in image data, it can be noticed that one differentiates between different locations and also between different sizes of anatomical structures. Consequently, it is reasonable to incorporate spatial as well as structure size information into the 2D TF generation. For this purpose, we have developed the SSE histogram – a 2D histogram that uses structure size information in addition to the gray value. Furthermore, spatial information is added for classifying the 2D bins.

2.1 Structure size estimation

Each voxel in a 3D image data set (except those at the boundaries of the data) has 26 direct neighbors. The difference vector between the reference voxel's position P_{ref} and the positions P_n of each of its neighbors defines 26 direction vectors. Starting from P_{ref}, for each direction the number of steps that can be done satisfying a threshold condition is counted. A step is possible if the gray value I_{curr} at the new position falls within the range $[I_{\text{ref}} - \tau \cdot I_{\text{max}}, I_{\text{ref}} + \tau \cdot I_{\text{max}}]$, where I_{ref} is the gray value at P_{ref}, I_{max} is the gray value maximum in the data set, and $\tau \in (0, 0.5)$ is a tolerance value.

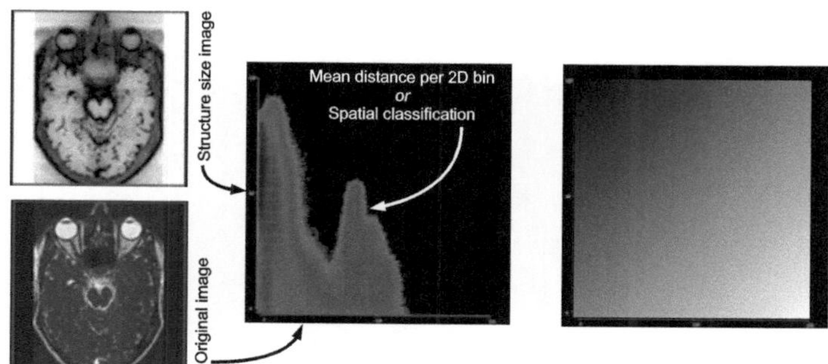

Fig. 1. The SSE histogram uses gray value information and the output of the structure size estimator as input (*left*). A non-classified SSE histogram is shown with color coding according to the bin population: *red* = low to *blue* = high. Distance map information can be used for a coarse classification, or spatial information à la Roettger [9] for an alternative classification approach (*center*). The opacity distribution that is used for an automatic TF initialization (white = 100% opaque, black = 0% opaque (*right*)).

Instead of defining the structure size as the sum of all counted voxels for all directions, we use a multi-scale approach that provides a more homogeneous *structure size image* with less artifacts compared to the simple voxel counting. For that, the algorithm checks for each of the 26 directions whether a certain number of steps $S_n, n = 1 \ldots N$ could be done. S_n we call the *scale* at which the structure size is examined. The largest scale S_N corresponds to half of the data set (the minimum size for (x, y, z)), and each subsequent scale is defined as $S_{n-1} = S_n/2$. In this work, we use $N = 8$ different scales. Consequently, for a data set of size $512 \times 512 \times 512$ isotropic voxels S_N equals to 256 voxels and S_1 to 1 voxel. For all 26 directions, we determine the largest value n such that we can do at least S_N steps, and the accumulation of all n gives the value for the structure size. Further improvement is achieved by taking into account only the largest value n for two opposite directions.

An interesting property of this structure size estimation is that very small values are assigned to boundaries, whereas large homogeneous regions receive a much higher value. If we associate high opacity with small structure size values and low opacity with large structure size values, we can achieve visualization effects similar to approaches based on gradient magnitude computation.

2.2 SSE histogram

The image generated by the structure size estimator serves as second input for our SSE histogram. In this 2D representation small structures are located in the bottom area whereas larger ones in the top region. Thus, interesting structures can be selected directly by means of manipulation widgets [4]. We implemented closed splines with an adjustable number of spline points for selecting regions of interest in the SSE histogram.

Furthermore, it is possible to specify a TF for opacity simply based on the 2D bin location in an automatic manner. In medical images, large regions with

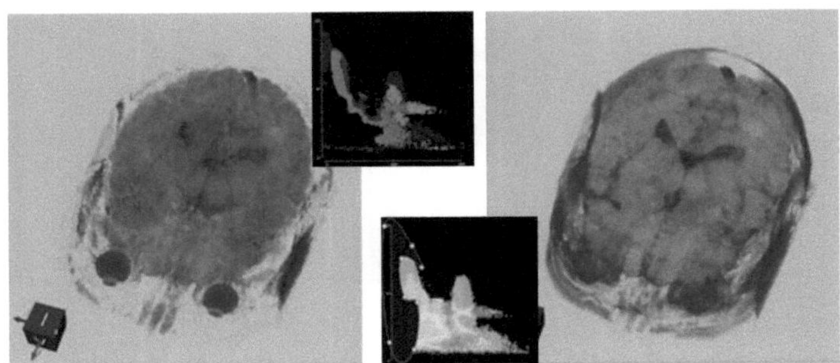

Fig. 2. Visualization of an MRI head data set employing a distance map for the SSE histogram classification. Only some (highlighted) classes have been picked(*left*). Color coding based on the mean distance for each 2D bin from a user given reference position – the center of the brain. The part belonging to low gray value values (red curve) has been masked out (*right*).

Fig. 3. CT data set of a foot. The classification method introduced by Roettger [9] has been used for creating 21 clusters, each labeled by a different color. Only some of the clusters are selected (highlighted structures), and the resulting 3D volume rendering is shown (*left*). CT data set showing an aortic stent in the abdominal region. The spline widet has been used to select the bins to be included in the 3D visualization (*right*).

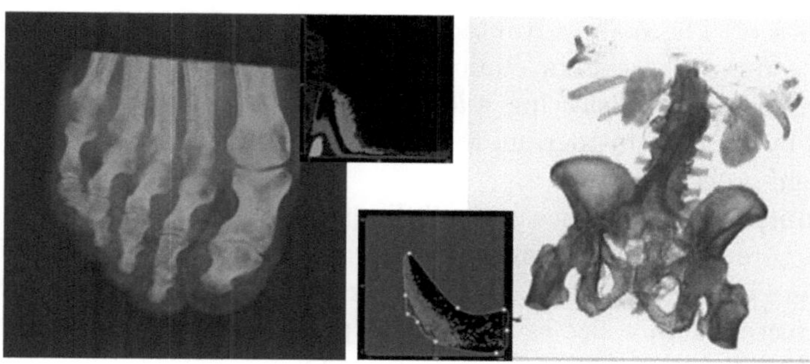

a low gray value (e.g. air) are mostly of low interest, and dark regions are often set to full transparency. We achieve a similar behavior by defining an opacity TF that increases with gray value and decreases with structure size (fig. 1).

2.3 Histogram classification

In many applications one is interested in a special structure and its surroundings. For the purpose of a coarse classification of the 2D bins, we use a distance map that contains information about the Euclidean distance from the reference position that has to be provided by the user. For each 2D bin we can compute the mean distance and display it using a color look-up table. This enables the user to select a region in the SSE histogram with a close spatial relationship (fig. 2).

As an alternative, we have also implemented the spatial classification introduced by Roettger et al. [9] with a random assignment of colors to the classes in the SSE histogram (fig. 3). In contrast to their implementation, here the selection of a 2D bin only affects 2D bins of the same class if they are connected to the one selected in the SSE histogram. This avoids selection/deselection of regions that have a spatial relationship but are very different in gray value and/or structure size. In any case, we use the colors that are shown in the SSE histogram also for the definition of a color TF for the subsequent volume visualization.

3 Results

We used the SSE histogram for an automatic TF specification for visualizing MRI and CT data sets (figs. 2 and 3). A simple point-and-click selection of regions in the SSE histogram was possible in cases where there was a large cluster of 2D bins with the same classification label. If there were too much small class regions, we preferred the closed 2D spline for selecting the regions.

4 Discussion

In this work we have presented a new type of 2D histogram and shown its application to TF specification. Instead of using gradient magnitude as second input, we employ an image that represents the estimated size of all structures in the data set. The main advantage of our approach is its intuitiveness. In contrast to computer scientists, clinicians are often not familiar with the concept of gradient magnitude. Selecting *a large region with medium gray value*, which is provided by the SSE histogram, is much easier to grasp by non-experts in the field of image processing.

The quality and significance of the SSE histogram depends on the correctness of the structure size estimation. Our current approach is a trade-off between exactness and computing time. Future work will focus on faster algorithms for a more correct structure size estimation. A possible extension of our technique is the usage of distance maps with multiple reference points [10].

The specification of TFs based on the SSE histogram is highly automated and leads to visualization results that are comparable to those of existing approaches. We see the main advantage of our work in its high degree of comprehensibility, especially for non-experts in medical image processing.

References

1. Preim B, Bartz D. Visualization in Medicine. Theory, Algorithms, and Applications. 1st ed. Series in Computer Graphics. Morgan Kaufmann; 2007.
2. Bajaj CL, Pascucci V, Schikore DR. The contour spectrum. Procs IEEE Vis. 1997; p. 167–173.
3. Pekar V, Wiemker R, Hempel D. Fast detection of meaningful isosurfaces for volume data visualization. Procs IEEE Vis. 2001; p. 223–230.
4. Kniss J, Kindlmann G, Hansen C. Multidimensional transfer functions for interactive volume rendering. IEEE TVCG. 2002;8(3):270–285.
5. Pfister H, Lorensen B, Bajaj C, et al. The transfer function bake-off. IEEE CG&A. 2001;21(3):16–22.
6. Botha CP, Post FH. New technique for transfer function specification in direct volume rendering using real-time visual feedback. Procs SPIE. 2002;4681:349–356.
7. Sereda P, Bartroli AV, Serlie IWO, et al. Visualization of boundaries in volumetric data sets using LH histograms. IEEE TVCG. 2006;12(2):208–218.
8. Birchfield ST, Rangarajan S. Spatiograms Versus Histograms for Region-Based Tracking. Procs IEEE CVPR. 2005;2:1158–1163.
9. Roettger S, Bauer M, Stamminger M. Spatialized transfer functions. Procs EUROVIS. 2005; p. 271–278.
10. Reitinger B, Zach C, Bornik A, et al. User-centric transfer function specification in augmented reality. Procs WSCG. 2004; p. 355–362.
11. Tappenbeck A, Preim B, Dicken V. Distance-based transfer function design: Specification methods and applications. Procs SimVis. 2006; p. 259–274.

Analysis and Visualization of Nerve Vessel Contacts for Neurovascular Decompression

Jochen Süßmuth[1], Alexander Piazza[1], Frank Enders[1,2], Ramin Naraghi[2], Günther Greiner[1], Peter Hastreiter[1,2]

[1]Computer Graphics Group, University of Erlangen-Nuremberg, Germany
[2]Dept. of Neurosurgery, Neurocenter, University of Erlangen-Nuremberg, Germany
suessmuth@informatik.uni-erlangen.de

Abstract. Neurovascular compression syndromes are caused by a pathological contact between cranial nerves and vascular structures at the surface of the brainstem. Aiming at improved pre-operative analysis of the target structures, we propose calculating distance fields to provide quantitative information of the important nerve-vessel contacts. Furthermore, we suggest reconstructing polygonal models for the nerves and vessels. Color-coding with the respective distance information is used for enhanced visualization. Overall, our new strategy contributes to a significantly improved clinical understanding.

1 Introduction

The detailed understanding of the complex anatomical relationships between nerves and vessels at the surface of the brainstem is of major importance for the understanding of neurovascular compression (NVC) syndromes [1]. Associated with diseases such as trigeminal neuralgia (TN) and hemifacial spasm (HS), they are characterized by a pathological contact between vessels and the root entry or exit zone of cranial nerves. Its correct assessment is crucial for diagnosis and therapy planning.

Visualization of strongly T2 weighted MR (magnetic resonance) images based on the CISS (constructive interference in steady state) sequence has been shown to be a powerful tool for the analysis of NVC syndromes [2, 3]. In order to overcome problems related to imaging artifacts, previous work suggested to consider vascular information from MR angiography (MRA) as additional source of information [4]. Based on the fusion of MRA and MR-CISS, advanced visualization was achieved [5]. The rendering quality was further improved with volume splatting and 2D transfer functions [6]. In a more recent contribution, polygonal reconstruction of neurovascular relationships and differentiation of arteries and veins based on additional MR imaging was suggested [7]. However, a software based detailed analysis of the nerve-vessel relationships is missing so far.

Aiming at an improved analysis of the nerve-vessel contacts in NVC syndromes, we suggest the computation of distance fields which store the spacing to the closest vascular structure. As input data, we use a combination of registered

MR-CISS and MRA-TOF (time of flight) volumes. For enhanced visualization, we reconstruct polygonal models of the target structures, which are color-coded with the information retrieved from the distance field. As a general achievement, our approach results in a considerably improved qualitative analysis and allows for a precise detection and evaluation of the nerve-vessel contacts in NVC syndomes.

2 Materials and methods

2.1 Data acquisition and preprocessing

All data sets consisted of $512 \times 512 \times 144$ voxels with a size of $0.39 \times 0.39 \times 0.4$ mm^3. As illustrated in figure 1, MR-CISS data shows a high degree of contrast between hyperintense CSF (cerebrospinal fluid) and hypointense cranial nerves. On the other hand, the representation of the larger vessels is ambiguous due to flow artifacts. This drawback is circumvented by additionally considering vascular information obtained from MRA-TOF. In a preprocessing step, the volumes are rigidly registered using an implementation based on normalized mutual information [5]. Then, we use a semi-automatic segmentation to extract subvolumes of the cranial nerves and the brainstem from the MR-CISS data [2] (Fig. 1(*right*)).

2.2 Polygonal reconstruction of nerves and vessels

For improved analysis and subsequent visualization, we compute polygonal models of the vascular structures, the brainstem and the cranial nerves. This is achieved by extracting iso-surfaces for the vessels from the MRA-TOF data and for the nerves and the brainstem from the segmented MR-CISS data using marching cubes.

To reduce the typical aliasing artifacts introduced by the marching cubes algorithm, we apply a series of smoothing steps to the extracted meshes of the nerves and vessels. Our experiments showed that the second order umbrella-operator $U^2(\mathbf{p})$ introduced by Kobbelt et al. [8] yields the best results. It minimizes the thin plate energy of the mesh and produces smooth surfaces while causing less volume shrinkage in thin areas compared to other algorithms.

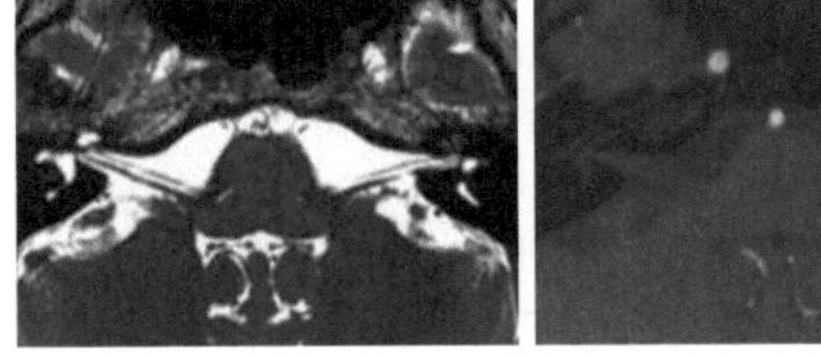
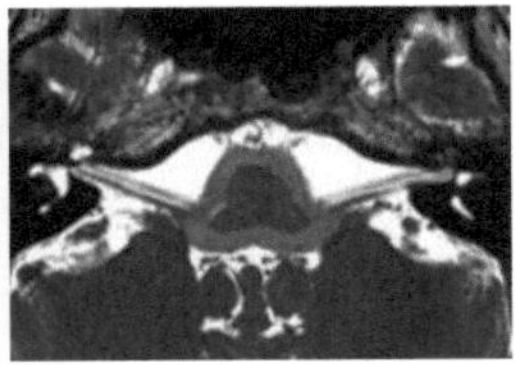

Fig. 1. Corresponding CISS (*left*), TOF (*middle*) and segmented CISS (*right*) slices

Fig. 2. Error-bounded smoothing. From left to right: original polyline; close-up of the constrained smoothing step; smoothed polyline.

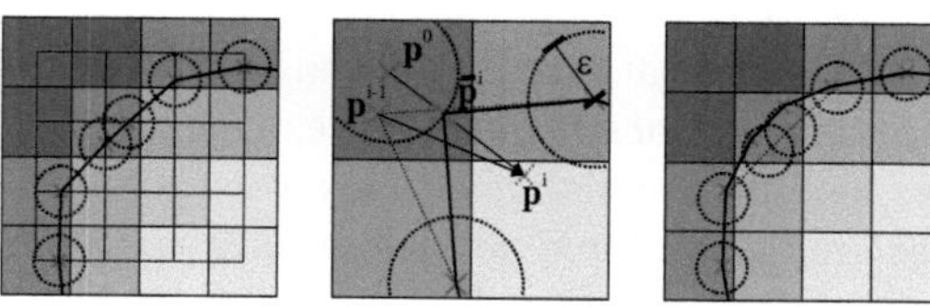

In order to bound the error introduced by mesh smoothing, we constrain vertex movement to a small sphere (we use a diameter of $\epsilon = 0.3$ mm in our implementation) around the initial vertex positions $\mathbf{p}_j^0$ as depicted in figure 2: During each smoothing iteration, we compute the position $\mathbf{p}_j^i$ satisfying the second order umbrella equation for each vertex $\mathbf{p}_j$. If $\mathbf{p}_j^i$ lies outside the ϵ-ball of $\mathbf{p}_j^0$, the vertex is projected back onto the sphere along the line from $\mathbf{p}_j^0$ to $\mathbf{p}_j^i$.

2.3 Distance field computation

To enable distance computations between nerves and vessels, we compute a distance field for the vascular structures. For this purpose, we create a discrete distance volume data set $\mathcal{D}$ the size of the MR-TOF volume and initialize all voxels v with distance $\mathcal{D}(v) = \infty$. Then, we compute the voxels of $\mathcal{D}$ that are intersected by the arteries mesh and assign them the distance zero (Fig. 3a) and put all *zero-distance* voxels into a queue (*active front*). For each voxel in *active front* we store the closest *zero-distance* voxel.

In the next step, we propagate the distance information of each voxel v in *active front* to its 27 direct neighbors n_i: If the current distance value $\mathcal{D}(n_i)$ of a neighbor voxel n_i is larger than the distance d between n_i and the nearest *zero-distance* voxel of v, $\mathcal{D}(n_i)$ is set to d and n_i is added into the active front. After all neighbors of v have been processed, v is removed from the *active front* queue. This step is iterated until the queue *active front* is empty (Fig. 3).

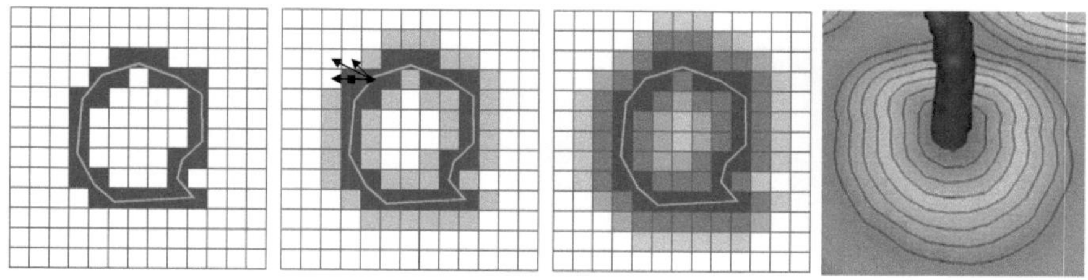

Fig. 3. Distance field computation. From left to right: *zero-distance* voxels; *active front* (green) and distance propagation; final distance volume; slice of a 3-D example.

2.4 Visualization

We render the previously extracted polygonal models using standard mesh rendering techniques. The visualization of potential nerve-vessel contacts is further improved by *color-coding* the mesh of the nerves (Figs. 4, 5): for each vertex of the nerves' mesh, we look up the distance to the vessels' mesh using the distance field $\mathcal{D}$. The vertices are then colored according to the respective distances. Values smaller than 1 mm are rendered in dark gray, distances between 1 and 3 mm are colored red to yellow and distances larger than 3 mm are colored yellow.

3 Results

The presented methods were so far used for pre-operative planning in 6 cases (4 $\times$ TN, 2 $\times$ HS). Data processing and analysis took roughly 2 hours: MR imaging (25 min), segmentation (1 hour), registration (10 min), mesh extraction, smoothing and distance field computation (15 min). The proposed polygonal visualization ensures interactive rendering even on workstations without high-end graphic cards. Renderings are shown for two of the examined cases in figure 4 and figure 5. In all cases, the identified contact locations were verified during surgery.

4 Discussion

The presented technique improves diagnosis of nerve-vessel contacts and leads to a more precise localization and quantitative analysis in pre-operative planning. Compared to traditional direct volume visualization (e.g. 3D-texture-slicing) (Fig. 4(left)), the perception of distances and spatial relationships is significantly improved by rendering color-coded polygonal models of the related structures.

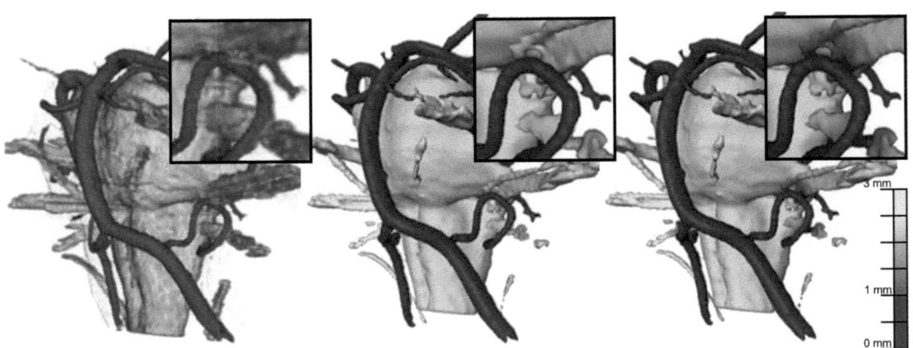

Fig. 4. Comparing rendering quality: conventional volume rendering of fused CISS-TOF volume (*left*), rendering polygonal models only (*middle*) and polygonal models with color-coded distance information (*right*).

Fig. 5. Case of hemifacial spasm: intraoperative photo (*left*) and rendering in the same viewing direction showing the offending artery (1) and the related nerve (2) (*right*).

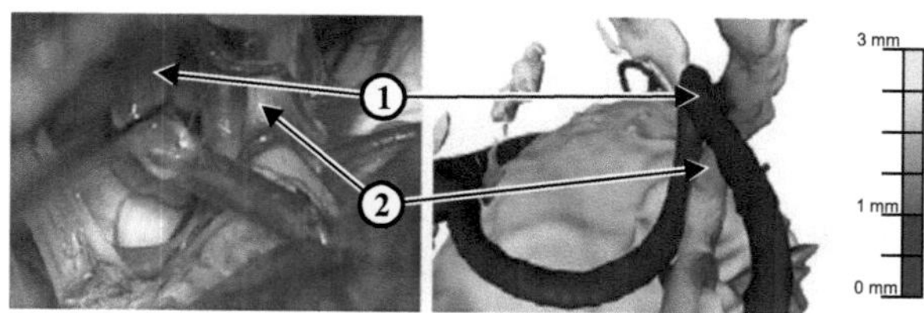

Our approach provides an excellent overview of the target area and allows easy interaction with the delineated structures. Furthermore, it offers the opportunity of non-invasive exploration and classification of the critical nerve-vessel contacts causing NVC syndromes.

During surgery, unnecessary manipulations with the risk of collateral damages leading to neurological deficits can be considerably reduced because of a more straight forward approach to the lesion. Furthermore, this technology can be very useful in large scale epidemiological studies on NVC syndromes. In consequence, the presented technique can support a further classification of neurovascular contacts. Other application fields include the improved information of the patient before the intervention as well as the use in education.

References

1. Jannetta P. Neurovascular compression in cranial nerve and systemic disease. Ann Surg. 1980;192:518–525.
2. Hastreiter P, Naraghi R, Tomandl B, et al. 3D-visualization and registration for neurovascular compression syndrome analysis. Procs MICCAI. 2002; p. I,396–403.
3. Naraghi R, Hastreiter P, Tomandl B, et al. Three dimensional visualization of neurovascular relationship in the posterior fossa: Technique and clinical application. J Neurosurg. 2004;100(6):1025–35.
4. Akimoto H, Nagaoka T, Nariai T, et al. Preoperative evaluation of neurovascular compression in patients with trigeminal neuralgia by use of three-dimensional reconstruction from two types of high-resolution magnetic resonance. Neurosurgery. 2002;51(4):956–61.
5. Hastreiter P, Vega-Higuera F, Tomandl B, et al. Advanced and standardized evaluation of neurovascular compression syndromes. Procs SPIE. 2004;5:267–274.
6. Vega-Higuera F, Hastreiter P, Fahlbusch R, et al. High performance volume splatting for visualization of neurovascular data. Procs IEEE Vis. 2005; p. 271–278.
7. Miller J, Acar F, Hamilton B, et al. Preoperative visualization of neurovascular anatomy in trigeminal neuralgia. J Neurosurg. 2008;108(3):477–82.
8. Kobbelt L, Campagna S, Vorsatz J, et al. Interactive multi-resolution modeling on arbitrary meshes. Procs SIGGRAPH. 1998; p. 105–114.

Evolutionäres Graphmatching zur Handknochen-Identifikation

Benedikt Fischer, Armin Fritsche, Christian Thies, Thomas M. Deserno

Institut für Medizinische Informatik, RWTH Aachen
bfischer@mi.rwth-aachen.de

Kurzfassung. Im medizinischen Umfeld ist häufig eine Identifikation lokaler Bildinhalte (z.B. Organe) erforderlich. Dazu lassen sich Bildinhalte als Graphstruktur abstrahieren und mit für die jeweilige Anwendung statistisch ermittelten Strukturprototypen vergleichen. Die Identifikation unbekannter Inhalte zu den Prototypen entspricht dann einem Graphmatching. In dieser Arbeit wird dazu ein auf evolutionärer Spieletheorie basierender Ansatz verwendet. Die Praxistauglichkeit wird am Beispiel der Identifikation von 19 Handknochen in 96 Handradiographien evaluiert und mit weiteren Matchingverfahren verglichen. Bei durchschnittlich 2.300 hierarchisch segmentierten Regionen je Radiographie werden mit 34 regionalen und 12 relationalen Merkmalen Werte von bis zu 71,63%, 65,76% bzw. 64,08% für Recall, Precision bzw. F-Measure für 27 unterschiedliche Parametrierungen erzielt.

1 Einleitung

Zur Identifikation medizinischer Bildinhalte werden häufig Graphen verwendet, da diese eine abstrakte relationale Strukturbeschreibung erlauben [1, 2, 3]. Dies ist insbesondere hilfreich, wenn eine punktweise Registrierung wenig erfolgversprechend ist, z.B. bei multimodalen Bilddaten mit unterschiedlicher Semantik der Bildkanäle, verschiedenen Skalierungen, oder auch Verformung und Verschiebungen beispielsweise durch Atmung oder Bewegung. Der Vergleich der Graphen wird über Graphmatching-Verfahren durchgeführt, wie sie auch in vielen Anwendungsdisziplinen außerhalb der Medizin eingesetzt werden [4].

Um die für eine Anwendung typischen Strukturen zu generalisieren, lassen sich Strukturprototypen definieren [3]. Diese repräsentieren Objekte im Bild als Graphknoten und modellieren die anwendungstypischen Eigenschaften über die statistische Verteilung regionaler und relationaler Merkmale. Zu registrierende Bilder werden zunächst in einen hierarchischen attributierten Regionenadjazenzgraph (HARAG) überführt, der dann über Graphmatchingverfahren mit Prototypen verglichen wird (Abb. 1). Die in [3] verwendeten Graphmatching-Verfahren sind jedoch mit teils umfangreichen Parametersätzen verbunden. Mit [5] ist dagegen ein evolutionärer Graphmatcher für das Matching von Gefäßbäumen bekannt, der lediglich wenige Parameter erfordert [1]. Allerdings werden in [5] zwei identische Graphtypen verglichen, welche die Prototypabstraktion und die generalisierende Struktur des HARAG unberücksichtigt lassen. Im Rahmen dieser

Arbeit wird deshalb der evolutionäre Graphmatcher für diese Zwecke angepasst und exemplarisch evaluiert.

2 Material und Methoden

Zum Vergleich der Graphen wird oft auf Assoziationsgraphen zurückgegriffen, bei denen jeder Graphknoten einer Zuordnungshypothese zwischen zwei Knoten aus den zu vergleichenden Graphen entspricht [3, 5]. Einzelne Hypothesen können durch Kanten bestärkt oder gehemmt werden. Die Suche nach dem optimalen Matching entspricht der nach einer maximalen Clique, wofür die Methodik aus [6] zum Einsatz kommt. Diese kann jedoch nicht direkt auf den Assoziationsgraphen für Prototypen und HARAGs angewendet werden. Zum einen operiert das Verfahren aus [6] nur auf kantengewichteten Graphen ohne Knotengewichtung, wodurch sämtliche regionalen Merkmale entfallen würden. In dieser Arbeit werden die regionalen Merkmale daher mit in die Kantengewichtung integriert. Zum anderen werden in [6] für die Verwendung eines Strafterms bei Mehrfachzuordnungen positive Kantengewichte voraussetzt. In dieser Arbeit wird statt dessen ein Benefit eingesetzt, der eine Unterscheidung zwischen unähnlichen Relationen (d.h. Kantenmerkmalen) und sich widersprechenden Hypothesen gewährleistet. Der entsprechend angepasste Assoziationsgraph ist wie folgt definiert:

Definition 1. *(angepasster Assoziationsgraph)*
Für zwei Graphen $G = (V_G, E_G)$ und $H = (V_H, E_H)$ mit

- *Knotenmarkierung $\ell_G(x_i)$ für $x_i \in V_G$ bzw. $\ell_H(y_k)$ für $y_k \in V_H$,*
- *Kantenmarkierung $\ell_G(x_i, x_j)$ für $x_i, x_j \in V_G$ bzw. $\ell_H(y_k, y_l)$, für $y_k, y_l \in V_H$,*
- *Ähnlichkeitsfunktionen σ_V bzw. σ_E für die Knoten- bzw. Kantenähnlichkeit,*
- *Schwellwerten θ_V bzw. θ_E für σ_V bzw. σ_E*

wird der angepasste Assoziationsgraph $A = (V_A, E_A)$ wie folgt konstruiert:

- $V_A = \{(x_i, y_k) : x_i \in V_G \text{ und } y_k \in V_H \text{ und } \sigma_V(\ell_G(x_i), \ell_H(y_k)) \geq \theta_V\}$,
  d.h. für jedes Knotenpaar der Ausgangsgraphen mit hinreichender regionaler Ähnlichkeit wird ein Hypothesenknoten erzeugt.
- *Die Knoten werden nicht markiert.*
- *$((x_i, y_k), (x_j, y_l)) \in E_A$ gdw. $i \neq j$ und $k \neq l$*
  d.h. zwischen allen nicht widersprüchlichen Matchinghypothesen wird eine Kante erzeugt.
- $\ell_A((x_i, y_k), (x_j, y_l)) = \begin{cases} ben + \frac{s_{i,k}+s_{j,l}}{2} + \frac{s_{ij,kl}}{2} & falls \frac{s_{ij,kl}}{2} > \theta_E \\ ben & falls \frac{s_{ij,kl}}{2} \leq \theta_E \end{cases}$
  d.h. alle hinreichend ähnlichen Kanten werden mit der angepassten Kantengewichtung markiert. Unähnliche, aber nicht in Widerspruch zu anderen Hypothesen stehende Kanten erhalten eine Markierung mit der Benefitgewichtung.

Zusammen mit der in [3] über eine gewichtete Mahalanobis-Distanz definierten Ähnlichkeit wird die angepasste Kantengewichtung für nichtnegative Kanten aus der lokalen Ähnlichkeit $s_{i,k}$, der relationalen Ähnlichkeit $s_{ij,kl}$ der beiden Hypothesen sowie einem Benefitwert *ben* gebildet:

$$s_{i,k} = \sigma_V(\ell_G(x_i), \ell_H(y_k)) \tag{1}$$

$$s_{ij,kl} = \sigma_E(\ell_G(x_i, x_j), \ell_H(y_k, y_l)) + \sigma_E(\ell_G(x_j, x_i), \ell_H(y_l, y_k)) \tag{2}$$

Zum einen lassen sich auf diese Weise die Knotengewichtungen in Kantengewichtungen überführen. Zum anderen können über *ben* die sich nicht widersprechenden Zuordnungshypothesen belohnt werden. Die Adjazenzmatrix des wie obig konstruierten Assoziationsgraphen bietet nun eine korrekte Eingabe für das Verfahren aus [6]. Neben dem obig eingeführten Parameter *ben* müssen außerdem zwei für den Evolutionsabbruch erforderliche Parameter gesetzt werden. Zunächst wird über den so genannten ϵ-Support [1] geprüft, ob die Bewertungen aller nicht-ausgestorbenen Hypothesen größer als ein Parameter ϵ sind. Weiter wird über eine Variable Δ_ϵ beobachtet, ob sich der ϵ-Support über eine bestimmte Anzahl von Generationen nicht mehr ändert. Aus [7] ist bekannt, dass die Größe des ϵ-Supports monoton fallend ist, wenn ϵ klein genug gewählt wurde.

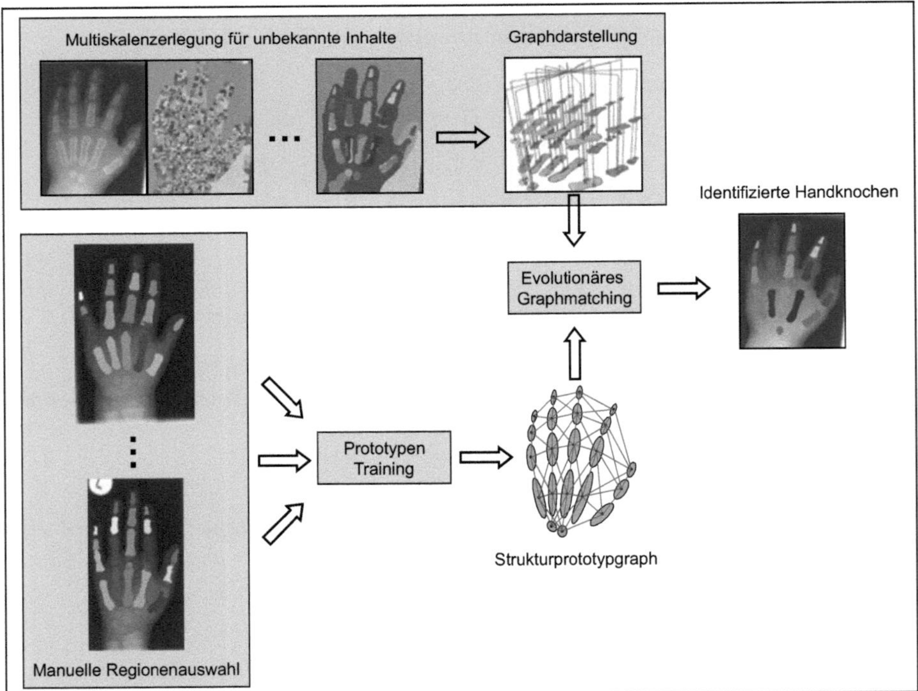

Abb. 1. Prinzip der Handknochenidentifkation: Bilder unbekannten Inhalts werden durch eine hierarchische Segmentierung in Graphen überführt. Diese werden mit Strukturprototypgraphen, die aus manueller Regionenauswahl synthetisiert werden, über den evolutionären Graphmatcher verglichen und die relevanten Regionen als Handknochen identifiziert.

Ist ϵ zu groß gewählt, könnte eine Hypothese die nur kurzzeitig geschwächt wird (etwa bis eine andere Hypothese ausstirbt) zu früh als ausgestorben definiert werden. Die Wahl Δ_ϵ hat ebenfalls Einfluss auf das Verfahren. Ist der Wert zu klein gewählt, ist es möglich, dass später noch weitere Hypothesen aussterben. Ist der Wert zu hoch gewählt, so kann es „nur" zu längeren Laufzeit führen.

Die Praxistauglichkeit des evolutionären Matchings zur Objektidentifikation wird anhand von Experimenten zur Identifizierung von Handknochen experimentell ermittelt. Dazu wurden 96 Radiographien von linken Händen in sechsfacher Kreuzvalidierung mit Strukturprototypen verglichen. Zur Validierung liegt zu jedem Matching eine von Hand erstellte Groundtruth vor. Ein Matching für eine Region wird als korrekt gewertet, wenn die zugeordnete Region mit der Region aus der Groundtruth zu mindestens 85% überlappt. Diese Einschränkung ist erforderlich, da durch die hierarchische Segmentierung teilweise mehrere übereinander liegende Regionen als korrekt angesehen werden können, allerdings nur eine davon in der Groundtruth markiert ist. Zur Evaluation werden die Standardwerte *Recall*, *Precision* und *F-Measure* sowie die Laufzeiten ausgewertet. Die Laufzeiten wurden auf einem Linux Rechner mit 2.8 GHz Intel Xeon Prozessor und 2 GB RAM ermittelt. Die Berechnung erfolgte mit jeweils drei Parameterwerten ($\{1, 2, 3\}$, $\{0, 10^{-5}, 10^{-2}\}$, bzw. $\{25, 50, 100\}$) für die drei Parameter *ben*, ϵ, und Δ_ϵ, so dass insgesamt 27 Parameterkombinationen getestet wurden. Um die Ergebnisse beurteilen zu können, werden sie mit den jeweiligen Werten der beiden besten Verfahren aus [3] verglichen.

3 Ergebnisse

Die verwendeten Bildgraphen enthalten jeweils zwischen 1.000 und 6.000 Knoten, durchschnittlich 2.300 und insgesamt 221.615 Knoten. Die jeweils aus den Trainingsdaten der Kreuzvalidierung erzeugten Handstrukturprototypen besitzen 19 Knoten zur Repräsentation der Phalanx- und Metakarpalknochen. Über alle getesteten Parametereinstellungen gemittelt ergeben sich für den evolutionären Matcher 60,37%, 60,63% und 60,49%, bzw. 1,17s für Recall, Precision und F-Measure bzw. für die mittlere Laufzeit. Die besten erzielten Werte mit jeweils eigenen Parametersätzen für Recall, Precision, F-Measure bzw. Laufzeit sind 71,63%, 65,76%, 64,08% bzw. 0,46 Sekunden. Die besten Ergebnisse hinsichtlich Recall im Vergleich zu den beiden besten Verfahren aus [3] sind in Tabelle 1 zusammengefasst.

4 Diskussion

Das hier untersuchte Verfahren stellt in allen Belangen eine Verbesserung zu den bisher eingesetzten Verfahren aus [3] dar. Wie Tabelle 1 belegt, konnte der Recall um 1,6% bzw. 2,6% in Bezug auf den Hopfield-Matcher bzw. Similarity Flooding gesteigert werden. Noch deutlicher ist der gleichzeitige Zugewinn der Precision (18,9% bzw. 10,4%), F-Measure (11,9% bzw. 7%) und Laufzeit (Reduktion um mindestens 78,9% bzw. 12%). Sofern die Parameter nicht wie in Tabelle 1 auf

Tabelle 1. Ergebnisse des Matchingverfahrens im Vergleich mit den beiden in Bezug auf Recall besten Verfahren aus [3]. Die besten Werte sind **fett** markiert. *Werte nicht genau bekannt.

Verfahren	Recall [%]	Precision [%]	F-Measure [%]	Laufzeit [s]
evolutionäres Graphmatching	**71,63**	**55,00**	**62,22**	**4,23**
Hopfieldmatcher NNGM aus [3]	70,50	46,26	55,58	20 - 50*
Similarity Flooding aus [3]	69,83	49,84	58,16	5,41

maximalen Recall sondern für die anderen Gütemerkmale optimiert werden, fällt die jeweilige Verbesserung noch stärker aus. Vor dem Hintergrund des schlechten Signal-Rausch-Verhältnisses von ca. 19 Handknochen: 2.300 Regionen = 0,008 wird der Erfolg noch deutlicher.

Insgesamt konnte also für die Objektidentifikation ein bislang schon in anderen Kontexten angewendetes Verfahren für die Verwendung mit Strukturprototypen angepasst werden. Die bisherigen Ergebnisse wurden in allen Gütekriterien deutlich verbessert obwohl gleichzeitig die Anzahl der relevanten Verfahrensparameter auf lediglich drei gesenkt werden konnte.

Für zukünftige Arbeiten gilt es die Segmentierungs- und damit auch die Trainingsqualität zu steigern. Zudem kann eine Einteilung in verschiedene geschlechtsabhängige Altersklassen sinnvoll sein, da sich die Ausprägung der Handknochen und damit die aus den Röntgenbildern extrahierten Textur- und Formmerkmale entsprechend stark unterscheiden [8]. Bislang wurde auch noch keinerlei Vorverarbeitung in Bezug auf Histogrammanpassung oder Bildausrichtung unternommen, wodurch weitere Verbesserungen zu erwarten sind. Letztendlich gilt es noch, neben der Identifikation von Handknochen weitere Anwendungsgebiete mit dem Verfahren zu testen.

Literaturverzeichnis

1. Metzen J, Krüger T, Schenk A, et al. Matching von Baumstrukturen. Proc BVM. 2007; p. 116–120.
2. Braumann UD, Franke H, Hengstler J, et al. Graph-based quantification of astrocytes. Proc BVM. 2006; p. 379–383.
3. Fischer B, Sauren M, Güld M, et al. Scene analysis with structural prototypes for content-based image retrieval in medicine. Procs SPIE. 2008;6914.
4. Conte D, Foggia P, Sansone C, et al. Thirty years of graph matching in pattern recognition. Intern J Pattern Recognit Artif Intell. 2004;18(3):265–298.
5. Pelillo M. Matching free trees, maximal cliques and monotone game dynamics. IEEE Trans PAMI. 2002;24(11):1535–1531.
6. Pavan M, Pelillo M. Generalizing the Motzkin-Straus theorem to edge-weighted graphs, with applications to image segmentation. LNCS. 2003; p. 485–500.
7. Bomze I. Evolution towards the maximum clique. J Glob Opt. 1997; p. 143–164.
8. Greulich W, Pyle S. Radiographic atlas of skeletal development of the hand and wrist. Palo Alto, CA, USA: Stanford University Press; 1959.

Präzise Messungen kleiner Durchmesser intrakranieller Gefäße in DSA-Bildern

Volker Aurich[1], Andreas Beck[1], Bernd Turowski[2]

[1]Institut für Informatik, Heinrich-Heine-Universität Düsseldorf
[2]Institut für Diagn. Radiologie/Neuroradiologie, Universitätsklinikum Düsseldorf
aurich-bvm2009@acs.uni-duesseldorf.de

Kurzfassung. Bei einigen Krankheitsbildern wie Vasospasmen nach Subarachnoidalblutungen ist es wichtig, sehr geringe Änderungen des Durchmessers von Gefäßen frühzeitig zu erkennen. Es werden zwei Messmethoden dafür vorgestellt, die leicht anwendbar sind. Anhand von Phantomen wird experimentell nachgewiesen, dass sie herkömmlichen Verfahren bezüglich der Reproduzierbarkeit und teilweise auch der Genauigkeit überlegen sind.

1 Einleitung

Durch die Injektion von Kontrastmittel kann man Blutgefäße in einem Röntgenbild deutlich sichtbar machen. Um andere, störende Strukturen wie Knochen zu eliminieren, wird bei der digitalen Subtraktionsangiographie (DSA) von dem Röntgenbild ein zuvor ohne Kontrastmittel aufgenommens Röntgenbild subtrahiert. Die DSA ist der Goldstandard für die klinische Analyse von intrakraniellen Gefäßen. Sie liefert eine höhere Auflösung als CT oder MRT [1]. Intravaskuläre Ultraschallmessungen sind invasiv und im intrakraniellen Bereich mit einem unverantwortbar hohen Risiko verbunden.

Üblicherweise bestimmt man in DSA-Bildern Gefäßdurchmesser, indem man einfach die Gefäßränder visuell schätzt und dann ihren Pixelabstand durch Abzählen ermittelt. Häufig wird versucht, die Genauigkeit dadurch zu erhöhen, dass man das DSA-Bild auf eine höhere Pixelauflösung interpoliert oder durch Änderung der Abbildunggeometrie vergrößert [2]. Im klinischen Einsatz kennt man die Parameter der durch die Zentralprojektion gegebenen Abbildung nicht sehr genau, so dass ohne Kalibrierung keine Absolutmessungen, sondern lediglich Vergleichsmessungen möglich sind. Schwierig ist es, bei Messungen in größeren Zeitabständen eine hohe, reproduzierbare Genauigkeit innerhalb weniger Prozent zu erreichen [3].

2 Material und Methoden

Bei allen Verfahren geht man davon aus, dass das Kontrastmittel homogen im Gefäß verteilt ist. Weil ein DSA-Bild nur eine Projektion auf zwei Dimensionen ist, kann man prinzipbedingt nicht die tatsächliche Gestalt des Gefäßquerschnitts bestimmen. Wenn man von Durchmesser spricht, nimmt man implizit immer einen kreisförmigen Querschnitt an. Bei der Abbildung eines kleinen Volumenbereichs in der Größenordnung der Gefäßdurchmesser ist die eigentlich vorliegende Zentralprojektion von einer Parallelprojektion kaum zu unterscheiden; deshalb wird im Folgenden bei lokalen Betrachtungen von einer Parallelprojektion ausgegangen. Außerdem sollen nur Gefäßstücke vermessen werden, die nahezu parallel zur Bildebene verlaufen und im DSA-Bild nicht von anderen überlappt werden.

2.1 Das Verfahren VESSEL

Auf unterschiedlichen Geraden senkrecht zu dem Gefäßstück variiert die Gestalt des Helligkeitsprofils meist sehr stark (Abb. 1), so dass damit die Gefäßränder nicht präzise zu bestimmen sind. Deshalb lässt ein menschlicher Betrachter seinen Blick längs des Gefäßes schweifen und führt damit implizit eine Art von Mittelung längs des Gefäßes durch. Diese Beobachtung ist die Grundlage des Verfahrens VESSEL. Der Benutzer gibt im DSA-Bild mit zwei Mausklicks die Endpunkte einer Strecke S in Richtung des Gefäßes an. Auf jeder Parallelen zu S werden die Grauwerte gemittelt und daraus das gemittelte Helligkeitsprofil P senkrecht zu S erstellt. Dabei werden Werte in Subpixelpositionen durch bilineare Interpolation berechnet. Im Idealfall eines Gefäßes mit kreisförmigen Querschnitt und ohne Rauschen ist P eine Halbellipse, deren horizontale Halbachse der mittlere Gefäßdurchmesser ist. Deshalb wird P bestmöglich durch eine Halbellipse approximiert und die Länge ihrer horizontalen Halbachse als Schätzwert genommen. Das Verfahren funktioniert auch für gekrümmte Gefäßstücke, indem der Benutzer ihre Richtung durch einen Polygonzug angibt.

2.2 Das Verfahren ANGIOTUX

G sei das Lumen eines kleinen Gefäßstücks. Ein Koordinatensystem sei so gewählt, dass die x-y-Ebene parallel zur Bildebene ist und die z-Achse in Richtung der Röntgenstrahlen weist, die wir wegen der geringen Größe von G als parallel annehmen. Die Angiographieabbildung ist dann einfach die Projektion in

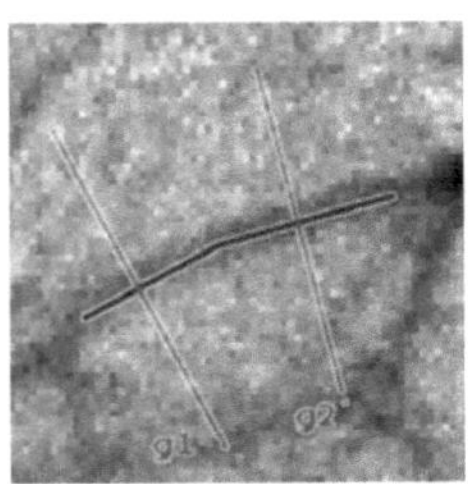

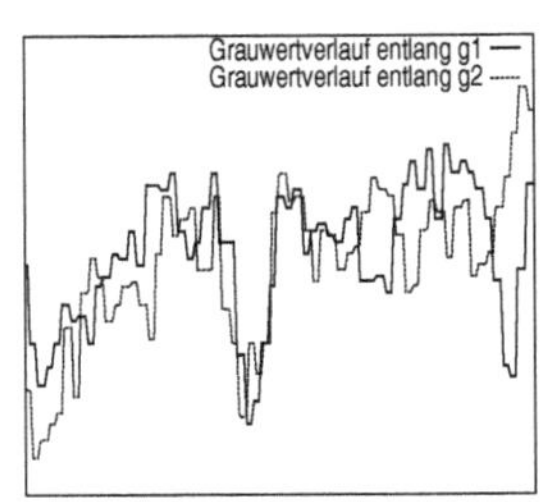

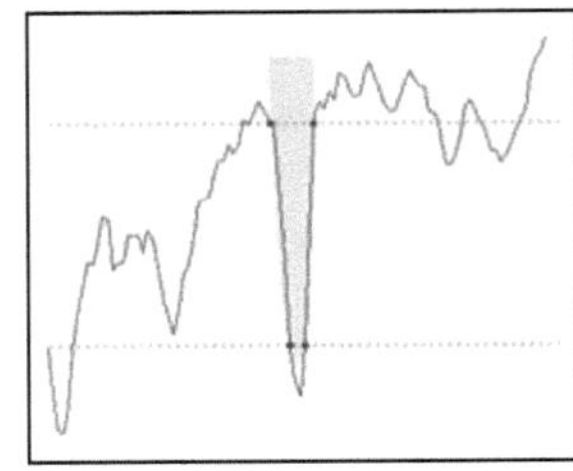

Abb. 1. DSA-Bild eines dünnen Gefäßstücks, Grauwertprofile auf zwei dazu quer verlaufenden Strecken $g1$ und $g2$ und Anpassung einer Ellipse an das gemittelte Helligkeitsprofil P senkrecht zum eingezeichneten Streckenzug.

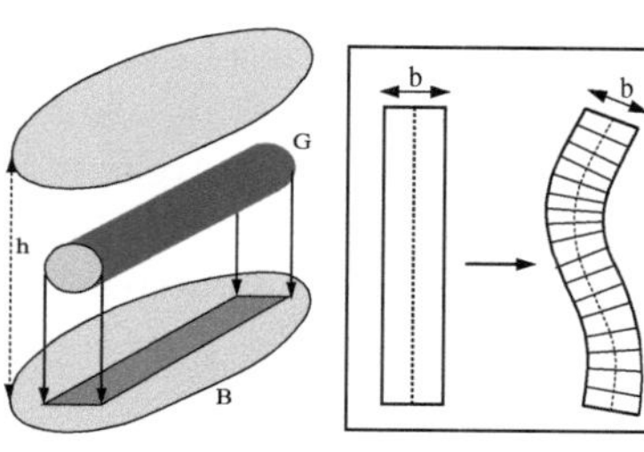

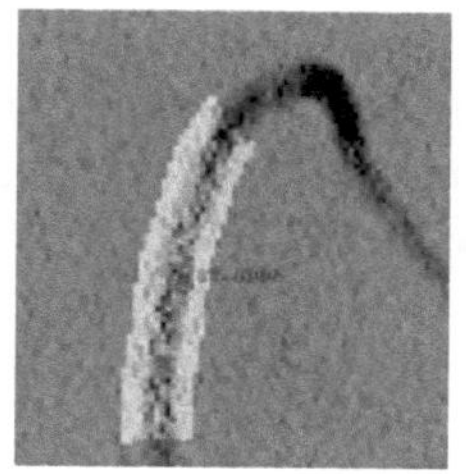

Abb. 2. Projektion eines Gefäßes, Verbiegung einer Tubenumgebung und mit rundem Pinsel angemaltes Gefäßstück

z-Richtung einer Zylindermenge $Q = B \times [0, h]$, die G enthält, auf ihre Basis B in der x-y-Ebene. $a_0(x, y, z)$ sei der Röntgenabsorptionskoeffizient an der Stelle (x, y, z) vor der Kontrastmittelinjektion. Die Helligkeit $f_0(x, y)$ des Pixels (x, y) des Angiographiebildes ist proportional zum Logarithmus der Abschwächung des Röntgenstrahls durch (x, y), also nach dem Lambert-Beerschen Absorptionsgesetz proportional zum Integral $\int_0^h a_0(x, y, z)\, dz$. Wenn das Gefäß homogen mit Kontrastmittel gefüllt ist, ergibt sich die Absorptionsfunktion $a_K = a_0 + \alpha\chi_G$ mit einem $\alpha > 0$ und die Angiographiebildhelligkeit $f_K(x, y) = \int_0^h a_K(x, y, z)\, dz$.

Bestimmung von Volumenverhältnissen. Es gilt

$$\begin{aligned} \mathrm{vol}(G) \sim \alpha \int_G dxdydz &= \int_Q (a_K - a_0\,)dxdydz \\ &= \int_B \int_0^h (a_K - a_0\, dz)dxdy = \int_B (f_K - f_0)\, dxdy \end{aligned}$$

Weil $f_K - f_0$ die Grauwertfunktion des DSA-Bildes ist, kann somit das Volumenverhältnis zweier Gefäßstücke G_1 und G_2 bestimmt werden. In der Praxis ergibt die Subtraktion der Bilder mit und ohne Kontrastmittel außerhalb der Gefäße nicht exakt den Wert 0; außerdem wird die Helligkeit des Bildhintergrundes zur besseren Betrachtung meist künstlich angehoben. Dieser Hintergrundwert wird durch Mittelung über einen Bildbereich ohne Gefäße ermittelt und abgezogen.

Bestimmung von Längenverhältnissen. Sind die G_j Zylinder mit Längen L_j und kreisförmigen Querschnitten der Durchmesser d_j, so gilt $\mathrm{vol}(G_j) = \frac{\pi}{4} d_j^2 L_j$, und somit könnte man das Verhältnis $d_1/d_2 = \sqrt{L_2 \mathrm{vol}(G_1)}/\sqrt{L_1 \mathrm{vol}(G_2)}$ bestimmen, wenn man die Längen L_1 und L_2 kennen würde. Um die Länge eines Gefäßstücks G aus seinem DSA-Bild berechnen zu können, müssen wir voraussetzen, dass es parallel zur Bildebene ist, so dass sein DSA-Bild die gleiche Länge hat (Abb. 2).

Robuste Längenmessung. Für die Längenmessung von Gefäßen im DSA-Bild wurde ein Ansatz gewählt, der die Approximation infinitesimaler Größen vermeidet. Ein rechteckiger Streifen mit Fläche A und Breite b hat die Länge $L = \frac{A}{b}$. Diese Beziehung gilt auch noch, wenn man den Streifen verbiegt, solange nur die Krümmung der Mittelkurve so klein bleibt, dass die dazu senkrechten Gräten sich nicht überschneiden, also im mathematischen Sinne eine sogenannte Tubenumgebung vorliegt (Abb. 2); zum Beweis man muss nur den Integraltransformationssatz auf die Deformierung anwenden. In der praktischen Anwendung fährt man wie in einem Malprogramm mit einem kreisrunden Pinsel dem Gefäßstück entlang, wobei die Dicke b des Pinsels so gewählt ist, dass das Gefäß ganz in dem vom Pinsel angemalten Bereich S liegt. Die Enden des Streifens S begradigt man noch (Abb. 2 rechts). Der Quotient (Anzahl der Pixel in S)/b ist ein Schätzwert für die Länge des Gefäßstückes, der sehr gut reproduzierbar ist, auch wenn die gewählte Pinselbreite b und der Benutzer variieren.

2.3 Messungen am Phantom

Zur experimentellen Auswertung wurde ein Phantom aus 5 Glaskanülen gebaut, die mit einem parallelen Ein- und Abfluss versehen sind. Unter dem Phantom wurde eine Schale mit einer 2cm tiefen Wasserschicht platziert, um Gewebe zu simulieren. Während der Messung wurden die Kanülen wie sonst die Gefäße mit Kontrastmittel gefüllt. Die Innendurchmesser der Kanülen 1 bis 5 betrugen 1.31 mm, 1.2 mm, 0.94 mm, 0.92 mm und 0.41 mm. Die Messungen wurden mit der bei DSA-Aufnahmen des Gehirns üblichen Vorgehensweise mit dem Angiographiegerät Integris Allura von Philips mit einer 1024×1024-Matrix bei kleinem Fokus, 60 kV und 300 ms vorgenommen.

Verglichen wurden 5 Messverfahren: 1. das Standardverfahren, also Vergrößerung des DSA-Bildes mit bikubischer Interpolation und visuelle Bestimmung der Gefäßränder und ihrer Pixelentfernung mit Hilfe der Software OSIRIS (Version 4.19 der Universität Genf); 2. dieselbe Methode, jedoch wurde das Bild durch Änderung der Abbildungsgeometrie um den Faktor 3.3 vergrößert; 3. das Verfahren VESSEL in einer Implementierung, die im Rahmen einer Bachelorarbeit entstanden ist [4] ; 4. das Verfahren ANGIOTUX; 5. eine weiter unten erklärte Variante, die wir ANGIOTUX-2 nennen; beide sind als spezielle Anwendung der ECCET-Plattform realisiert [5].

Alle Messungen wurden von zwei erfahrenen Radiologen unabhängig voneinander vorgenommen. Beide nahmen mit jeder der 5 Messmethoden je 15 Messungen vor; jedesmal wurde die gesamte Messprozedur neu durchgeführt.

Die von dem Angiographiegerät gelieferten Subtraktionsbilder enthalten eine leichte Kantenüberhöhung, die die visuelle Inspektion erleichtern soll, die jedoch bei dem Verfahren Angiotux zu einem prinzipbedingten Fehler führt. Deshalb wurden aus dem Angiographiegerät die Originalbilder ausgelesen und auf einem externen Rechner subtrahiert. Dieses so modifizierte Verfahren wird in den Resultatdiagrammen ANGIOTUX-2 genannt.

3 Ergebnis

Für jede der 5 Kanülen werden mit jeder der 5 Methoden in den 2×15 Messungen die zu den Durchmessern proportionalen Messwerte $d_1, \dots, d_5$ bestimmt. Da ja nur Relativmessungen betrachtet werden, wählt man jeweils den Wert d_1 der dicksten Kanüle 1 als Referenzwert und betrachtet nur noch die Quotienten $\frac{d_2}{d_1}, \dots, \frac{d_5}{d_1}$. In Abb. 3 ist für jede Methode aufgetragen, wie stark der Mittelwert dieser Quotienten vom wahren Durchmesserverhältnis abweicht und wie groß die Standardabweichung der Messungen ist.

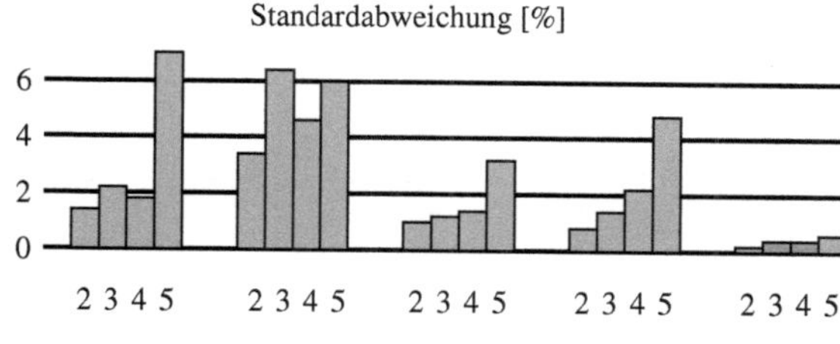

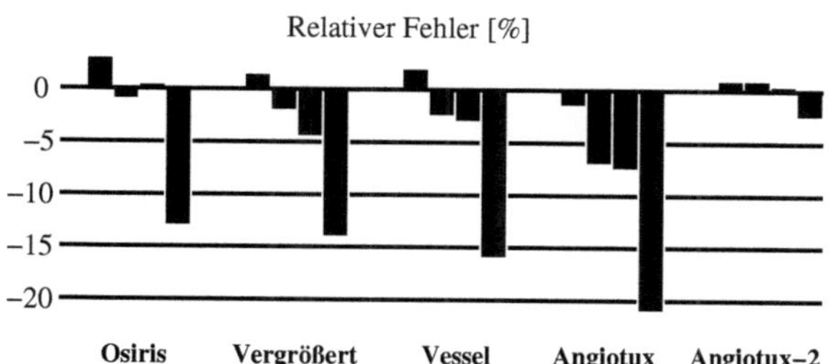

Abb. 3. Standardabweichung und relativer Fehler der Durchmesser der Kanülen 2, 3, 4, 5 im Verhältnis zur Kanüle 1. Man beachte die geringere Streuung der Verfahren Vessel und Angiotux.

4 Diskussion

Wenn man etliche Einzelmessungen durchführen und mitteln kann, so liefern alle Verfahren außer Angiotux ähnlich große Fehler; nur bei der dünnste Kanüle ist Angiotux-2 deutlich besser. Da in der klinischen Routine meist nur eine Messung vorgenommen wird, ist es wichtig, die Streuung gering zu halten. Das ist bei Angiotux-2 am besten erfüllt. Zudem ist es einfach anzuwenden und erfordert vom Benutzer keinerlei kritische Entscheidungen wie die präzise Erkennung von Gefäßrändern. Es ermöglicht, an einer Standard-Angiographieanlage Durchmesserverhältnisse intrakranieller Gefäße mit hoher und reproduzierbarer Präzision auf klinischen Routine-Aufnahmen zu messen, und es ist sogar unempfindlich gegenüber leichten Bewegungsartefakten.

Literaturverzeichnis

1. Yoon D, Choi C, Kim K, et al. Multidetector row CT angiography of cerebral vasospasm after aneurismal subarachnoid hemorrhage: Comparison of volume-rendered images and digital subtraction angiography. AJNR. 2006;27(2):370–377.
2. Luedemann W, Brinker T, Schuhmann M, et al. Direct magnification technique for cerebral angiography in the rat. Invest Radiol. 1998;33:421–424.
3. Turowski B, du Mesnil de Rochemont R, Beck J, et al. Assessment of changes in cerebral circulation time due to vasospasm in a specific arterial territory: Effect of angioplasty. Neuroradiology. 2005;47(2):134–143.
4. Kopp W. Bestimmung von Gefäßdurchmessern in Angiographiebildern. Bachelorarbeit: Institut für Informatik der Heinrich-Heine-Universität Düsseldorf; 2007.
5. `http://www.eccet.de`; 2008.

Estimating Blood Flow Velocity in Liver Vessels

Michael Müller[1], René Keimling[1], Sascha Lang[1], Josef Pauli[1], Uta Dahmen[2], Olaf Dirsch[2]

[1]Informatik und Angewandte Kognitionswissenschaft, Uni Duisburg-Essen
[2]Klinik für Allgemein-, Viszeral- und Transplantationschirurgie, Uniklinikum Essen
michael_mueller@uni-due.de

Abstract. Orthogonal polarization spectroscopy (OPS) is a technique for taking images to finally characterise microcirculation. Current image analysis algorithms have limitations when applied to image sequences obtained from the liver. We developed an automatic analysis tool which enables detection of liver vessels, measurement of vessel diameters, and determination of blood flow velocities with sparse user interactions. For validation purpose, data was analysed with our proposed algorithm and compared with manual results by experienced users. Related to commercial products, the needed time for analysis is reduced from more than 30 minutes to less than 2 minutes with comparable results for accuracy.

1 Introduction

This article covers the problem field of automatic characterisation of blood flow through the liver, i.e. liver perfusion, which is important for the assessment of regeneration after parial liver resection [1]. Orthogonal Polarization Spectroscopy (OPS) is a non-extensive technology, avoiding radiation, enabling high spatial and temporal resolution. It is useful for noninvasive in vivo measurements of hepatic microcirculation in small liver vessels (sinusoids) of the same individual repeatedly [2]. OPS-based commercial products like CapiScope [3] or MicroScan [4] need continual time-consuming user interactions, e.g. for vessel detection. Recently, an academic OPS-based system for the analysis of sublingual or cardiac microcirculation has been published [5], but no experiments were reported for liver perfusion which would have to cope with higher densities of vessels and lower signal-to-noise ratios. We aimed at developing an OPS-based tool allowing an automated analysis of liver perfusion with a minimum of user interactions.

2 Materials and methods

We first describe the sensing device for taking image sequences, then describe the methods for sinusoid detection, including image preprocessing, foreground/background separation, and skeletonisation, and finally describe the methods relevant for velocity measurement in a sinusoid, including also width analysis of sinusoids and the placing of virtual sensors in sinusoid sections.

OPS visually records the blood flow in microscopical scale within the liver tissue at 0.5mm beneath the surface. Polarised green light is sent towards the target tissue and the reflections are perceived by a CCD camera. At the surface a part of the light is reflected, within the tissue the remaining light is dispersed by most of the cells and absorbed by the red blood-cells (erythrocytes). Using an additional orthogonally oriented polarisation filter, the light from the surface is suppressed and only the light dispersed from the tissue interior will reach the camera. A lens is used for magnification leading to a spatial resolution of approximately 450 pixel/millimeter. The flow of erythrocytes appear as moving dark blobs and surrounding tissue as bright. Typically, image sequences of 375 images are taken in a period of 15 seconds with a refreshing rate of 50 fields/second. Problems with image processing originate from low signal-to-noise ratio, unbalanced illumination, and motion blur. The latter is due to unavoidable, external movement of the hand-held camera as well as respiratory and cardiac actions of the animal. In our work, image sequences from the liver tissue of rats are analysed in the context of experimental surgery.

Four steps treat the problems with illumination and noise (Fig. 1a). Histogram equalisation is applied to each image individually in order to increase the contrast. Then, the mean gray levels of all images are measured, the global mean brightness is computed, and the mean gray levels of all images are adjusted to that global mean. Next, noise is removed from each image using a median filter, that does not affect image structures too much. Finally, different gray levels in various image parts, caused by unbalanced illumination, are nomalised using a maximum filter for shading correction.

The set of sinusoids is defined as foreground and the remaining tissue as background. Apart from clearly visible sinusoids there are additional sinusoids which are hardly detectable in a single image. But the motion of erythrocytes encodes additional information concerning presence of sinusoids. This finding is included in the binarisation process which consists of five steps. a) All images of the sequence are combined into one aggregated image using a special median filter that operates on corresponding pixels in the temporal context (rather than spatial). b) The resultant aggregate image is binarised using local histograms for adaptive thresholding. c) Artefacts at the image border, caused by the limited aperture, are removed by image clipping to a circular shape. d) Salt-

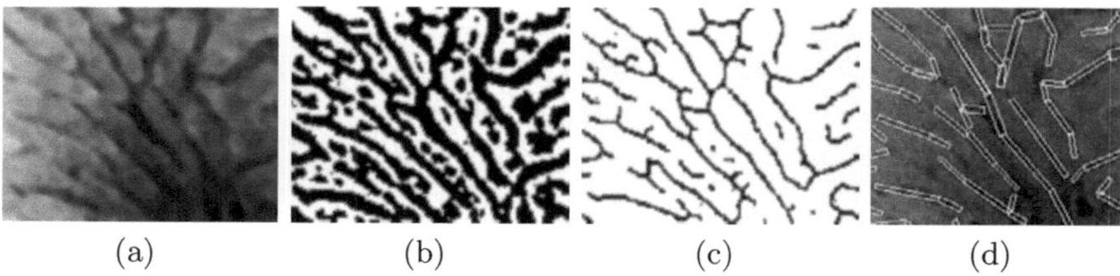

(a) (b) (c) (d)

Fig. 1. (a) Original image with unbalanced illumination. (b) Binarised image of sinusoids and some artefacts. (c) Removal of artefacts and skeletonisation. (d) Rectangular sinusoid areas for placing virtual sensors.

and-pepper noise is removed by morphological opening and closing operations: e) Non-sinusoid regions are detected and removed, using morphological hit-or-miss operations which consider the region shapes and the local background. The remaining regions are candidate areas for sinusoids (Fig. 1b).

A further hit-or-miss operation is applied repeatedly for a skeletonisation of this candidate regions, leading to curved center lines. Occasionally, this basic procedure will remove important parts of the network of lines, which in turn have to be recovered again. The line end points are detected and Gestalt laws like smooth continuation and neighborhood are applied. Further methods are responsible for treating splitting, converging, or crossing lines (Fig. 1c).

By counting the number of iterations during skeletonisation, also the width of the sinusoid regions can be obtained. For the subsequent method of analysing velocities, so-called virtual sensors are placed into sinusoid sections. A virtual sensor is a small area (e.g. square) of pixels from which the gray levels are recorded. Two such sensors are treated as pair and placed at a certain offset in the sinusoid. Rectangular areas are embedded into sinusoid sections, wherein to place the sensor pairs and thereby making sure that both sensors are nearby and from the same sinusoid. From the skeleton curves, straight line segments of maximal lengths are constructed respectively, whose end points lie on the curve and whose intermediate points lie completely within the width of the considered part of the sinusoid region. These straight line segments are used in combination with the stored diameters to create the rectangular areas (Fig. 1d).

The flow of erythrocytes in sinusoids is observable as movement of dark blobs surrounded by slightly brighter pixels. However, the gray values of the pixels in the image sequence are exposed to intense noise. An explicit blob extraction would be unreliable and time-consuming and is therefore avoided. Instead, the gray values of a virtual sensor area are combined to a scalar value using an adequate filter (e.g. median or Gaussian), and recorded in the course of time, leading to a one-dimensional signal. From a pair of sensors in a sinusoid section we obtain two similar, time-shifted signals. Based on normalised cross-correlation of the two signals we compute the time-shift more reliably. It is obtained as maximum correlation value for a certain time-shift value. Auto-correlation is used for normalisation.

For increasing the reliability of velocity measurement the following strategy is applied: a) Based on prior experiments the optimal sensor configuration is chosen in the rectangular area of a sinusoid. b) A cross-correlation value related to a sensor pair is only accepted if a certain threshold is exceeded. c) The percentage of accepted cross-correlation values must exceed a further threshold, and these set of values are fused alternatively by two types of algorithms, i.e. computing the mean or the median (MeanCCA or MedCCA).

3 Results

The automatic detection has been validated with measures of precision ($\frac{TP}{TP+FP}$) and recall ($\frac{TP}{TP+FN}$), which consider true positives (TP), false positives (FP),

Sequ.	TP	FP	FN	Precision	Recall
1	10500	2800	3100	78,95%	77,21%
2	11200	1200	2800	90,32%	80,00%
3	10500	1700	3600	86,07%	74,47%
4	10500	2600	3300	80,15%	76,09%
5			mean value	83,87%	76,94%
6	standard deviation			9,19%	4,03%

Table 1. Results for sinusoid detection, including precision and recall values for four image sequences, mean values and standard deviations.

and false negatives (FN). TP is the number of pixels of the skeleton curves of sinuisoids both extracted automatically and manually, FP is the number of pixels extracted only automatically, FN is the number of pixels extracted only manually. Fig. 2 shows exemplary an overlay of automatic and manual sinusoid detection (green for TP, red for FP, blue for FN). The precision value should exceed a certain threshold, otherwise too many measurements are taken in non-sinusoid areas. Also the recall value must exceed a certain threshold, otherwise too many sinusoids are not considered for velocity measurements. In average, precision and recall is about 84 % and 77 % with a standard deviation of 9% and 4%, respectively (Tab. 1).

Considering a sinusoid, the ground truth of velocity of blood flow has to be compared with the results of automatic estimation. However, the ground truth is initially unknown and will be estimated manually. For this purpose a graphical user interface is used to place a dynamic black-white pattern in the image near to a real sinusoid and then to adjust the velocity of the movable black squares to finally be synchronous with the velocity in the sinusoid (Fig. 3). For the automatic estimation several measurements from different pairs of sensors are combined by computing the mean or median cross-correlation. For velocity estimation, several image sequences were treated, several sinusoids were considered therein, the manual estimations of the experienced users were logged, and the algorithm with median cross-correlation was applied (Tab. 2). Ground truth estimation is done by 10 users leading to a coefficient of variation 0.22. For the results produced by the algorithm this coefficient is 0.37.

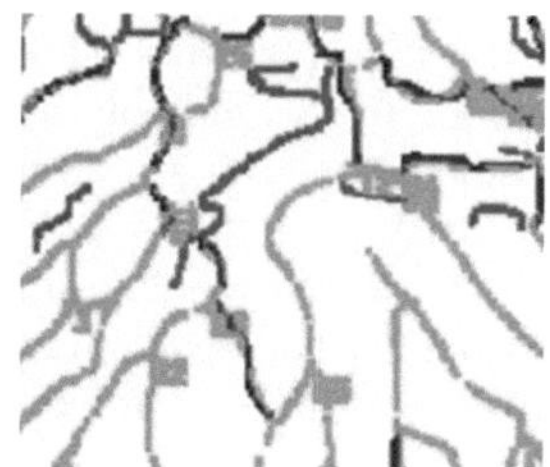

Fig. 2. Overlay of automatic and manual sinusoid detection.

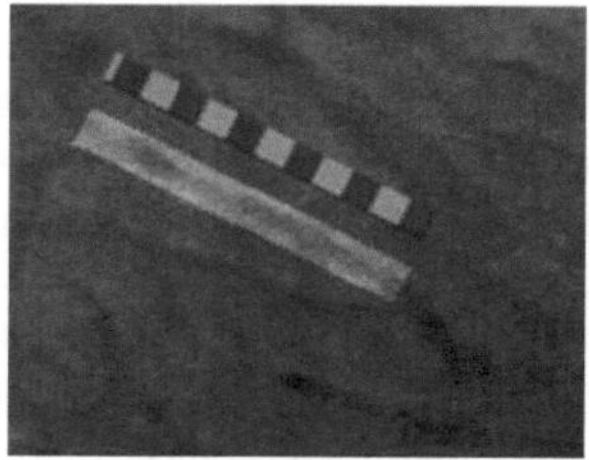

Fig. 3. Sinusoid section, dynamic pattern to estimate velocity ground truth.

Table 2. Typical velocity estimations for four image sequences by an experienced user and by the two types of the algorithm.

Sequ.	Manually [mm/sec]	MeanCCA [mm/sec]	MedCCA [mm/sec]
1	0.60	0.60	0.50
2	0.65	0.75	0.70
3	0.30	0.35	0.25
4	0.40	0.45	0.40

4 Discussion

The algorithm automatically detects sinusoids, selects the relevant and reliable ones, and estimates the blood flow velocity therein. For the purpose of reproducibility we refer to the theses of Keimling and Lang [6] for details like binarisation thresholds, morphological structure elements, correlation thresholds, and other parameters. Evaluations have shown acceptable precision and recall values (84% and 77%) for sinusoid detection. Concerning velocity estimations, manual and automatic responses are similar, but the coefficient of variance is still larger for the algorithm (0.37 versus 0.22). Due to the automatisation of sinusoid detection and selection, the liver perfusion can be characterised in less than 2 minutes, as opposed to more than 30 minutes by formerly used systems [3, 4]. Currently, we conduct more systematic experiments and evaluations in order to find out the degree of acceptability by relevant medical experts. Future work may be devoted to a further improvement of the accuracy of velocity estimations, and to the automatic selection of unblurred sections in image sequences.

References

1. Fogli L, Gorini P, Cappellari L, et al. Effect of partial hepatectomy and liver regeneration on portal pressure in rats. Surgical Research Comm. 1990;6:159–166.
2. Puhl G, Schaser K, Vollmar B, et al. Noninvasive in vivo analysis of the human hepatic microcirculation using OPS imaging. Transplantation. 2003;75:756–761.
3. KKTechnology. Cam1 and CapiScope User Manual. Honiton, Devon, England; 2004. http://www.kktechnology.com/help/book1.html, visited 02.01.2009.
4. MicroVisionMedical. MicroScan. Amsterdam, Netherlands; 2007. http://www.microvisionmedical.com/images/microscan2.pdf, visited 02.01.2009.
5. Dobbe J, Streekstra G, Atasever B. Measurement of functional microcircularity geometry and velocity distributions using automated image analysis. Medical and Biological Engineering and Computing. 2008;46:659–670.
6. Keimling R, Lang S. Bildfolgenanalyse in der Transplantationsmedizin am Beispiel der Leberperfusion mit orthogonaler Polarisationsspektroskopie. Lehrstuhl Intelligente Systeme, Universität Duisburg-Essen. Duisburg; 2008. Diploma Theses, http://www.uni-due.de/is, visited 02.01.2009.

Probabilistic Tracking and Model-Based Segmentation of 3D Tubular Structures

Stefan Wörz, William J. Godinez, Karl Rohr

University of Heidelberg, BIOQUANT, IPMB, and DKFZ Heidelberg,
Dept. Bioinformatics and Functional Genomics, Biomedical Computer Vision Group
s.woerz@dkfz.de

Abstract. We introduce a new approach for tracking-based segmentation of 3D tubular structures. The approach is based on a novel combination of a 3D cylindrical intensity model and particle filter tracking. In comparison to earlier work we utilize a 3D intensity model as the measurement model of the particle filter, thus a more realistic 3D appearance model is used that directly represents the image intensities of 3D tubular structures within semi-global regions-of-interest. We have successfully applied our approach using 3D synthetic images and real 3D MRA image data of the human pelvis.

1 Introduction

Accurate segmentation and quantification of 3D tubular structures is crucial in many biomedical applications. Examples of such structures are blood vessels, airways, or the spinal cord. In particular, the accurate quantification of human blood vessels is indispensable for diagnosis, treatment, and surgical planning. In clinical practice, the human vascular system is typically imaged by 3D magnetic resonance angiography (MRA) or computed tomography angiography (CTA).

Previous work on the automatic segmentation of tubular structures from 3D images can be divided into two main classes of approaches, one based on two-step centerline segmentation schemes and the other based on incremental tracking schemes. In two-step centerline segmentation schemes, first a local vesselness measure or a binary segmentation is determined. In the second step, the centerline of a tubular structure is constructed based on the results of the first step. Such approaches are, e.g., based on differential measures [1], minimal cost paths [2], or region growing with subsequent skeletonization [3]. A disadvantage of two-step approaches is that often only the centerline is computed and, thus, an additional step is required to estimate the local vessel shape (e.g., radius) [3].

In contrast, incremental tracking schemes segment vessels by incrementally proceeding along a vessel. In each increment, the image information of a vessel is analyzed locally, and a prediction of the centerline position of the next increment is generated. Incremental tracking schemes differ w.r.t. the used measurement model and the prediction method. Concerning the prediction, three different methods are typically used. Often, a simple forward propagation method is utilized where the predicted position of the next increment is directly based on the segmentation result of the current increment, usually proceeding a short distance along the local direction of a vessel (e.g., [4]). A more robust prediction method is the Kalman filter, which assumes a linear measurement model (e.g., [5, 6]). A promising alternative method are particle filters, which are more general than the Kalman filter (e.g., inclusion of a nonlinear measurement model) and exploit more effectively the image information (e.g., [7, 8, 9]). Regarding the measurement model, for tracking schemes based on forward propagation or a Kalman filter, typically contour information (e.g., [6]) or intensity information (e.g., [4, 5]) is used. For approaches employing particle filters, different measurement models have been used, e.g., based on circular shortest path search [7], gradient-based shape detection [9], or maximization of the image contrast [8]. However, these approaches utilize only relatively coarse appearance models based on mean intensity levels [7, 8, 9]. Also, these approaches often analyze tubular structures in 2D planes orthogonal to the centerline, i.e., the full 3D information is not exploited.

In this contribution, we introduce a new approach for the segmentation of 3D tubular structures, which is based on a combination of 3D parametric intensity models and particle filter tracking. In contrast to previous approaches based on particle filters (e.g., [7, 8, 9]), our approach relies on a 3D cylindrical intensity model as the measurement model in conjunction with a model fitting scheme. This 3D appearance model directly represents the image intensities of 3D tubular structures within semi-global regions-of-interest (ROIs). Thus, we utilize an advanced and more realistic appearance model. Also, since we directly exploit the 3D intensity information, a segmentation step or computation of image gradients is not required. Moreover, we directly quantify the tubular structure (e.g., centerline and local shape) based on the integrated model fitting scheme.

2 Materials and methods

In our approach, we use a 3D parametric intensity model which represents the shape and the image intensities of a tubular structure, and which serves as the appearance model of the particle filter. The model consists of an ideal sharp 3D cylinder convolved with a 3D Gaussian and incorporates, for example, the blurring effect of the image formation process. This cylindrical model comprises parameters for the width of the tubular structure (radius R) and the image blur σ, and is well-suited to represent tubular structures of different widths. Since the exact solution of a Gaussian smoothed cylinder cannot be expressed in closed form, we use an accurate approximation g_{Cylinder}, which is defined as the weighted superposition of two approximations for thin and thick cylinders [5].

Moreover, we incorporate the intensity levels a_0 (surrounding tissue) and a_1 (vessel) as well as a 3D rigid transform $\mathcal{R}$ with rotation parameters $\boldsymbol{\alpha} = (\alpha, \beta, \gamma)$ and translation parameters $\mathbf{x_0} = (x_0, y_0, z_0)$. This results in the parametric model $g_{M,\text{Cylinder}}(\mathbf{x}, \mathbf{p}) = a_0 + (a_1 - a_0)\, g_{\text{Cylinder}}(\mathcal{R}(\mathbf{x}, \boldsymbol{\alpha}, \mathbf{x_0}), R, \sigma)$ where $\mathbf{x} = (x, y, z)$ and $\mathbf{p} = (R, a_0, a_1, \sigma, \alpha, \beta, \gamma, x_0, y_0, z_0)$. To segment a certain vessel segment, we use a model fitting approach based on least-squares fitting of the

3D model to the image intensities $g(\mathbf{x})$ within a ROI:

$$\sum\nolimits_{\mathbf{x}\in\mathrm{ROI}} \left(g_{M,\mathrm{Cylinder}}\left(\mathbf{x},\mathbf{p}\right) - g\left(\mathbf{x}\right)\right)^2 \rightarrow \min. \tag{1}$$

For 3D vessel segmentation, we use a particle filter approach where tracking is formulated as a Bayesian sequential estimation problem. We represent the configuration of a vessel by a state vector $\boldsymbol{\theta}_k$ and assume that the measurement $\mathbf{z}_k$ reflects the true state of $\boldsymbol{\theta}_k$. At the increment k, the aim is to estimate the state $\boldsymbol{\theta}_k$ given a sequence of measurements $\mathbf{z}_{1:k}$. By modeling the state's evolution via a dynamical model $p(\boldsymbol{\theta}_k|\boldsymbol{\theta}_{k-1})$ and incorporating measurements derived from the images via a measurement model $p(\mathbf{z}_k|\boldsymbol{\theta}_k)$, a Bayesian filter estimates the posterior distribution $p(\boldsymbol{\theta}_k|\mathbf{z}_{1:k})$ via stochastic propagation and Bayes' theorem:

$$p(\boldsymbol{\theta}_k|\mathbf{z}_{1:k}) \propto p(\mathbf{z}_k|\boldsymbol{\theta}_k) \int p(\boldsymbol{\theta}_k|\boldsymbol{\theta}_{k-1})\, p(\boldsymbol{\theta}_{k-1}|\mathbf{z}_{1:k-1})\, d\boldsymbol{\theta}_{k-1} \tag{2}$$

An estimate of $\boldsymbol{\theta}_k$ can be obtained from the posterior $p(\boldsymbol{\theta}_k|\mathbf{z}_{1:k})$, which, in our case, is determined using a particle filter. The main idea of this algorithm is to employ a set $\{\boldsymbol{\theta}_k^i; w_k^i\}_{i=1}^{N_s}$ of N_s weighted random samples $\boldsymbol{\theta}_k^i$ (the 'particles') to approximate the posterior distribution.

Based on the particle filter framework we have developed two different tracking schemes. In the first scheme, the state vector is defined by the position $\mathbf{x}_0$ of the 3D tubular model $g_{M,\mathrm{Cylinder}}$ and by its velocity vector, thus $\boldsymbol{\theta}_k = (x_{0,k}, x'_{0,k}, y_{0,k}, y'_{0,k}, z_{0,k}, z'_{0,k})$. For the dynamical model $p(\boldsymbol{\theta}_k|\boldsymbol{\theta}_{k-1})$ we adopt a constant velocity model. Measurements for $p(\mathbf{z}_k|\boldsymbol{\theta}_k)$ are computed based on the difference between the predicted position and the measured position $\mathbf{z}_k = \hat{\mathbf{x}}_{0,k}$, which is obtained by fitting the 3D tubular model based on (1).

In our second tracking scheme, the parameters $\mathbf{p}$ including the position $\mathbf{x}_0$ of the 3D tubular model $g_{M,\mathrm{Cylinder}}$ constitute the state $\boldsymbol{\theta}$. For the dynamical model $p(\boldsymbol{\theta}_k|\boldsymbol{\theta}_{k-1})$ we assume that the radius R, intensity levels a_0 and a_1, the image blur σ, and the rotation parameters $\boldsymbol{\alpha}$ follow independent Gaussian random walk dynamics. For the position $\mathbf{x}_0$, the dynamical model is defined by

$$\mathbf{x}_{0,k}^i = \mathbf{x}_{0,k-1}^i + \mathcal{R}^{-1}\big((0,0,l)^T, \boldsymbol{\alpha}_{k-1}^i, \mathbf{0}\big) + \mathbf{n}_k^i, \tag{3}$$

where l denotes the magnitude of the displacement vector and $\mathbf{n}$ is a noise vector comprising independent zero-mean Gaussian noise statistics. Our measurement model $p(\mathbf{z}_k|\boldsymbol{\theta}_k)$ quantifies the probability that the measured image intensities $\mathbf{z}_k$ of the image g conform to the predicted state $\boldsymbol{\theta}_k$ within a 3D ROI.

3 Results

We have applied our new approach to different 3D synthetic images as well as 3D MRA image data. In the first part of the experiments, we have used 3D synthetic images containing different tubular structures (straight and curved structures) with a spectrum of different widths, curvatures, and noise levels.

From the experiments we found that our two tracking schemes generally yield accurate results for the centerline and shape of the tubular structures. As an example, we have used tubular spirals which comprise several short low contrast parts along the spiral to simulate vessels with poor local contrast (see Fig. 1, left). Both tracking schemes performed well for a range of different noise levels. In the case of a relatively high noise level (normal contrast $a = 50$, low contrast $a_{low} = 10$, and added Gaussian noise with standard deviation $\sigma_n = 30$), it turned out that the first tracking scheme terminates in the third winding. In comparison, the second tracking scheme, which directly employs the cylindrical appearance model, is able to segment the full spiral (seven windings) despite the poor signal-to-noise ratio. Fig. 1 shows the segmentation result represented by the centerline (center) and shape (right). It can be seen that the spiral including the highly curved inner part has been fully tracked and generally well segmented. In contrast, a previous approach based on a Kalman filter [5] failed to segment the full spiral, and terminated even earlier than the first tracking scheme based on a particle filter (see the marked termination points in Fig. 1, left). To quantify the results, we have computed the maximal error $e_{R,\max}$ of the estimated radius. For the first 1000 voxels along the centerline (about two windings), which have

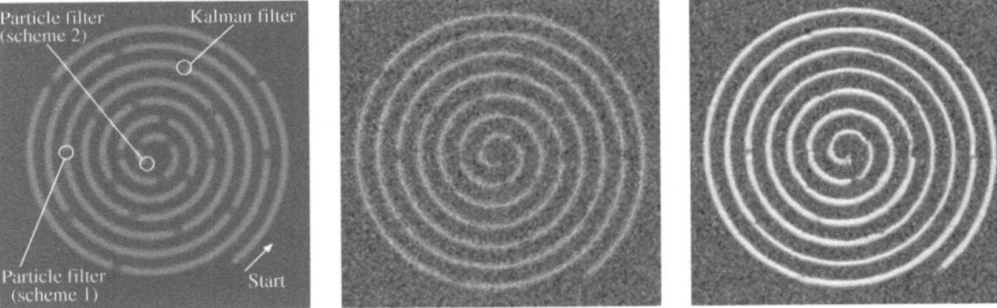

Fig. 1. 3D spiral with low contrast parts and indicated end points for the tracking schemes based on the Kalman filter and both particle filter schemes (left) as well as segmentation result of our new approach using the second tracking scheme represented by the centerline (center) and shape (right).

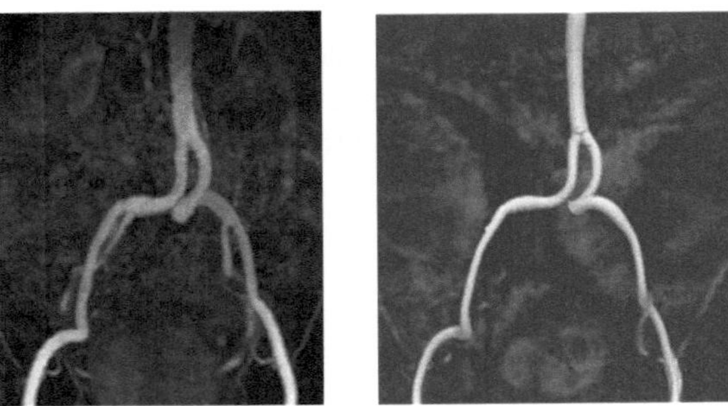

Fig. 2. Maximum intensity projection of a 3D MRA of a human pelvis (left) and segmentation result for two arteries using the second particle filter tracking scheme (right).

been segmented by all three approaches, we found that the new approach yields a maximal error of $e_{R,\max} = 1.12$ and $e_{R,\max} = 0.87$ voxels for the first and second tracking scheme, respectively, and the Kalman filter yields $e_{R,\max} = 1.28$ voxels.

Moreover, we have also applied the new approach using both tracking schemes to 3D MRA images. For example, Fig. 2 shows the maximum intensity projection of the MRA of a human pelvis (left) as well as the 3D segmentation result using the second tracking scheme (right). It can be seen that arteries of varying sizes and high curvatures have been well segmented.

4 Discussion

We introduced a new approach for tracking-based segmentation of 3D tubular structures. The approach is based on a combination of a 3D cylindrical intensity model and particle filter tracking. In comparison to earlier work we utilize a 3D intensity model as the measurement model of the particle filter, thus a more realistic appearance model is used that directly represents the image intensities of 3D tubular structures within semi-global regions-of-interest. We have successfully applied our approach using 3D synthetic images and real 3D MRA image data.

Acknowledgement. This work has been funded by the Deutsche Forschungsgemeinschaft (DFG) within the project QuantVessel (RO 2471/6-1).

References

1. Frangi AF, Niessen WJ, Vincken KL, et al. Multiscale vessel enhancement filtering. Proc MICCAI. 1998; p. 130–137.
2. Wink O, Niessen WJ, Viergever MA. Multiscale vessel tracking. IEEE Trans Med Imaging. 2004;23(1):130–133.
3. Volkau I, Ng TT, Marchenko Y, et al. On geometric modeling of the human intracranial venous system. IEEE Trans Med Imaging. 2008;27(6):745–51.
4. Noordmans HJ, Smeulders AWM. High accuracy tracking of 2D/3D curved line structures by consecutive cross-section matching. Pattern Recogn Lett. 1998;19(1):97–111.
5. Wörz S, Rohr K. Segmentation and quantification of human vessels using a 3-D cylindrical intensity model. IEEE Trans Image Process. 2007;16(8):1994–2004.
6. Guerrero J, Salcudean SE, McEwen JA, et al. Real-time vessel segmentation and tracking for ultrasound imaging applications. IEEE Trans Medical Imaging. 2007;26(8):1079–1090.
7. Florin C, Paragios N, Williams J. Globally optimal active contours, sequential Monte Carlo and on-line learning for vessel segmentation. Proc ECCV. 2006; p. 476–489.
8. Schaap M, Manniesing R, Smal I, et al. Bayesian tracking of tubular structures and its application to carotid arteries in CTA. Proc MICCAI. 2007; p. 562–570.
9. Lesage D, Angelini ED, Bloch I, et al. Medial-based bayesian tracking for vascular segmentation: Application to coronary arteries in 3D CT angiography. Proc IEEE ISBI. 2008; p. 268–271.

Automatische Segmentierung der zerebralen Gefäße aus 3D-TOF-MRA-Bildsequenzen mittels Fuzzy-Methoden

Nils Daniel Forkert[1], Dennis Säring[1], Karolin Wenzel[2], Jens Fiehler[2], Till Illies[2], Dietmar Möller[3], Heinz Handels[1]

[1]Institut für Medizinische Informatik, Universitätsklinikum Hamburg-Eppendorf
[2]Klinik und für Neuroradiologie, Universitätsklinikum Hamburg-Eppendorf
[3]AB Technische Informatiksysteme, Department Informatik, Universität Hamburg
n.forkert@uke.uni-hamburg.de

Kurzfassung. Im Rahmen dieses Beitrages wird eine automatische Methode zur Extraktion des zerebralen Gefäßsystems aus 3D-Time-of-Flight (TOF)-MRA-Bildsequenzen vorgestellt. Hierbei wird zunächst in einem Vorverarbeitungsschritt das Gehirn von den nicht-zerebralen Gewebeklassen befreit. In einem weiteren Schritt wird aus dem TOF-Datensatz ein Vesselness- und Maximum-Parameterbild berechnet. Diese werden dann unter Verwendung eines Fuzzy-Inferenzsystems mit dem TOF-Datensatz kombiniert. In dem daraus resultierenden Datensatz heben sich sowohl kleine als auch pathologisch veränderte Gefäße deutlicher vom restlichen Gewebe ab. Abschließend wird das Gefäßsystem unter Verwendung des Fuzzy-Connectedness-Regionenwachstums extrahiert. Eine erste Evaluation der vorgestellten Methode zeigte, dass sich die Ergebnisse im Bereich des Inter-Observer-Vergleichs befinden.

1 Einleitung

Bei Vorliegen einer zerebralen Gefäßmissbildung ist ein genaues Verständnis der individuellen Gefäßanatomie von großer Bedeutung für Diagnose, Risikoeinschätzung und Therapie. Zerebrale Gefäße stellen ein äußerst komplexes System dar, dessen Verständnis durch eine schichtweise Darstellung von 3D-Angiographie Bilddaten ein hohes Maß an räumlichem Vorstellungsvermögen sowie anatomisches Fachwissen verlangt. Eine 3D-Darstellung des zerebralen Gefäßsystems ermöglicht eine verbesserte und einfachere visuelle Beurteilung. Eine detailierte Segmentierung erlaubt, gegenüber Volume-Rendering Techniken, nicht nur eine verbesserte Visualisierung mittels Oberflächenmodellen, sondern darüber hinaus auch eine Quantifizierung von pathologischen Veränderungen der Gefäße.

Zur Segmentierung des zerebralen Gefäßsystems wurde eine Vielzahl von Methoden publiziert. Für einen umfassenden Überblick wird an dieser Stelle auf die Arbeit von Suri et al. [1] verwiesen. Viele vorgeschlagene Methoden zeichnen sich dadurch aus, dass Modellwissen in Form von typischen Grauwertverteilungen [2] oder typischen Eigenschaften der Gefäßtopologie [3] verwendet wird. Bei pathologischen Veränderungen der Gefäße, wie z.B. bei der arteriovenösen Malformation, ist das verwendete Modellwissen jedoch nicht mehr zwingend erfüllt und kann daher zu Segmentierungsfehlern führen.

2 Material und Methoden

2.1 TOF-MRA-Bildsequenzen und Vorverarbeitung

Die zur Verfügung stehenden MRA-Datensätze wurden mit einem 3 Tesla Trio Scanner der Firma Siemens aufgenommen. Die verwendeten TOF-Bildsequenzen weisen 156 Schichten mit einer Voxelgröße von $0{,}47 \times 0{,}47 \times 0{,}5\ \text{mm}^3$ auf.

Time-of-Flight-MRA-Daten werden häufig überlappend blockweise aufgenommen (Multi-Slab-Aufnahmetechnik). Im Bereich der Überschneidungen der einzelnen Schichtblöcke kommt es jedoch häufig zu einem Abfall der Amplitude (Slab Boundary Artefakt). Da dieses bei einer intensitätsbasierten Weiterverarbeitung zu Problemen führt, wurden diese Intensitätsinhomogenitäten automatisch mittels dem von Kholmovski et al. [4] vorgestellten Verfahren reduziert.

Nicht-zerebrale Gewebeklassen, wie Fett und Knochenmark, weisen eine der Gefäße ähnliche Intensitätsverteilung auf und können bei der Weiterverarbeitung zu Übersegmentierungen führen. Daher werden diese in einem abschließenden Vorverarbeitungsschritt nach der Methode von Forkert et al. [5] ausgeschlossen.

2.2 Fuzzy Gefäßsegmentierung

Zur Segmentierung des zerebralen Gefäßsystems wird auf Basis des TOF-MRA-Datensatzes T zunächst ein Parameterbild V unter Verwendung des von Sato et al. [6] vorgeschlagenen Vesselnessfilters generiert. Hierbei wird jedem Voxel,

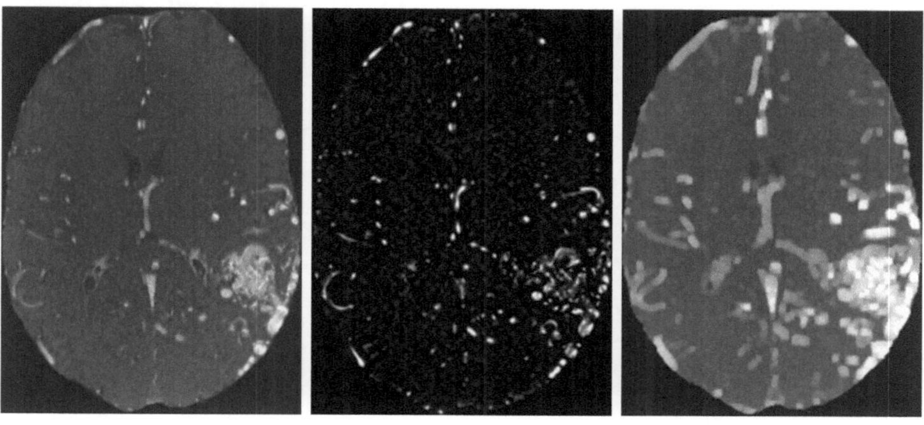

Abb. 1. Schicht aus einem TOF-Datensatz (links), Ergebnis des Vesselnessfilter (Mitte), Ergebnis des Maximum-Filter (rechts).

unter Berücksichtigung einer typischen Gefäßtopologie, ein Wert für dessen Gefäßähnlichkeit zugewiesen. Dieses führt dazu, dass auch kleine Gefäße, die sich durch geringe Intensitäten auszeichnen, durch den Filter gegenüber dem Hintergrund hervorgehoben werden. Auf Grund der implizit verwendeten Forminformation führt der Vesselnessfilter bei pathologischen Gefäßveränderungen jedoch zu unbefriedigenden Ergebnissen (Abb. 1 (mitte)). In einem weiteren Schritt wird ein zweites Parameterbild M unter Verwendung eines Maximalwertfilters generiert (Abb. 1 (rechts)). Hierbei wird jedem Voxel der maximal auftretende Intensitätswert innerhalb einer definierten 3D-Nachbarschaft zugeordnet. Dieser Datensatz dient im Folgenden dazu, Intensitätsinformationen der Nachbarschaft eines Voxels mit in die Fuzzy-Kombination einzubeziehen.

Nach Berechnung der Parameterbilder können diese unter Verwendung eines Fuzzy-Inferenzsystem mit dem TOF-MRA-Datensatz voxelweise kombiniert werden. Wesentlicher Vorteil eines Fuzzy-Inferenzsystems ist, dass eine nichtlineare Kombination der einzelnen Parameter möglich ist. Darüber hinaus kann so unsicheres Wissen in den Inferenzmechanismus integriert werden. Für eine ausführliche Einführung in Fuzzy-Inferenzsysteme sei an dieser Stelle auf [7] verwiesen.

Der erste Schritt der Kombination der Parameter mittels eines Fuzzy-Inferenzsystems besteht darin, die scharfen Eingangswerte zu fuzzyfizieren. Im Rahmen dieser Arbeit wurden die auftretenden Signale der drei Eingänge durch jeweils 3 Zugehörigkeitsfunktionen fuzzyfiziert. Hierbei wurden Dreiecksfunktionen als Zugehörigkeitsfunktionen für die linguistischen Terme „niedrig", „mittel" und „hoch" verwendet. Abbildung 2 zeigt die Zugehörigkeitsfunktionen exemplarisch für die auftretenden Signale eines TOF-Datensatzes. Der jeweils obere und untere Schwellwert der Zugehörigkeitsfunktionen wird dabei datensatzspezifisch für jeden Parameter auf Basis der dazugehörigen Histogramme extrahiert.

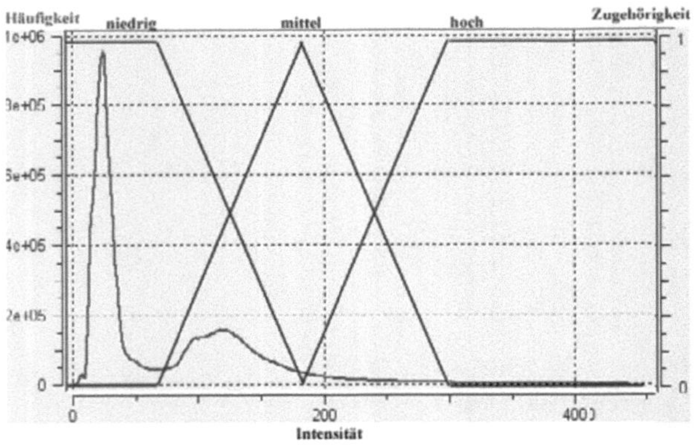

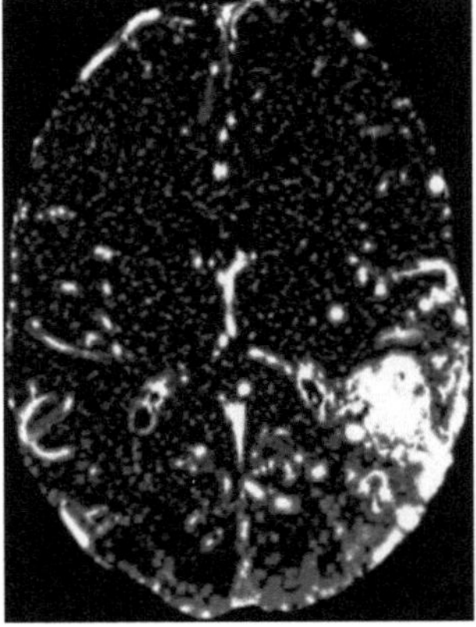

Abb. 2. Histogramm des TOF-Datensatz (rot) und Fuzzyfizierung (blau) des TOF-Eingangs (links), Ergebnis der Fuzzy-Kombination (rechts).

Für die Fuzzy-Inferenz wurde eine Regelbasis mit insgesamt 27 (3 Eingänge mit je 3 liguistischen Termen) empirisch bestimmten Regeln definiert. Diese Regeln ordnen jeder Kombination von linguistischen Termen eine von 5 Konklusionen (Gefäßwahrscheinlichkeit: sehr gering, gering, mittel, hoch, sehr hoch) zu, welche wiederum durch Dreiecks-Zugehörigkeitsfunktionen beschrieben wurden. Die Fuzzy-Inferenz wurde im Rahmen dieser Arbeit durch einen Maximum-Operator für die Akkumulation und einen Minimum-Operator für die Implikation implementiert. Das Ergebnis der Auswertung aller Regeln für ein Voxel durch den Inferenzmechanismus liefert eine Fuzzymenge. Um hieraus den benötigten scharfen Ausgabewert für das Fuzzy-Parameterbild zu gewinnen (Defuzzyfizierung) wurde die Center-of-Gravity Methode [8] verwendet.

Die Idee bei der Definition der 27 Regeln war es, bei der Wahl der Konklusion die Antwort des Vesselnessfilter stärker zu gewichten, wenn der Maximumfilter nur eine schwache Antwort geliefert hat und den TOF-Eingang stärker, wenn der Maximumfilter ein starkes Signal ausgegeben hat. Das Resultat der Fuzzy-Kombination ist ein Datensatz, in dem sich sowohl kleine als auch pathologische Gefäße deutlich vom umliegenden Gewebe abheben (Abb. 2).

Um das Gefäßsystem aus dem Fuzzy-Parameterdatensatz zu extrahieren, wird zunächst eine Schwellwertoperation mit nachfolgender Zusammenhangsanalyse auf diesen angewendet. Für jede extrahierte Komponente werden dann Mittelwert und Standardabweichung für die dazugehörigen Fuzzy-Werte berechnet. Abschließend wird das von Udupa vorgeschlagene Fuzzy-Connectedness-Regionenwachstum [8] verwendet, um das Gefäßsystem, unter Verwendung der zuvor bestimmten Parameter, aus dem Fuzzy-Parameterdatensatz zu segmentieren. Als Saatpunkt hierfür dient das Voxel der jeweiligen Komponente mit dem höchsten Fuzzy-Wert. Die Segmentierungsergebnisse der einzelnen Komponenten werden abschließend mittels Disjunktion zu einem Endergebnis verknüpft.

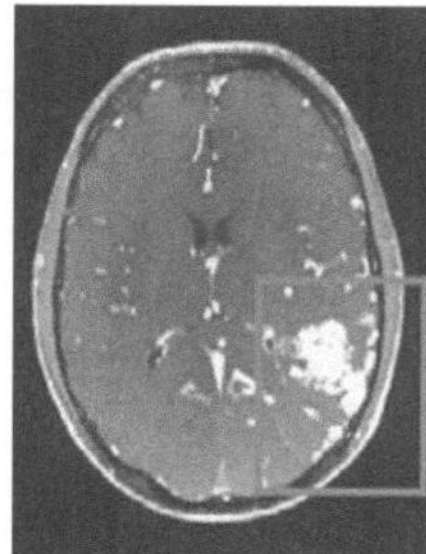
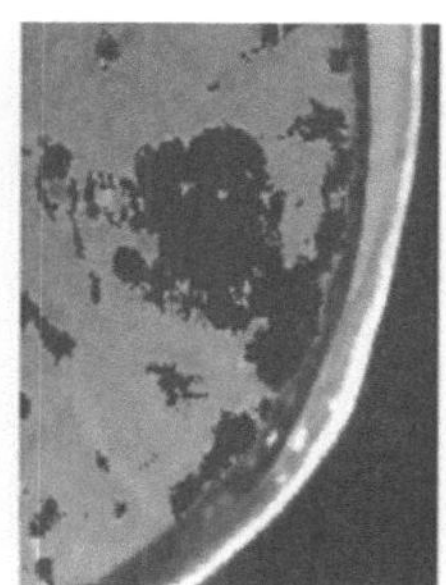
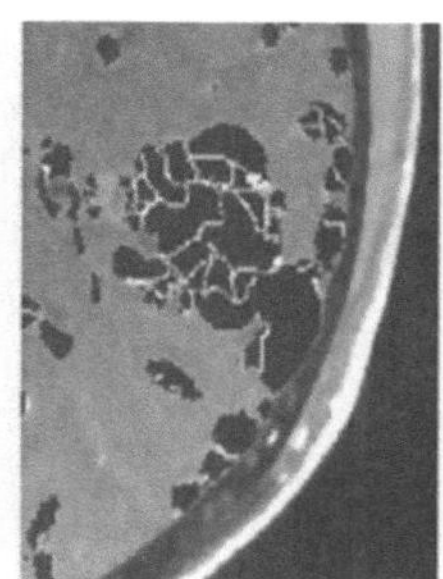
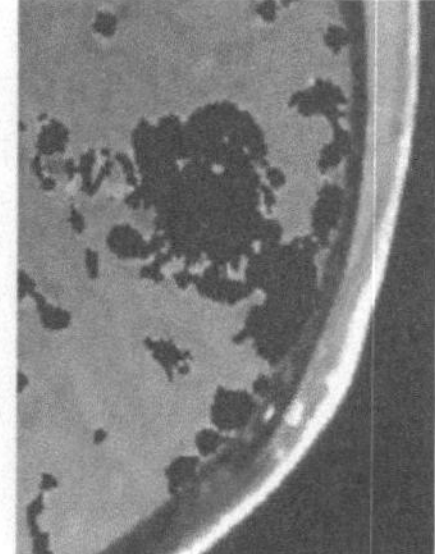

Abb. 3. Ergebnis der Segmentierungen im grün dargestellten Bereich für eine TOF-Schicht (links): Manuelle Segmentierungen von 2 Experten (mitte) und Fuzzy-Segmentierung (rechts).

3 Ergebnisse

Zur ersten Evaluation der vorgeschlagenen Methode zur Segmentierung des zerebralen Gefäßsystems stand ein TOF-Datensatz von einem Patienten mit einer zerebralen arteriovenösen Malformation zur Verfügung. Als Goldstandard dienten Segmentierungen von zwei medizinischen Experten, die unabhängig voneinander unter Verwendung von Volume Growing und manueller Nachkorrektur das zerebrale Gefäßsystem extrahiert haben. Zur quantitativen Evaluation wurde der Dice-Koeffizient [5] verwendet, wobei Werte nahe 1 auf eine gute Übereinstimmung hinweisen. Ein Vergleich der beiden manuellen Segmentierungen ergab einen Dice-Koeffizient von 0.8154. Bei dem Vergleich der automatischen zu den manuellen Segmentierungen ergab sich ein Dice-Koeffizient von 0.8116 und 0.8219 (∅ 0.8168). Das gute quantitative Ergebniss wurden durch eine visuelle Begutachtung von erfahrenen Neuroradiologen bestätigt (Abb. 3). Im Gegensatz zur manuellen Segmentierung, für die, je nach Komplexität des Gefäßsystems, zwischen 6 und 10 Stunden benötigt werden, beträgt die Berechnungszeit für die automatische Segmentierung ca. 1 Stunde, währenddessen keine Benutzerinteraktion nötig ist.

4 Diskussion

Im Rahmen dieses Beitrages wurde ein Ansatz, basierend auf Fuzzy-Methoden, zur Segmentierung des zerebralen Gefäßsystems aus TOF-MRA-Bildsequenzen vorgestellt. Eine erste Evaluation anhand eines vollständig segmentierten Datensatzes ergab, dass die vorgestellte Methode gute Ergebnisse im Bereich des Inter-Observer-Vergleichs erzielt. Eine visuelle Begutachtung zeigte, dass sowohl gesunde als auch missgebildete Gefäße, sofern sie sich hinreichend gut vom Hintergrund abheben, durch das vorgestellte Verfahren extrahiert werden konnten.

Eine weitergehende Evaluation der Fuzzy-Gefäßsegmentierung anhand einer größeren Anzahl an Datensätze ist derzeit in der Vorbereitung. In diesem Rahmen soll auch ein quantitativer Vergleich mit anderen bereits etablierten Methoden zur Gefäßsegmentierung erfolgen.

Danksagung. Diese Arbeit wurde von der Deutschen Forschungsgemeinschaft gefördert (Ha2355/10-1).

Literaturverzeichnis

1. Suri J, Liu K, Reden L, et al. A review on MR vascular image processing algorithms: Skeleton versus nonskeleton approaches: Part II. IEEE Trans Inf Technol Biomed. 2002;6(4):338–350.
2. Hassouna MS, et al. Cerebrovascular segmentation from TOF using stochastic models. Med Image Anal. 2006;10(1):2–18.
3. Lorigo L, et al. Curves: Curve evolution for vessel segmentation. Med Image Anal. 2001;5:195 – 106.

4. Kholmovski E, Alexander A, Parker D. Correction of slab boundary artifact using histogramm matching. J Magn Reson Imaging. 2002;15:610–617.
5. Forkert N, et al. Fully automatic skull-atripping in 3D time-of-flight MRA image sequences. In: Visual Computing for Biomedicine; 2008. p. 159 –165.
6. Sato Y, et al. Three-dimensional multi-scale line filter for segmentation and visualization of curvelinear structures in medical images. Med Image Anal. 1998;2(2):143–168.
7. Tizhoosh H. Fuzzy Bildverarbeitung - Einführung in Theorie und Praxis. Springer; 1998.
8. Udupa JK, Samarasekera S. Fuzzy connectedness and object definition: Theory, algorithms, and applications in image segmentation. Graph Models. 1996;58(3):246–261.

Segmentation of the Knee for Analysis of Osteoarthritis

A Robust Algorithm for the Definition of Subchondral Evaluation Regions

Peter Zerfass[1], Oleg Museyko[1], Valérie Bousson[2], Jean-Denis Laredo[2], Willi A. Kalender[1], Klaus Engelke[1]

[1]Institute of Medical Physics, Friedrich-Alexander-University Erlangen-Nürnberg
[2]Service de Radiologie Ostéo-Articulaire, Hôpital Lariboisière, Paris, France
peter.zerfass@imp.uni-erlangen.de

Abstract. Osteoarthritis changes the load distribution within joints and also changes bone density and structure. Within typical timelines of clinical studies these changes can be very small. Therefore precise definition of evaluation regions which are highly robust and show little to no inter- and intra-operator variance are essential for high quality quantitative analysis. To achieve this goal we have developed a system for the definition of such regions with minimal user input.

1 Introduction

Our task is to evaluate changes in bone mineral density (BMD) and bone structure in patients with osteoarthritis based on CT datasets. Usually MRI scans and radiographs of the joint gap are used as diagnostic imaging procedures. However, CT is better suited for the quantification of changes in BMD and bone structure which may add significant information for the diagnosis of osteoarthritis.

The aim is to define evaluation regions largely independent of the user perfoming the analysis. To achieve this we need to automatically identify at least one salient anatomical feature.

One such feature is the growth plate. During development of the foetus the epiphyses and diaphyses of tibia and femur are initiated as separate structures which are joined during growth. This process causes a visible break in the texture of the cancellous bone called the growth plate. Even though the trabecular structure and shape of the bone change during lifetime, the texture change at the growth plate does not. Our system first segments the growth plate. A further step restricts the volumes of interest (VOIs) to areas adjacent to the joint gap between tibia and femur, since we anticipate the biggest BMD changes in the subchondral bone VOIs.

Together with the eigenvectors of the moments of inertia of the anatomical structure we can define position and orientation of our VOIs in a robust and repeatable manner.

2 Materials and methods

CT data for this study were acquired on a Siemens Somatom Sensation 64 scanner at 120 kV and 255 mAs. Each scan includes a calibration phantom which allows for quantitative analysis once the segmentation steps are complete. Images are reconstructed with 434 slices and 512 by 512 pixels with an isotropic resolution of 0.5 mm and a medium U40u kernel.

Step 1: Automatic detection of the calibration phantom. We segment the periosteal and endosteal areas of the femur and tibia using an adaptation of an algorithm described in [1, 2].

Step 2: To segment the growth plate (Fig. 1) we have implemented a new segmentation algorithm which combines statistical gray value information and a constraint on the shape of the growth plate.

The user sets one seed point somewhere in the central region of the growth plate. Relative to this point we define a band of voxels with a width of 60 slices in the z-direction of the image. The algorithm divides this band further into individual columns oriented in z-direction. In each column we find the voxel whose gray value deviates most from its neighbors within a given distance (Fig. 3(a)).

The seed point is transformed into the first link from which we grow a chainmail data structure as described in [3]. Each point or "link" in the chainmail has 4 neighbors whose maximum and minimum distances are limited by the data structure. We iteratively search for the closest point found in step one of the algorithm. If there is a point within reach then a new link is added and its position fixed. If no point is found to be close enough then a link is added but left 'floating free'. Free floating links add their mobility when they are processed so their neighboring links are able to connect to points further away. In a post processing step the position of floating points is interpolated between neighboring links. Then the edges are trimmed because the growth plate is only visible in the center region of the bone (Fig. 3(b)).

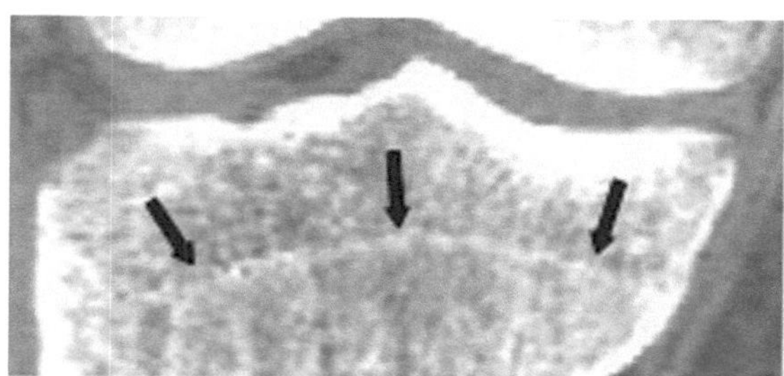

Fig. 1. The tibia growth plate (indicated by arrows)

Fig. 2. Growth plate segmentation (window level adjusted for better contrast)

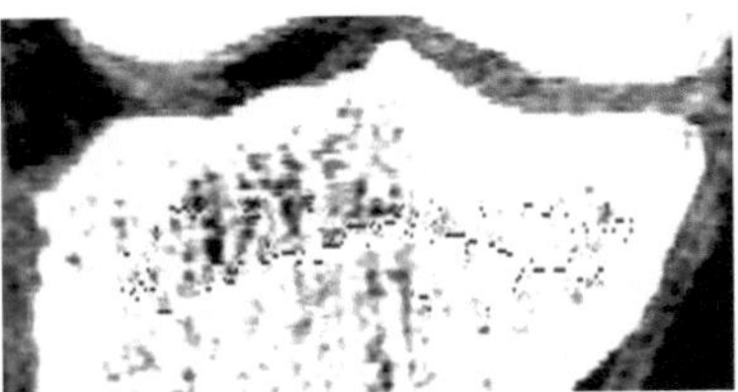

(a) Voxels of greatest gray value deviation (dark dots).

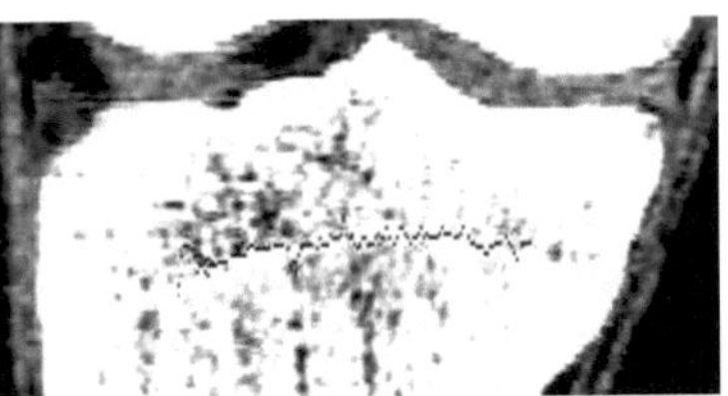

(b) After chainmailing, relaxation and trimming.

Step 3: To define the VOIs we also segment the joint gap by calculating distance maps for the femur and tibia. Then we perform two walks: One starting from the surface voxels of the femur to the tibia and one in the opposite direction.

We define a voxel as belonging to the joint gap if during both walks it has the following property: All neighboring points, which are farther away from the starting anatomical structure than the voxel under consideration are equally close (or closer) to the target structure.

Step 4: VOIs are defined between the periosteal surface bordering the joint gap and the growth plate which is extended by a plane. This plane is fitted through the mass center of the growth plate (Fig. 3).

3 Results

Preliminary results were evaluated from analysis and comparison of the results of the same datasets by three operators (inter-operator variability) and also by repeated analysis of single datasets by one operator (intra-operator variability). The only possible variation is the seed point of the growth plate, since the bone and joint gap segmentation are done fully automatic. Thus only the variation of

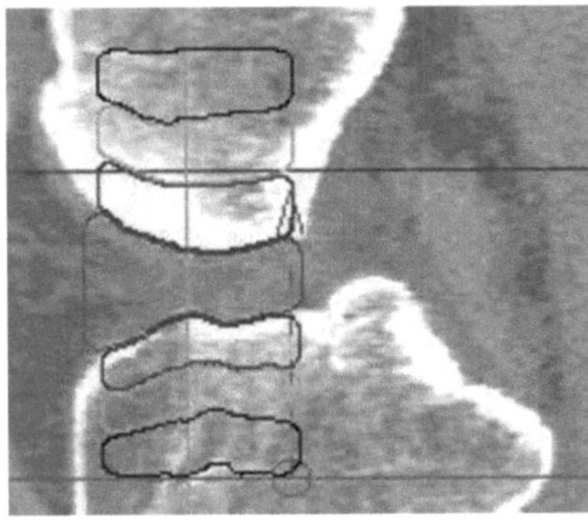

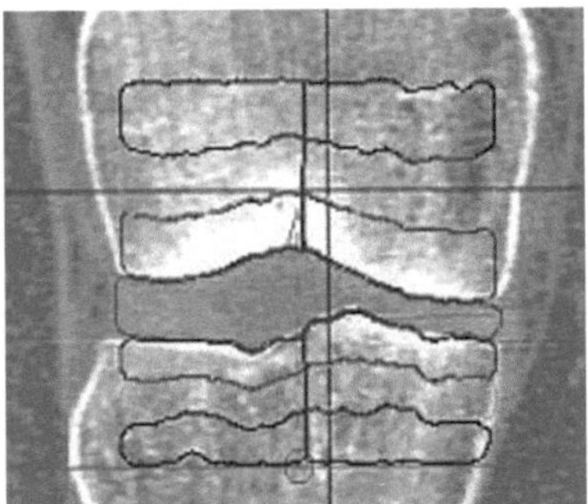

Fig. 3. Joint gap and three subchondral VOIs per structure (lateral and coronal view)

the center of mass of the growth plate enters as an operator dependent variable into the positioning of the VOIs.

In both experimental setups deviation of the center of mass averaged 1 ± 0.8 voxels. Thus we conclude that the definition of the VOIs as described above is repeatable and robust.

4 Discussion

We have demonstrated a way to define VOIs within the knee in a robust and repeatable way using a novel segmentation algorithm for 'noisy' structures. The center of mass of the growth plate coupled with the eigenvectors of the moments of inertia of the anatomical structures provide salient features for the attachment of the VOIs.

Together with the fully automatic definition of the joint gap we have managed to decouple the positioning of the VOIs largely from the dependence of operator input.

In the future we will perform more extensive precision analysis with more datasets and larger number of operators. We will add evaluation algorithms, which will perform e.g. trabecular morphology analyzes within the defined VOIs. Due to the high precision the developed methodology seems a promising tool for the analysis of osteoarthritis induced bone changes in longitudinal studies.

Acknowledgement. This project was supported in part by Servier, France.

References

1. Kang Y. 3D Quantitative Computed Tomography (QCT) of the Proximal Femur. Erlangen: Institut der Medizinischen Physik der Friedrich-Alexander-Universität Erlangen-Nürnberg; 2000.
2. Mastmeyer A. Segmentierung der Wirbelsäule und Definition anatomischer Kordinatensysteme für Quantitative Computertomographie (QCT). Erlangen: Institut der Medizinischen Physik der Friedrich-Alexander-Universität Erlangen-Nürnberg; 2006.
3. Gibson S. 3D chainmail: A fast algorithm for deforming volumetric objects. Procs Symp Interactive 3D Graph. 1997; p. 149 ff.

Zweistufige Segmentierung des Tracheobronchialbaums mittels iterativen adaptiven Bereichswachstumsverfahren

Ingmar Gergel[1], Ingmar Wegner[1], Ralf Tetzlaff[2], Hans-Peter Meinzer[1]

[1]Abt. Medizinische und Biologische Informatik, Deutsches Krebsforschungszentrum
[2]Abt. Radiologie, Deutsches Krebsforschungszentrum
i.gergel@dkfz-heidelberg.de

Kurzfassung. Die Segmentierung des Tracheobronchialbaums aus medizinischen Bilddaten ist essentiell für unterschiedliche Anwendungen, beispielsweise der navigierten Bronchoskopie. Hierbei liegt das Hauptaugenmerk auf einer möglichst detaillierten Segmentierung der Bronchien bei möglichst geringer Laufzeit des Algorithmus. Dieser Beitrag beschreibt ein Verfahren, welches in zwei Schritten den Tracheobronchialbaum anhand eines adaptiven Bereichswachstumsverfahrens aus CT-Aufnahmen segmentiert. Im ersten Schritt werden die großen Atemwege und im zweiten Schritt die kleinen Atemwege getrennt segmentiert. Insgesamt wird dadurch die Anzahl der Voxel, die von rechenaufwändigeren Algorithmen (bspw. Gefäß-Tracking) verarbeitet werden müssen, verringert. Die Ergebnisse zeigen bei minimaler Laufzeiterhöhung eine deutliche Steigerung der Anzahl sowie Tiefe der segmentierten Bronchien.

1 Einleitung

Die Segmentierung von verschiedenen Objekten aus medizinischen Bilddaten stellt eine zentrale Komponente in der Bildverarbeitung dar, meist dient Sie als initialer Schritt für weitere Bearbeitungsprozesse. In Abhängigkeit vom Anwendungsbereich und der Zielsetzung kommen unterschiedliche Segmentierungsalgorithmen zum Einsatz. In der medizinischen Bildverarbeitung liegt unter anderem ein Fokus auf der Segmentierung von tubulären Strukturen, wie sie beispielsweise in Blutgefäßen oder im Tracheobronchialbaum vorliegen.

Statistische Verfahren wie das Bayesian Tracking [1] oder aktive Formmodelle [2] werden als äußerst robust beschrieben, gehen jedoch mit einer erhöhten Rechenzeit einher. Diese sollte jedoch für die Akzeptanz in der klinischen Routine möglichst gering gehalten werden. Ein viel genutzter Algorithmus zur Segmentierung von komplex zusammenhängenden Strukturen ist das Bereichswachstumsverfahren, das sich durch eine geringe Laufzeit auszeichnet. Speziell bei der Segmentierung des Bronchialbaums resultiert das Bereichswachstumsverfahren jedoch oft in einem Auslaufen ins Lungenparenchym, dass heißt aufgrund der durch das CT-Auflösungsvermögen begrenzten Dicke der Bronchialwände entstehen Löcher über die der Wachstumsprozess das Innere der Bronchien verlässt und außerhalb liegende Strukturen mitsegmentiert. Durch einen adaptiven

Schwellwertansatz im Bereichswachstumsverfahren lässt sich die Stelle des Auslaufens automatisch detektieren und die Segmentierung vorher stoppen [3]. Das Ergebnis entspricht jedoch nicht der maximal möglichen Segmentierung mittels Bereichswachstumsverfahren, da peripher liegende Bronchien mit Grauwerten außerhalb des einen automatisch gefundenen Grauwertintervalls nicht mehr hinzu segmentiert werden können. Diese Grenze ist jedoch gegebenenfalls nur auf einen Bronchus optimiert. Für die verbleibenden Bronchialäste liese sich ein größeres Grauwertintervall ansetzen. Diesen Punkt aufgreifend beschreibt der vorliegende Beitrag ein Verfahren, welches nach der primären Segmentierung des Bronchialbaumes, an den ermittelten Endpunkten der Bronchien das adaptive Schwellwert-Bereichswachstumsverfahren erneut durchführt, um weitere Bronchialäste zu erfassen. Hierbei wurde ein automatisierter Ablauf gewählt um die Laufzeit so gering wie möglich zu halten.

2 Material und Methoden

Zur Implementierung des Verfahrens wurde die quelloffene C++ Klassenbibliothek Medical Imaging Interaction Toolkit (MITK) verwendet [4]. Die Primär-Segmentierung wird im Gegensatz zum reinen Bereichswachstum nicht über ein festes Grauwertintervall gebildet. Vielmehr wird während der Segmentierung sukzessive das Grauwertintervall vergrößert, so dass festgehalten wird, bei welchem Intervall ein Voxel in die Segmentierung aufgenommen wurde. So kann auch nach der Berechnung die gewünschte Schwelle automatisch gefunden oder interaktive gewählt werden [3, 5]. Auf den Enden (Blättern) dieser Segmentierung aufbauend erfolgen weitere Segmentierungen, welche ebenfalls durch einen automatisierten Abbruchmechanismus gesteuert werden.

In dem von den Autoren entwickelten Verfahren werden zwei Modi für den Abbruchmechanismus unterschieden: Die initiale Segmentierung der großen Atemwege (*Grob-Segmentierung*) und die blattbasierte Segmentierung der kleinen Atemwege(*Fein-Segmentierung*). Die Tatsache, dass bei dem Schritt, in dem die Segmentierung ins Lungenparenchym ausläuft, signifikant mehr Voxel integriert werden als in den vorherigen Schritten, stellt das Abbruchkriterium der Grob-Segmentierung dar.

Aus dem Ergebnis der initialen Grob-Segmentierung wird über ein Skelettierungsalgorithmus die Baumstruktur mit zugehörigen Endblattknoten berechnet [6]. Die ermittelten Blattknoten dienen den anschließenden Fein-Segmentierungen als Saatpunkte. Dabei wird überprüft ob der Grauwert des jeweiligen Saatpunktes noch innerhalb der definierten Schwelle liegt. Außerhalb liegende Punkte werden anhand einer Kostenfunktion, bestehend aus Grauwert und Abstand zum Original-Saatpunkt innerhalb eines definierten Volumens, neu gesetzt. Somit wird sichergestellt, dass die Position der Saatpunkte optimiert wird, da der Skelettierungsalgorithmus keine Grauwertunterschiede berücksichtigt.

Der Abbruchmechanismus der Fein-Segmentierung basiert auf der Annahme, dass im zweiten Segmentierungsschritt im Verhältnis zum ersten nur ein Bruchteil an Voxel hinzugefügt wird, da lediglich einzelne Bronchialäste und

Tabelle 1. Übersicht der Segmentierungsergebnisse: Die Anzahl an Blätter entspricht der Anzahl an segmentierten Bronchien aus der Grob-Segmentierung. In der dritten Spalte ist die Anzahl an weiterverfolgten Bronchien durch die Fein-Segmentierung aufgelistet. Spalte vier zeigt die an den weiterverfolgten Bronchien maximal hinzugewonnene Segmentierungstiefe in mm an; Spalte fünf die durchschnittliche Segmentierungstiefe.

ID	# Blätter	# weiterverfolgt	Zuwachs max.	⊘ (mm)	CT-Auflösung (mm)
1.	89	58 (65%)	35,6	10,2	$0,57 * 0,57 * 1,25$
2.	32	17 (53%)	18,9	5,3	$0,723 * 0,723 * 1$
3.	56	46 (82%)	38,1	11,2	$0,742 * 0,742 * 1$
4.	21	8 (38%)	9,9	2,5	$0,702 * 0,702 * 1$
5.	36	17 (47%)	26,8	10,7	$0,552 * 0,552 * 1$
6.	60	27 (45%)	27,56	7,6	$0,354 * 0,354 * 0,4$

nicht mehr der gesamte Bronchialbaum erfasst werden. Sobald die Anzahl der neueingeschlossenen Voxel eine bildspezifische Grenze überschreitet greift das Abbruchkriterium. Zusätzlich gilt weiterhin das Abbruchkriterium der Grob-Segmentierung.

Über eine Maskierung des Ausgangsbildes mit dem Ergebnis der Grob-Segmentierung wurde gewährleistet, dass die anschließende Fein-Segmentierung Bereiche, die bereits im ersten Schritt erfasst wurden, nicht erneut aufnimmt. Folglich werden tatsächlich nur neue Strukturen (Bronchialäste) segmentiert, die nicht in der Grob-Segmentierung lagen.

Abschließend erfolgt die Addition der Segmentierungsergebnisse aus dem initialen und blattbasierten Lauf hin zur Gesamt-Segmentierung, die als Ausgang für weitere, rechenintensivere Segmentierungsalgorithmen, wie das in [3] beschriebene Pattern-Matching, dienen kann.

3 Ergebnisse

Die iterative Segmentierung wurde erfolgreich auf bisher sechs CT-Datensätzen durchgeführt. In Abhängigkeit der Qualität des Eingangsdatums wurden Bronchien bis maximal zur siebten Generation verfolgt. Insgesamt konnte das neue Verfahren an 55% der Blattknoten den vorliegenden Bronchialast weiter segmentieren. Allein das Verfahren der automatischen Saatpunktkorrektur konnte die Anzahl an weiterverfolgten Bronchien um bis zu 17% erhöhen. Da die Saatpunktkorrektur die Laufzeit nur marginal erhöhte, wurde das Verfahren standardmäßig bei allen Saatpunkten außerhalb des Grauwertintervalls angewandt. In Tabelle 1 sind die Ergebnisse der Segmentierungen detailiert aufgelistet. Zum Vergleich der Ergebnisse der einzelnen Datensätze untereinander sind zusätzlich die CT-Auflösungen angegeben. Insgesamt lag der Anteil falsch positiv erkannter Äste bei unter 4%.

Die initiale Grob-Segmentierung benötigt, wieder in Abhängigkeit der Auflösung und Größe des Eingangsbildes, ca. 15-30 Sekunden inklusive Benutzerinteraktion zur evtl. Anpassung des automatisch detektierten Schwellenintervalls. Die anschließende Fein-Segmentierung benötigt im vollautomatischen Modus ca. eine bis zwei Minuten, alternativ können die Ergebnisse der Fein-Segmentierung, im manuellen Modus einzeln angezeigt und gegebenenfalls wie im ersten Schritt angepasst werden (ca. 8 Minuten, abhängig von der Anzahl der Blattknoten). Sämtliche Berechnungen erfolgten auf einem Standard-PC: Intel P4 Quad Core 2,4 Ghz; 4 GB RAM. Insgesamt lässt sich somit die erweiterte Segmentierung innerhalb weniger Minuten berechnen und als interaktive 3D-Baumstruktur oder als 3D-Oberfläche anzeigen. Weiterhin können falsch positiv erkannte Bereiche in der Baumdarstellung ausgewählt und respektive gelöscht werden.

4 Diskussion

Es wurde ein Verfahren entwickelt welches in zwei Schritten anhand eines adaptiven Bereichswachstumsalgorithmus den Tracheobronchialbaum in kurzer Zeit segmentiert. Die Evaluation zeigt, dass die Fein-Segmentierung zusätzliche Bronchialäste in der Peripherie aufnehmen konnte (Abb. 1) und stellenweise eine Erhöhung der Segmentierungstiefe pro Bronchus um mehr als drei cm erzielte. Ein Vergleich der Ergebnisse mit denen anderer Algorithmen gestaltet sich als schwierig, da es keinen Goldstandard wie die manuelle Segmentierung gibt und die Qualität der Ergebnisse stark von dem jeweiligen Eingangsbild abhängt [7]. Dennoch zeigt der direkte Vergleich auf demselben Eingangsbild mit dem in [3] verwendeten Pattern-Matching Algorithmus, dass ähnlich gute Ergebnisse in kürzerer Laufzeit erzielt werden. Gleichzeitig läuft das Verfahren ohne zu-

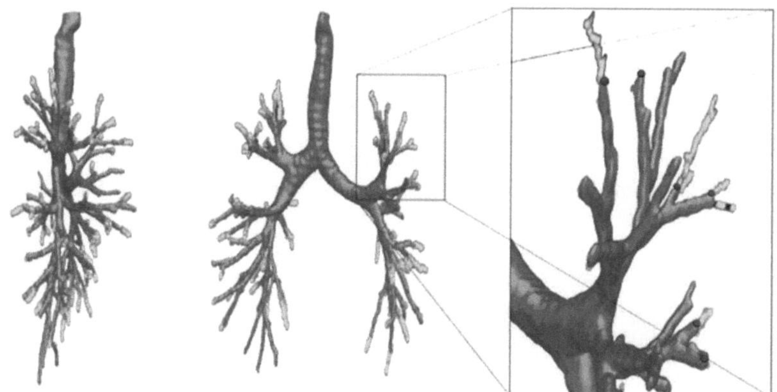

Abb. 1. Segmentierungsergebnis des Tracheobronchialbaums aus einem CT-Datum. Die durch die Fein-Segmentierung erweiterte Segmentierung ist gelb hervorgehoben, links in sagitaler und mittig in coronaler Ansicht. Der rechte Teil des Bildes zeigt den vergrößerten Ausschnitt des linken Oberlappens; die roten Punkte repräsentieren hierbei durch das Verfahren optimierte Saatpunkte.

sätzliche Parameter, welche wiederum für das Pattern-Matching vom Benutzer gewählt werden müssen.

Durch die Verwendung einer Maske (das Ergebnis der Grob-Segmentierung) konnte zum Einen unnötige redundante Rechenzeit minimiert werden, da das Verfahren bereits segmentierte Bereiche nicht noch einmal erfasst. Zum Anderen wurde sichergestellt, dass die anschließenden blattbasierten Segmentierungen nicht an derselben Stelle wie in der Grob-Segmentierung ins Lungenparenchym auslaufen und folglich immer ein eigenes Grauwertintervall haben. Des Weiteren wird das Gesamt-Segmentierungsergebnis schnell genug erstellt um anschließend weitere, rechenaufwändigere Algorithmen, an den neuen Blattknoten anzusetzen. Zukünftige Pläne sehen die Steigerung der Segmentierungstiefe durch ein statistisches Verfahren im Anschluss vor.

Ein zusätzlicher Vorteil, der durch den blattbasierten Segmentierungsansatz entsteht, ist die Möglichkeit zur Auslagerung der einzelnen Segmentierungen in Threads, wodurch eine weitere Rechenzeitverkürzung erwartet wird.

Danksagung. Diese Arbeit wurde von der DFG im Rahmen des Projektes „Navigierte Bronchoskopie“ (ME 833/13-1) gefördert.

Literaturverzeichnis

1. Schaap M, Smal I, Metz C, et al. Bayesian tracking of elongated structures in 3D images. Inf Process Med Imaging. 2007;20:74–85.
2. de Bruijne M, van Ginneken B, Viergever M et al. Adapting active shape models for 3D segmentation of tubular structures in medical images. Procs IPMI. 2003;2723:136–147.
3. Wolber P, Wegner I,Heiman T, Puderbach M, Wolf I, Meinzer HP. Tracking und Segmentierung baumförmiger,tubulärer Strukturen mit einem hybriden Verfahren. Procs BVM. 2008; p. 242–246.
4. Wolf I, Vetter M, Wegner I et al. The medical imaging interaction toolkit. Med Image Anal. 2005;9(6):594–604.
5. Hojjatoleslami S, Kittler J. Region growing: A new approach. Department of Electronic & Electrical Engineering, University of Surrey, Guildford, UK; 1995.
6. Schoebinger M, Thorn M, Vetter M et al. Robuste Analyse von Gefäßstrukturen auf Basis einer 3D-Skelettierung. Procs BVM. 2003; p. 76–80.
7. Tschirren J, Hoffman E A, McLennan G et al. Segmentation and quantitative analysis of intrathoracic airway trees from computed tomography images. Proc Am Thorac Soc. 2005;2:484–487.

Contrast Enhancement with Dual Energy CT for the Assessment of Atherosclerosis

Stefan C. Saur[1], Hatem Alkadhi[2], Luca Regazzoni[1], Simon Eugster[1], Gábor Székely[1], Philippe Cattin[1,3]

[1]Computer Vision Laboratory, ETH Zurich, Switzerland
[2]Institute of Diagnostic Radiology, University Hospital Zurich, Switzerland
[3]Medical Image Analysis Center, University of Basel, Switzerland
saur@vision.ee.ethz.ch

Abstract. A drawback of the commonly used single source computed tomography systems (CT) is that different materials might show very similar attenuation at any selected radiation energy. However, the assessment of atherosclerosis requires good differentiation between vessel lumen, calcium, adipose, and surrounding tissue. Dual energy CT (DECT) simultaneously measures attenuations at two energies and therefore can improve the differentiation to some extent. A tissue cancelation and enhancement algorithm for dual energy data was already proposed in 1981 and evaluated on experimental settings with a stationary X-ray source. For this study, we adapted this algorithm for DECT and propose its usage as a pre-processing step for the assessment of atherosclerosis. On clinical DECT patient data and with fixed parameters we could show a simultaneous contrast enhancement between 8% and 67% among all targeted tissues.

1 Introduction

Each material has a characteristic X-ray attenuation depending on its atomic number, density and the incident energy of the X-ray beam. Single source computed tomography systems (CT) characterize tissues with only one value such that different materials might show very similar attenuation. For the assessment of atherosclerosis, however, a precise differentiation between different tissues is needed: Calcified hard plaques are detected by differentiating calcium from the vessel lumen (blood/iodine), whereas for non-calcified soft plaques, vessel lumen, adipose and surrounding tissue must be distinguished.

A dual energy CT system (DECT) has two X-ray sources and therefore allows to simultaneously measure the X-ray attenuation at low and high energy levels such that two attenuation values are present for each volume element (voxel). This additional dimension can be used for better material discrimination. Dual energy X-ray acquisitions have been discussed and evaluated on basic phantoms since the early 1980s [1, 2, 3] until the first commercial DECT system was introduced 2005 [4]. On this DECT system, Eusemann et al. [5] evaluated different blending techniques to combine the low and high energy images into one improved single image whereas Johnson et al. [6] used unpublished algorithms to estimate the iodine content of each voxel from the low and high energy images.

In 1981, Lehmann et al. [1] proposed a tissue cancelation algorithm by decomposing the low and high energy images into two basis material images and combining them afterwards into a single projection image. Depending on a single parameter, the algorithm cancels out the contrast between two materials to enhance a third one, or it enhances the contrast between materials - both demonstrated on experimental settings with a stationary X-ray source. We adapted this algorithm for clinical DECT and propose its usage as a pre-processing step for the assessment of atherosclerosis. We applied the method on clinical dual-energy (DE) data and measured the contrast enhancement and signal to noise ratio between several tissues of interest. With one fixed parameter setting we could simultaneously enhance the contrast between all targeted tissues.

2 Methods

The principle of the tissue cancelation algorithm by Lehmann et al. [1] is summarized in Fig. 1 and described below in detail. First, the original low and high energy images are decomposed into two basis material images to map the density distribution of two arbitrarily chosen basis materials. Then, the two bases are combined in a cancelation step into a single projection image.

The two attenuation coefficients $\mu(low)$ and $\mu(high)$ obtained by DECT for each voxel are decomposed into a basis pair ρ_A and ρ_B of two chosen basis materials A and B by

$$\rho_A = \frac{1}{\alpha}\left[\mu(high)\mu_B(low) - \mu(low)\mu_B(high)\right] \tag{1}$$

$$\rho_B = \frac{1}{\alpha}\left[\mu(low)\mu_A(high) - \mu(high)\mu_A(low)\right] \tag{2}$$

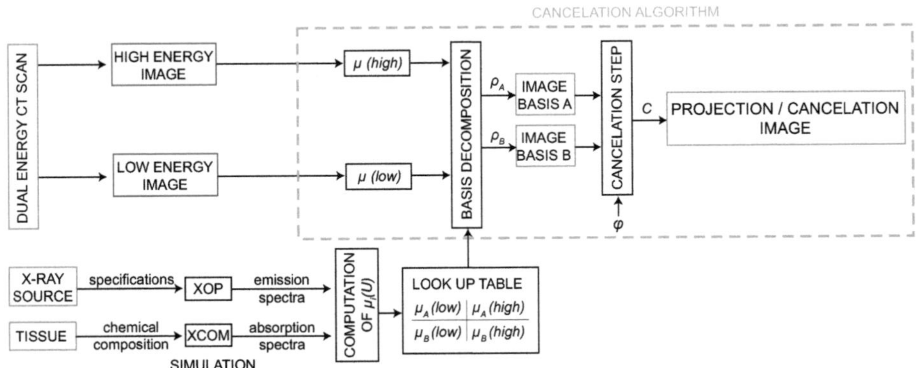

Fig. 1. Workflow of the tissue cancelation algorithm proposed by Lehmann et al. [1]

Table 1. For each possible material combination of lumen, tissue, adipose, and calcium, we determined the cancelation angle $\varphi_{\max}$ that maximized the mean contrast enhancement factor ($\overline{\text{CEF}}$) measured between the cancelation image and the 140 kV acquisition over all data sets.

	lumen	tissue	adipose	calcium
max $\overline{\text{CEF}}$ ($\varphi_{\max}$) lumen	-	1.58 (0.81)	2.82 (0.84)	1.30 (0.81)
max $\overline{\text{CEF}}$ ($\varphi_{\max}$) tissue	1.58 (0.81)	-	1.16 (0.80)	1.38 (0.81)
max $\overline{\text{CEF}}$ ($\varphi_{\max}$) adipose	2.82 (0.84)	1.16 (0.80)	-	1.48 (0.81)
max $\overline{\text{CEF}}$ ($\varphi_{\max}$) calcium	1.30 (0.81)	1.38 (0.81)	1.48 (0.81)	-

with $\alpha = \mu_B(low)\mu_A(high) - \mu_B(high)\mu_A(low)$. The attenuation coefficient $\mu_i(U)$ of the basis material i at the tube voltage U is calculated by $\mu_i(U) = \frac{\int_0^\infty N_U(E)\mu_i(E)dE}{\int_0^\infty N_U(E)dE}$ where $N_U(E)$ is the photon energy distribution at tube voltage U and $\mu_i(E)$ is the attenuation spectrum for material i. We used [7] to compute $N_U(E)$ of a Tungsten X-ray tube (5 mm Al filter) and for $\mu_i(E)$ we used a photon cross sections database [8]. For this study, we considered all possible basis material pair combinations between iodine, calcium, water, polymethyl methacrylate, adipose and blood.

The projection, or cancelation, image is computed by $C = \rho_A \sin(\varphi) + \rho_B \cos(\varphi)$ with φ, the cancelation angle, as a parameter.

For the assessment of atherosclerosis, a good contrast between vessel lumen, soft tissue, adipose, and calcium is desired. Therefore, we manually selected a region R_i within a data set for each material i ($i = 1..4$). The mean intensity $\bar{I}_i$ and standard deviation σ_i are computed within each R_i for every data set. The cancelation angle φ is varied between $-\pi$ and $+\pi$ with a step of 0.01. For each selected φ, the contrast enhancement factor (CEF) between material i and j is computed as

$$\text{CEF}_{ij} = \frac{|\bar{I}_{c_i} - \bar{I}_{c_j}|}{\bar{I}_{c_i} + \bar{I}_{c_j}} \bigg/ \frac{|\bar{I}_{h_i} - \bar{I}_{h_j}|}{\bar{I}_{h_i} + \bar{I}_{h_j}}, \tag{3}$$

where CEF represents the enhancement ratio of the contrast in the cancelation image (index c) and the original high energy image (index h). Hence, a CEF>1 should be achieved. Further, the signal to noise ratio $SNR_i = \bar{I}_i/\sigma_i$ is measured for each material i in the low and high energy, and cancelation image, respectively.

The cancelation angle is only dependent on the materials to be enhanced [1] such that we expected different optimal cancelation angles for the various targeted tissues which, however, should be universally applicable for all patient images. We evaluated this by measuring the CEF and SNR in dependence on φ. Further, we determined the optimal angles maximizing the contrast between two targeted tissues.

Table 2. We measured the mean (±std) contrast enhancement factor ($\overline{\text{CEF}}$) for the cancelation image ($\varphi = 0.79$) against the high energy 140 kV acquisition for each possible material combination. Further, the mean (±std) signal to noise ratio ($\overline{SNR}$) in the cancelation, the 80 kV, and the 140 kV images was measured.

	lumen	tissue	adipose	calcium
$\overline{\text{SNR}}$ cancelation	61.6 (±28.2)	39.6 (±17.8)	60.9 (±23.5)	11.3 (±1.6)
$\overline{\text{SNR}}$ 140kV	51.4 (±11.7)	37.8 (±10.9)	56.7 (±15.5)	14.7 (±6.3)
$\overline{\text{SNR}}$ 80kV	42.9 (±22.2)	27.3 (±14.2)	40.4 (±18.3)	9.5 (±0.7)
$\overline{\text{CEF}}$ lumen	-	1.27 (±0.06)	1.67 (±0.34)	1.16 (±0.03)
$\overline{\text{CEF}}$ tissue	1.27 (±0.06)	-	1.08 (±0.08)	1.19 (±0.03)
$\overline{\text{CEF}}$ adipose	1.67 (±0.34)	1.08 (±0.08)	-	1.23 (±0.04)
$\overline{\text{CEF}}$ calcium	1.16 (±0.03)	1.19 (±0.03)	1.23 (±0.04)	-

3 Results

The presented method was evaluated on five abdominal DE scans showing both lipid and calcified plaques in the descending aorta. The data sets were acquired on a Siemens Definition DECT scanner (Siemens Medical Solutions, Forchheim, Germany). The study was approved by the local ethics committee. A clinical abdominal DE protocol was used with a tube voltage of 80 kV for the low and 140 kV for the high energy image, respectively. The in-plane resolution and slice spacing ranged between 0.68-0.87 mm with a slice thickness of 2 mm.

In each patient, a region for lumen and tissue (both $7 \times 7 \times 9$ voxels), for adipose ($5 \times 5 \times 1$ voxels), and for calcium ($3 \times 3 \times 1$ voxels) was selected by an experienced reader. Among all basis material combinations, the pair calcium-adipose showed the best results in terms of magnitude and robustness for the intended contrast enhancement such that this basis pair was used for this study.

Figure 3(a) exemplarily shows the CEF between adipose and calcium in dependence of φ for all data sets. Our initial expectation regarding patient independent characteristics could be justified. The mean $\overline{\text{CEF}}$ and mean $\overline{\text{SNR}}$ over all data sets were computed and for each possible tissue combination, we determined an optimal cancelation angle $\varphi_{\max}$ that maximized $\overline{\text{CEF}}$ (Table 1).

As all $\varphi_{\max}$ were very similar, we decided to determine one single optimal angle φ^* that simultaneously enhances the contrast among all targeted tissues. Based on one data set, we chose the optimal angle $\varphi^* = 0.79$ that maximized the CEF among all tissue combinations but also showed a good SNR for each material (Fig. 3(b)). A higher CEF would have been possible with a slightly larger φ but that would have resulted in a worse SNR. The optimal angle φ^* was then fixed and applied on all data sets. The contrast between all targeted tissues could be simultaneously enhanced between 8% and 67% (Table 2). Except for calcium, the SNR in the cancelation image was also higher for the materials than the SNR measured in the 80 kV and 140 kV data sets, respectively.

Fig. 2. (a) Contrast enhancement factor (CEF) between adipose and calcium in dependence on the cancelation angle φ for all data sets. The selected φ^* (dashed) simultaneously enhanced the contrast among all targeted tissues in the cancelation image compared to the 140 kV image - exemplarily shown in (b) and (c).

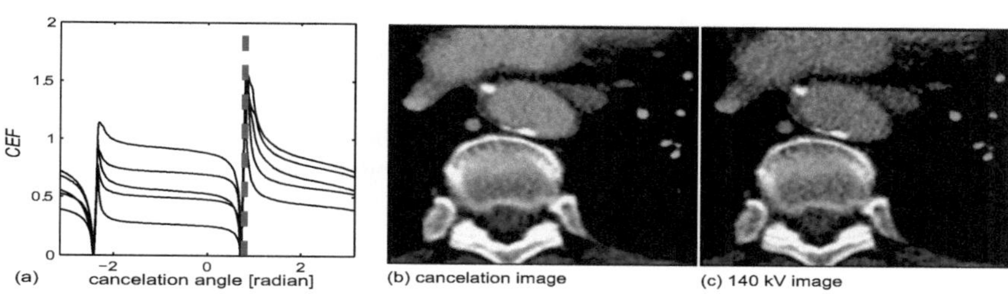

4 Discussion and conclusion

This study evaluated for the first time the performance of a tissue cancelation algorithm on real DECT patient data for contrast enhancement. We propose to use this procedure as a pre-processing step for the assessment of atherosclerosis to improve the robustness of both the manual reading and intensity-based detection algorithms. We could show by measuring the contrast enhancement between targeted tissues that there is one fixed, patient-independent optimal angle for the assessment of atherosclerosis as it enhances the contrast between all targeted tissues. Future work will concentrate on incorporating this contrast enhancement into radiological workstations and into algorithms for automatic detection and quantification of atherosclerosis.

Acknowledgement. This work has been supported by the CO-ME/NCCR research network of the Swiss National Science Foundation.

References

1. Lehmann LA, Alvarez RE, Macovski A, et al. Generalized image combinations in dual KVP digital radiography. Med Phys. 1981;8(5):659–667.
2. Marziani M, Taibi A, Tuffanelli A, et al. Dual-energy tissue cancellation in mammography with quasi-monochromatic x-rays. Phys Med Biol. 2002;47(2):305.
3. Taibi A, Fabbri S, Baldelli P, et al. Dual-energy imaging in full-field digital mammography: A phantom study. Phys Med Biol. 2003;48(13):1945–1956.
4. Flohr T, McCollough C, Bruder H, et al. First performance evaluation of a dual-source CT (DSCT) system. Eur Radiol. 2006;16(2):256–268.
5. Eusemann C, Holmes III DR, Schmidt B, et al. Dual energy CT: How to best blend both energies in one fused image? Procs SPIE. 2008;6918(1):691803–8.
6. Johnson T, Krauß B, Sedlmair M, et al. Material differentiation by dual energy CT: Initial experience. Eur Radiol. 2007;17(6):1510–1517.
7. del Rio MS, Dejus RJ. XOP: Recent developments. Procs SPIE. 1998;3448(1):340–345.
8. Berger MJ, Hubbel JH. XCOM: Photon Cross Sections Database. National Institute of Standards and Technology; 1998.

Effiziente automatische Bestimmung interventionsrelevanter Entfernungsmaße

Ivo Rössling[1,2], Christian Cyrus[1], Lars Dornheim[1,2], Bernhard Preim[1]

[1]Otto-von-Guericke-Universität Magdeburg
[2]Dornheim Medical Images*
iroess@isg.cs.uni-magdeburg.de

Kurzfassung. Bei der Operationsplanung sind quantitative Aussagen zu räumlichen Verhältnissen essentiell für die präoperativen Risikoabklärung. Tumorausdehnung und Abstände zu Risikostrukturen entscheiden über die Art der Therapierbarkeit. Eine manuelle Erhebung solcher Maße ist aufwändig und fehlerbehaftet. Automatische Verfahren sind derzeit oft ungenau und geben keine klare Zusicherung zur Ergebnisgüte. Ausgehend von einer gegebenen Segmentierung in Form eines Dreiecksnetzes stellen wir ein Verfahren vor, das den kürzesten Abstand zwischen zwei anatomischen Strukturen bestimmt. Zur Berechnung werden dabei nicht nur die Punkte sondern alle Primitive herangezogen und in einer speziellen räumlichen Baumstruktur effizient organisiert. Das Verfahren erlaubt durch Austausch des Zielkriteriums auch andere relevante Maße wie den Durchmesser eines Objekts zu bestimmen. In empirischen Tests stellte sich unser Verfahren als das derzeit effizienteste heraus. Zudem können wir bzgl. der gegebenen Oberflächennetze ein geometrisch korrektes Ergebnis garantieren und erhalten auch die jeweils definierenden geometrischen Primitive.

1 Einleitung

In der chirurgischen Diagnostik und Therapieplanung spielt die Beurteilung anatomischer und pathologischer Strukturen mittels bildgebender Verfahren eine tragende Rolle. Nicht immer jedoch erlaubt die visuelle Darstellung eine zuverlässige Einschätzung. Der Arzt benötigt dann zusätzliche quantitative Angaben, auf die er seine Entscheidungen stützen kann, wie z.B. die Größe eines Tumors, den Durchmesser einer Blutgefäßstenose oder den Abstand einer krankhaften Veränderung zur nahe liegenden Risikostruktur.

Eine manuelle Ermittlung solcher Maße ist nicht nur aufwändig, sondern fehleranfällig und nur begrenzt genau. Basierend auf einer Segmentierung (z. B. als Oberflächendreiecksnetz) der relevanten Strukturen können bestimmte Maße vollautomatisch ermittelt werden. Dies schafft Sicherheit, Objektivität und Reproduzierbarkeit. Trotz ihres Potentials scheint die Thematik der automatischen Vermessung segmentierter Strukturen jedoch in der Literatur der medizinischen

* Gefördert durch EXIST, BMWi und ESF

Bildverarbeitung bis dato stark unterrepräsentiert. Insbesondere ist uns für die automatische Bestimmung kürzester Abstände nur ein publiziertes Verfahren in der medizinischen Anwendung [1] bekannt. In der Algorithmischen Geometrie und der Robotik wurde diese Fragestellung dagegen bereits verstärkt untersucht. In letzterem Falle jedoch eher mit Interesse an reiner Kollisionserkennung oder Approximation, weshalb sich dortige Erkenntnisse nur eingeschränkt auf das vorliegende Szenario übertragen lassen. Während die Verfahren sich lange Zeit nur auf konvexe Objekte beschränkt haben (z.B. [2, 3]), wird zunehmend auch das nicht-konvexe Szenario betrachtet. Neben rein analytischen Ansätzen (z.B. [4]), die sich nur bedingt in der Praxis durchgesetzt haben, finden hierarchie-basierte Verfahren am häufigsten Anwendung. Die Hierarchie kann dabei aus verschiedenen Detailstufen (LOD) des Objektes selbst aufgebaut sein (Hierarchical Object Models, z.B. [5]). Oder sie besteht aus einer Sammlung von simplen Hüllkörpern, die aufeinander aufbauend immer größere Teile des Objektes überdecken (Bounding Representations). Auch das in [1] beschriebene Verfahren zur Abstandsberechnung anatomischer Strukturen basiert auf Bounding Representations. In Anlehnung an [6] wurden in diesem Falle Kugeln als Hüllkörper gewählt, was im Hinblick auf die Laufzeit nicht optimal ist.

2 Material und Methoden

Wir nutzen Segmentierungen in Form von Dreiecksnetzen, da selbige besonders effiziente, exakte und generische Abstandsmessungen erlauben. Voxelbasierte Segmentierungen können in diesem Zusammenhang ohne komplexitätsmäßigen Mehraufwand in äquivalente Dreiecksnetze überführt werden.

Als Vorverarbeitung wird für jedes Dreiecksnetz einmalig eine geometrische Datenstruktur in Form eines spatialen Suchbaumes aufgebaut. Die Bestimmung eines Kennwertes, wie z.B. des kürzesten Abstandes, stellt dann jeweils eine Anfrage an die Suchstruktur dar. Dabei ermöglicht die separate Wahl für Parameter und Zielfunktion die Berechnung einer Fülle unterschiedlicher Maße mit nur einer Struktur. Diese Punkte werden in den folgenden Abschnitten näher erläutert.

2.1 Aufbau des Suchbaumes für ein Dreiecksnetz

1. In einem initialen Schritt werden von allen geometrischen Primitiven des Dreiecksnetzes die Schwerpunkte bestimmt und ihnen zugewiesen.
2. Für den Suchbaum wird ein Wurzelknoten angelegt und ihm die gegebene Menge an Primitiven zugewiesen. Dabei werden die Grenzen der minimalen achsenparallelen Bounding-Box sowie der Schwerpunkt der Menge bestimmt und ebenfalls diesem Knoten zugewiesen. Für den Schwerpunkt werden hierzu alle Primitive gewichtet gemittelt (Punkt=1, Segment=2, Dreieck=3).
3. Als Split bezeichnen wir den Vorgang, die in einem Knoten K gespeicherte Menge an Primitiven zu zerlegen und auf Kind-Knoten aufzuteilen. Dabei wird für jeden der acht durch den Schwerpunkt von K definierten Oktanden ein korrespondierender Kind-Knoten angelegt. Beim Durchlaufen der in K

gespeicherten Primitive ergibt ein Koordinatenvergleich des Schwerpunktes von K mit dem jeweiligen Schwerpunkt des Primitivums, in welchem Kind-Knoten selbiges hinzugefügt wird. Analog zu Schritt 2 werden bei diesem Aufteilen für jeden Kindknoten die Bounding-Box sowie der Schwerpunkt aller assoziierten Primitive ermittelt und ihm zugewiesen. Sollte der aktuelle Knoten nur noch ein Primitivum enthalten, so wird nicht weiter gesplittet.

Der Split kann an zwei Stellen initiiert werden: Entweder wird der Wurzelknoten nach Erzeugung rekursiv gesplittet, bis die Baumstruktur vollständig aufgebaut ist (Full Split). Oder er wird lediglich angelegt und die Such-Funktion triggert Splits On Demand für jeden Knoten, von dem aus sie weiter absteigen will.

2.2 Suchanfrage für den kürzesten Abstand

1. S und T sind zwei Suchbäume, wie eben beschrieben. Es wird eine Prioritäts-Warteschlange angelegt, deren Elemente jeweils aus einem Paar (A, B) von Bäumen (bzw. Wurzelknoten) zusammen mit einer zugehörigen Priorität bestehen. Diese Priorität ist eine untere Schranke für den kürzesten Abstand zwischen den in A und den in B gespeicherten Primitiven. Initial wird das Paar (S, T) der beiden gegebenen Suchbäume in die Prioritäts-Warteschlange eingehängt, wobei diesem Element als Priorität der kleinstmögliche Abstand zwischen den Bounding-Boxen von S und T zugewiesen wird.
2. Nun wird das vorderste Element (A, B) der Prioritäts-Warteschlange entnommen. Für den Baum mit der größeren Bounding-Box (o. B. d. A.: B) werden die acht Kind-Knoten $B_1 ... B_8$ genommen und zusammen mit dem anderen Baum als neue Paare $(A, B_1)...(A, B_8)$ in die Warteschlange wieder einsortiert, wobei als Priorität jeweils der kürzeste Abstand zwischen der Bounding-Box von A und der von B_i verwendet wird.
3. Die Schritte 1 und 2 werden nun solange wiederholt, bis der Prioritäts-Warteschlange an vorderster Stelle ein Paar zweier Primitive entnommen wird. Diese beiden definieren dann den kürzesten Abstand.

2.3 Vielseitigkeit der Methode

Das beschriebene Verfahren erlaubt uns bereits, den kürzesten Abstand zweier segmentierter anatomischer Strukturen zu bestimmen. Ein Vergleich dieses Wertes mit 0 zeigt an, ob eine Infiltration vorliegt. Wird statt einer zweiten anatomischen Struktur eine Skelettierung ersterer verwendet, so kann der minimale Abstand zu dieser Skelettierung bestimmt werden, also z.B. der kleinste Durchmesser einer Blutgefäßstenose. Würden von einer anatomischen Struktur (z.B. Blutgefäß, Organ oder Knochen) separate Segmentierungen für innere und äußere Oberfläche vorliegen, so ließe sich damit effizient die minimale Wanddicke bestimmen.

Wird bei einer Suchanfrage die Bildung des Minimums durch das Maximum ersetzt, so wird der größte Abstand zweier anatomischer Strukturen berechnet.

Wird auch hier statt einer zweiten Struktur erneut dieselbe gewählt, so liefert dies die größte Ausdehnung dieser anatomischen Struktur.

Da die Warteschlange des vorgestellten Algorithmus die Primitiven-Paare ihrem Abstand nach sortiert enthält, können nach dem ersten auch alle weiteren sich schneidenden Primitiven-Paare zurückgeben werden. Dies ergäbe den Umriss eines Infiltrationsrandes. Für diesen ließe sich ebenfalls die größte Ausdehnung effizient ermitteln.

3 Ergebnisse

Zur Evaluation des vorgestellten Algorithmus wurde eine Testumgebung erstellt. Als Eingabedaten dienten Segmentierungen des Halses in Form von Oberflächendreiecksnetzen unterschiedlicher Komplexität. Für ausgewählte Paare von ihnen wurde als Referenzmaß mit dem in [1] beschriebenen Verfahren der kürzeste Abstand bestimmt. Anschließend wurde er mit unserem Verfahren auf vier Arten erneut bestimmt: Die Varianten ergaben sich zum einen aus einer Unterscheidung der Interpretation der Eingabedaten als Punktmengen wie in [1] oder als Dreiecksmengen, zum anderen aus einer Unterscheidung der Splitting-Strategie in Full Split und On Demand. Für jede derartige Kombination wurde die Laufzeit über 20 Durchläufe gemittelt auf einem Intel Pentium 4 mit 3,2 GHz und 1 GB RAM gemessen. Die Ergebnisse sind in Abb. 1 festgehalten.

Den Werten lässt sich entnehmen, dass bei Full Split erwartungsgemäß eine hohe Aufbauzeit und eine niedrige Testzeit auftritt. Beim On Demand Split verhält es sich erwartungsgemäß entgegengesetzt. Weiterhin zeigte sich bei unserer Methode, dass die beiden auf Dreiecken basierenden Varianten langsamer als ihre auf Punkten basierenden Gegenspieler waren. Solange die Anzahl der Eckpunkte beider Segmentierungen jeweils im einstelligen Tausenderbereich lag, waren kaum Laufzeiten messbar. Für diese Größenordnung können alle Verfahren daher als hinreichend effizient bezeichnet werden. Je größer die Anzahl der Eckpunkte jedoch wird, desto schlechter war die Methode aus [1] relativ zu allen anderen. Im Fall der größten Dreiecksnetze (letzte Tabellenzeile) waren alle unsere Varianten deutlich schneller, was die Effizienz unseres Verfahrens bei großen Datenmengen unterstreicht.

4 Diskussion

Nach unseren Tests ist das hier vorgestellte Verfahren zur automatischen Berechnung von Abständen und Ausdehnungen auf Basis von Segmentierungen und Organbeschreibungen als Dreicksnetzen das derzeit effizienteste im medizinischen Umfeld. Zudem liefert es geometrische exakte Ergebnisse, da es die zu Verfügung stehenden geometrischen Primitive komplett einbezieht (Punkte, Kanten und Dreiecke), statt wie sonst üblich, nur die Punktmengen zu betrachten und ihre Konnektivität zu vernachlässigen. Dadurch ist es auch zum ersten mal möglich, Durchdringungen und Infiltrationen zu entdecken und zu vermessen. Weiterhin werden durch die direkte Rückgabe der geometrischen Primitive,

Abb. 1. Bestimmung kürzester Abstände: Laufzeiten in ms (J.=Jugularis, C.=Carotis, KoZ=Knochen ohne Zungenbein, l/r=links/rechts, jeweils original (obere Tableauhälfte) und reduziert (untere Tableauhälfte), A=Aufbau, T=Test)

Algorithmus			nach [1]		Punkte				Dreiecke			
					Full-Split		On-Demand		Full-Split		On-Demand	
Objekt	Anzahl Punkte	Anzahl Dreiecke	A	T	A	T	A	T	A	T	A	T
C. (l) C. (r)	3620 3120	7232 6210	2.0	27.8	9.6 7.8	0.2	1.6 1.6	7.2	31.4 18.0	18.0	7.2 5.0	37.6
C. (l) J. (l)	3620 3142	7232 6276	2.0	29.0	9.6 6.6	0.4	2.0 1.4	11.4	30.6 16.6	10.4	6.4 4.4	36.2
C. (l) KoZ	3620 222079	7232 445348	60.2	2670.6	9.2 1579.3	1.0	1.6 275.8	448.0	29.8 1790.5	381.6	7.0 358.6	1210.3
C. (l) C. (r)	1807 1558	3616 3104	1.0	0.8	3.6 3.4	<0.1	1.0 0.8	3.2	11.0 7.8	10.4	2.6 2.4	18.4
C. (l) J. (l)	1807 1567	3616 3137	0.8	10.8	4.0 3.0	0.8	0.8 0.4	5.0	11.4 8.4	163.0	2.8 2.0	176.8
C. (l) KoZ	1807 110452	3616 222674	29.4	704.4	4.0 741.2	1.0	1.0 137.8	229.8	11.4 864.9	628.2	3.0 176.2	1050.1
Haut KoZ	129099 110452	258348 222674	60.0	78600.1	878.5 725.2	44.6	159.8 129.6	1241.9	1920.7 866.1	14475.7	384.4 168.0	17320.1

zwischen denen z. B. ein Abstand gemessen wurde, bessere Möglichkeiten für eine genaue Abstandsvisualisierung gerade im Nahbereich geschaffen.

Die methodische Stärke des Verfahrens liegt neben der Exaktheit und Effizienz vor allem in seiner Vielseitigkeit, da sich – ohne Anpassung der Datenstruktur – durch kleine Variationen an Argumenten und Zielfunktion eine Fülle wichtiger Kennwerte (Abstände, Durchmesser, Wanddicken, etc.) ermitteln lassen. Sogar zur Kollisionserkennung, z. B. bei der virtuellen Endoskopie, lässt es sich auf Grund seiner Effizienz hervorragend einsetzen. Dies ist auch der Grund, warum das Verfahren direkt für den Anwendungseinsatz im klinischen Umfeld geeignet ist, denn es ist auch für erwartungsgemäß zukünftig immer größere Datenmengen noch schnell genug und vollautomatisch.

Literaturverzeichnis

1. Preim B, Tietjen C, Hindennach M, et al. Integration automatischer Abstandsberechnungen in die Interventionsplanung. Proc BVM. 2003; p. 259–263.
2. Lin MC, Canny JF. A fast algorithm for incremental distance calculation. Proc IEEE ICRA. 1991;2:1008–1014.
3. Bobrow JE. A direct minimization approach for obtaining the distance between convex polyhedra. Int J Rob Res. 1989;8(3):65–76.
4. Gilbert EG, Johnson DW. A fast procedure for computing the distance between complex objects in three space. IEEE J Rob Autom. 1988;4(2):193–203.
5. Faverjon B. Hierarchical object models for efficient anti-collision algorithms. Proc IEEE ICRA. 1989;1:333–340.
6. Quinlan S. Efficient distance computation between non-convex objects. Proc IEEE ICRA. 1994;4:3324–3329.

Trajektoriendichte bei Magnetic Particle Imaging

Tobias Knopp[1], Timo Sattel[1], Sven Biederer[1], Jürgen Weizenecker[2], Bernhard Gleich[2], Jörn Borgert[2], Thorsten M. Buzug[1]

[1]Institut für Medizintechnik, Universität zu Lübeck, Lübeck
[2]Philips Technologie GmbH Forschungslaboratorien, Hamburg
knopp@imt.uni-luebeck.de

Kurzfassung. Magnetic Particle Imaging ist ein neues bilgebendes Verfahren zur Darstellung der räumlichen Verteilung von magnetisierbaren Nanopartikeln. In einer Simulationsstudie wurde zuletzt das Auflösungsvermögen und die Sensitivität dieser Methode untersucht. Die Abtasttrajektorie wurde dabei so gewählt, dass der Messbereich deutlich überabgetastet wurde. In dieser Arbeit wird in einer Simulationsstudie untersucht, welchen Einfluss die Dichte der Trajektorie auf die Bildqualität der rekonstruierten Bilder hat. Es wird gezeigt, dass die Auflösung in den rekonstruierten Bildern durch die Feldstärke des angelegten Magnetfeldes und die Trajektoriendichte beschränkt ist. Die Trajektorie kann bei konstanter Feldstärke bis zu einem gewissen Grad ausgedünnt werden. Der Simulation liegt dabei ein Model zu Grunde, welches das Signal entsprechend der Langevin-Theorie des Paramagnetismus approximiert.

1 Einleitung

Magnetic Particle Imaging (MPI) ist ein neues bilgebendes Verfahren, das es ermöglicht, super-paramagnetische Nanopartikel, sogenannte SPIOs, direkt abzubilden [1]. Das Verfahren verspricht dabei zugleich eine hohe räumliche und zeitliche Auflösung und eine hohe Sensitivität [2]. Mit diesen Eigenschaften hat MPI daher das Potential, Anwendungen in der quantitativen Bildgebung oder bei der Visualisierung des Blutflusses (z.B. in der Kardiographie) zu finden. Das Verfahren kommt dabei ohne ionisierende Strahlung aus.

Die Grundidee von MPI besteht in der Nutzung der nichtlinearen Magnetisierungskurve der Nanopartikel. Das Verfahren nutzt dazu zwei überlagerte Magnetfelder: ein statisches Selektionsfeld und ein dynamisches Wechselfeld (Anregungsfeld). Werden die Nanopartikel in das Wechselfeld gebracht, erfahren sie eine nichtlineare Magnetisierung, die mit einer Empfangsspule gemessen werden kann. Aufgrund der Nichtlinearität enthält das gemessene Signal Harmonische des Anregungssignals, also Schwingungen, deren Frequenzen jeweils ein ganzzahliges Vielfaches der Grundfrequenz sind. Nach Separation dieser Harmonischen vom ebenfalls aufgenommenen Grundsignal kann die Konzentration der Nanopartikel ermittelt werden. Zur räumlichen Kodierung wird das statische Selektionsfeld verwendet, dessen Feldstärke nur an einer bestimmten Stelle, dem sogenannten feldfreien Punkt (FFP), gleich Null und ansonsten groß ist. Da die Magnetisierung der Nanopartikel schon bei geringen Feldstärken in die Sättigung gelangt (ca. 2 mT bei 50 nm Partikeldurchmesser), antworten nur Nanopartikel in direkter Nachbarschaft des FFPs auf das Anregungsfeld. Somit kann die gemessene Konzentration einem bestimmten Punkt im Raum zugeordnet werden. Das Grundprinzip von MPI ist in Abb. 1 dargestellt.

In [3] wurde in einer Simulationsstudie gezeigt, dass das Auflösungsvermögen des neuen Verfahrens von der angelegten Feldstärke, der Partikelkonzentration, dem Partikeldurchmesser und der Messzeit abhängt. In dieser Arbeit wird erstmals die Abhängigkeit der Auflösung von der verwendeten Trajektoriendichte untersucht.

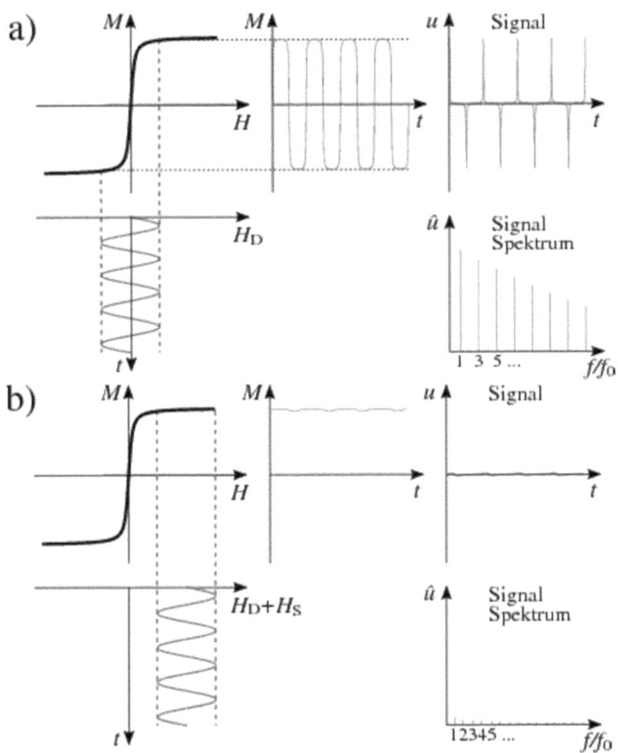

Abb. 1. Grundprinzip von MPI. a) Die super-paramagnetischen Nanopartikel werden in ein Anregungsfeld $H_D(t)$ gebracht. Aufgrund der Nichtlinearität der Magnetisierungkurve $M(H)$ enthält die resultierende zeitliche Magnetisierung $M(t)$ und die induzierte Spannung $u(t)$ nicht nur die Anregungsfrequenz, sondern zusätzlich höhere Harmonische, die für die Bildgebung genutzt werden können. b) Wird das Anregungsfeld $H_D(t)$ mit einem statischen Selektionsfeld H_S überlagert, verbleiben die Partikel in Sättigung. Da die resultierende Magnetisierung fast konstant ist, wird kein messbares Signal in der Empfangsspule induziert.

2 Material and Methoden

Im Folgenden wird das verwendete Simulationsmodel vorgestellt. Aufgrund des Induktionsgesetzes, kann die Beziehung zwischen der Partikelkonzentration c an einer Position $\boldsymbol{r}$ und dem induzierten Signal u zum Zeitpunkt t durch

$$u(t) = -\mu_0 \int_\Omega \frac{\partial}{\partial t} \widehat{\boldsymbol{M}}(\boldsymbol{H}(\boldsymbol{r},t)) \cdot \boldsymbol{p}(\boldsymbol{r}) c(\boldsymbol{r})\, \mathrm{d}\boldsymbol{r}, \tag{1}$$

modelliert werden. Dabei bezeichnet μ_0 die Permeabilitätskonstante im Vakuum, $\boldsymbol{p}(\boldsymbol{r})$ das ortsabhängige Sensitivitätsprofil der Empfangsspule und $\widehat{\boldsymbol{M}}$ das magnetische Moment eines Partikels, das von der magnetischen Feldstärke $\boldsymbol{H}(\boldsymbol{r},t)$ abhängt. Für die Modellierung der Nanopartikel wird die Langevin-Theorie des Paramagnetismus [4] verwendet. Zur Berechnung der magnetischen Feldstärke wird das Gesetz von Biot-Savart genutzt. Zum simulierten Spannungssignal $u(t)$ wird modelliertes Patientenrauschen addiert, wie in [3] beschrieben.

Neben dem zuvor beschriebenen Partikelsignal, induziert auch das angelegte Wechselfeld ein Signal in der Empfangsspule, welches mehrere Größenordnungen höher ist. Um das Partikelsignal vom Anregungssignal zu separieren, wird das empfangene Signal in eine Fourier-Reihe enwickelt, wobei die Fourierkoeffizienten durch

$$\hat{u}_k = -\mu_0 \int_\Omega \left(\int_{-\frac{T}{2}}^{\frac{T}{2}} \frac{\partial}{\partial t} \widehat{\boldsymbol{M}}(\boldsymbol{H}(\boldsymbol{r},t)) \cdot \boldsymbol{p}(\boldsymbol{r}) \mathrm{e}^{2\pi \mathrm{i}kt/T} \mathrm{d}t \right) c(\boldsymbol{r})\, \mathrm{d}\boldsymbol{r} \tag{2}$$

gegeben sind. Anschließend werden nur die Frequenzen zur Rekonstruktion verwendet, welche nicht im Signal des Anregungsfeldes vorkommen.

Zur numerischen Verarbeitung wird das kontinuierliche Model (2) an Ortspunkten $\boldsymbol{r}_\rho$, $\rho = 0, \ldots, N-1$ und Zeitpunkten t_κ, $\kappa = 0, \ldots, K-1$ diskretisiert, wobei die Ortspunkte auf einem Gitter der Größe 180×90 liegen und eine Abtastrate von 20 MS/s verwendet wird. Das diskrete Model kann als lineares Gleichungssystem in Matrix-Vektor-Form

$$\boldsymbol{Gc} = \hat{\boldsymbol{u}}, \tag{3}$$

geschrieben werden. Zum Lösen dieses linearen Gleichungssystems, wird eine Singulärwertzerlegung mit Tikhonov-Regularizierung verwendet [5].

In der Simulation wird als MPI-Messaufbau dieselbe Spulenkonfiguration wie in [3] verwendet (Abb. 2). Um die Dichte der Abtasttrajektorie zu variieren, werden die Anregungsfrequenzen modifiziert. Die Trajektorie kann als Funktion $\boldsymbol{\psi}(t)$ definiert werden, die jedem Zeitpunkt t die Position des FFPs zuordnet. Für die Bewegung des FFPs in y-Richtung wird eine sinusförmige Anregung mit einer Grundfrequenz von $f_0 = 25$ kHz genutzt. In x-Richtung wird eine leicht unterschiedliche Frequenz $f_1 = \frac{N_P+1}{N_P} f_0$ verwendet, woraus sich eine Lissajous-Figur mit dem kommensurablen Frequenzverhältnis $\frac{N_P+1}{N_P}$ als Trajektorie ergibt. Dabei bezeichnet N_P die Anzahl an Grundfrequenzen pro Periodenlänge $T_\mathrm{R} = N_P/f_0$ (Repetitionszeit). Die Dichte der Trajektorie steigt mit N_P und damit auch die Repetitionszeit. Um das Signal-zu-Rausch-Verhältnis (SNR) des gemessenen Signals zu verbessern, können mehrere Messungen wiederholt und die Ergebnisse aufsummiert werden. Dabei bezeichnet T_{AQ} die Gesamtmesszeit. Um für verschiedene Trajektoriendichten dasselbe SNR zu gewährleisten, wird die Gesamtmesszeit in dieser Arbeit mit $T_{\mathrm{AQ}} = 40$ s konstant gehalten. Das verwendete Phantom (Abb. 2) besteht aus Kreisen mit unterschiedlichen Durchmessern, befüllt mit Partikeln mit einem Kerndurchmesser von 50 nm und einem Eisengehalt von 774 μmol/l. Die Auflösung in den rekonstruierten Bildern wird als kleinster Abstand definiert, bei dem zwei Kreise gleicher Größe noch klar unterscheidbar sind.

3 Ergebnisse

Die rekonstruierten Bilder sind mit den verwendeten Abtasttrajektorien in Abb. 3 dargestellt. Wie deutlich erkennbar ist, verbessert sich die Bildqualität mit steigender Abtastdichte. Während für ein Frequenzverhältnis von 11/10 eine Auflösung von 1.2 mm in y-Richtung und 1.6 mm in x-Richtung erreicht wird, ist mit Hilfe des verwendeten Phantoms für ein Frequenzverhältnis von 101/100 eine Auflösung von 0.5 mm in y-Richtung und 0.8 mm in x-Richtung feststellbar.

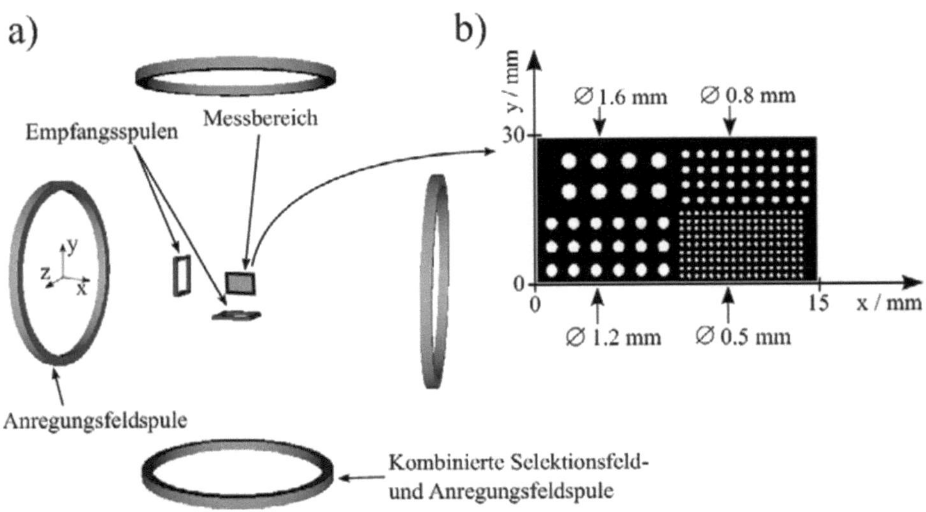

Abb. 2. Messaufbau eines zweidimensionalen MPI Scanners. Kombinierte Selektionsfeld- und Anregungsfeld-Spulen, die in y-Richtung zeigen, sind symmetrisch mit einem Abstand von 0.5 m zum Zentrum plaziert. Ein zweites Anregungsfeld-Spulenpaar zeigt in x-Richtung mit demselben Abstand zum Zentrum. Quadratische Empfangsspulen mit einer Seitenlänge von 10 cm sind 15 cm (x-Richtung) und 10 cm (y-Richtung) entfernt vom Zentrum angebracht. Der Messbereich ist 32×16 mm^2 groß und liegt zentrisch. Rechts ist das für die Simulation verwendete Phantom abgebildet, das aus mehreren Kreisen unterschiedlicher Durchmesser besteht.

Abb. 3. Rekonstruktionsergebnisse für verschiedene Abtastdichten, angegeben durch das Frequenzverhältnis.

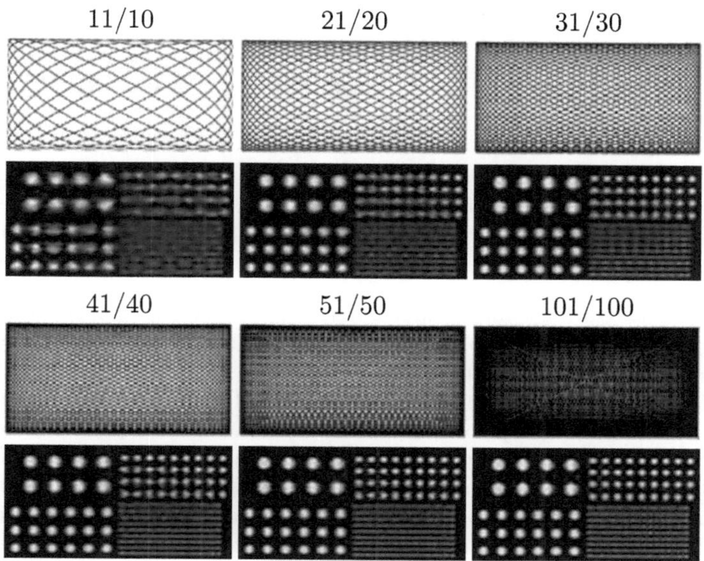

4 Diskussion

In der vorliegenden Arbeit wurde der Einfluss der Abtasttrajektoriendichte auf die erreichte Bildqualität in Magnetic Particle Imaging untersucht. Die Auflösung in den rekonstruierten Bildern nahm dabei mit der Trajektoriendichte zu. Allerdings wurde die beste Auflösung schon bei einem Frequenzverhältnis von 51/50 erreicht, während sich die Bildqualität bei einem Frequenzverhältnis von 101/100 nur unmerklich verbesserte. Von der nominellen Auflösung von 0.17 mm ist die erreichte Auflösung von 0.5 mm allerdings weit entfernt. Das zeigt, dass die zu erwartende Auflösung dieses neuen bildgebenden Verfahrens eine vielschichtige Größe ist, die von der Trajektoriendichte, der Voxelgröße, der Akquisitionszeit und insbesondere von der Stärke der angelegten Magnetfelder abhängt.

Literaturverzeichnis

1. Gleich B, Weizenecker J. Tomographic imaging using the nonlinear response of magnetic particles. Nature. 2005;435:1214–1217.
2. Gleich B, Weizenecker J, Borgert J. Experimental results on fast 2D-encoded magnetic particle imaging. Phys Med Biol. 2008;53:N81–N84.
3. Weizenecker J, Borgert J, Gleich B. A simulation study on the resolution and sensitivity of magnetic particle imaging. Phys Med Biol. 2007;52:6363–6374.
4. Chikazumi S, Charap S. Physics of Magnetism. New York: Wiley; 1964.
5. Knopp T, Biederer S, Sattel T, et al. Singular value analysis for magnetic particle imaging. Proc IEEE Nuc Sci Symp Med Im Conf. 2008; p. 5.

Extracting a Purely Non-rigid Deformation Field of a Single Structure

Stefanie Demirci[1], Frode Manstad-Hulaas[2], Nassir Navab[1]

[1]Computer Aided Medical Procedures (CAMP), TU München,
[2]Department of Surgery, St. Olavs Hospital, NTNU Trondheim
demirci@cs.tum.edu

Abstract. During endovascular aortic repair (EVAR) treatment, the aortic shape is subject to severe deformation that is imposed by medical instruments such as guide wires, catheters, and the stent graft. The problem definition of deformable registration of images covering the entire abdominal region, however, is highly ill-posed. We present a new method for extracting the deformation of an aneurysmatic aorta. The outline of the procedure includes initial rigid alignment of two abdominal scans, segmentation of abdominal vessel trees, and automatic reduction of their centerline structures to one specified region of interest around the aorta. Our non-rigid registration procedure then only computes local non-rigid deformation and leaves out all remaining global rigid transformations. In order to evaluate our method, experiments for the extraction of aortic deformation fields are conducted on 15 patient datasets from endovascular aortic repair (EVAR) treatment. A visual assessment of the registration results were performed by two vascular surgeons and one interventional radiologist who are all experts in EVAR procedures.

1 Introduction

An abdominal aortic aneurysm (AAA) is an enlargement of the abdominal aorta, resulting from weakened arterial walls. During Endovascular aortic repair (EVAR), an aortic prosthesis (stent graft) is inserted via an introducer system through one femoral artery into the aneurysmatic aorta excluding the aneurysm sack from the circulation and reducing the pressure/strain on the aortic wall.

Organ deformation in general can be measured by non-rigidly registering the preoperative to the postoperative CT scan [1]. In the case of abdominal aortic aneurysms, however, this task is associated with several problems and challenges. The overall deformation in the abdominal region includes breathing deformation and specific motion of several organs, each different and not comparable. Hence, true deformation fields of the aorta can only be obtained by registering segmentations of the pre- and postoperative structures. However, in contrasted CT scans, a segmentation of the entire vessel tree may include regions that are again subject to different types of deformations. Additionally, the implanted stent graft separates parts of the enlarged aorta from blood flow which would be computed as a shrinking deformation by the registration algorithm. As we are interested in the true deformation of the aorta, our method has to narrow down the vessel tree segmentation to a region of interest around the aorta and also eliminate any additional information such as shrinking and rigid body transformations due to different patient positioning.

We propose a method for extracting specific deformation of the aorta during and after EVAR. It segments both preoperative and postoperative aortic structures with minimal user interaction and automatically extracts the region of interest around the aneurysm. To this end, the centerlines of both structures are extracted and reduced to the region of interest around the aorta. After an initial rigid registration, non-linear registration of the structures provides pure deformation fields of the aorta. Our method was tested by evaluating 15 datasets of patients that were treated by EVAR.

2 Materials and methods

2.1 Rigid registration

A rigid registration problem can be formulated as the maximization of a similarity measure using image information over a possible range of transformation parameters:

$$\mathbf{T}_{\text{opt}} = \arg\max_{\mathbf{T}} \mathcal{D}_1(\mathbf{I}^F, \mathbf{T} * \mathbf{I}^M) \tag{1}$$

where $\mathbf{I}^F$ and $\mathbf{I}^M$ are the fixed and the moving volume respectively, $\mathbf{T}$ a rigid transformation matrix and $\mathcal{D}_1$ a certain similarity measure that is to be maximized. As our two CTA volumes contain severe dissimilarity introduced by the high intensities of the stent graft, an appropriate similarity measure needs to be chosen carefully. Given a segmentation of the stent graft, the adapted normalized cross correlation (A-NCC)[2] measure only evaluates those voxels that are not part of the segmentation. In our case, a rough segmentation of the stent graft can be easily extracted from the postoperative scan by thresholding. The resulting optimal transformation $\mathbf{T}_{\text{opt}}$ that maximizes A-NCC, describes the overall rigid body transformation. For our following explanations, we set $\mathbf{I}^M := \mathbf{T}_{\text{opt}} * \mathbf{I}^M$.

2.2 Segmentation and preprocessing

We segment the contrasted vessel tree out of the preoperative as well as the postoperative volume using the connected threshold segmentation method provided by ITK[1]. Given this segmentation S of the abdominal vessel tree and a point bif for the aortic bifurcation, topological thinning is processed onto S resulting in a centerline structure C for the entire abdominal vessel tree. Then, the root *seed* of the aortic centerline is calculated. Here, the biggest connected component of segmented pixels in the first slice of the segmentation image is computed by counting neighboring pixels of value other than 0. The centerline voxel nearest

[1] Insight Toolkit, http://www.itk.org

to the center of mass of the biggest component (assumed to be the aortic lumen) is then taken as seed point. In order to further narrow the information down to the region of interest around the aorta, the centerline structure C is processed by an adapted wave front propagation algorithm. It adapts the wave propagation approach of Zahlten *et al.* [3] by stepping down the aortic centerline from a given seed point *seed* in region growing manner until the indicated bifurcation bif is reached. At all other bifurcations, our algorithm automatically finds the path belonging to the aorta by comparing the different angles between the connecting parts. The aortic path usually continues in the direction that forms the smallest angle with the previous direction. The branching paths are included into the aortic centerline data only up to the next bifurcation respectively. Thereby, we ensure a fully three-dimensional tree structure T which can be used to cover a full transformation including rotation. Finally, we compute a Danielsson distance map [4] $\mathbf{D}$ on the reduced centerline data.

2.3 Non-rigid registration

The preprocessing steps narrow down the scatter of the abdominal vessel tree to one centerline including the aorta and small parts of all branching vessels. We can now employ a non-rigid registration in order to obtain the deformation of the aorta. Non-rigid registration consists of deforming a source image $\mathbf{I}^M$ to best match a target image $\mathbf{I}^F$. Using similar formulation as before, this can be expressed as

$$\mathbf{V}_{\text{opt}} = \arg\min_{\mathbf{V}} \mathcal{E}(\mathbf{I}^F, \mathbf{I}^M, \mathbf{V}) \tag{2}$$

There energy functional $\mathcal{E}$ is defined as

$$\mathcal{E}(\mathbf{I}^F, \mathbf{I}^M, \mathbf{V}) = \mathcal{D}_2(\mathbf{I}^F, \mathbf{V} + \mathbf{I}^M) + \alpha\mathcal{S}(\mathbf{V}) \tag{3}$$

Here, $\mathbf{V} = \{\mathbf{V}_x, \mathbf{V}_y, \mathbf{V}_z\}$ gives the deformation or displacement field that warps image $\mathbf{I}^M$. $\mathcal{D}$ is a certain distance or dissimilarity measure and $\mathcal{S}$ a certain diffusion regularization term which ensures smooth resulting deformations, by penalizing high gradients of the displacement fields. The positive scalar α controls the influence of the regularization terms. In order to define the dissimilarity measure $\mathcal{D}_2$ for centerlines, correspondences of pre- and postoperative centerline points are required. Except of the bifurcation points, it is highly costly to establish correspondences for the other points on the centerlines. We avoid the necessity of correspondences by computing distance maps $\mathbf{D}^F, \mathbf{D}^M$ on the reduced centerline images and computing the sum of absolute differences

$$\mathcal{D}(\mathbf{D}^F, \mathbf{V} + \mathbf{D}^M) = \sum_x |\mathbf{D}^F(x) - \mathbf{V} + \mathbf{D}^M(x)| \tag{4}$$

as dissimilarity measure. As smoothing term for the energy functional (3), we use diffusion regularization[5].

With initial rigid registration and final non-rigid-registration, we have obtained the linear and non-linear part of the overall transformation of the abdominal aorta. However, according to Zikic *et al.* [6], deformation fields that are computed by a local nonlinear registration algorithm, still contain a linear transformation $\mathbf{T}_{\text{local}} = \mathbf{T}_{\text{linear}} \circ \mathbf{T}_{\text{nonlinear}}$. In order to obtain a pure non-linear deformation field, the authors suggest to minimize the norm of the displacement field $\mathbf{V}$ of the nonlinear component $\mathbf{T}_{\text{nonlinear}}$ with respect to the linear transformation $\mathbf{T}_{\text{linear}}$.

$$\min_{p} \mathcal{E}(\mathbf{T}_{\text{linear}}) = \min_{p} \frac{1}{n} \sum_{i=1}^{n} \| \mathbf{X}_i - \mathbf{T}_{\text{linear}}^{-1}(\mathbf{Y}_i) \|^2 \tag{5}$$

where $\mathbf{X}$ defines a control point grid of size n over $\mathbf{T}_{\text{global}}(\mathbf{I}^M)$ and $\mathbf{Y} = \mathbf{X} + \mathbf{V}$ presents the deformed control point grid. As we are only interested in the deformation of the aortic shape, the optimizer needs only to evaluate those displacement positions that belong to the aorta. Once the optimal linear transformation $\mathbf{T}_{\text{linear}}$ is computed, we obtain the corresponding minimal displacement field by

$$\mathbf{V}_{\text{minimal}}(\mathbf{X}) = \mathbf{T}_{\text{linear}}^{-1}(\mathbf{Y}) - \mathbf{X} \tag{6}$$

3 Results

Experiments have been conducted on 15 patient datasets each consisting of one preoperative and one postoperative CT angiography (CTA) scan. All images were acquired by a Siemens Somatom Sensation 64 scanner at our partner clinic. The reconstructed image resolution is 0.54 x 0.54 x 1.00 mm.

As we deal with real medical images, there is no ground truth data available that could be used for the assessment of the registration accuracy. Therefore, we reconstruct centerlines out of the deformed distance maps and evaluate these to the preoperative and postoperative lines. Next to a visual evaluation of the registration error, we choose to use the euclidean distance between the centerlines before and after non-rigid registration.

Table 1 shows the evaluation results. For each of the 15 datasets the *initial distance* and *final distance* each presented by their maximal and mean value. Additionally, the initial and final values for the mean μ, variance σ^2, and standard deviation σ over all datasets are given. Our method results in reduced values (*final distance*) for the distance in between the respective shapes. This states that the deformed centerline fits better to the entire shape of the postoperative centerline after non-rigid registration.

The visual assessment of registration accuracy was performed by three experts from our partner medical centers (two interventional radiologists and one vascular surgeon). They were asked to evaluate four different visualizations of the non-rigid registration results and compare these to visualizations given by existing rigid registration frameworks [2]. All experts found our visualizations as highly beneficial for assessing and quantifying the aortic deformation. In contrast to the vascular surgeon to whom the branching vessels were of no importance, the interventional radiologists were also interested in the accuracy of especially the renal arteries as these are often included within the stent graft

Table 1. Evaluation results

	initial distance		final distance		bifurcation distance			
	max	mean	max	mean	bif1	bif2	bif3	bif4
Dataset 1	11,56	3,46	5,22	1,14	6,91	-	6,90	5,45
Dataset 2	14,13	5,41	4,35	1,41	4,97	3,29	7,08	12,90
Dataset 3	29,68	5,27	6,77	1,50	2,89	3,99	4,39	11,61
Dataset 4	15,46	4,17	2,15	1,32	5,45	4,69	3,67	5,45
Dataset 5	16,96	5,41	4,73	1,14	10,32	9,92	7,37	3,38
Dataset 6	10,35	4,46	3,42	1,31	1,02	2,33	4,50	12,84
Dataset 7	11,21	4,27	4,11	1,60	12,45	11,10	11,13	5,92
Dataset 8	12,26	4,17	3,10	1,32	3,06	5,48	4,32	20,32
Dataset 9	17,44	4,46	3,56	1,24	15,78	12,95	11,52	3,05
Dataset 10	19,91	3,41	4,05	1,41	14,10	10,09	9,64	4,12
Dataset 11	26,00	5,27	7,41	1,50	13,77	10,14	10,58	2,43
Dataset 12	15,60	3,17	2,09	1,22	5,09	7,55	6,32	8,88
Dataset 13	9,55	3,46	4,45	1,14	3,01	4,99	4,12	13,83
Dataset 14	16,22	5,11	4,07	1,51	1,45	4,50	3,77	9,82
Dataset 15	13,08	5,27	3,10	1,50	3,78	6,32	4,51	10,74
μ	15,96	4,45	4,17	1,35	6,93	6,97	6,65	8,68
σ	5,66	0,81	1,47	0,15	4,99	3,34	2,83	5,06
σ^2	32,01	0,66	2,17	0,02	24,92	11,17	8,03	25,61

as side branches. However, as our approach highly concentrates on the aortic trunk and only takes small parts of branching vessels into account for rotational orientation purposes, branching vessels might not be accurately aligned.

4 Discussion

In this paper, we address the challenging task of extracting the intraoperative aortic deformation out of pre- and postoperative CT scans. We believe due to constraining the given image information to the region of interest around the aorta, it is possible to only extract aorta specific displacement fields. The method was successfully tested on 15 datasets of patient that had been treated by EVAR in the abdomen.

In the near future, we plan to optimize the non-rigid registration algorithm by establishing correspondences in order to give branching and bifurcation points more weight. Moreover, we intent to apply this method to preoperative CTA and intraoperative rotational angiography volumes in order to display electromagnetically tracked catheter positions within a combined volume.

References

1. Crum WR, Hartkens T, Hill DLG. Non-rigid image registration: Theory and practice. Br J Radiol. 2004;77:S140–S153.
2. Demirci S, Kutter O, Manstad-Hulaas F, et al. Advanced 2D-3D registration for Endovascular Aortic Interventions: Addressing Dissimilarity in Images. Proc SPIE. 2008; p. 69182S–69182S–8.
3. Zahlten C, Juergens H, Peitgen HO. Reconstruction of branching blood vessels from ct data. In: Eurographics Workshop of Visualization in Scientific Computing. Springer; 1994. p. 161–168.
4. Danielsson PE. Euclidean Distance Mapping. Computer Graph Image Process. 1980;14(3):227–248.
5. Modersitzki J. Numerical Methods for Image Registration. Oxford University Press; 2004.
6. Zikic D, Sass Hansen M, Glocker B, et al. Computing Minimal Deformations: Application to Construction of Statistical Shape Models. Proc IEEE Conf: Computer Vision and Pattern Recognition. 2008; p. 1–8.

Reduktion der Invasivität bei nadelbasierter Bewegungskompensation für navigierte Eingriffe im Abdomen

L. Maier-Hein[1], A. Tekbas[2], A. M. Franz[1], R. Tetzlaff[1,4], S. A. Müller[2], F. Pianka[2], I. Wolf[1], H.-U. Kauczor[3,4], B. M. Schmied[2], H.-P. Meinzer[1]

[1]German Cancer Research Center, Div. of Medical and Biological Informatics
[2]University of Heidelberg, Dept. of General, Abdominal and Transplant Surgery
[3]University of Heidelberg, Dept. of Diagnostic Radiology
[4]German Cancer Research Center, Dept. of Radiology
l.maier-hein@dkfz-heidelberg.de

Kurzfassung. Diese Arbeit stellt eine in-vivo Genauigkeitsstudie über das Kombinieren interner und externer Marker für die Bewegungskompensation bei Leberinterventionen vor. Abhängig von der Anzahl und Anordnung der verwendeten Marker sowie der angewandten Echtzeittransformation wurde bei kontinuierlicher Atmung eine Schätzgenauigkeit der Zielposition zwischen 1 und 5 mm erreicht. Das Hinzufügen einer einzigen Hilfsnadel zu einer Menge von Hautmarkern führte zu einer Fehlerreduktion von über 50%. Die Ergebnisse dieser Studie können in der Praxis verwendet werden, um basierend auf dem Tradeoff zwischen geringer Invasivität und hoher Genauigkeit eine geeignete Kombination von internen und externen Markern für eine gegebene Fragestellung zu wählen.

1 Einleitung

Aktuellen Studien zufolge lösen minimal-invasive Verfahren zur Krebsdiagnose und -therapie (z.B. Biopsie, Ablationsverfahren) offene Verfahren aufgrund ihres schonenden Charakters in der klinischen Routine zunehmend ab. Diese Eingriffe erfordern typischerweise das Einführen eines nadelförmigen Instrumentes in das vom Krebs befallene Organ. Dabei hängt der Erfolg der Intervention nachweislich von der Genauigkeit der Instrumenteninsertion ab. Computergestützte Systeme für die Nadelinsertion in Weichgewebe benutzen meist das Prinzip der Atemtriggerung für die notwendige Kompensation der intra-interventionellen Organbewegung. Bei Spontanatmung müssen die Patienten in der Lage sein, einen bestimmten Zustand im Atemzyklus wiederholt zu reproduzieren, was insbesondere in stressbehafteten Situation eine Herausforderung ist.

In Vorarbeiten [1] haben wir ein nadelbasiertes Navigationskonzept für CT-gesteuerte Punktionen der Leber vorgestellt, bei der die Position einer anatomischen Struktur kontinuierlich aus der Lage von getrackten Hilfsnadeln berechnet wird. Bei Insertion von drei Hilfsnadeln wurde zwar eine hohe Systemgenauigkeit erreicht, allerdings führt die erhöhte Invasivität im Vergleich zu Hautmarkern auch zu einem potentiell höheren Komplikationsrisiko für den Patienten. Um navigierte Punktionen unter Spontanatmung durchführen zu können und gleichzeitig die Invasivität des Eingriffs zu minimieren, schlagen wir das Kombinieren interner und externer Marker vor und evaluieren die Schätzgenauigkeit (engl: Target registration error [TRE]) für verschiedene Anzahlen von Hautmarkern (externe Marker) und von nadelförmigen Markern (interne Marker).

2 Material und Methoden

Diese vom Regierungspräsidium Karlsruhe genehmigte Studie wurde an zwei anästhesierten und intubierten Schweinen durchgeführt. Das optische Trackingsystem MicronTracker 2, Modell H40 (Claron Technology, Inc.; Toronto, Ontario, Canada) wurde zum Tracken der verwendeten Instrumente (*Tools*) benutzt. Als interne Marker wurden kommerziell erhältliche Sonden für die Radiofrequenzablation [RFA] (LeVeen® CoAccess™ Electrode System; Boston Scientific Corp., Marlborough, MA, USA) benutzt, welche mit einer trackbaren Vorrichtung versehen wurden. Durch die regenschirmförmigen "Anker" (Abb. 1a) können die Nadeln im Gewebe befestigt werden. Für die externen Marker wurde das vom Hersteller vorgeschlagene Design für Hautmarker übernommen.

Für jedes Tier S_i $(i = 1, 2)$ wurden drei *Markerkonfigurationen* K_j $(j = 1, 2, 3)$ untersucht, wobei eine Konfiguration eine Anordnung von drei nadelförmigen Markern und vier Hautmarkern repräsentiert wie exemplarisch in Abb. 1b dargestellt. Für jede Konfiguration (S_i, K_j) wurde der folgende Arbeitsablauf durchgeführt:

1. Die Hautmarker $E = \{e_1, \ldots, e_4\}$ wurden mittels Mastix Hautkleber auf der Haut des Tiers befestigt wie in Abb. 1b gezeigt.
2. Die internen Marker $I = \{i_1, i_2, i_3\}$ wurden so in die Leber eingebracht, dass sie ungefähr parallel zur kraniokaudalen Achse angeordnet waren und das Trackingsystem freie Sicht auf alle Tools hatte.
3. Ein CT wurde akquiriert, um sicherzustellen, dass sich alle Nadeln in der Leber befinden.

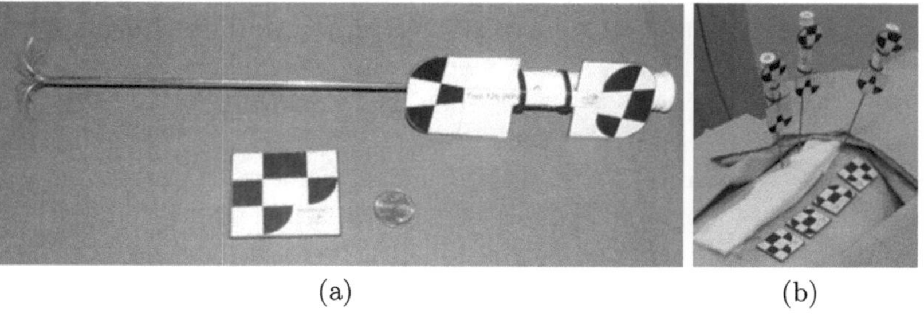

(a) (b)

Abb. 1. Interne und externe Marker (a) und exemplarische Markerkonfiguration (b)

4. Beginnend in voller Ausatmung wurden die Toolpositionen über sieben Atemzyklen aufgezeichnet.

Zur Verarbeitung der Daten für eine Konfiguration (S_i, K_j), eine Zielnadel $i^{\text{target}} \in I$, eine Menge von Markern $M \subset I \backslash \{i^{\text{target}}\} \cup E$ sowie eine Transformation $\Phi_{\text{def}} \in \{\text{RIGIDE, AFFIN, TPS}\}$ (TPS: thin-plate spline Transformation) wurde der folgende Arbeitsablauf durchgeführt:.

1. *Initialisierung:* Die Spitze von i^{target} zum Zeitpunkt $t = 0$ (erstes aufgenommenes Sample) wurde als Ziel t^0 definiert. Zur Speicherung der initialen Markerposition wurde eine Menge von Landmarken $L^0 = \{\boldsymbol{l}_1^0, \ldots \boldsymbol{l}_n^0\}$ vom ersten aufgenommenen Sample extrahiert: Drei Landmarken von jedem Hautmarker und zwei Landmarken von der Achse jeder Hilfsnadel (plus einer weiteren Landmarke, falls nur eine Hilfsnadel ohne Hautmarker für die Bewegungskompensation genutzt wurde). Das Deformationsmodell Φ_{def} wurde dann mit L^0 initialisiert.
2. *Echtzeitschätzung:* Die Intervention wurde durch die letzten fünf Atemzyklen repräsentiert. Für jedes Sample k wurde das Deformationsmodell mit den aktuellen Kontrollpunktpositionen $L^k = \{\boldsymbol{l}_1^k, \ldots \boldsymbol{l}_n^k\}$ zu $\Phi_{\text{def}}^{0\to k}$ aktualisiert. Anschließend wurde die Zielverschiebung δ_{target}^k und der TRE berechnet:

$$\delta_{\text{target}}^k = \left\|t^k - t^0\right\|_2 \tag{1}$$

$$TRE^k = \left\|t^k - \Phi_{\text{def}}^{0\to k}(t^0)\right\|_2 \tag{2}$$

wobei t^k die Position des Ziels zum Zeitpunkt k repräsentiert ($\|.\|_2$: Euklidische Norm).

Für die Datenanalyse wurde jedes Sample k mit dem zugehörigen Zustand im Atemzyklus $\text{state}(k) \in \{\text{expiration, inspiration}\}$ annotiert und der RMS TRE in $\{\text{TRE}^k\}$ sowie in $\{\text{TRE}^k | \text{state}(k) = \text{expiration}\}$ bestimmt. Um die Methoden auf einer maximalen Datenmenge zu evaluieren, wurde die Zielnadel sowie (wenn möglich) die Marker permutiert.

3 Ergebnisse

Wie in Tabelle 1 gezeigt, hatte die Anzahl n_i interner Marker bei kontinuierlicher Atmung mit einem mittleren quatratischen Fehler von $4,8 \pm 1,1$ mm ($n_i = 0$), $2,0 \pm 0,9$ mm ($n_i = 1$) und $1,7 \pm 0,8$ mm ($n_i = 2$) ermittelt aus verschiedenen Markerplatzierungen ($n = 18, 36, 18$) den grössten Einfluss auf die Genauigkeit (Anzahl externer Marker n_e: 4). Das Hinzufügen einer einzigen Hilfsnadel zu einer Menge von Hautmarkern führte zu einer Fehlerreduktion von über 50%.

Aus Abb. 2 ist zu erkennen, dass der TRE drastisch sinkt, wenn interne und externe Marker kombiniert werden gegenüber dem Fall, wenn nur ein Markertyp verwendet wird. Die Experimente zeigten des weiteren, dass die Platzierung der Hilfsnadeln eine wichtige Rolle spielt: Wurden für $n_i = 2$ interne Marker nur diejenigen Markerkombinationen gewählt, bei der die Hilfsnadeln die Zielnadel

Tabelle 1. RMS TRE (in mm) für verschiedene Deformationsmodelle und Anzahlen n_i von internen Markern während kontinuierlicher Atmung (TRE) sowie in Exspiration (TRE(exp)) gemittelt über alle möglichen Permutationen in zwei Schweinen. Alle Hautmarker wurden zur Bewegungskompensation verwendet ($n_e = 4$). Anm: Affine Transformationen und TPS werden bei $n_i = 0$ Hilfsnadeln nicht angewandt, da die Hautmarker eine Ebene approximieren.

		$n_i = 0$	$n_i = 1$	$n_i = 2$
TRE	RIGIDE	**4,8 ± 1,1**	3,8 ± 1,1	3,4 ± 1,2
	AFFIN	-	**2,0 ± 0,9**	1,8 ± 0,9
	TPS	-	2,1 ± 1,0	**1,7 ± 0,8**
TRE(exp)	RIGIDE	**1,1 ± 0,3**	**0,9 ± 0,2**	**0,8 ± 0,2**
	AFFIN	-	1,0 ± 0,4	0,9 ± 0,3
	TPS	-	1,0 ± 0,4	0,8 ± 0,3

in kraniokaudaler Richtung umschlossen wie in [1] vorgeschlagen, ergab sich eine Fehlerreduktion von 34% von $1,8 \pm 0,9$ (n = 18) auf $1,2 \pm 0,5$ (n = 6) (affine Transformation, $n_e = 4$). Dies könnte jedoch zu einem großen Teil auf die Zielposition selbst zurückzuführen sein: Wurden bei $n_i = 0$ bzw. 1 internen Markern nur die kraniokaudal umschlossenen Nadeln als Ziel gewählt, wurden Fehlerreduktionen von 12% bzw. 20% erzielt. Die Lage der Hautmarker hingegen hatte keinen großen Einfluss auf die Genauigkeit, d.h., bei Permutation der externen Marker (für $n_e < 4$) wurden ähnliche Genauigkeiten erreicht. Wie in Abb. 2 gezeigt, war die Genauigkeit bei $n_e = 2, 3$ and 4 Hautmarkern vergleichbar.

Laut Tabelle 1 ist die Performanz affiner Transformationen und TPS bei kontinuierlicher Atmung wesentlich besserer als die rigider Transformationen, während in Exspiration ähnliche Ergebnisse erzielt wurden.

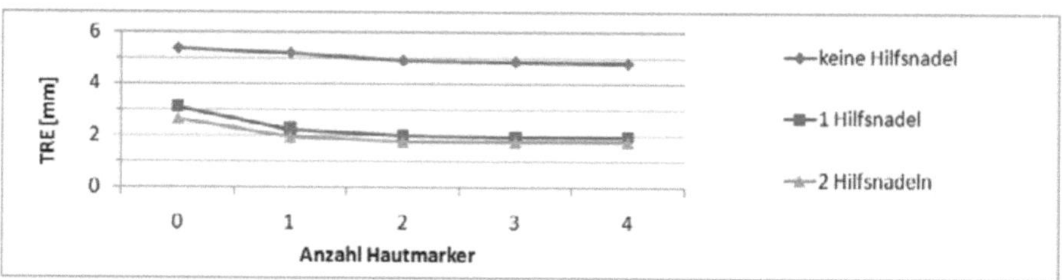

Abb. 2. RMS TRE für verschiedene Kombinationen von externen und internen Markern. Das Deformationsmodell war affin, wenn beide Markertypen verwendet wurden und andernfalls rigide. Für $n_i = n_e = 0$ ist die RMS Verschiebung des Ziels aufgeführt.

4 Diskussion

Weichgewebenavigation mit internen Markern gewinnt zunehmende Aufmerksamkeit in der Literatur. Einer der ersten Ansätze wurde von Schweikard *et al.* [2] vorgestellt, welcher Echtzeit-Tracking von Hautmarkern mit gelegentlicher Röntgenkontrolle implantierter interner Marker für die Radiotherapie kombinierte. Zhang *et al.* [3] untersuchten die Verwendung einer Hilfsnadel in Kombination mit Hautmarkern zur Verbesserung der initialen Registrierung ihres Navigationssystems. Da die Marker jedoch nicht getrackt wurden, konnte keine Analyse über den Atemzyklus durchgeführt werden. Unsere Arbeit ist am ehesten vergleichbar mit den kürzlich von Krücker *et al.* [4] publizierten Studie. Dort wurde die Verwendung einer Menge von externen *oder* internen Marker für die Bewegungskompensation untersucht. Ähnlich wie wir stellten die Autoren fest, dass Atembewegungskompensation mit einer einzigen Hilfsnadel möglich ist. Unseres Wissens nach sind wir jedoch die Ersten, die das kontinuierliche Tracken einer Kombination der verschiedenen Markertypen für die Bewegungskompensation bei Leberinterventionen in-vivo untersucht haben.

In dieser Studie haben wir uns auf den Vergleich verschiedener Markerkombinationen und Transformationen konzentriert. Zukünftige Arbeiten sollten sich mit geeigneten Platzierungsstrategien beschäftigen. Für den Fall rigider punktbasierter Registrierung konnte bereits gezeigt werden, dass der TRE von (1) dem Fehler zur Lokalisation der Kontrollpunkte (hier: Marker), (2) der Anordnung der Marker und (3) der Zielposition relativ zu den Markern abhängt [5].

Abschließend stellen wir fest, dass die Ergebnisse dieser Studie in der Praxis genutzt werden können, um basierend auf dem Tradeoff zwischen geringer Invasivität und hoher Genauigkeit eine geeignete Kombination von internen und externen Markern für eine gegebene Fragestellung zu wählen.

Literaturverzeichnis

1. Maier-Hein L, Müller SA, Pianka F, et al. Respiratory motion compensation for CT-guided interventions in the liver. Comp Aid Surg. 2008;13(3):125–38.
2. Schweikard A, Glosser G, Bodduluri M, et al. Robotic motion compensation for respiratory movement during radiosurgery. Comp Aid Surg. 2000;5:263–277.
3. Zhang H, Banovac F, Cleary K. Increasing registration precision for liver movement with respiration using electromagnetic tracking. Proc CARS. 2005 May;1281:571–576.
4. Krücker J, Xu S, Glossop N, et al. Evaluation of motion compensation approaches for soft tissue navigation. Proc SPIE. 2008;6918:691814.
5. Fitzpatrick JM, West JB, Maurer CR. Predicting error in rigid-body point-based registration. IEEE Trans Med Imaging. 1998;17(5):694–702.

VR-Trainingssimulator für Lumbal- und Aszitespunktionen mit elastischer Nadelverbiegung

Thorsten Dahmke[1,2], Matthias Färber[1], Christian-Arved Bohn[2], Heinz Handels[1]

[1]Department of Medical Informatics, University Medical Center Hamburg-Eppendorf
[2]Computergraphics & Virtual Reality, University of Applied Sciences Wedel
tdahmke@freenet.de

Kurzfassung. Es wird ein VR-Trainingssimulator zum Erlernen von Lumbal- und Aszitespunktionen vorgestellt. Dieser stellt vielseitige visuelle Hilfsmittel, sowie eine Evaluationskomponente, die dem Benutzer Auskunft über das Ergebnis seiner Punktion gibt, zur Verfügung. Ein haptisches Ein-/Ausgabegerät ermöglicht die Steuerung der virtuellen Nadel und das Erfühlen von Strukturen während der Punktion. Über die Koppelung der durch ein bewegliches Rotationsfedermodell repräsentierten Nadel mit einem Multiproxy-Ansatz wird die Simulation von Nadelverbiegungen ermöglicht.

1 Einleitung

Lumbalpunktionen dienen der Entnahme von Rückenmarksflüssigkeit und Aszitespunktionen der Entnahme von Bauchwasser. Im Rahmen der medizinischen Ausbildung findet das Erlernen dieser Punktionseingriffe in der Regel direkt am Patienten unter Anleitung durch einen Facharzt statt. Dieses Vorgehen erhöht das Verletzungsrisiko beim Patienten und stellt eine zusätzliche Belastung für den Medizinstudenten dar.

In dieser Arbeit wird ein Virtual-Reality-Trainingssystem vorgestellt, welches die Möglichkeit bietet diese Punktionen in virtuellen Körpern zu erlernen. Im Gegensatz zu anderen Ansätzen zur Punktionssimulation (bspw. [1, 2]) in denen haptische Geräte mit drei Freiheitsgraden zur Kraftausgabe (3DOF) verwendet werden, wird in dieser Arbeit ein 6DOF Gerät verwendet, um auch die Ausgabe von Drehmomenten zu ermöglichen, wodurch unnatürliche seitliche Nadelbewegungen verhindert werden können. In Erweiterung zu [3] wurde die Simulation von Nadelverbiegungen integriert und die Simulation von Aszitespunktionen ermöglicht. Ansätze zur Nadelverbiegung bilden neben Finite-Elemente-Methoden (FEM) [4, 5] auch die Angular Spring Method [5]. Dieser 2D-Ansatz ist effizienter und effektiver als FEM und daher für eine haptische Echtzeit-Anwendung besser geeignet [5].

2 Material und Methoden

Im Folgenden werden die drei Kernkomponenten des Simulators, die haptische Komponente, die visuelle Komponente und die Evaluationskomponente, vorgestellt. Dabei wird noch einmal gesondert auf die Berechnung der Nadelverbiegung eingegangen.

2.1 Haptische Komponente

Den Kern der haptischen Komponente bildet ein proxybasiertes haptisches Volumenrendering, durch das Kräfte und Drehmomente erzeugt werden [3, 6]. Die haptische Ein- und Ausgabe erfolgt mittels des Phantom Premium 1.5 mit 6DOF. Die an das haptische Gerät zurückzugebenen Kräfte und Drehmomente ergeben sich aus den Nadelspitzen- und den Nadelschaftkräften. Zu den Nadelspitzenkräften zählen die Durchdringbarkeit der Oberfläche, die Oberflächenreibung und die Viskosität. Die Nadelschaftkräfte werden aus den Nadelschaftreibungs-, Transversal- und Rotationskräften gebildet.

Im Folgenden wird nun die Erweiterung des bisher verwendeten Ansatzes zu einem Multiproxy-Ansatz beschrieben. Zur Berechnung der Nadelspitzenkräfte wird dabei die Spitze der Nadel x_n über ein virtuelles Federelement mit einem Proxy (Stellvertreter) x_{p_n} verbunden. Der Proxy wird in seiner Bewegung, wie in [6, 7] beschrieben, durch virtuelle Oberflächen beschränkt, wodurch über das Hookesche Gesetz

$$\boldsymbol{f} = -k \cdot \boldsymbol{d}; \boldsymbol{d} = \boldsymbol{x_n} - \boldsymbol{x}_{p_n} \tag{1}$$

eine Kraft ausgeübt wird. Der Multiproxy-Ansatz entsteht durch die Verknüpfung des Nadelmodells mit weiteren Proxies entlang des Nadelschafts (Abb. 1, Abschnitt 2.2). Durch die Beschränkung der Bewegung dieser Proxies gemäß

$$\boldsymbol{x}'_{p_i} = \begin{cases} \boldsymbol{x}_i + F/k \cdot \boldsymbol{d}^0, & \text{wenn } |\boldsymbol{d}| > F/k \\ \boldsymbol{x}_{p_i}, & \text{sonst} \end{cases} \tag{2}$$

kann die Nadelschaftreibung ermittelt werden. Die Berechnung der Transversalkräfte erfolgt durch die Projektion sämtlicher Proxys auf den Einstichsvektor. Die Rotationskräfte werden über die Drehmomente simuliert (Abschnitt 2.2). Die an das Gerät zurückgegebene Kraft und das zurückgegebene Drehmoment ergeben sich aus der Summe der im Nadelmodell auftretenden Kräfte und Drehmomente.

$$\boldsymbol{f}_{\text{feedback}} = \sum_{0}^{n} \boldsymbol{f}_i \tag{3}$$

$$\boldsymbol{m}_{\text{feedback}} = \sum_{0}^{n} \boldsymbol{m}_i \tag{4}$$

2.2 Nadelverbiegung

Basis für die Nadelverbiegung bildet eine 3D-Adaption der Angular Spring Method [5]. Ausgehend von den auf die Rotationsfedern wirkenden Kräften $\boldsymbol{f}_i$ können mittels

$$\boldsymbol{m}_i = \sum_{j>i}^{n} \boldsymbol{l}_{ij} \times \boldsymbol{f}_j \tag{5}$$

die Drehmomente $\boldsymbol{m}_i$ an den jeweiligen Federn x_i berechnet werden. $\boldsymbol{l}_{ij}$ stellt dabei den Hebelarm zwischen den Rotationsfedern x_i und x_j dar. Diese Drehmomente dienen dazu, das vom Gerät ausgehende Drehmoment zu berechnen (Formel 4) und die Orientierung der Rotationsfedern über

$$\mathbf{angles}_i = \boldsymbol{m}_i / k. \tag{6}$$

zu ermitteln. Dabei besteht der Vektor **angles** aus drei Winkeln α, β, γ, die die Orientierung der Feder im Raum beschreiben. Auf Basis dieser Winkel kann die auf eine Rotationsfeder x_i jeweils nachfolgenden Rotationsfeder x_{i+1} entsprechend der Formel

$$\boldsymbol{x}_{i+1} = \boldsymbol{x}_i + \begin{pmatrix} 0 \\ 0 \\ \text{Segmentlänge} \end{pmatrix} \cdot M_{\text{gerät}} \cdot M_{\text{angles}} \tag{7}$$

neu positioniert werden, wobei $M_{\text{gerät}}$ die Orientierung des haptischen Gerätes und die Rotationsmatrix M_{angles} die Rotation um die aufsummierten Winkel der Rotationsfedern x_0 bis x_i beschreiben. Zudem kann über die Winkel geprüft werden, ob die Nadel zerbrochen ist. Hierzu wurde ein maximaler Winkel $\alpha_{\max}$ definiert. Wird dieser von einem der Winkel an den Rotationsfedern überschritten, so gilt die Nadel an dieser Feder als zerbrochen.

2.3 Visuelle Komponente

Den Kern der Visualisierung bilden ein 3D-Viewer, in dem ein auf den manuell segmentierten CT-Daten des Patienten basierendes 3D-Modell und ein 3D-Modell der Nadel dargestellt werden und drei SliceViewer, in denen wahlweise aus den CT- oder den manuell segmentierten Daten orthogonale 2D-Schichtbilder in Abhängigkeit von der aktuellen Nadelposition generiert werden (Abb. 2). Die Nadelverbiegung wird innerhalb des 3D-Viewers durch ein Mapping der OpenGL-Vertices des Polygonmodells der Nadel auf die Positionen und Orientierungen der Rotationsfedern realisiert.

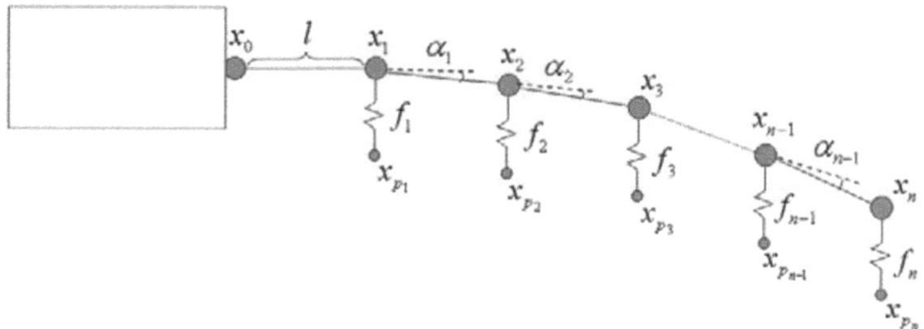

Abb. 1. Das Nadelmodell für den Multiproxy-Ansatz und die Nadelverbiegung. x_i: Rotationsfeder zur Berechnung der Kräfte und der Verbiegung. x_{p_i}: Feder x_i zugeordneter Proxy. f_i: Die aus $-k \cdot (x_i - x_{p_i})$ resultierende Kraft. α_i: Der Verbiegungswinkel an Rotationsfeder x_i.

2.4 Evaluationskomponente

Die Evaluationskomponente dient dazu, dem Benutzer ein bewertetes Feedback über seine virtuell durchgeführten Punktionen in Form von quantitativen Scoringwerten zu geben, Fehler aufzuzeigen und Verbesserungsvorschläge zu unterbreiten. Hierzu wird die Punktion aufgezeichnet und anhand von verschiedenen Kriterien, die nach Expertenaussagen eine gelungene Punktion ausmachen, analysiert und bewertet. Zudem besteht die Möglichkeit die Evaluationergebnisse automatisch im csv-Format speichern zu lassen, um Lernfortschritte später beurteilen zu können. Für die Aszitespunktion sind diese Kriterien das Erreichen der Zielstruktur, das Verletzen von Risikostrukturen wie z.B. Knochen, Gefäße oder innere Organe und die Dauer der Punktion. Für die Bewertung von Lumbalpunktionen wird zusätzlich die Übereinstimmung des Einstichs mit von Experten bestimmten optimalen Einstichpfaden quantifiziert. Hierbei werden der Abstand, die Winkeldifferenz sowie die Eindringtiefe im Vergleich zu den optimalen Pfaden bewertet.

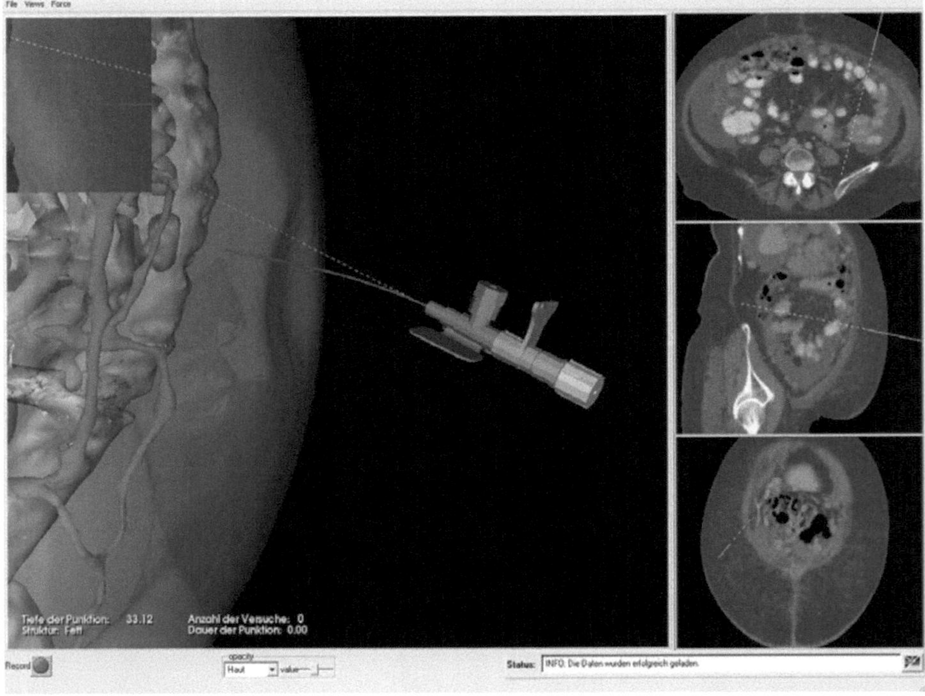

Abb. 2. GUI des Punktionssimulators. Mittig: Der 3D-Viewer. Oben links: Zweiter Viewer mit seitlicher Ansicht auf die Nadel. Rechts: Die SliceViewer zur Darstellung der 2D-Schichtbilder.

3 Ergebnisse

Der entwickelte Simulator ermöglicht die Durchführung von virtuellen Punktionen in Echtzeit. Auf einem Intel Xeon (3GHz, 2GB DDR2 RAM, Nvidia Quadro FX 4400) werden bei einem Rotationsfedermodell mit 20 Federn haptische Framerates von fast 2000 fps erreicht, so dass die Anbindung eines haptischen Gerätes problemlos möglich ist. In einer ersten Evaluation wurden Aszites- und Lumbalpunktionen von Medizinstudenten an unterschiedlichen virtuellen Patienten durchgeführt. Hierbei hat sich gezeigt, dass die Intuitivität der Benutzerinterkation durch den Multiproxy-Ansatz und den Verbiegungsalgorithmus verbessert werden konnte.

4 Diskussion und Ausblick

Der hier vorgestellte Punktionssimulator bietet die Möglichkeit Lumbal- und Aszitespunktionen an virtuellen Körpern zu erlernen. Durch vielfältige Visualisierungsmöglichkeiten bietet der Simulator zusätzliche Hilfestellungen beim Durchführen der Punktion und ermöglicht während der Durchführung der Punktion Einblick in die Anatomie des Patienten zu nehmen. Durch die Evaluationskomponente des Simulators ist eine objektive Bewertung des Eingriffes mittels quantitativer Scoringwerte möglich. Fehler werden aufgezeigt und Verbesserungsvorschläge gemacht.

Als zukünftige Weiterentwicklungen ist die Integration eines deformierbaren Körpermodells und die Erweiterung des Simulators auf weitere Punktionseingriffe geplant.

Literaturverzeichnis

1. Ra JB, Kwon SM, Kim JK, et al. Spine needle biopsy simulator using visual and force feedback. Comput Aided Surg. 2002;7(6):353–363.
2. Gorman P, Krummel T, Webster R, et al. A prototype haptic lumbar puncture simulator. Stud Health Technol Inform. 2000;70:106–109.
3. Färber M, Hoeborn E, Dalek D, et al. Training and evaluation of lumbar punctures in a VR-environment using a 6DOF haptic device. Stud Health Technol Inform. 2008;132:112–114.
4. DiMaio SP, Salcudean SE. Interactive simulation of needle insertion models. IEEE Trans Biomed Eng. 2005;52(7):1167–1179.
5. Dehghan E, Goksel O, Salcudean SE. A comparison of needle bending models. Med Image Comput Comput Assist Interv Int Conf Med Image Comput Comput Assist Interv. 2006;9(Pt 1):305–312.
6. Färber M, Heller J, Handels H. Simulation and training of lumbar punctures using haptic volume rendering and a 6DOF haptic device. Proc SPIE. 2007;6509:0F1–0F8.
7. Lundin K, Ynnerman A, Gudmundsson B; United Kingdom University of Edinburgh. Proxy-based haptic feedback from volumetric density data. Proc Eurohaptic Conf. 2002; p. 104–109.

Der Telemanipulator daVinci als mechanisches Trackingsystem
Bestimmung von Präzision und Genauigkeit

Johannes Kast[1], Jochen Neuhaus[1], Felix Nickel[2], Hannes Kenngott[2], Markus Engel[1], Elaine Short[1], Michael Reiter[2], Hans-Peter Meinzer[1], Lena Maier-Hein[1]

[1]Abteilung für Medizinische und Biologische Informatik, DKFZ Heidelberg
[2]Universitätsklinikum Heidelberg
j.kast@dkfz-heidelberg.de

Kurzfassung. Der Telemanipulator daVinci (Intuitive Surgical, Sunnyvale, Kalifornien) ist ein Master-Slave System für roboterassistierte minimalinvasive Chirurgie. Da er über integrierte Gelenksensoren verfügt, kann er unter Verwendung der daVinci-API als mechanisches Trackingsystem verwendet werden. In dieser Arbeit evaluieren wir die Präzision und Genauigkeit eines daVinci mit Hilfe eines Genauigkeitsphantoms mit bekannten Maßen. Der ermittelte Positionierungsfehler liegt in der Größenordnung von 6 mm und ist somit für einen Großteil der medizinischen Fragestellungen zu hoch. Zur Reduktion des Fehlers schlagen wir daher eine Kalibrierung der Gelenksensoren vor.

1 Einleitung

Chirurgische Eingriffe werden immer häufiger mit Navigationssystemen unterstützt. Dabei haben sich vor allem optische und magnetische Trackingsysteme durchgesetzt. Mechanische Trackingsysteme werden auf Grund ihres Platzbedarfs selten eingesetzt, obwohl sie viele Vorteile der optischen und magnetischen Tracker vereinen [1]. Der Telemanipulator daVinci (Intuitive Surgical, Sunnyvale, Kalifornien) ist ein Master-Slave System für roboterassistierte minimalinvasive Chirurgie. Da er über integrierte Gelenksensoren verfügt, kann er als mechanisches Trackingsystem genutzt werden, so dass zusätzliche Trackinghardware im Operationssaal entfallen kann. Die Daten für die Positionsberechnung liefert die API-Schnittstelle des Telemanipulators [2]. Da die Freischaltung der API bislang nur für wenige Institute vorgenommen wurde (u.a. [3, 4]), gibt es bisher lediglich eine Arbeitsgruppe, die sich mit der Genauigkeit und Präzision des Telemanipulators beschäftigt hat [4, 5]. Bei Industrierobotern gibt es bekanntermaßen Fertigungstoleranzen zwischen verschiedenen Geräten eines Modelles. Daher führen wir in dieser Arbeit eine weitere Genauigkeitsstudie durch. Wir arbeiten dabei mit einem Genauigkeitsphantom, welches annähernd das gesamte Arbeitsvolumen des Telemanipulators abdeckt.

2 Material und Methoden

Die Position der Instrumentenspitze eines Manipulatorarms zu einem festen Bezugspunkt wird mit der Vorwärts-Kinematik nach der Denavit-Hartenberg Konvention berechnet [6]. Die dafür notwendigen aktuellen Winkelstellungen der Manipulatorarme sendet der Telemanipulator über eine Netzwerkschnittstelle. Die Anbindung an die von Intuitive Surgical freigeschaltene Schnittstelle wurde in das Medical Imaging Interaction Toolkit (MITK) [7] integriert.

Zur Bestimmung der Präzision und Genauigkeit des daVinci wurde ein Phantom gebaut, welches die Positionierung eines Manipulatorarms auf insgesamt 27 Referenzpunkte in einem 3 x 3 x 3 Gitter mit den Kantenlängen 17 x 17 x 12 cm ermöglicht und somit nahezu das gesamte Arbeitsvolumen in einer Grundgelenkstellung (engl.: Setup-Joints [2]) des daVinci abdeckt (siehe Abb. 1). Die folgenden Abschnitte beschreiben die durchgeführten Experimente.

Experiment zur Bestimmung der Präzision. Zur Bestimmung der Präzision wurde jeder Gitterpunkt des Phantoms mit einem Manipulatorarm manuell in drei Durchgängen angefahren (Abb. 2) und die Position erfasst. Die Präzision ist hier als das quadratische Mittel (engl.: root mean square (RMS)) der Distanzen von allen gemessenen Positionen $\boldsymbol{p}_{jl}$ (j: Position) zu ihrem über alle Durchgänge l bestimmten Schwerpunkt $\boldsymbol{s}_j$ definiert.

$$\text{Präzision}_{\text{RMS}} = \sqrt{\frac{1}{81}\sum_{j=1}^{27}\sum_{l=1}^{3}||\boldsymbol{m}_{jl} - \boldsymbol{s}_j||^2} \tag{1}$$

Evaluation der Genauigkeit. Das Phantom wurde mit dem optischen Trackingsystem Polaris (NDI, Waterloo, Kanada) mit Hilfe des Zeiger-Instruments *NDI 4-Marker Passive Probe* vermessen. Die Genauigkeit des daVinci wurde mittels

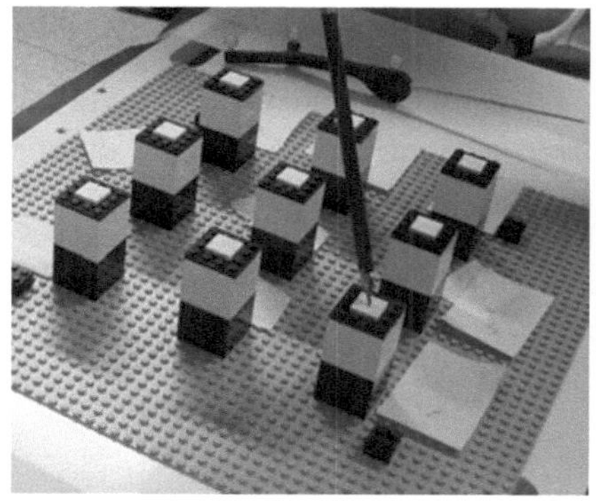

Abb. 1. Eine von drei Ebenen des vermessenen Phantoms, im Hintergrund Zeiger für optisches Tracking.

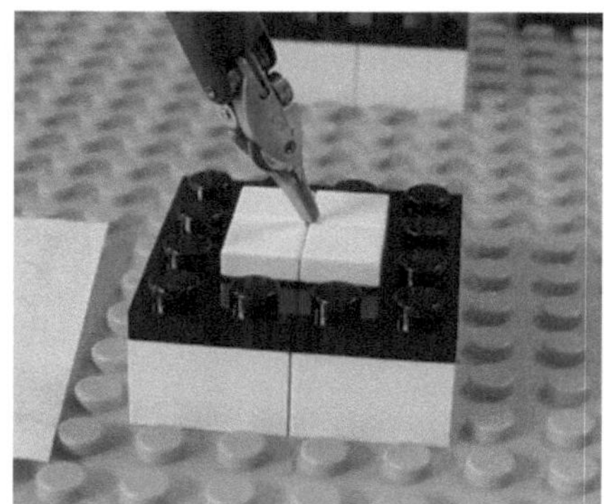

Abb. 2. Ein mit dem daVinci Manipulator angefahrene Phantomposition in der unteren Ebene.

punktbasierter rigider Registrierung der gemessenen Positionen $\boldsymbol{m}_{jl}$ (j: Position; l: Durchgang) mit den korrespondierenden Referenzpunkten $\boldsymbol{r}_j$ im Phantomkoordinatensystem bestimmt. Dazu wurde mittels der Methode der kleinsten Quadrate [8] diejenige rigide Transformation Φ ermittelt, die den zugehörigen Registrierungsfehler (engl.: Fiducial Registration Error (FRE))

$$\mathrm{FRE} = \sqrt{\frac{1}{81}\sum_{j=1}^{27}\sum_{l=1}^{3}||\boldsymbol{m}_{jl} - \Phi(\boldsymbol{r}_j)||^2} \tag{2}$$

minimiert. Der FRE der ermittelten Transformation Φ dient als Maß für die Positionierungsgenauigkeit.

Um zu Untersuchen wie exakt der daVinci eine Position treffen kann, die nicht in eine Registrierung mit eingegangen ist, werden k Referenzpositionen mit $\{f_1, ..., f_k\} \subset \{r_1, ..., r_{27}\}$ ausgewählt. Danach wird die Transformation Φ mit den der Auswahl zugeordneten, gemessenen und über die Durchgänge gemittelten Positionen $\{z_1, ..., z_k\} \subset \{\bar{m}_1, ..., \bar{m}_27\}$ wieder über eine punktbasierte rigide Registrierung berechnet. Alle nicht ausgewählten Referenzpositionen werden als Zielpunkte $\boldsymbol{t}_j$ (engl.: Targets) definiert. Der RMS der Distanzen von den mit Φ transformierten Zielpunkten zu korrespondierenden, gemessenen und gemittelten Positionen $\{\bar{g}_1, ..., \bar{g}_j\} = \{\bar{m}_1, ..., \bar{m}_{27}\}\backslash\{z_1, ..., z_k\}$ ist der Target Registration Error (TRE). Dieser wurde für alle kombinatorischen Möglichkeiten von vier bis 26 Referenzpositionen berechnet. Für k Referenzpositionen existieren somit $\binom{27}{27-k}$ RMS Werte die mit folgender Formel berechnet wurden.

$$\mathrm{TRE}_{\mathrm{RMS}} = \sqrt{\frac{1}{k}\sum_{j=1}^{27-k}||\bar{\boldsymbol{g}}_j - \Phi(\boldsymbol{t}_j)||^2} \tag{3}$$

Aus den $\binom{27}{27-k}$ RMS Werten wurde für jedes k der Mittelwert und die Standardabweichung gebildet.

Abhängigkeit der Genauigkeit von der Grundgelenkstellung. Um die Abhängigkeit der Genauigkeit des daVinci von der Grundgelenkstellung zu bestimmen, wurde das erste Experiment für vier weitere Grundgelenkstellungen durchgeführt. Jede Position wurde zwei mal angefahren. Unmittelbar nach jeder daVinci Positionsbestimmung wurde die entsprechende Position optisch nachgemessen. Der FRE wurde analog zum ersten Versuch der Genauigkeitsbestimmung, der TRE mit Mittelwert und Standardabweichung für $k = 26$ berechnet.

3 Ergebnisse

Der erste Versuch ergibt eine Präzision von 0,64 mm RMS (Min: 0,04 mm, Max: 1,63 mm) sowie einen FRE von 7,6 mm. Der Mittelwert des TRE sinkt für eine steigende Anzahl von Referenzpositionen von 9,0 mm auf 7,6 mm. Die Standardabweichung der berechneten Mittelwerte ist dabei in den Randbereichen erhöht

Tabelle 1. Fiducial Registration Error (FRE) und Mittelwert und Standardabweichung des Target Registration Error (TRE) jeweils für unterschiedliche Grundgelenkstellungen (Pose).

	Pose 1	Pose 2	Pose 3	Pose 4
FRE [mm]	6,7	6,2	6,2	6,5
TRE [mm]	6,6 ±2,4	6,1 ±2,3	6,1 ±2,1	6,4 ±2,3

(Abb. 3). Im Versuch mit verschiedenen Grundgelenkstellungen variiert der FRE zwischen 6,2 mm und 6,7 mm. Die berechneten Mittelwerte des TRE für $k = 26$ liegen zwischen 6,1 ±2,1 mm und 6,6 ±2,4 mm (Tabelle 1). Im Mittel über alle fünf untersuchten Grundgelenkstellungen ist der FRE 6,5 ±0,4 mm und der TRE 6,6 ±0,4 mm.

4 Diskussion

In dieser Arbeit wurde die Präzision und Genauigkeit des daVinci Telemanipulators untersucht. Der ermittelte TRE fällt wie erwartet mit einer steigenden Anzahl von Referenzpositionen. Er ist trotzdem immer größer als 6 mm und damit für die meisten medizinischen Anwendungen zu hoch. Die steigenden Werte für die Standardabweichung in den Randbereichen und insbesondere für $k = 26$ lassen sich damit erklären, dass sich Ausreißer (Abb. 4) bei wenigen RMS Werten stärker bemerkbar machen. Eine Abhängigkeit von der Grundgelenkstellung konnte nicht festgestellt werden.

Unsere Arbeit orientierte sich an der von Kwartowitz *et al.* [4] publizierten Studie. Dort wurde ebenfalls ein Genauigkeitsphantom mit optisch vermessenen Referenzpunkten verwendet, um den FRE und TRE mittels landmarkenbasier-

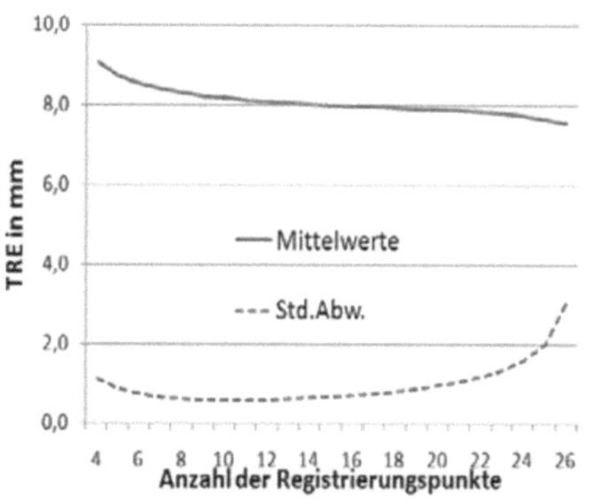

Abb. 3. Target Registration Error (TRE) über unterschiedliche Referenzpositionenanzahl.

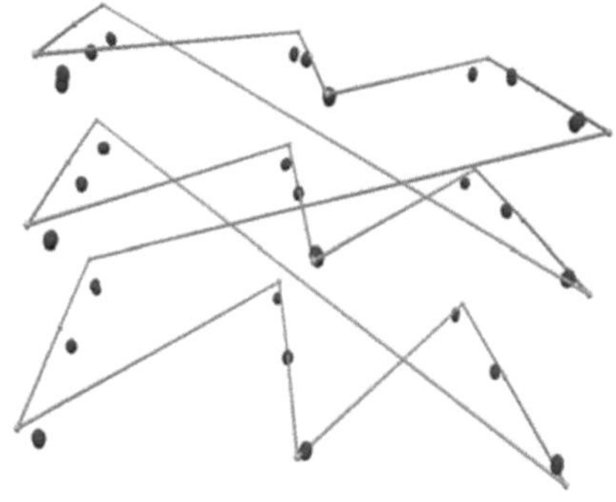

Abb. 4. Visualisierung einer Registrierung: gemessene daVinci Positionen als rote Punkte, Referenzpositionen in gelb durch Linien verbunden.

ter Registrierung zu bestimmen. Allerdings basierte die Messung auf lediglich elf Punkten in einem kleineren Messvolumen. In Abhängigkeit der Anzahl der für die Registrierung verwendeten Referenzpositionen lag der TRE zwischen 1,9 mm und 2,4 mm und somit deutlich unter unseren Werten. Bei Nutzung aller Referenzpositionen wurde dort ein FRE in der Größenordnung von 1,6 mm erreicht.

Im Allgemeinen wird der TRE von folgenden Faktoren beeinflusst:

1. Lokalisierungsfehler von zugeordneten Positionen: Korrespondierende Punkte müssen im Phantom- und im daVinci Koordinatensystem akkurat lokalisiert werden. Ein Fehler resultiert aus der Positionierungsgenauigkeit des daVinci, dem Ansteuerungsfehler und dem optischen Vermessungsfehler.
2. Lage und Anordnung der Referenzpunkte relativ zum Zielpunkt: Bekanntermaßen steigt der TRE bei punktbasierter rigider Registrierung i.d.R. mit sinkender Anzahl von Referenzpositionen sowie steigendem Abstand des Zielpunktes vom Schwerpunkt der Referenzpositionen.

Da die Präzision im Submillimeterbereich liegt obwohl sie zusätzlich den Benutzerfehler enthält, vermuten wir, dass sich die Unterschiede im ermittelten TRE auf Fehler in der Gelenksensorik zurückführen lässt [9]. Die Sensoren geben eine sehr exakte Winkelveränderung wieder, haben jedoch in ihrer Nullstellung einen Versatz. Dieser setzt sich durch die komplette kinematische Kette fort und führt zu einem systematischen Positionierungsfehler. Gelingt es die Sensorfehler zu identifizieren, ist es denkbar, hinreichende Positionierungsgenauigkeiten zu erreichen. Derzeit wird an einer solchen Kalibrierung der Sensoren gearbeitet. Erste Berechnungen geben Hinweise auf eine deutliche Reduktion des TRE.

Literaturverzeichnis

1. Yaniv Z, Cleary K. Image-Guided Procedures: A Review. Computer Aided Interventions and Medical Robotics; 2006.
2. DiMaio SP, Simon P, Hasser C. The daVinci Research Interface. Procs MICCAI Workshop. 2008.
3. Wang DA, Bello F, Darzi A. Augmented reality provision in robotically assisted minimally invasive surgery. Int J CARS. 2004;1268:527–532.
4. Kwartowitz DM, Herrell DS, Galloway RL. Toward image-guided robotic surgery: determining intrinsic accuracy of the daVinci robot. Int J CARS. 2006;1(3):157–165.
5. Kwartowitz DM, Herrell DS, Galloway RL. Update: Toward image-guided robotic surgery: determining the intrinsic accuracy of the daVinci-S robot. Int J CARS. 2007;1(5):301–304.
6. Denavit J, Hartenberg S. A Kinematic notation. for lower pair mechanisms based on matrices. J Appl Mech. 1955;22:215–219.
7. Wolf I, Vetter M, Wegner I, et al. The medical imaging interaction toolkit. Med Image Anal. 2005 Dec;9(6):594–604.
8. Horn BKP. Closed-form solution of absolute orientation using unit quaternions. J Opt Soc Am. 1987;4:629–642.
9. Beyer L. Genauigkeitssteigerung von Industrierobotern - Insbesondere mit Parallelkinematik. Universität der Bundeswehr Hamburg; 2004.

Camera Augmented Mobile C-arm
Towards Real Patient Study

Lejing Wang[1], Simon Weidert[2], Joerg Traub[1], Sandro Michael Heining[2], Christian Riquarts[2], Ekkehard Euler[2], Nassir Navab[1]

[1]Chair for Computer Aided Medical Procedures (CAMP), TU Munich, Germany
[2]Trauma Surgery Department, Klinikum Innenstadt, LMU Munich, Germany
wangle@in.tum.de

Abstract. The Camera Augmented Mobile C-arm (CamC) system that extends a regular mobile C-arm by a video camera provides an X-ray and video image overlay. Thanks to the mirror construction and one time calibration of the device, the acquired X-ray images are co-registered with the video images without any calibration or registration during the intervention. It is very important to quantify and qualify the system before its introduction into the OR. In this communication, we extended the previously performed overlay accuracy analysis of the CamC system by another clinically important parameter, the applied radiation dose for the patient. Since the mirror of the CamC system will absorb and scatter radiation, we introduce a method for estimating the correct applied dose by using an independent dose measurement device. The results show that the mirror absorbs and scatters 39% of X-ray radiation.

1 Introduction

Mobile C-arms are an everyday tool to acquire X-ray images in the operating room during surgery. The Camera Augmented Mobile C-arm (CamC) system that extends a regular mobile C-arm by a video camera was proposed by Navab et al. [1] for X-ray and video image overlay. Thanks to the mirror construction and one time calibration of the device, the acquired X-ray images are co-registered with the video images without any further calibration or registration during the intervention. The CamC system can support a wide range of potential clinical applications, such as needle guidance [2], interlocking of intramedullary nails [3], and pedicle screw placement [4]. However, it is very important to quantify and qualify the system before its introduction into the operating room for the real patient study. Every clinically used mobile C-arm has a dose-area product (DAP) meter permanently built into the x-ray tube housing to measure the radiation dose to air. The overall measured DAP values must be recorded for each patient, and these DAP values allow to determine the patient exposition and eventually the effective dose which is related to the cancer risk of the procedure [5]. However, one mirror of the CamC system is placed between the DAP meter and the patient. Thus, it is partially absorbing and scattering radiation, and the patient will receive less dose than the reading from the built-in DAP meter. Both the accuracy of the video and X-ray image overlay and the correct applied dose to the patient by using the CamC system are clinically important parameters. Therefore, we extended the performed overlay accuracy analysis of the CamC system by the evaluation of the percentage of absorbed and scattered radiation of the mirror. This value can be then used to estimate the correct applied dose to the patient.

2 Materials

Our Camera Augmented Mobile C-arm system is composed of a mobile C-arm, Siremobile Iso-C 3D, from Siemens Healthcare and an optical video camera, Flea, from Point Grey Research Inc. A double mirror construction is attached to the housing of the X-ray source to virtually align the camera center with the X-ray source. Figure 1 shows the system setup of our dose evaluation experiments. One standard mirror of the CamC system is placed between the built-in DAP meter and the image intensifier. For evaluation of the applied radiation dose for the patient, we employed an independent dose measurement device (see figure 1), which consists of the Unfors Xi R/F Detector and the Unfors Xi Base Unit, from Unfors Instruments GmbH, Germany. The Unfors Xi R/F Detector can measure the X-ray radiation dose in the range from 10 nGy - 9999 Gy with the uncertainty of 5%. This detector is connected to the Unfors Xi Base Unit which displays and records the measured results. It is used to evaluate the percentage of absorbed and scattered radiation by the mirror.

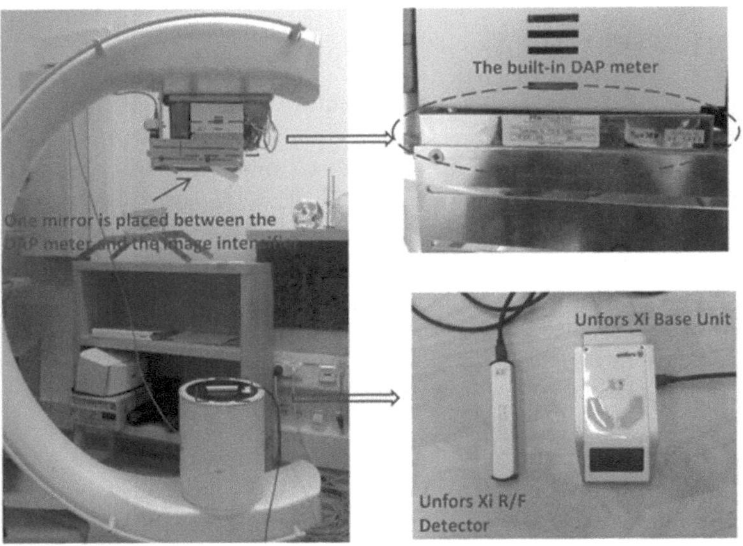

Fig. 1. The left shows the CamC system, the right top is the built-in DAP meter, and the right bottom shows our dose measurement device (Unfors Xi).

3 Evaluation

To determine the accuracy of the image overlay for the guidance of medical instruments using CamC, we performed a set of experiments to compute the difference of corresponding feature points between the video image and the overlaid X-ray image. Futhermore, to determine the correct applied dose to the patient, we introduced a method by using an independent dose measurement device for finding the percentage of absorbed and scattered radiation by the mirror. This value will eventually allow to correct the values given by the built-in DAP meter.

3.1 Overlay accuracy

We performed the experiments to evaluate not only the accuracy of the image overlay for the instrument guidance, but also the influence of the orbital and angular rotation on the overlay accuracy. A pattern that is generally used for geometrical X-ray calibration and distortion measurements is attached to the image intensifier. The markers of the pattern are visible in both X-ray and video image at the same time. The centroids of the markers are extracted in both views with subpixel accuracy and used to compute the overlay error which is the distance between corresponding point pairs. We performed the proposed calibration of [1] and then computed the difference of the centroid in the video image and overlaid X-ray image. The mean error was found to be 1.59 ± 0.87 pixels with a maximum error of 5.02 pixels. The same experiment with the attached calibration phantom was also conducted with different angular and orbital rotations. In all angular and orbital poses we analysed the overlay accuracy with and without an online estimation of a new homography. The mean overlay error was found to be constant during orbital and angular rotation of the C-arm if a re-estimation of the homography is performed at the specific C-arm orientation. In the cases where the homography was not re-estimated, i.e. the homography was estimated in the original position of the C-arm with no orbital and angular rotation and applied for other poses of the C-arm, the mean error of the points increased with an increase in the rotation angle.

3.2 Dose estimation

Since the Unfors Xi R/F Detector can not intercept the entire area of the X-ray beam on any plane perpendicular to the beam central axis between the X-ray housing and the image intensifier, we can not directly measure the total dose. Thus, the property of the dose distribution on the plane has to be known to derive the total dose in our case. Generally, the dose distribution of the C-arm Cone-Beam on the plane perpendicular to the beam central axis is homogenous. However, we conducted an experiment to check the dose distribution in both cases of with mirror and without mirror. We placed the dosimeter, Unfors Xi R/F Detector, on the image intensifier in three different positions. For each of the three positions (see figure 2), we took 3 shots with the mirror and another 3 shots without the mirror. Through the whole experiment, we used the single shot

Table 1. The measured dose(μGy) of each shot by the Unfors Xi R/F Detector with the fixed tube voltage(64 kV).

Mirror	position A			position B			position C			Mean±std
Without	27.04	25.82	25.85	26.00	26.00	26.25	26.54	26.05	26.17	26.1911 ± 0.3862
With	15.36	14.41	15.71	14.93	16.06	16.00	15.46	15.62	15.08	15.4033 ± 0.5302

Table 2. The average measured dose (μGy) for three different tube voltage settings, 64 kV, 70 kV and 77 kV. Rate refers to "Percentage of absorbed and scattered radiation".

Mirror	64 kV (Mean±std)	70 kV (Mean±std)	77 kV (Mean±std)
Without	26.0833 ± 0.1443	33.6200 ± 0.1572	96.6167 ± 0.5369
With	15.6633 ± 0.6358	20.5467 ± 0.3656	60.1967 ± 1.7923
Rate	39.95%	38.89%	37.70%

mode (DR-mode) with fixed radiation time and the tube voltage (64 kV) in order to produce constant radiation doses for each shot on the level of the x-ray tube. The dose values measured by the unfors dosimeter are shown in Table 1. For each case, the standard deviation is relatively small. This means dose distribution on the detector level is homogenous with and without the mirror. Therefore, the percentage of the absorbed and scattered radiation estimated for the partial area of the X-ray beam corresponds to the entire X-ray beam. In order to investigate the influence of the tube voltage on the percentage of absorbed and scattered radiation, we performed another experiment. In this experiment, we used the DR-mode of the C-arm and a fixed dosimeter position (Position B) for all shots. In each of the three different tube voltage settings, 64 kV, 70 kV and 77 kV, we took 5 shots with mirror and another 5 shots without mirror. Table 2 shows the average dose values for each case. The percentage of absorbed and scattered radiation by the mirror was found to be almost constant for the different tube voltage settings. Knowing the total applied dose (DAP) from the C-arm's built-in DAP meter, we can apply 39% as the percentage of the absorbed and scattered radiation by the mirror to estimate the correct applied dose for the patient according to our experiments.

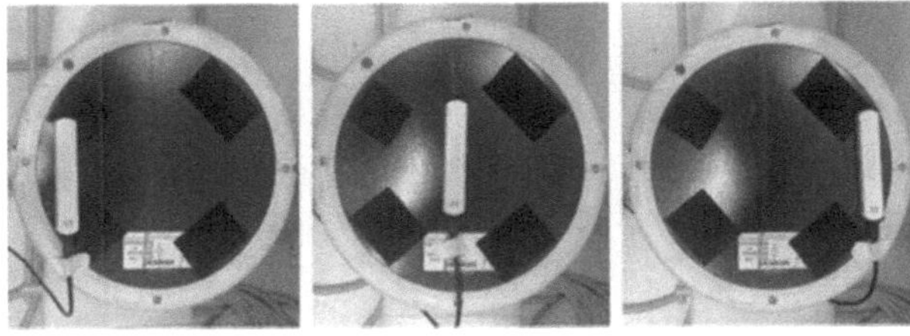

Fig. 2. The positions of the Unfors Xi R/F Detector in our experiments. From the left to the right, they are position A, position B and position C.

4 Discussion and conclusion

The CamC system proposed by Navab et al. [1] can support a wide range of potential clinical applications as shown by their cadaver studies of [2], [3] and [4]. Since the mirror of the CamC system will absorb and scatter radiation, the applied dose (DAP) from the C-arm is on longer valid for the patient. Before the introduction of the CamC system in the OR for patient studies, it is required to quantify and qualify the system not only for the technical accuracy, but also for the correct applied dose to the patient and estimation of the scattered radiation. In this paper, we extended the previously performed overlay accuracy analysis by estimating the percentage of the absorbed and scattered radiation by the mirror. The results show that the mirror absorbs and scatters 39% of X-ray radiation. The applied dose was adjusted such that the dose with the mirror construction matches the dose without the mirrors resulting in no change of the X-ray image quality. The housing of the radiation source was covered by lead foil to reduce the effect of scattered radiation for surgical staff. To correct the overlay after a deviation of the C-arm from the calibrated orientation (e.g. gravity effects on C-arm structure), we will adapt the idea of a virtual detector plane proposed by [6] and attach at least four X-ray markers on the back of the mirror. Last but not least, an X-ray and video visible marker is employed for patient motion detection since the overlay will not be valid if the patient and the C-arm have a relative motion. In case the marker in the X-ray image and the video image are not aligned, a new X-ray image must be acquired. The CamC system provides a promising solution for image guided surgery which could lead to a considerable reduction of radiation dose for patients and surgical staff in the future.

Acknowledgement. Thank to Unfors for providing the dose measurement device.

References

1. Navab N, Mitschke M, Bani-Hashemi A. Merging visible and invisible: Two camera-augmented mobile C-arm (CAMC) applications. Procs IWAR. 1999; p. 134–141.
2. Mitschke M, Banihashemi AH, Navab N. Interventions under video-augmented x-ray guidance: Application to needle placement. Procs MICCAI. 2000.
3. Heining SMM, Wiesner S, Euler E, et al. Locking of intramedullary nails under video-augmented flouroscopic control: First clinical application in a cadaver study. Proc CAOS. 2006.
4. Heining SM, Wiesner S, Euler E, et al. Pedicle screw placement under video-augmented fluoroscopic control: First clinical application in a cadaver study. Int J Computer Assist Radiol Surg. 2006;1(Supplement 1):189–190.
5. Schultz FW, Zoetelief J. Dose conversion coefficients for interventional procedures. Radiat Prot Dosimetry. 2006;117(6):225–230.
6. Navab N, Mitschke M. Method and apparatus using a virtual detector for three-dimensional reconstruction form x-ray images. Patent US 6236704.

Estimation of Inner Lung Motion Fields by Non-linear Registration

An Evaluation and Comparison Study

René Werner[1], Jan Ehrhardt[1], Alexander Schmidt-Richberg[1], Florian Cremers[2], Heinz Handels[1]

[1]Department of Medical Informatics,
[2]Department of Radiotherapy and Radio-Oncology,
University Medical Center Hamburg-Eppendorf
r.werner@uke.uni-hamburg.de

Abstract. Detailed analysis of breathing dynamics, as motivated by radiotherapy of lung tumors, requires accurate estimates of inner lung motion fields. We present an evaluation and comparison study of non-linear non-parametric intensity-based registration approaches to estimate these motion fields in 4D CT images. In order to cope with discontinuities in pleura and chest wall motion we restrict the registration by applying lung segmentation masks and evaluate the impact of masking on registration accuracy. Furthermore, we compare diffusive to elastic regularization and diffeomorphic to non-diffeomorphic implementations. Based on a data set of 10 patients we show that masking improves registration accuracy significantly. Moreover, neither elastic or diffusive regularization nor diffeomorphic versus non-diffeomorphic implementation influence the accuracy significantly. Thus, the method of choice depends on the application and requirements on motion field characteristics.

1 Introduction

Respiratory motion is a main problem in radiation therapy of lung cancer. Various authors emphasize the need of further analysis and quantification of breathing dynamics [1]. At present, such analysis is mostly based on 4D(=3D+t) image data. Within this field of research non-linear registration has become increasingly important, since it allows to estimate respiratory motion fields between the 3D images representing the patient's anatomy at different breathing phases. The motion fields form the basis of motion analysis and modeling issues. Thus, motion field estimates are required to be feasible and as accurate as possible. Though a wide variety of registration approaches has been proposed to estimate respiratory motion fields in 4D image sequences, there exists a substantial lack of evaluation and comparison studies for those methods [2].

Representing the few existing studies, in [2], [3], and [4] conceptually different registration approaches are compared in order to estimate inner lung motion fields (biomechanical modeling, surface models, landmark-based registration, parametric registration, non-parametric registration). On the one hand, our paper aims to complement these studies. On the other hand, we pursue a slightly different strategy: We focus on a non-linear, non-parametric, intensity-based registration scheme which we want to optimize in order to estimate inner lung motion fields. Therefore we define and evaluate different modifications of the registration scheme.

2 Materials and methods

The study is based on 4D CT data sets of 10 lung cancer patients. Spatial resolution of the CT data is between $0.78\times0.78\times1.5$ mm^3 and $0.98\times0.98\times1.5$ mm^3; image sequences consist of 10 to 14 CT images reconstructed at different breathing phases. Due to memory and computation time restrictions, the 3D data are downsampled to a spatial resolution of $1.5\times1.5\times1.5$ mm^3/voxel. For evaluation purposes we focus on the breathing phases of end-expiration (EE), mid-inspiration (MI), end-inspiration (EI), and mid-expiration (ME).

2.1 Registration approaches

Image registration can be seen as finding a transformation φ minimizing a distance between the transformed target image I_j (here: $j \in \{\text{EE, MI, ME}\}$) and a reference image I_i (here: $i = \text{EI}$) with respect to a desired smoothness of φ (represented by a regularization term). As distance measure we choose an adaptation of Thirion's demons approach, which is suitable for registration of low contrast structures like inner lung structures; for details see [5, 6]. In previous studies we used a diffusive approach for regularization, which has the advantage of an efficient implementation (time complexity of $O(n)$ [5]). Though time complexity is $O(n \log n)$, several authors propose elastic regularization in case of lung motion estimation [3]. This is due to the assumption that lungs behave like an elastic medium during respiration. Here we compare the diffusive smoothing approach (method m_1) and an elastic regularization (method m_2).

Additional requirements arise on deformation field characteristics when faced with advanced analysis and modeling issues. For instance, the generation of lung motion atlases and its use for model-based motion prediction requires the motion fields to be invertible [7]. To ensure invertibility, we adapt a diffeomorphic and a symmetric-diffeomorphic registration method [6] to our registration scheme (methods m_3 and m_4).

From a perspective of physiology, discontinuities in respiratory motion between the lung surface and the chest wall occur [4]. One approach to handle the discontinuities is to restrict force computation to the lungs by applying lung segmentation masks (here: segmented lungs at EI). The impact of masking on inner lung registration accuracy is therefore also evaluated here.

2.2 Evaluation methods

As two quality measures of the deformation fields, we determine the number of voxels with negative values of the Jacobian and analyze the symmetry properties of the fields. Voxels with negative values of the Jacobian indicate unwanted singularities of the field (deformation locally non-invertible). Analyzing symmetry means to check $\varphi_{i\to j\to i} := \varphi_{i\to j} \circ \varphi_{j\to i}$ which is ideally the identity vector field. To obtain $\varphi_{j\to i}$, the registration is performed with target and reference image being interchanged when compared to the computation of $\varphi_{i\to j}$.

Quantitative evaluation of the registration accuracy is based on 80 inner lung landmarks identified by a medical expert in each CT data set considered. To gain insights to strengths and weaknesses of the different registration methods we differentiate landmarks located in the middle of the lung (40 landmarks), near the lung borders (30 landmarks), and close to the tumor (10 landmarks). The landmark displacements between EI and the target image breathing phase (MI, EE, ME) as observed by the expert are compared to the landmark displacements obtained by applying the motion field estimates to the EI CT data and the EI landmark positions, respectively. Then, we determine the mean difference between the observed displacements and the displacements predicted by the model (mean target registration error, TRE). To check whether two registration approaches behave equivalently we apply a paired t-test [2].

2.3 Study design

Before applying the registration to the 10 patient data sets considered for this study, parameters (such as the regularization weight and step size) are optimized in order to achieve a good trade-off between a minimal number of voxels with negative Jacobian values and a small TRE. Optimization is based on a separate data set. The study itself consists of three steps where each step is a competitive study between different registration methods or adaptations of a method:

1. *masked vs. non-masked registration:* Masked and non-masked registration are compared with each other using method m_1 as registration technique and focusing on the TRE. If it cannot be shown that masking improves registration accuracy significantly, registration applied in steps 2 and 3 will be unmasked because this is the commonly used registration approach.
2. *diffusive vs. elastic regularization:* The influence of the regularization approach on registration accuracy and qualitative measures is evaluated using methods m_1 and m_2. If elastic regularization does not improve motion field estimation significantly, we will choose the diffusive approach in step 3 due to lower computational costs (Sec. 2.1).
3. *diffeomorphic vs. non-diffeomorphic registration:* The diffeomorphic registration approaches m_3 and m_4 are compared to the corresponding non-diffeomorphic registration m_1 or m_2 (depending on step 1 and 2 results).

3 Results

Registrations are performed using a bi-processor system with 3 GHz Intel Xeon dual-core processors and 16 GB RAM. Computation times for a 3D-3D registration are approximately $\frac{1}{2}$ h for m_1, $1\frac{1}{2}$ h for m_3, and 3 h for m_2 and m_4. Subsequent TRE values should be compared against the mean landmark motion of

6.82 ± 5.42 mm (EI-EE registration), 5.02 ± 3.48 mm (EI-MI), and 2.55 ± 1.97 mm (EI-ME), and the intraobserver variability of approx. 1 voxel.

3.1 Evaluation of the estimated motion fields

In Step 1 (masked vs. non-masked registration), masking of force computation turns out to improve the registration accuracy. Averaged over all landmarks, the mean TRE decreases from 2.07 ± 2.32 mm for unmasked to 1.55 ± 1.26 mm for masked EI-EE registration (EI-MI: 1.68 ± 1.20 to 1.57 ± 0.98 mm; EI-ME: 1.46 ± 0.94 to 1.45 ± 0.92 mm). This is mostly due to an increased registration accuracy for landmarks close to the lung borders (see fig. 1). The improvement can be shown to be significant (e.g., $p<0.05$ for all patients for EI-EE registration).

Step 2 (diffusive vs. elastic regularization) shows that elastic and diffusive regularization (here: masked registration) behave almost equivalently in terms of registration accuracy and motion field quality measures. For m_2, i.e., elastic regularization, the mean TRE values are 1.55 ± 1.21 mm (EI-EE), 1.51 ± 0.91 mm (EI-MI), and 1.46 ± 0.94 mm (EI-ME). TRE differences between m_1 and m_2 are significant for none of the patients (EI-EE), 4 patients (EI-MI; m_2 better in each case), and 2 patients (EI-ME; m_1 better). Mean symmetry errors are 0.88 ± 0.24 mm, 0.55 ± 0.11 mm, and 0.30 ± 0.07 mm for m_2 vs. 0.94 ± 0.33 mm, 0.62 ± 0.11 mm, and 0.34 ± 0.04 mm for m_1. For both m_1 and m_2 the number of voxels with negative Jacobian is negligible ($\ll 0.01\%$ of the lung voxels).

Step 3 (diffeomorphic vs. non-diffeomorphic registration) is based on diffusive regularization due to the preceding results. The mean TRE is 1.57 ± 1.26 mm (EI-EE), 1.58 ± 1.00 mm (EI-MI), and 1.46 ± 0.99 mm (EI-ME) for m_3, and 1.59 ± 1.28 mm, 1.57 ± 1.00 mm, and 1.46 ± 0.97 mm for m_4. Comparison of m_3 and m_1 yields that TRE differences are statistical significant for 4 patients (EI-EE; $3\times$ m_1 better than m_3, $1\times$ vice versa), 2 patients (EI-MI, $1\times$ m_1 better, $1\times$ m_3 better), and 1 patient (EI-ME, m_1 better). m_1 shows a significantly decreased TRE compared to m_4 for 4 patients (only in EI-EE registration). TRE values of m_3 are significantly lower than for m_4 for one data set (EI-ME). In short, registration accuracy is almost the same for m_1, m_3, and m_4. For the diffeomorphic implementations no negative Jacobian values are observed. In terms of the symmetry error the symmetric-diffeomorphic registration is superior to the non-diffeomorphic and the diffeomorphic implementation; the mean symmetry errors for m_4 are 0.36 ± 0.10 mm, 0.20 ± 0.04 mm, and 0.10 ± 0.02 mm. Corresponding values for m_3 are 1.18 ± 0.48 mm, 0.67 ± 0.13 mm, and 0.35 ± 0.04 mm.

4 Discussion

In summary, neither the elastic or diffusive regularization nor diffeomorphic vs. non-diffeomorphic implementation can be shown to influence registration accuracy significantly. For the given application diffusive regularization tends to be superior to elastic regularization due to a better time complexity. Furthermore, the symmetric-diffeomorphic registration tends to be superior to the other

Fig. 1. Left: Landmark motion and TRE values for registration of I_{EI} and I_{EE}. Right: Visualization of the arc differences between EI-EE motion field estimates for patient 02 obtained by method m_1 with and without masking of force computation.

	Landmark motion [mm]	Target registration error [mm]				
		no mask	masked registration			
		m_1	m_1	m_2	m_3^*	m_4^*
Pat. 1	6,29	2,06	1,48	1,45	1,49	1,54
Pat. 2	5,45	1,87	1,59	1,62	1,64	1,57
Pat. 3	6,19	1,70	1,55	1,61	1,57	1,57
Pat. 4	6,44	1,65	1,41	1,47	1,44	1,46
Pat. 5	4,31	1,44	1,37	1,38	1,37	1,36
Pat. 6	10,76	3,07	1,52	1,47	1,62	1,60
Pat. 7	6,40	2,85	1,99	2,00	1,91	2,01
Pat. 8	6,06	1,52	1,19	1,22	1,24	1,28
Pat. 9	7,98	2,09	1,62	1,58	1,60	1,61
Pat. 10	8,32	2,47	1,80	1,71	1,89	1,94
mean	**6,82**	**2,07**	**1,55**	**1,55**	**1,58**	**1,59**

*) diffusive regularization

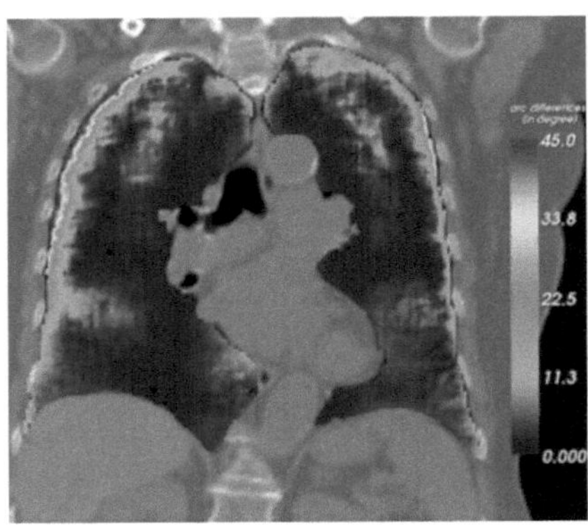

methods since it minimizes the symmetry error. However, computational costs of symmetric-diffeomorphic registration are higher. Thus, if computing time is a crucial issue, non-diffeomorphic or diffeomorphic diffusive registration can be considered as better choices (depending on whether invertibility is required).

As an essential result we show that masking significantly improves registration accuracy. This demonstrates that integrating a-priori knowledge about physiological processes (here: behavior of pleura and chest wall during breathing) to registration schemes has potential to improve registration accuracy.

Acknowledgments: This work is supported by German Research Foundation (DFG, HA 2355/9-1). We thank D. Low and W. Lu from the Washington University School of Medicine, St. Louis (USA), for providing the CT data.

References

1. Li XA, et al. Point/counterpoint: Respiratory gating for radiation therapy is not ready for prime time. Med Phys. 2007;34(3):867–70.
2. Sarrut D, et al. A comparison framework for breathing motion estimation methods from 4-D imaging. IEEE Trans Med Imaging. 2007;26(12):1636–48.
3. Vik T, et al. Validation and comparison of registration methods for free-breathing 4D lung-CT. Procs SPIE. 2008;6914:2P1–10.
4. Werner R, et al. Validation and comparison of a biophysical modeling approach and non-linear registration for estimation of lung motion fields in thoracic 4D CT data. Procs SPIE. 2009.
5. Modersitzki J. Numerical Methods for Image Registration. Oxford University Press; 2003.
6. Vercauteren T, et al. Symmetric log-domain diffeomorphic registration: A demons-based approach. Procs MICCAI. 2008.
7. Ehrhardt J, et al. Generation of a mean motion model of the lung using 4D-CT image data. Procs VCBM. 2008; p. 69–76.

Landmark-Based 3D Elastic Registration of Pre- and Postoperative Liver CT Data

An Experimental Comparison

Thomas Lange[1], Stefan Wörz[2], Karl Rohr[2], Peter M. Schlag[3]

[1]Experimental and Clinical Research Center, Charité–Universitätsmedizin Berlin
[2]University of Heidelberg, BIOQUANT, IPMB, and DKFZ Heidelberg,
Dept. Bioinformatics and Functional Genomics, Biomedical Computer Vision Group
[3]Charité Comprehensive Cancer Center, Charité–Unversitätsmedizin Berlin
thomas.lange@charite.de

Abstract. The qualitative and quantitative comparison of pre- and postoperative image data is an important possibility to validate computer assisted surgical procedures. Due to deformations after surgery a non-rigid registration scheme is a prerequisite for a precise comparison. Interactive landmark-based schemes are a suitable approach. Incorporation of a priori knowledge about the anatomical structures to be registered may help to reduce interaction time and improve accuracy. Concerning pre- and postoperative CT data of oncological liver resections the intrahepatic vessels are suitable anatomical structures. In addition to using landmarks at vessel branchings, we here introduce quasi landmarks at vessel segments with anisotropic localization precision. An experimental comparison of interpolating thin-plate splines (TPS) and Gaussian elastic body splines (GEBS) as well as approximating GEBS on both types of landmarks is performed.

1 Introduction

The validation of new computer-assisted surgical procedures in oncological liver surgery like preoperative planning [1] and intraoperative navigation [2] is challenging. The main question is, how accurate a resection plan has been implemented in the operating room. Besides complete tumor removal it is very important to resect exactly the planned parts of the liver vessels to ensure blood supply and drainage of the remaining liver tissue. The comparison of planned and resected tissue volumes [3] is only a coarse and unspecific validation possibility. A more detailed validation by determining the remaining vessel parts can be obtained based on pre- and postoperative CT data (Fig. 1a, b). The aim is to visualize and quantify those vessel parts, which have been resected as planned and those, which have been accidentally removed (Fig. 1c). Due to deformations of the liver between pre- and postoperative CT acquisitions non-rigid registration algorithms are needed. The challenge of this intra-patient registration task is due to the fact that significant parts of the liver are missing in the postoperative images.

Although some publications exist dealing with liver registration only few work has been published on non-rigid registration of pre- and postoperative image data. In some publications image data of the brain before and during/after resection of tumors [4, 5] are compared. In the case of the liver only the evolution of tumors of the same patient based on two different image acquisitions, but not the resection of tumors has been considered [6]. The algorithm of Charnoz et al. [6] finds corresponding vessel center lines via tree matching, but until now the method has been validated only on one clinical data set.

Our approach is based on interactively chosen corresponding point landmarks using different interpolation and approximation schemes based on splines. Besides the natural choice of landmarks at vessel branchings we introduce a special kind of landmarks adapted to vessel segments.

2 Materials and methods

2.1 Non-rigid landmark-based registration

In landmark-based non-rigid registration methods usually a smooth displacement function $u : \mathbb{R}^3 \rightarrow \mathbb{R}^3$ is searched, which maps n landmark positions p_i of a source image exactly to their corresponding positions q_i of the target image. This means, u has to fulfill the interpolation conditions $q_i = u(p_i)$, $i = 1, \ldots, n$. A function u can be defined to be smooth, if it minimizes a smoothing functional $S[u]$. The very common functional S^{tps} represents the bending energy of a thin plate leading to so called thin plate spline (TPS) interpolation functions [7]. The S^{tps} functional represents a relatively coarse deformation model, because transverse contraction does not lead to longitudinal dilation (see also [8]). In comparison, Gaussian elastic body splines (GEBS) [5] are derived from the Navier equation, which describes the deformation of homogeneous elastic materials leading to the corresponding smoothing functional $S^{\text{elas}}[u]$.

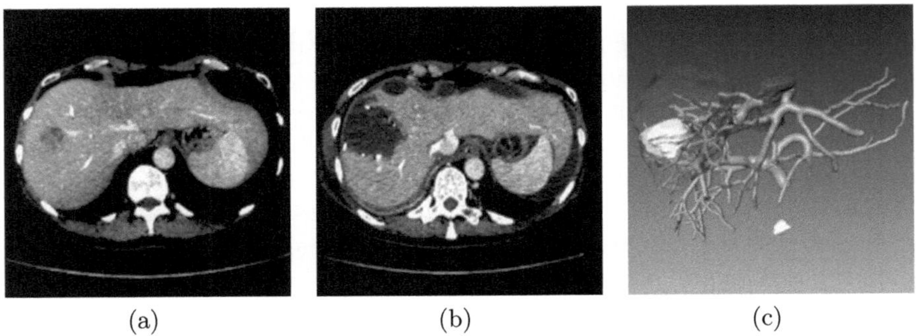

(a) (b) (c)

Fig. 1. a) Preoperative CT, b) Postoperative CT, c) Preoperative 3D model of liver vessels with tumor. The parts of the vessels, which have been resected as planned (green) and unnecessarily (red) have been determined by a registered postoperative 3D model. The resected tissue part is illustrated in brown.

Interpolating thin-plate splines (iTPS) and interpolating Gaussian elastic body splines (iGEBS) are analytic solutions of the following constrained optimization problem:

$$J[u] = S[u] \overset{u}{\rightarrow} \min \quad \text{subject to} \quad u(p_i) - q_i = 0, i = 1, \ldots, n \tag{1}$$

Both *interpolation* schemes above ignore that landmark localization is generally prone to errors. Therefore, to take into account landmark errors, *approximation* schemes have been proposed (e.g., [8]). The localization uncertainties are characterized by weight matrices Σ_i representing anisotropic errors. Based on those matrices a weighted landmark distance functional can be formulated:

$$P[u] = \frac{1}{n} \int \sum_{i=1}^{n} f(x - p_i)(q_i - u(x))^T \Sigma_i^{-1}(q_i - u(x))dx \tag{2}$$

with a Gaussian function $f(x) = (\sqrt{2\pi}\sigma)^{-3}\exp(-\frac{\|x\|^2}{2\sigma^2})$ controlling the local influence of the landmarks on the transformation.

Instead of a constrained optimization problem like in (1), approximating GEBS (aGEBS) are formulated as an unconstrained optimization problem by adding the landmark distance functional to the smoothness functional with a weighting factor $\lambda_A \in \mathbb{R}^+$:

$$J^{\text{aGEBS}}[u] = S^{\text{elas}}[u] + \lambda_A P[u] \overset{u}{\rightarrow} \min \tag{3}$$

2.2 Different types of landmarks for liver registration

We now describe how the presented landmark registration schemes can be applied to the registration of pre- and postoperative contrast-enhanced CTs of the liver. The main structures which are identifiable inside the liver are vessels. The vessel center lines and local radii r are usually provided by the planning process [1]. Besides landmarks at branching points of the vessel center lines, alternatively landmarks along vessels between two branchings can be used. With the latter landmarks the localization uncertainty is high along the vessel, but low perpendicular to it (Fig. 2a, b). In the following the two types of landmarks are called *branching* and *segment* landmarks. For the branching landmarks we assumed no localization uncertainty in the interpolating schemes and for the approximating scheme we assume isotropic errors $\Sigma_i = aI_3$, with $a \in \mathbb{R}$. The anisotropic error matrices of the segment landmarks can be modeled via their eigenvectors and eigenvalues. The first eigenvector $v_{i,1}$ points in the direction of the center line at the position of the landmark, the other two eigenvectors $v_{i,2}, v_{i,3}$ are perpendicular to the center line. As the localization uncertainty is high in the direction of the vessel and low perpendicular to it depending on the area of the vessel cross section, the eigenvalues are chosen as $\lambda_{i,1} = \text{const} \gg \max r_i^2, \lambda_{i,2} = r_i^2, \lambda_{i,3} = r_i^2$. With $D_i = \text{diag}(\lambda_{i,1}, \lambda_{i,2}, \lambda_{i,3})$ and $R_i = (v_{i,1}, v_{i,2}, v_{i,3})$ the uncertainty matrices are defined as $\Sigma_i = R_i^T D_i R_i$.

2.3 Design of experimental comparison

The different registration methods were compared on clinical pre- and post-operative contrast-enhanced CT data sets of 13 different patients, which have undergone oncological liver resections. For comparison we used a weighted Euclidean distance between dense point correspondences on the vessel center lines [9]. The weighting in the direction of a vessel is set to zero such that only the distance perpendicular to the vessel is measured. 5 sets of landmarks for each patient were interactively chosen as follows: 1. As many as possible branching landmark pairs (p_i^B, q_i^B), 2. a comparable number of segment landmarks on vessel segments between the branching landmarks (p_i^S, q_i^S), 3. a combination of the branching and segment landmarks (p_i^C, q_i^C), 4. a reduced number of 12 branching landmark pairs $(p_i^{B_{12}}, q_i^{B_{12}})$ and 5. a reduced number of 12 segment landmark pairs $(p_i^{S_{12}}, q_i^{S_{12}})$.

3 Results

The iTPS and iGEBS non-rigid registration approaches have been applied to landmark sets 1 and 4 which only include branching landmarks, but the aGEBS approximation was applied to all five landmark sets. The resulting average weighted Euclidean distances for each patient was determined (Fig. 2 c). On average over all patients we obtained a weighted distance of 4.9mm after rigid registration. iGEBS and aGEBS using branching landmarks decrease the average distance down to 1.7 and 1.5mm, respectively. aGEBS using segment landmarks and iTPS using branching landmarks yield comparable results and lead to 1.4mm average distance. By using a combination of segment and branching landmarks the best results of 1.0mm average distance were achieved using approximating GEBS.

Because interactive determination of landmarks is tedious and time-consuming we also performed a validation based on a reduced set of 12 landmarks.

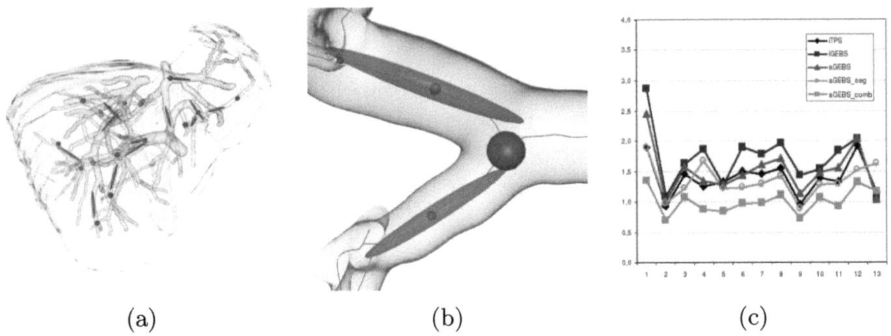

(a) (b) (c)

Fig. 2. a) Different types of landmarks at vessel branchings (isotropic error spheres) and segments (anisotropic error ellipsoids). b) Detailed view. c) Mean weighted Euclidean distances (in mm) after registration at vessel center lines of all 13 patients.

In this case we obtained 2.5mm for iGEBS, 2.3 mm for iTPS and aGEBS on branching landmarks and the best result of 2.0mm for aGEBS on segment landmarks.

4 Discussion

For the first time interpolating and approximating landmark-based methods have been proposed for non-rigid registration of pre- and postoperative CT data of the liver. Besides the natural choice of landmarks at vessel *branchings* also landmarks with anisotropic localization errors have been adapted to the tube-like structure of liver vessel *segments*. In an experimental comparison it turns out that the *segment* landmarks using approximating GEBS provide registration accuracies as good as *branching* landmarks and can improve the accuracy if combined with *branching* landmarks. *Segment* landmarks are even superior for a low number of landmarks. Hence segment landmarks are a promising alternative and/or extension to branching landmarks. They offer an additional flexibility in interactive landmark registration allowing an intuitive and efficient registration workflow. The registration accuracy of 2.0mm for only 12 landmarks is promising as a basis of an algorithm which automatically identifies parts of the vessel trees, which have been removed during the surgical procedure (Fig. 1c).

References

1. Selle D, Preim B, Schenk A, et al. Analysis of vasculature for liver surgical planning. IEEE Trans Med Imaging. 2002;21(11):1344–1357.
2. Beller S, Hünerbein M, Lange T, et al. Image-guided surgery of liver metastases by 3D ultrasound-based optoelectronic navigation. Brit J Surg. 2007;94(7):866–875.
3. Lemke A, Brinkmann M, Schott T, et al. Living donor right liver lobes: Preoperative CT volumetric measurement for calculation of intraoperative weight and volume. Radiology. 2006;240(3):736–742.
4. Ferrant M, Nabavi A, Macq B, et al. Serial registration of intraoperative MR images of the brain. Med Image Anal. 2002;6(4):337–359.
5. Kohlrausch J, Rohr K, Stiehl HS. A new class of elastic body splines for nonrigid registration of medical images. J Math Imaging Vis. 2005;23:253–280.
6. Charnoz A, Agnus V, Malandain G, et al. Design of robust vascular tree matching: Validation on liver. Lect Note Comp Sci. 2005;3566:443–455.
7. Bookstein FL. Principal warps: Thin-plate splines and the decomposition of deformations. IEEE Trans Pattern Anal Mach Intell. 1989;11(6):567–585.
8. Wörz S, Rohr K. Physics-based elastic registration using non-radial basis functions and including landmark localization uncertainties. Computer Vis Image Underst. 2008;111(3):263–274.
9. Lange T, Lamecker H, Hünerbein M, et al. Validation metrics for non-rigid registration of medical images containing vessel trees. Procs BVM. 2008; p. 82–86.

Binary Segmentation Masks for Registration of Bone Structures in CT Images

Oleg Museyko[1], Fabian Eisa[1], Andreas Hess[2], Peter Zerfass[1], Willi Kalender[1], Klaus Engelke[1]

[1]Institut für Medizinische Physik, Friedrich-Alexander Universität Erlangen-Nürnberg
[2]Institut für Pharmakologie und Toxikologie, Universität Erlangen-Nürnberg
oleg.museyko@imp.uni-erlangen.de

Abstract. Rigid registration of bone structures in stacks of CT images can be improved by using a binary segmentation mask for the registration compared to using the segmented grey values directly. Three criteria are applied to the different reference and template datasets in order to quantify registration results. For all three criteria a statistically significant superiority of the technique using the binary segmentation masks is demonstrated. First results for a multimodal registration of a μCT with μMR dataset also show better results if binary segmentation masks are used for the registration.

1 Introduction

The accurate rigid registration of serial 3D CT datasets of the spine and the hip to determine for example longitudinal changes of geometry or bone mineral density requires an initial segmentation to separate individual vertebrae or the femur from the acetabulum. Otherwise the different relative position of multiple bones in baseline and follow-up image stacks will result in inadequate registration results. In this contribution we investigated whether the registration result can be improved by using a binarized segmentation mask instead of the segmented grey value structures. This is an important question, in particular in the presence of high noise levels as the segmentation may be less affected by noise than the registration process. Also the registration of multimodal datasets may benefit from the use of binarized segmentation masks. While for bone various registration [1, 2, 3] and segmentation [4, 5] methods exist, to our knowledge this problem has never been investigated.

2 Materials and methods

We used the 3D rigid intensity based registration method implemented in ITK. Specifically, for all registrations a gradient flow algorithm was used to find the (local) extremum of a registration energy function, sum of squared differences (SSD) for monomodal registration and Mattes mutual information (MMI) for multimodal registration. The multiresolution 3D versor-based rigid body registration was applied.

2.1 Spine and femur CT datasets

Pairs of CT datasets from the proximal femur and the lumbar spine from 30 human subjects each were acquired at baseline (reference) and after 12 months (template). All CT datasets were segmented by a combination of global and adaptive local thresholds followed by morphological operations as reported by Kang et al. [4] for the femur and by Mastmeyer for the vertebrae [5]. For example, Fig. 1 shows two orthogonal multiplanar reformations (MPRs) of a segmented femur. Fig. 2 shows the segmentation result in an axial MPR along with a binarized mask. Registration was performed using grey value segmentations (reg1) and binary masks (reg2).

Figure 3 shows axial MPRs of the 3D difference datasets (template minus reference) for the two registrations (reg1 and reg2). Three criteria were used to quantify the registration accuracy: the normalized (i.e. divided by the volume of the union) symmetric difference of binary reference and template mask (XOR), which equals the relative number of voxels that are not in the intersection of the two datasets; the values of the registration criterion itself (mean sum of squared differences, SSD); and the mean sum of absolute differences (SAD), computed in the union of corresponding template and reference binary datasets.

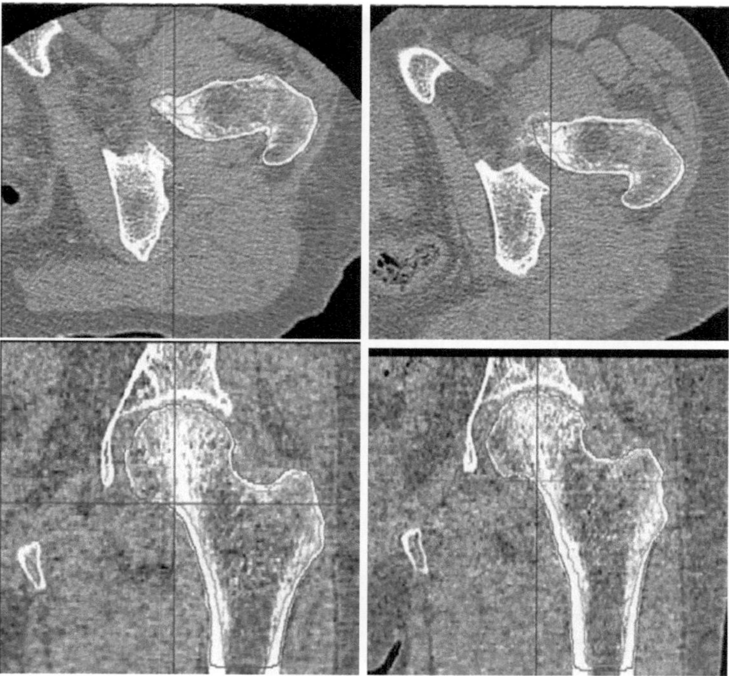

Fig. 1. Baseline (left) and follow-up (right): MPRs of the femur with periosteal and endosteal segmentation results. Note that patient positioning slightly differed between the two scans.

Table 1. Femur and spine: difference Δ between reg1 and reg2 for SSD, SAD and XOR(%) (non-parametric Wilcoxon test, number of experiments 30).

	Femur			Spine		
Criterion	ΔSSD	ΔSAD	ΔXOR(%)	ΔSSD	ΔSAD	ΔXOR(%)
Positive ranks sum	445	447	275.5	389	329.5	256
Negative ranks sum	-20	-18	-24.5	-76	-105.5	-69
p-value	$3.5 \cdot 10^{-7}$	$2.4 \cdot 10^{-7}$	$5 \cdot 10^{-5}$	0.0004	0.007	0.0053

2.2 μCT and μMR datasets

Figure 4 demonstrates reg1 and reg2 for multimodal 3D registration of a μMR ($78 \times 78 \times 156\mu$m) and a μCT (40μm isotropic) dataset from a rat knee.

3 Results

For each of the 30 spine and hip datasets the two registrations, reg1 and reg2, were compared by first computing each quality criterion separately in the two image stacks resulting from reg1 and reg2. Then the difference Δ for each quality criterion was determined for all 30 datasets. Table 1 summarizes the results for ΔSSD, ΔSAD, and ΔXOR(%) for the proximal femur and the spine. The significance of the difference of the two registrations reg1 and reg2 was verified using a one-side Wilcoxon test, which is a non-parametric test (parametric tests are not suitable for these quality values).

In all cases the registration based on the binary masks lead to better results: p-values < 0.05 indicate significant differences. The advantage of binary masks for registration holds also for the multimodal registration (μMR to μCT) for the example in Fig. 4, where the growth plate and the trabecular structure indicate better registration results with binary masks.

4 Discussion

We have demonstrated that for clinical CT datasets the registration of binary segmentation masks is superior to the registration of grey value based segmentations. Of course this procedure requires an adequate segmentation technique.

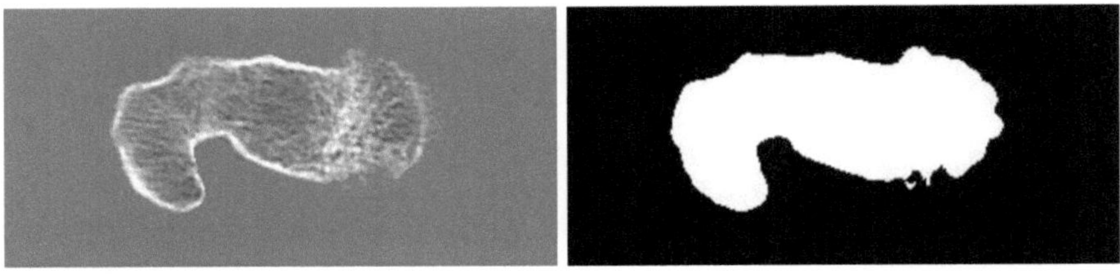

Fig. 2. Left: grey value segmentation results; right: binary segmentation mask

This effect is also very important for small animal imaging in cases such as μCT - μMR registration where the spatial resolution of the two datasets may be different. Our results still have to be statistically confirmed for this multimodal application but we have shown the statistical significance for CT–CT applications of the spine and the proximal femur. The comparison of the values of the registration criterion for the two registrations shows that the registration of grey value images converges to a local minimum, which is different from the more optimal solution obtained with reg2. This suggests that the structural differences in a pair of images are strong enough to deteriorate the registration, but do not have that influence on the segmentation. Thus, the binarization of the bone images improves the efficiency of the registration optimization algorithm. We have also shown that the results were largely independent of the quantitative criteria used for the measurement of the registration quality.

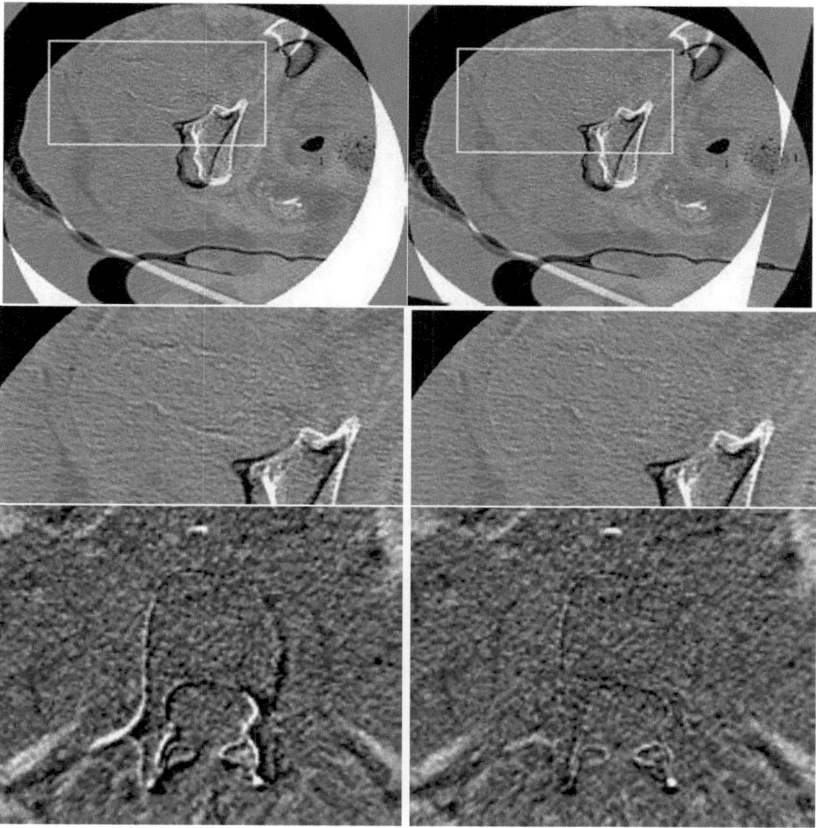

Fig. 3. CT-CT registration. Difference images (reference minus template), left: registration using grey value segmentation; right: improved registration with binary segmentation masks. Top: femur; center: femur regions of interest enlarged; bottom: spine.

Fig. 4. Multimodal image registration for small animal imaging. Upper left: μMR dataset; upper right: μCT dataset. Bottom: blended MPRs (a reference with a registered template), left: registration using grey value 3D image stacks (reg1); right: improved registration when using binary segmentation mask for μCT (reg2).

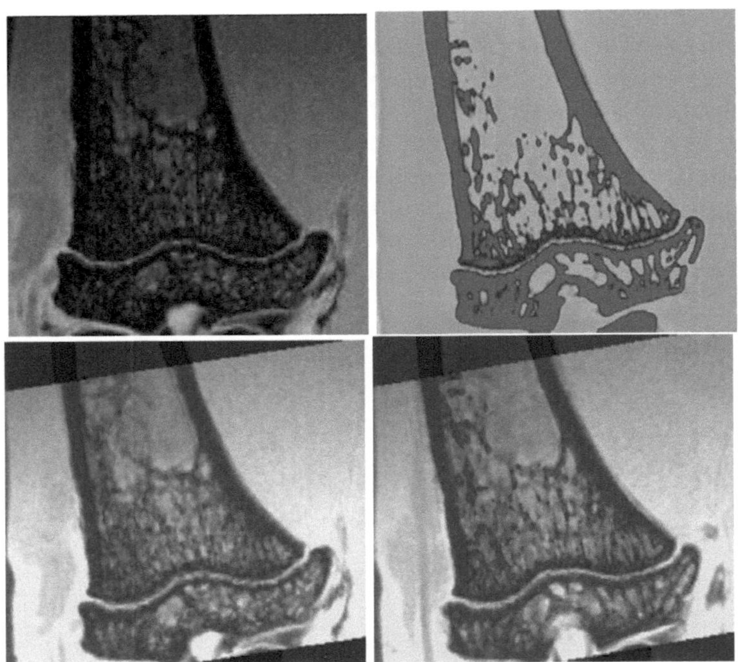

References

1. Hajnal JV, Hill DLG, Hawkes DJ, editors. Medical Image Registration. CRC; 2001.
2. Wang L, Greenspan M, Ellis R. Validation of bone segmentation and improved 3D registration using contour coherency in CT data. IEEE Trans Med Imaging. 2006;25(3):324–334.
3. Yezzi A, Zöllei L, Kapur T. A variational framework for integrating segmentation and registration through active contours. Med Image Anal. 2003;7:171–185.
4. Kang Y, Engelke K, Kalender WA. A new accurate and precise 3D segmentation method for skeletal structures in volumetric CT data. IEEE Trans Med Imaging. 2003;22(5):586–598.
5. Mastmeyer A, Engelke K, Fuchs C, et al. A hierarchical 3D segmentation method and the definition of the vertebral body coordinate system for QCT of the lumbar spine. Med Image Anal. 2006;10:560–577.

Image Registration Using Tensor Grids for Lung Ventilation Studies

Heike Ruppertshofen[1,2], Sven Kabus[2], Bernd Fischer[1]

[1]Institut für Mathematik, Universität zu Lübeck, Wallstraße 40, 23560 Lübeck
[2]Philips Research Europe - Hamburg, Röntgenstraße 24-26, 22335 Hamburg
heike.ruppertshofen@philips.com

Abstract. In non-parametric image registration it is often not possible to work with the original resolution of the images due to high processing times and lack of memory. However, for some medical applications the information contained in the original resolution is crucial in certain regions of the image while being negligible in others. To adapt to this problem we will present an approach using tensor grids, which provide a sparser image representation and thereby allow the use of the highest image resolution locally. Applying the presented scheme to a lung ventilation estimation shows that one may considerably save on time and memory while preserving the registration quality in the regions of interest.

1 Introduction

One possible way to assess lung ventilation is to evaluate the result of non-parametric image registration of thorax CT scans at different stages of the breathing cycle [1]. For this evaluation a dense deformation vector field is needed that maps one phase of the breathing cycle onto another, providing information about the motion of the lung and therefore about the gas exchange. However, finding this deformation field in a non-parametric registration approach is a challenging task mainly due to the size of the images. For a typical thorax CT scan of size $512^2 \times 141$ voxels a linear system of equations with more than 10 million unknowns needs to be solved in each iteration step inducing a challenge in both time and memory.

A general approach to speed up computations is to embed the registration algorithm into a multi-level setting, which in addition enhances the likelihood of bypassing local minima. By omitting the highest level(s) of resolution the problem of memory can be solved as well. Often, results on a lower level are satisfying. However, Cook et al. [2] stated that the impact of the image resolution on the registration result depends locally on the anatomy. For ventilation studies the information contained in diseased regions (e.g. trapped-air regions) is especially important but often lost after the first downsampling. Thus an approach using adaptive grids should be favored.

An adaptive scheme based on octrees has been presented by Haber et al. [3]. Here the computational grid is automatically chosen based on image gradient information, leading to a sparse but computationally tricky representation of the problem. Papenberg et al. [4] developed a multi-level approach, where the field of view becomes smaller with every level, hence focusing only on a certain region and not the entire lung.

In this contribution we will introduce an approach using tensor grids, which are straightforward to implement and offer a sparse but meaningful representation of the images. These grids are fine in user chosen regions of interest (ROI), while being coarser in the remaining image domain, yielding a deformation field for the complete field of view. To our best knowledge, tensor grids have not been used in a registration framework before.

2 Materials and methods

2.1 Material

For the evaluation the POPI-Data provided by Vandemeulebroucke et al. [5] were used. The dataset consists of 10 breathing related 3D thorax CT images covering the whole breathing cycle. The images were acquired on a Philips Brilliance CT Big Bore Oncology with an isotropic in-slice resolution of 0.98 mm and a slice thickness of 2 mm. Furthermore, the CT images are equipped with 41 landmarks, 37 of which are located in the lung and were used for evaluation. The landmarks were annotated by medical experts.

2.2 Elastic registration

The non-parametric registration algorithm [6] applied here uses a standard variational approach. The aim is to minimize a functional $\mathcal{J}$ consisting of a regularizer $\mathcal{S}$ and a similarity measure $\mathcal{D}$. For $\mathcal{D}$ the sum of squared differences is chosen, since monomodal images are used. The regularizer is based on the Navier-Lamé equation. Taking the Gâteaux-derivative of $\mathcal{J}$ results in the following system of non-linear partial differential equations

$$\mu\Delta u + (\mu + \lambda)\nabla\nabla\cdot u = \nabla T_u(R - T_u), \tag{1}$$

where R and T_u stand for the reference and the deformed template image, u is the deformation vector field and μ and λ are material properties appearing in the Navier-Lamé equation that characterize the elastic behavior.

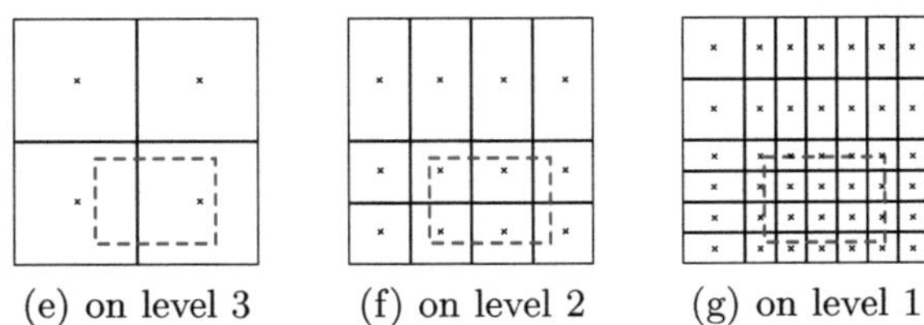

(e) on level 3 (f) on level 2 (g) on level 1

Fig. 1. Tensorgrid pyramid with three levels. In this example only two levels of resolution are allowed. The ROI chosen for the refinement is shown as a dashed rectangle.

Eq. 1 is discretized by a finite difference scheme with Neumann boundary conditions, which will be explained in more detail in the next section. The discretized system is solved using a time-marching algorithm and the method of conjugate gradients (CG). The method applies a multi-level strategy combined with an affine pre-registration.

2.3 Tensor grid

The tensor grid of a three dimensional image is defined by vectors x_1, x_2, x_3 containing the coordinates of the voxel centers in the three dimensions. The grid is constructed by forming the tensor product of these vectors.

For the multi-level setting the tensor grid is built by starting on an equidistant grid on the coarsest level and bisecting the grid elements on each level where the grid lines pass through one of the ROIs. Depending on the application the tensor grid can be further refined. Since we are aiming for a rather good deformation of the whole image, only three consecutive levels of resolution are allowed in one image, thus on higher levels the regions outside the ROI will be refined as well. An example of a tensor grid for a multi-level setting can be seen in Fig. 1.

Eq. 1 is discretized on this grid using standard stencils for the elastic regularizer. Note that since the grid is not equidistant the grid spacing has to be included in the stencil, so that neither the stencil nor the resulting matrix is symmetric. However, this matrix can be symmetrized by multiplying each row with a factor that depends on the grid spacing, so that Eq. 1 can still be solved with the CG-method.

3 Results

The maximum-inhale and -exhale phase (i.e. phase1 and phase7) were chosen for a first demonstration of the algorithm. In regions with distinctive structures that can still be well distinguished on lower resolution levels we do not expect the tensor grid approach to be superior to the standard approach. The ROI was therefore placed in the lower left lung enclosing six of the landmarks. A coronal view of phase7 together with the landmarks and the ROI can be seen in Fig. 2.

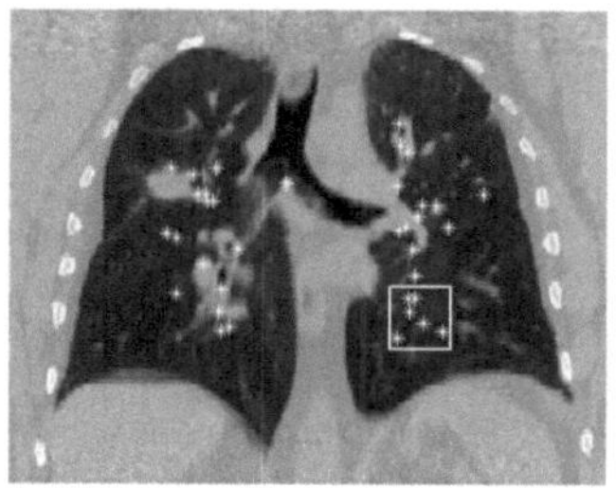

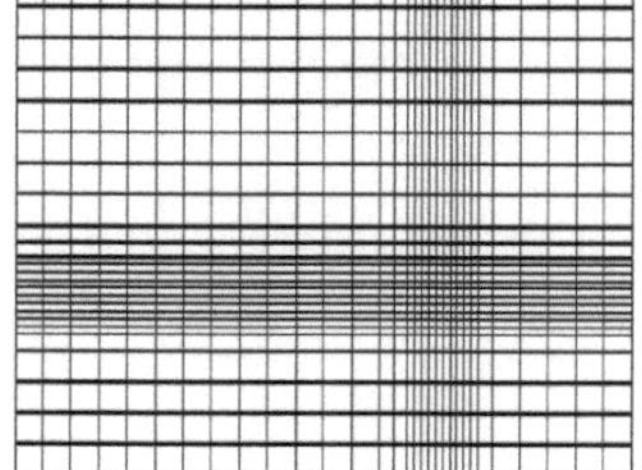

Fig. 2. Coronal view of the lung together with the ROI and the landmarks (left). Same view of the tensor grid used for the computations on level 3 (right).

Table 1. Landmark error in mm before and after registration using the two different grids. The values are in the order: mean±std (max).

landmarks	before registration	using equidistant grids	using tensor grids
all (37)	5.7±2.5 (14.0)	1.8±1.2 (6.0)	1.7±1.3 (5.6)
in ROI (6)	6.4±1.9 (8.1)	1.3±0.5 (1.9)	0.9±0.6 (1.7)
not in ROI (31)	5.5±2.6 (14.0)	1.9±1.3 (6.0)	1.8±1.3 (5.6)

The registration of the two phases was run twice, once with the tensor grid approach and once with the same implementation but using equidistant grids. The computation using the tensor grid was performed up to level 1 (image size: 352×288×128), while the equidistant grid stopped on level 3 (image size: 88×72×64). For the computations an Intel Dual Core with 2.4GHz and 2GB RAM was used. The algorithms were implemented in Matlab and are not yet optimized for speed.

The landmark error before and after registration using the tensor grid (tg) and the equidistant grid (eg) can be seen in Table 1. The error outside of the ROI is approximately the same for both grids since the coarse region of the tensor grid on level 1 has the same resolution as the equidistant grid on level 3. Inside the ROI the landmark error for the tensor grid is smaller due to the higher resolution.

Using the tensor grid approach the image size is reduced by up to 95%. This allows for computations on higher levels as can be seen in Table 2.

The ventilation V is evaluated using the Jacobian of the deformation [1]:

$$V(x) = \det(\nabla(x + u(x))) - 1. \tag{2}$$

A comparison of the ventilation images obtained with the registration using the two grids is given in Fig. 3. The tensor grid yields a result with more details within the ROI and its tails, which have been missed by the equidistant grid.

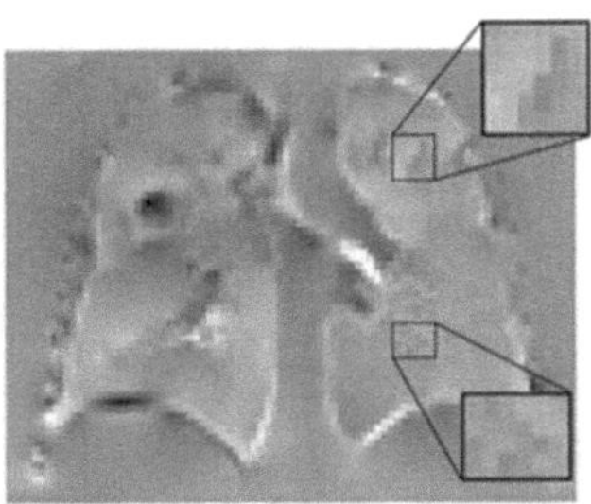
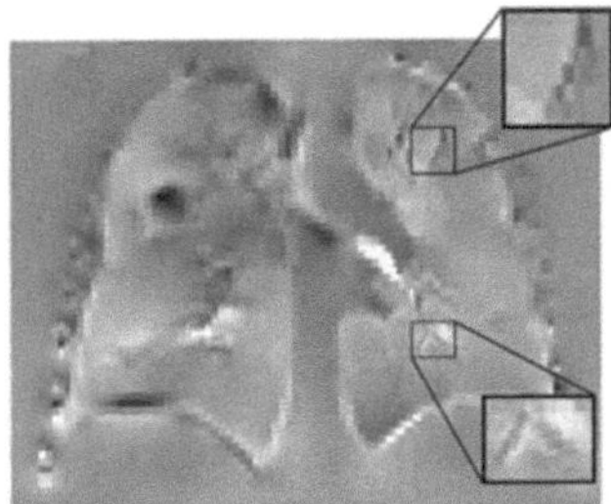

Fig. 3. Ventilation images computed from the registration result using the equidistant grid (left) and the tensor grid (right). Medium gray corresponds to volume preservation, while dark and light gray colors indicate contraction and expansion, respectively.

Table 2. Comparison of the processing time in minutes for each level given the number of voxels and the number of iterations. Level 1 is the original resolution.

	eg:	#voxels	#iterations	time	tg:	#voxels	#iterations	time
level 1		12976128	-	-		943056	100	86.80
level 2		3244032	-	-		164395	100	13.92
level 3		405504	100	9.91		23250	100	1.90
level 4		50688	92	0.65		4046	97	0.26

4 Discussion

In this paper we present an approach using tensor grids for non-parametric image registration. The advantage of this approach over equidistant grids is the possibility to use the highest resolution in user chosen regions of interest while keeping the original field of view. The sparser image representation results in a lower memory demand and a faster algorithm on each level of the multi-level setting. Considering the landmark error it turns out that the algorithms using the two different grids perform similar in the regions outside of the ROI while the tensor grid is reaching a better result within the ROI.

The tensor grid is especially useful for ventilation studies where an accurate registration of the complete lung is needed. Due to the size of the images the highest level of resolution is often omitted and thus details in diseased regions are easily lost. Furthermore, the tensor grid approach can be used for any application where one is interested in both a good registration of the complete image and certain regions in detail. It is also possible to define several ROIs in one image, which will be processed at once.

This first result of the new approach is very promising and will be followed by further tests using different datasets to proof its advantage. Moreover, more equally distributed landmarks in the lung need to be identified to allow a profound testing of the algorithm using different ROIs.

References

1. Kabus S, von Berg J, Yamamoto T, et al. Lung ventilation estimation based on 4D-CT imaging. Proc MICCAI Workshop: Pulmonary Image Analysis. 2008; p. 73–81.
2. Cook TS, Tustison N, Biederer J, et al. How do registration parameters affect quantitation of lung kinematics. In: Proc MICCAI; 2007. p. 817–824.
3. Haber E, Heldmann S, Modersitzki J. Adaptive mesh refinement for non-parametric image registration. SIAM J Sci Comp. 2007;Submitted.
4. Papenberg N, Modersitzki J, Fischer B. Registrierung im Fokus. Proc BVM. 2008; p. 138–142.
5. Vandemeulebroucke J, Sarrut D, Clarysse P. The POPI-model, a point-validated pixel-based breathing thorax model; 2007. ICCR, Toronto, Canada.
6. Modersitzki J. Numerical Methods for Image Registration. OUP; 2004.

Landmark Constrained Non-parametric Image Registration with Isotropic Tolerances

Nils Papenberg[1], Janine Olesch[1,3], Thomas Lange[2], Peter M. Schlag[4], Bernd Fischer[1]

[1] Institute of Mathematics, University of Lübeck
[2] Experimental and Clinical Research Center, Charité - Universitätsmedizin Berlin
[3] Graduate School for Computing in Medicine and Life Sciences, University of Lübeck
[4] Charité Comprehensive Cancer Center, Charité - Universitätsmedizin Berlin
papenber@math.uni-luebeck.de

Abstract. The incorporation of additional user knowledge into a non-rigid registration process is a promising topic in modern registration schemes. The combination of intensity based registration and some interactively chosen landmark pairs is a major approach in this direction. There exist different possibilities to incorporate landmark pairs into a variational non-parametric registration framework. As the interactive localization of point landmarks is always prone to errors, a demand for precise landmark matching is bound to fail. Here, the treatment of the distances of corresponding landmarks as penalties within a constrained optimization problem offers the possibility to control the quality of the matching of each landmark pair individually. More precisely, we introduce inequality constraints, which allow for a sphere-like tolerance around each landmark. We illustrate the performance of this new approach for artificial 2D images as well as for the challenging registration of preoperative CT data to intra-operative 3D ultrasound data of the liver.

1 Introduction

Non-rigid image registration is one of the key problems in computer-assisted liver surgery. Based on a pre-operative CT volume, interventions are planned by means of segmenting tumors and vessels and defining resection volumes. During the intervention the surgeon is guided by 3D ultrasound (US), which captures the actual shape and position of the liver [1]. The aim of registration is to compensate for liver deformations, such that the pre-operative planning can be directly used to guide the surgeon. Registration challenges are the homogeneous structure of the liver and its elastic behavior. Therefore the use of variational methods appears to be inevitable. In [2] a method is described which is based on an intensity driven registration of CT and US-data equipped with additional anatomical landmark information. The use of landmarks within this approach is twofold. They not only provide a good initial deformation field [3] but their preservation throughout the whole registration process, nicely guides the scheme to its final stage. However, the advantage of the approach - the simultaneous registration based on image gray values together with exact landmark matching - suffers from localization inaccuracies of the landmarks. These landmarks are set intra-operatively by the surgeon. Typical landmark positions are the junctions of the main vessels. However, due to the poor image quality, the location of these landmarks is inexact in general. Consequently, the assumption of exact landmarks appears to be not the correct modeling.

To avoid this drawback several other approaches are described in literature. The first one is an alternating optimization of a distance measure and a Gaussian elastic body spline (GEBS) based landmark registration with coupled displacement fields [4]. In this scheme anisotropic localization uncertainties of the landmarks are considered by a global penalty term. The second one is based on an additional penalty term [5, 6], that sums the local errors of the landmarks. This global error measure is added to the objective function and weighted by a corresponding parameter, so the landmark misfit is globally controlled. An individual landmark control is not possible. Secondly the penalty approach suffers from parameter tuning. Another approach is described in [7]. Here, a constrained optimization problem is invoked, which ensures small landmark errors without parameter tuning, but again only the global error is restricted.

Here we are presenting a new approach by considering individual landmark localization inaccuracies. For each landmark a tolerance estimating the localization error of the landmarks is defined. Similar to the CoLD-approach in [2], the new approach is formulated as a constraint optimization problem, this time however, with an inequality constraint for each individual landmark pair.

2 Methods

In the following we describe the above outlined new approach in more detail. Let R, T (US-) reference and (CT-) template volumes, with $R, T : \mathbb{R}^d \rightarrow \mathbb{R}$, continuous functions. Furthermore, let $y : \mathbb{R}^d \rightarrow \mathbb{R}^d$ the deformation in question. The landmarks are given by $r_j, t_j \in \mathbb{R}^d, j = 1, \ldots, m$ and the corresponding tolerated error distance of the landmarks r_j, t_j by $c_j \in \mathbb{R}$. The key term within the optimization problem is given by

$$\mathcal{P}_j(y) = c_j^2 - \|y(r_j) - t_j\|^2 .$$

Note that $\mathcal{P}_j(y) \geq 0$ ensures that the squared difference of the deformed j^{th} pair of landmarks is less than c_j^2. Altogether we arrive at the following constraint optimization problem

$$\min_y \mathcal{J}(y) = \mathcal{D}(y) + \alpha\mathcal{S}(y) \quad \text{s.t.} \qquad P_j(y) \geq 0, \quad j = 1, \ldots, m. \tag{1}$$

In contrast to [7] we do not summarize the differences of the landmarks, but handle each of them separately. As a consequence, we are able to guarantee an individual error for each pair of landmarks. The tolerance c_j may be interpreted as the radius of a sphere around the jth landmark. A deformed landmark will be accepted if it is located within this sphere, see Figure 1 (lower right). It should be noted, that the extension to anisotropic tolerance regions (e.g. an ellipsoid) [8] is straightforward. To keep the issues of interest clear, we only present the isotropic case, c.f. the tolerance region is a sphere.

The remaining terms of the functional $\mathcal{J}(y)$ are the well known normalized gradient field (NGF) distance measure [9]

$$\mathcal{D}(y) = \frac{1}{2} \int_{\Omega} \left(1 - \left(\frac{< \nabla T_y, \nabla R >}{\|\nabla T_y\| \cdot \|\nabla R\|} \right)^2 \right) \, dx,$$

which is well suited for multimodal problems and the elastic regularizer [10]

$$\mathcal{S}(y) = \frac{1}{2} \int_{\Omega} \sum_{l=1}^{3} \mu \|\nabla y_l\|^2 + (\mu + \lambda) \mathrm{div}^2 y \, dx.$$

Here $\lambda, \mu \in \mathbb{R}^+$ are the so called Navier-Lamé constants, which control the elastic behavior of the deformation.

For the optimization of (1) we use the first-discretize-then-optimize-approach. That means, the objective function as well as the constraints are discretized first to achieve a finite optimization problem. In particular, the constraints are approximated by means of linear interpolation as described in [7].

We solve the finite optimization problem by a generalized Gauss-Newton-method [11, 12]. Applying a pre-registration based on thin plate splines (TPS) [10], we arrive at a starting point for the optimization procedure that fulfills the constraints. Due to the constraints, the resulting linear system, known as KKT-system, is indefinite. Therefor we use the iterative solution technique MinRes [13] for these systems. All algorithms are implemented in Matlab.

3 Experiments

We demonstrate the applicability of the new method in two steps. First we start with artificial generated data. Afterwards we test it on real clinical data from liver surgery. In the upper left and middle images of Figure 1 we depict two dimensional reference and template test images. Also four pairs of corresponding landmarks are shown, where the second landmark is intentionally misplaced. The remaining images of Figure 1 demonstrate different registration results. To this end, the deformed template is overlaid by the boundaries of the reference, resulting in an easy visual validation. The upper right image shows the result of a TPS-based registration, while the lower left illustrates the solution of the CoLD-approach described in [2]. It should come as no surprise, that both methods suffer from the misplaced second landmark. Next we applied the CoLD-approach to the problem by completely ignoring the second landmark. Again the registration quality is poor which is apparent in the lower half of the image. Finally, we tested the new approach. For the second landmark we define a tolerance of $c_2 = 1$, (to compare, image domain is $\Omega = (15, 10)$) drawn as a green circle (Fig. 1, lower right). The overall result outperforms all other methods by generating a smooth and feasible deformation.

In a second step the algorithm was applied to real clinical data from a patient who underwent an oncological liver resection. The aim is to register pre-operative CT data to intra-operative 3D power Doppler ultrasound data. We defined eight landmarks interactively and intentionally moved one landmark by 2 mm. The contours of vessels from the registered CT data are shown after CoLD-registration with no tolerances (Fig. 2a) and with a tolerance of 2 mm at the moved landmark (Fig. 2b,c). Again, the new method shows a superior quality, even for this very challenging problem.

4 Discussion

We presented a non-rigid registration approach, which combines intensity-based registration with additional landmark constraints. The important contribution is the introduction of isotropic tolerances in order to be able to compensate for localization uncertainties of the landmarks. In clinical application these tolerances are set by the surgeon depending on the accuracy of the related landmark. We demonstrated the influence of an accidentally displaced landmark on the registration result and the satisfactory improvement by the new method. Furthermore, the outlined method exhibits success for real clinical data. In a forthcoming investigation we plan to evaluate the novel method for a large collection of clinical data sets.

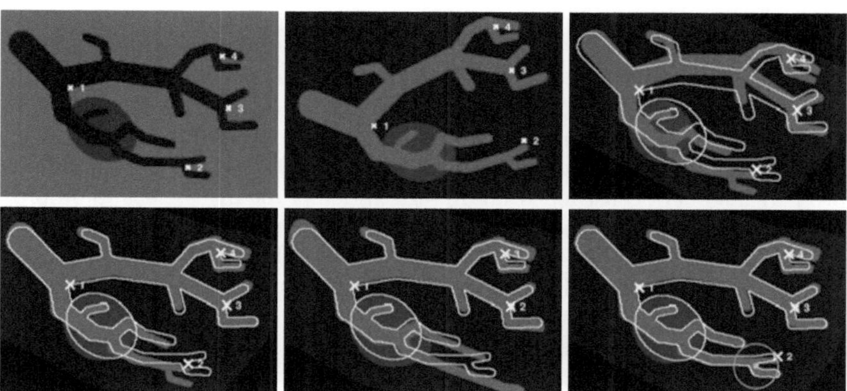

Fig. 1. 2D example; *upper left:* reference; *upper mid:* template both with landmarks; *upper right:* TPS-based registration; *lower left:* CoLD-registration; *lower mid:* CoLD-registration without misplaced landmark; *lower right:* new approach; green: given landmark tolerance.

Fig. 2. One slice of real clinical 3D ultrasound data (B-mode + power Doppler) with isolines of registered CT data is shown; *left:* Registered with correct (white) and moved landmark (black) with no tolerances; *mid:* with 2 mm tolerance for the moved landmark (black); *right:* Overview of the whole slice with moved landmark with 2 mm tolerance.

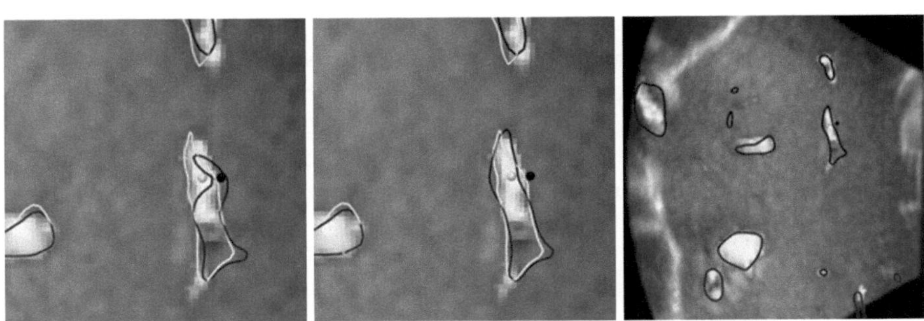

References

1. Beller S, Hünerbein M, Lange T, et al. Image-guided surgery of liver metastases by 3D ultrasound - based optoelectronic navigation. Brit J Surg. 2007;94(7):866–875.
2. Lange T, Papenberg N, Heldmann S, et al. 3D Ultrasound-CT Alignment of the Liver using Combined Landmark-Intensity Registration. Int J CARS. 2008; p. S107–S108.
3. Rohr K. Landmark-Based Image Analysis. vol. 21 of Computational Imaging and Vision. Springer; 2001.
4. Wörz S, Rohr K. Hybrid spline-based elastic image registration using analytic solutions of the Navier equation. Proc BVM. 2007; p. 151–155.
5. Sorzano COS, Thevenaz P, Unser M. Elastic registration of biological images using vector-spline regularization. IEEE Trans Bio Eng. 2005.
6. Papenberg N, Lange T, Modersitzki J, et al. Image registration for CT and intra-operative ultrasound data of the liver. Proc SPIE. 2008;6918(1):691808.
7. Olesch J, Papenberg N, Lange T, et al. Matching CT and ultrasound data of the liver by landmark constrained image registration. Proc SPIE. 2009; p. in press.
8. Rohr K, Stiehl H, Sprengel R, et al. Landmark-based elastic registration using approximating thin-plate splines. IEEE Trans Med Imag. 2001;20(6):526–534.
9. Haber E, Modersitzki J. Intensity gradient based registration and fusion of multi-modal images. Method Inform Med. 2007;46(3):292–299.
10. Modersitzki J. Numerical Methods for Image Registration. Oxford University Press; 2004.
11. Bock HG, Kostina E, Schlöder JP. Numerical methods for parameter estimation in nonlinear differential algebraic equations. GAMM Mitt. 2007;30(2):376 – 408.
12. Nocedal J, Wright SJ. Numerical Optimization. Berlin: Springer; 2000.
13. Golub GH, Van Loan CF. Matrix Computations. The Johns Hopkins University Press; 1996.

Hybrid Spline-Based Multimodal Registration Using a Local Measure for Mutual Information

Andreas Biesdorf[1], Stefan Wörz[1], Hans-Jürgen Kaiser[2], Karl Rohr[1]

[1]University of Heidelberg, BIOQUANT, IPMB, and DKFZ Heidelberg
Dept. Bioinformatics and Functional Genomics, Biomedical Computer Vision Group
[2]University Hospital, RWTH Aachen University, Department of Nuclear Medicine
a.biesdorf@dkfz.de

Abstract. We introduce a new hybrid approach for spline-based elastic registration of multimodal medical images. The approach uses point landmarks as well as intensity information based on local analytic measures for mutual information. The intensity similarity metrics are computationally efficient and can be optimized independently for each voxel. We have successfully applied our approach to synthetic images, brain phantom images, as well as real multimodal medical images.

1 Introduction

In modern radiology, image registration is important for diagnosis, surgical planning, and treatment control. A challenge is to cope with the broad range of applications as well as the large spectrum of imaging modalities. Previous approaches for image registration can be classified according to the transformation model and the used image information. Typical transformation models are rigid and elastic transformations. Regarding the used image information, registration schemes can be subdivided in landmark-based and intensity-based approaches. For intensity-based approaches, it is important to distinguish between monomodal and multimodal registration problems, as both classes require different types of similarity metrics. In monomodal registration, images from the same modality are aligned, which can be achieved by, e.g., using the sum of squared intensity differences (SSD). Registration of images of different modalities, however, requires multimodal similarity metrics such as mutual information (MI). In general, metrics for MI are computationally expensive because they require the estimation of probability density functions based on joint histograms (e.g., [1, 2]).

In recent years, increased attention has been paid to hybrid registration approaches that integrate landmark-based schemes with intensity-based schemes (e.g., [3, 4, 5, 6, 7]). However, only few hybrid approaches are designed for multimodal images (e.g., [3, 4, 5]) and, although MI is employed as similarity measure, often only application to monomodal images is reported. Furthermore, previous spline-based approaches typically use coarse physical deformation models such as B-splines (e.g., [3, 4]) or thin-plate splines (e.g., [5]), and incorporate intensity information using global, computationally expensive measures for MI.

In this contribution, we present a new hybrid approach for spline-based elastic registration of multimodal medical images. Our approach is formulated as an energy-minimizing functional that incorporates point landmarks and intensity information as well as a regularization based on Gaussian elastic body splines (GEBS) [8]. Moreover, the intensity information is evaluated locally based on analytic measures for MI. These measures are computationally efficient since they do not require the estimation of probability density functions.

2 Materials and methods

2.1 Hybrid spline-based registration

Our new hybrid approach for elastic registration of multimodal images is based on an energy minimizing functional J_{Hybrid} that incorporates both landmark and intensity information and a regularization term:

$$J_{\text{Hybrid}}(\mathbf{u}) = J_{\text{Data},I}(g_1, g_2, \mathbf{u}^I) + \lambda_I J_I(\mathbf{u}, \mathbf{u}^I) + \lambda_L J_{Data,L}(\mathbf{u}) + \lambda_E J_{El}(\mathbf{u}) \quad (1)$$

The first term $J_{\text{Data},I}$ describes the intensity-based similarity measure between the source and target image, g_1 and g_2, respectively. In the second term J_I the intensity-based deformation field $\mathbf{u}^I$ is coupled with the final deformation field $\mathbf{u}$ using a weighted Euclidean distance. The term $J_{\text{Data},L}$ incorporates the landmark information based on approximating GEBS. The fourth term J_{El} represents the regularization of the deformation field according to the Navier equation, which constrains the deformation field to physically realistic deformations. The overall functional J_{Hybrid} is minimized alternatingly w.r.t. $\mathbf{u}^I$ and $\mathbf{u}$. In previous work [7], $J_{\text{Data},I}$ was defined based on the sum of squared intensity differences, thus the approach was only applicable to monomodal registration. Here, we present a new formulation of $J_{\text{Data},I}$ for multimodal registration as well as a new scheme for minimizing J_{Hybrid} w.r.t. $\mathbf{u}^I$.

2.2 Multimodal registration using analytic expressions for MI

For the intensity-based similarity measure $J_{\text{Data},I}$, we suggest to use local analytic measures for MI. Let g be an image of dimension d over the continuous domain $\Omega \subset \mathbb{R}^d$, and $N_R(\mathbf{x})$ be the neighborhood of radius R around a point $\mathbf{x} \in \Omega$. For R being sufficiently small, the first order Taylor approximation $T_g(\mathbf{x}) \simeq \nabla g(\mathbf{x})^T \cdot \mathbf{x} + g_0(\mathbf{x})$ can be used as an approximation of $g(\mathbf{x})$ in the neighborhood of $\mathbf{x}$, where ∇g denotes the image gradient. The intensities $g(\mathbf{x})$ in the neighborhood $N_R(\mathbf{x})$ can be characterized by a random variable $\mathbf{g}$, which can be described by a probability density function. In [9] it was shown that for two images g_1 and g_2 the mutual information can then be approximated by

$$MI_{\text{orig}}(\mathbf{x}) : \quad \max\{c_d - \log_2 |\sin\theta|\}, \quad (2)$$

where θ represents the angle between $\nabla g_1(\mathbf{x})$ and $\nabla g_2(\mathbf{x})$, and c_d is a constant that depends on the dimension d. However, due to properties of the logarithm,

$MI_{\text{orig}}(\mathbf{x})$ yields very high values if the argument $|\sin\theta|$ is close to zero and thus leads to unstable results. In [9], MI is evaluated globally, i.e. the similarity for each voxel is integrated over the whole image. If at a single voxel $|\sin\theta|$ is zero or close to zero, the global measure yields a high value, since adding logarithmic terms is equivalent to the logarithm of the product of the arguments ($\sum_i \log_2 s_i = \log_2 \prod_i s_i$). To circumvent this problem, in [9] a simplified metric is used which omits the logarithm and replaces the sine by a squared cosine:

$$MI_{\text{simp}}(\mathbf{x}): \quad \max\{c_d - \log_2 |\sin\theta|\} \equiv \min\{-\cos^2\theta\} \tag{3}$$

Instead, we suggest an alternative to cope with this problem, where the logarithm is still included but a constant $\epsilon > 0$ is introduced. This measure is more similar to the original measure in (2) and allows robust computation:

$$MI_{\text{new}}(\mathbf{x}): \quad \max\{c_d - \log_2 |\sin\theta|\} \equiv \min\{\log_2 |\epsilon + \sin\theta|\} \tag{4}$$

In our approach, we use $MI_{\text{simp}}(\mathbf{x})$ and $MI_{\text{new}}(\mathbf{x})$ for $J_{\text{Data},I}$ in (1). Optimization of J_{Hybrid} is computed alternatingly w.r.t. $\mathbf{u}^I$ and $\mathbf{u}$. For minimization w.r.t. $\mathbf{u}^I$, $J_{\text{Data},I} + \lambda_I J_I$ has to be minimized. To this end we have derived analytic expressions for the partial derivatives of $MI_{\text{simp}}(\mathbf{x})$ and $MI_{\text{new}}(\mathbf{x})$. In contrast to [9], in our approach MI is evaluated locally, i.e., optimization of $\mathbf{u}^I$ is computed independently for each voxel, which improves the efficiency.

3 Results

We have applied the new registration scheme to synthetic images, to brain phantom images, and to real medical images. In a first experiment, we have applied the new registration scheme to different 3D synthetic images. Fig. 1 (left), for example, shows the case of a sphere and a cube. Note that the images have inverted contrast to simulate a multimodal registration problem. Thus, a registration scheme using SSD would fail. Eight landmarks were defined at the corners of the cube, and the registration is computed based on the metric MI_{new}. The other images in Fig. 1 show the results for pure landmark-based, pure intensity-based, and hybrid registration. For landmark-based registration, only the corners of the cube are aligned. Using the pure intensity-based registration approach, the faces of the sphere are aligned, but not the corners. The

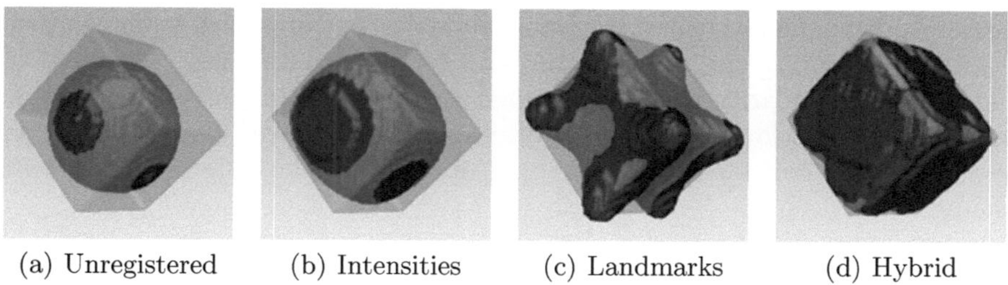

(a) Unregistered (b) Intensities (c) Landmarks (d) Hybrid

Fig. 1. 3D synthetic images: Registration of a sphere with a cube

Table 1. Registration of phantom images: Mean geometric error $\overline{e}_{\text{geom}}$ for different metrics using different types of image information.

Metric	Unregistered	Landmarks	Intensities	Hybrid
MI_{simp}	7.85	3.41	2.74	2.02
MI_{new}	7.85	3.41	2.41	1.61

best result is obtained using the hybrid approach, since both the faces and the corners are aligned.

To quantitatively evaluate the registration accuracy, we have used multi-modal phantom images (MRI-T1 and MRI-T2) from the BrainWeb database [10]. We have generated a deformation field $\mathbf{u}_{\text{orig}}$ based on eight landmarks using GEBS, which is applied to the MRI-T2 image to obtain a target image with known deformation. After registration, we compared the computed deformation $\mathbf{u}$ with the original deformation $\mathbf{u}_{\text{orig}}$ and quantified the registration accuracy by the mean geometric error $\overline{e}_{\text{geom}} = \overline{\|\mathbf{u}_{\text{orig}} - \mathbf{u}\|}$. Table 1 gives the results. Without registration, the mean error is $\overline{e}_{\text{geom}} = 7.85$ pixels. Using only landmarks, we have $\overline{e}_{\text{geom}} = 3.41$ pixels. Registration using intensities leads to a significant reduction of the registration error to $\overline{e}_{\text{geom}} = 2.74$ pixels for MI_{simp} and $\overline{e}_{\text{geom}} = 2.41$ pixels for MI_{new}. When using the hybrid scheme, we obtain the best result $\overline{e}_{\text{geom}} = 2.02$ pixels for MI_{simp} and $\overline{e}_{\text{geom}} = 1.61$ pixels for MI_{new}.

We have also applied the new registration scheme to real, clinically relevant medical images. In Fig. 2 (top), we show PET (left) and CT (right) images of the thorax. For registration, we placed three landmarks, and computed the registration using only intensities (b) and using the hybrid approach (c) based on MI_{new}. It can be seen that using the hybrid scheme, we obtain a significant improvement compared to the pure intensity-based scheme.

4 Discussion

We introduced a new hybrid spline-based approach for elastic registration of multimodal images which incorporates point landmarks, intensity information, as well as a physically-based regularization. Since the approach uses a local analytic measure for Mutual Information, the required derivatives can be calculated analytically, and optimization can be performed independently for each voxel. We have demonstrated the applicability of our approach using synthetic images, phantom images of the brain, and real medical images. It turned out that our new similarity measure is more accurate than a previously proposed measure. We also found that the hybrid approach achieves more accurate registration results compared to a pure intensity-based and a pure landmark-based scheme.

Acknowledgement. Support of the Deutsche Forschungsgemeinschaft (DFG) within the project ELASTIR (RO 2471/2) is gratefully acknowledged.

Fig. 2. Top: PET (left) and CT (right) images. Bottom: Edge overlay of a section before registration (a), after intensity-based registration (b), and hybrid registration (c).

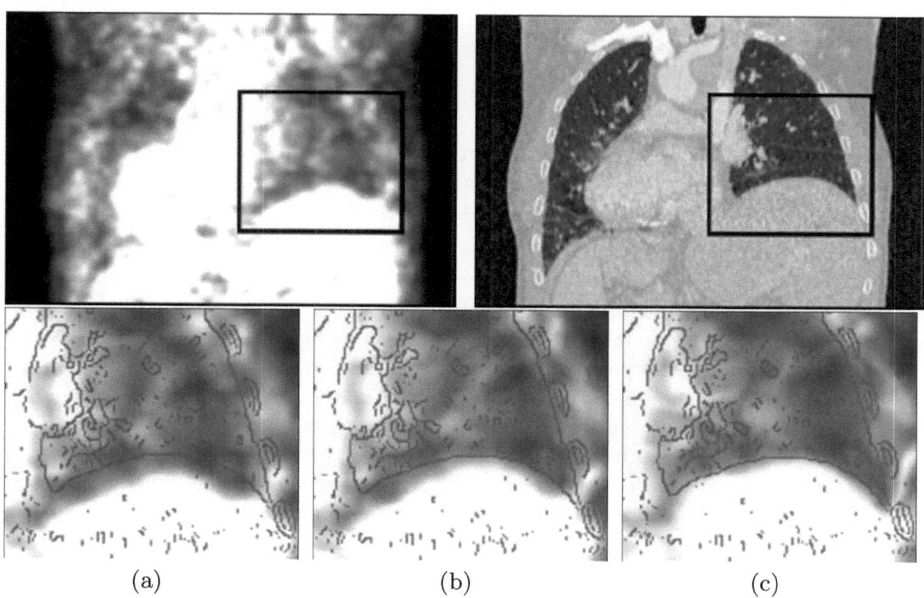

(a) (b) (c)

References

1. Viola P, Wells WM. Alignment by maximization of mutual information. Proc ICCV. 1995; p. 16–23.
2. Rueckert D, Sonoda LI, Hayes C, et al. Nonrigid registration using free-form deformations: Application to breast MR images. IEEE Trans Med Imaging. 1999;18(8):712–721.
3. Hartkens T, Hill D, Castellano-Smith A, et al. Using points and surfaces to improve voxel-based non-rigid registration. Proc MICCAI. 2002; p. 565–572.
4. Teng CC, Shapiro LG, Kalet I. Head and neck lymph node region delineation using a hybrid image registration method. Proc IEEE ISBI. 2006; p. 462–465.
5. Wang X, Feng DD. Automatic hybrid registration for 2-D CT abdominal images. Proc ICIG. 2004; p. 208–211.
6. Fischer B, Modersitzki J. Intensity-based image registration with a guaranteed one-to-one point match. Methods Inf Med. 2004;43:327–30.
7. Wörz S, Winz ML, Rohr K. Geometric alignment of 2D gel electrophoresis images. Proc BVM. 2008; p. 97–101.
8. Wörz S, Rohr K. Physics-based elastic registration using non-radial basis functions and including landmark localization uncertainties. Computer Vis Image Underst. 2008;111:263–274.
9. Karaçali B. Information theoretic deformable registration using local image information. Int J Computer Vis. 2007;72:219–237.
10. Kwan RKS, Evans AC, et al. MRI simulation-based evaluation of image-processing and classification methods. IEEE Trans Med Imaging. 1999;18(11):1085–1097.

Nichtrigide Bildregistrierung für die adaptive Strahlentherapie mittels Free Form Deformation

Gernot Wurst[1], Rolf Bendl[1,2]

[1]Abteilung Medizinische Physik in der Strahlentherapie, DKFZ Heidelberg
[2]Fakultät für Informatik, Hochschule Heilbronn
g.wurst@dkfz-heidelberg.de

Kurzfassung. Im Rahmen der Adaptiven Strahlentherapie müssen zum Behandlungszeitpunkt Abweichungen der aktuellen Patientengeometrie von den Planungsdaten bekannt sein, damit eine Anpassung des Bestrahlungsplans vorgenommen werden kann. State of the Art ist in diesem Zusammenhang die rigide Registrierung von Planungs- und Kontrolldaten. Hierbei werden jedoch komplexere, nichtrigide Deformationen nicht angemessen berücksichtigt. Daher wurde ein Verfahren entwickelt, das diese komplexen Deformationen durch ein Free Form-Deformationsmodell beschreibt. Die dafür vorzugebenden Translationsvektoren wurden durch Template Matching bestimmt. Es zeigte sich, dass die vorhandenen Deformationen weitgehend erkannt werden. Weiterhin ist das Verfahren aufgrund seines günstigen Laufzeitverhaltens prädestiniert für die Adaptive Strahlentherapie.

1 Einleitung

Die Kenntnis der Abweichungen der Patientengeometrie zum Bestrahlungszeitpunkt von den Planungsdaten ermöglicht eine Anpassung des Bestrahlungsplans. Bisher wird hierzu das Lagekontroll-CT rigide auf das Planungs-CT registriert. Da dabei jedoch komplexere nichtrigide Deformationen unberücksichtigt bleiben, wie sie etwa durch Gewichtsverlust oder Füllungsunterschiede von Hohlorganen entstehen, besteht Bedarf an alternativen Ansätzen. Von besonderer Relevanz ist in diesem Zusammenhang die Performance, weil zwischen Lagekontrolle und Bestrahlung möglichst wenig Zeit vergehen soll. Ein am DKFZ entwickelter, auf Template Matching und einer globalen Interpolation basierender Algorithmus [1] beschleunigt die Registrierung durch Verzicht auf iterative Optimierung, ist jedoch wegen der hohen Komplexität der globalen Interpolation bezüglich der möglichen Anzahl der Landmarken limitiert. Der hier realisierte Ansatz kombiniert daher Template Matching mit einem lokal interpolierten Free Form-Deformationsmodell, das ein lineares Laufzeitverhalten aufweist.

2 Material und Methoden

Gesucht ist ein Deformationsvektorfeld, das ein zu deformierendes Bild (Zielbild) an ein Referenzbild angleicht.

Prinzip der Free Form Deformation (FFD, [2]): Über den zu registrierenden Bereich des Zielbildes wird ein äquidistantes Gitter gelegt. Das Deformationsvektorfeld ist dann definiert durch Translationen der Gitterpunkte (Kontrollpunkte) sowie eine Interpolation.

Prinzip des Template Matchings: Für Überlagerungen einer Umgebung des Kontrollpunktes (Template) und einen größeren Bildausschnitt aus dem Referenzbild (Suchbereich) werden Werte eines Ähnlichkeitsmaßes berechnet. Aus der Translation des Templates hin zum Maximum dieser Ähnlichkeitswerte ergibt sich die Translation des Kontrollpunktes.

2.1 Gitteraufbau und Klassifikation der Gitterpunkte

Über einen vorzugebenden Bereich des Zielbildes wird ein äquidistantes Gitter gelegt. In einem zweiten Schritt werden anhand eines Gewebekantendichtemaßes diejenigen Gitterpunkte aussortiert, die sich in homogenen Bildbereichen befinden, da dort aufgrund mangelnder Bildinformation kein verwertbares Matchingergebnis zu erwarten ist. Die übrigen Punkte heißen Kontrollpunktkandidaten. Sie werden dem Matching zugeführt.

2.2 Matching und Bewertung der Matchingresultate

Da hier monomodale Registrierung von CT auf CT praktiziert wird, kommt als Ähnlichkeitsmaß die Kreuzkorrelation zum Einsatz. Sie ist im Unterschied zu der in diesem Fall ebenfalls populären SSD-Metrik (sum of squared differences) unabhängig von den absoluten Grauwerten und lässt sich unter Ausnutzung des Faltungssatzes und der Verwandtschaft zwischen Korrelation und Faltung besonders effizient berechnen.

Im Anschluss werden die gefundenen Matchings durch eine Korrelationsschwelle sowie hinsichtlich des Erfüllens der hinreichenden Bedingung für lokale Maxima bewertet [3]. Diejenigen Matchings, bei denen das Korrelationsmaximum zu niedrig ausfällt, werden verworfen, da mit dem Korrelationswert die Zuverlässigkeit des Matchings abnimmt [1]. Für die übrigen Matchings wird geprüft, ob ein ausgeprägtes Korrelationsmaximum vorliegt. Dies ist erforderlich, da es Fälle gibt, in denen die Translation in eine (z.B. parallel zu einem Röhrenknochen) oder zwei (z.B an größeren Oberflächen) Richtungen nicht eindeutig bestimmbar ist. In diesem Fall wird zur Entschärfung des Blendenproblems [1] ein erneutes Matching unter Verwendung eines größeren Bildbereiches durchgeführt und neu klassifiziert . Kann wieder kein ausgeprägtes Maximum gefunden werden, so wird der Kontrollpunktkandidat verworfen.

Kontrollpunktkandidaten, deren Templates erfolgreich gematcht wurden, wird die gefundene Translation zugeordnet. Sie sind nun FFD-Kontrollpunkte.

2.3 Aufbau des Translationsvektorfeldes

Die bei Free Form-Verfahren üblichen globalen Interpolationsverfahren wie etwa Thin Plate Splines [4] haben den Nachteil, dass der Rechenaufwand mit der Anzahl verwendeter Kontrollpunkte überproportional zunimmt. Unter der Annahme eines äquidistanten Gitters können jedoch auch schnelle lokale Verfahren mit linearer Laufzeit zum Einsatz kommen. Hier wurde mit Trikubischen Hermite-Splines (Trikubische Polynome mit Glattheitsbedingungen [5]) interpoliert. Da nach Abschluss des Matchings jedoch nur ein Teil des FFD-Gitters mit Kontrollpunkten besetzt und somit kein verwendbares äquidistantes Gitter vorhanden ist, wird dieses in einem Vorverarbeitungsschritt aufgefüllt. Dabei ergeben sich iterativ die fehlenden Translationsvektoren durch distanzgewichtete Linearkombinationen der Translationen benachbarter Kontrollpunkte.

2.4 Testdaten

Zum Testen der Registrierung wurden zwei Datensätze (P1: Prostatakarzinom, P2: Paraspinaltumor) herangezogen, die je aus einem Planungs- und einem rigide vorregistrierten Lagekontroll-CT sowie einem Satz manuell definierter Landmarkenkorrespondenzen für die quantitative Analyse des Registrierungsergebnisses bestehen. Die Auflösung beträgt 256×256 Pixel pro Schicht bei einem Pixelabstand von ca. 1,95 mm. Der Schichtabstand beträgt 3,00 mm. Bei P1 wurden 60 Schichten registriert, und es standen 60 Landmarken zur Verfügung, während es bei P2 73 Schichten und 56 Landmarken waren.

3 Ergebnisse

3.1 Funktionsweise

Die Bildfolge in Abb. 1 zeigt die Arbeitsweise sowie die Möglichkeiten und Grenzen des vorgestellten Verfahrens. Im Bereich und in der Umgebung des Wirbels sowie lateral wurden die Lageunterschiede gut korrigiert. Der Darm im oberen Bildbereich bleibt dagegen unregistriert. Dies ist darauf zurückzuführen, dass die

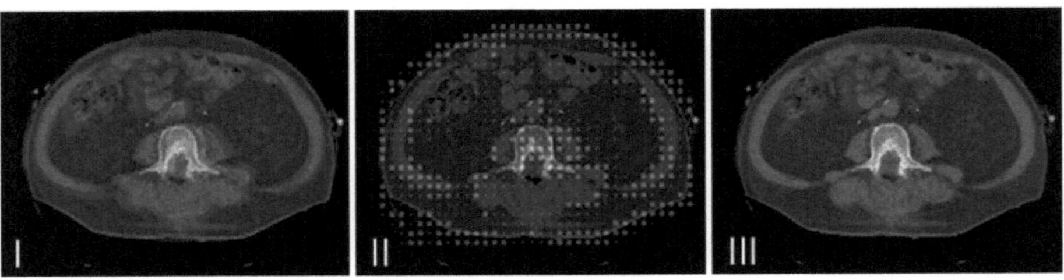

Abb. 1. Visualisierung der Situationen vor (I) und nach (III) einer Registrierung sowie einer FFD-Gitterebene (II) durch transversale Überlagerungsbilder von Datensatz P2. In grün dargestellt ist eine Schicht aus dem Planungs-CT. In (I) und (III) ist diese mit dem unregistrierten bzw. registrierten Lagekontrollbild in rot überlagert. (II) zeigt durch kleine Markierungen die Positionen der verworfenen Kontrollpunktkandidaten und durch große Markierungen die Positionen der gefundenen FFD-Kontrollpunkte.

Tabelle 1. Gegenüberstellung von FFD und Vergleichsalgorithmus (V)

	P1-FFD	P1-V	P2-FFD	P2-V
Dauer f. Auswahl der Landmarken (s)	18	29	15	24
Anzahl gewählter Landmarken	6207	3019	3926	2590
Dauer des Matchings (s)	322	176	200	139
Anzahl erfolgreicher Matchings	1953	1355	2017	1669
Matching-Erfolgsrate (%)	32	45	51	64
Dauer der Interpolation (s)	8	341	8	631
Gesamtdauer (s)	348	546	223	794

dort auftretenden schnellen Deformationsänderungen durch lokal-rigide Templates nicht erfassbar sind. (II) zeigt, dass in der Konsequenz keine Kontrollpunkte gefunden werden konnten und somit lokal Translationsinformation fehlt.

3.2 Performance

Für die Gegenüberstellung von FFD und dem vorhandenen Algorithmus von [1] (im Folgenden Vergleichsalgorithmus V genannt) wurden die gemeinsamen Parameter Templategröße (7×7×5 Pixel), Suchbereichsgröße (19×19×14 Pixel), Korrelationsschwelle für die Akzeptanz der Matchingergebnisse (0,8) und Anzahl zu registrierender Schichten (60 bzw. 73) identisch gewählt. Alle Registrierungen wurden auf einem PC mit P4-CPU (3 GHz) und 3 GB RAM berechnet. Offenbar hat sich (Tab. 1) der Rechenzeitbedarf für die Interpolation durch die Einführung der lokalen Interpolationsmethode vom Löwenanteil hin zur Vernachlässigbarkeit reduziert. Auf der anderen Seite hat sich der Aufwand für das Matching erhöht. Dies ist einerseits auf eine höhere Anzahl von Landmarken und andererseits auf eine geringere Matching-Erfolgsrate zurückzuführen. Die niedrigere Erfolgsrate kann dadurch erklärt werden, dass die Kontrollpunkte an FFD-Gitterpunktpositionen und nicht wie bei (V) direkt auf den Gewebekanten sitzen, wodurch das Matching etwas erschwert wird.

3.3 Qualitative Evaluierung

Für beide Datensätze standen von einem Radiologen manuell definierte Landmarkenkorrespondenzen zur Verfügung. Diese geben die nach der rigiden Vorregistrierung noch vorhandenen Lageunterschiede an. Durch Transformation der Landmarkenpositionen im Zielbild mit Translationslationsvektorfeldern aus der nichtrigiden Registrierung wurden neue Korrespondenzen hergestellt, die die verbleibenden Lageunterschiede nach der nichtrigiden Registrierung angeben.

Tabelle 2 zeigt, dass die mittleren Registrierungsungenauigkeiten für beide Algorithmen im Subvoxelbereich (x,y < 1,95 bzw. z < 3 mm) liegen. Beim FFD-Verfahren treten stets deutlich höhere Maxima auf, was vom teilweisen lokalen Fehlen von Translationsinformation herrührt. Aus dem Vergleich von Mittelwert und Median geht hervor, dass es sich hierbei um einige Ausreißer handelt.

Tabelle 2. Statistische Kenngrößen der Lageunterschiede zwischen Planungs- und Kontroll-CT nach rigider Vorregistrierung bzw. Registrierung mit FFD und Vergleichsalgorithmus V (Werte aus [1]) nach Raumrichtungen. Alle Angaben sind in mm.

	rigide			FFD			V		
	x	y	z	x	y	z	x	y	z
P1 Mittelwert	1,47	1,75	2,14	0,88	0,97	1,79	0,70	0,80	1,20
P1 Median	1,10	1,46	3,00	0,73	0,88	1,50	na	na	na
P1 Maximum	4,39	5,37	6,00	2,76	2,42	5,57	1,90	2,20	3,10
P2 Mittelwert	9,34	2,34	3,05	1,36	1,12	1,40	1,10	0,60	0,90
P2 Median	10,04	2,29	3,00	0,81	0,82	1,23	na	na	na
P2 Maximum	14,16	5,37	8,25	5,86	4,64	4,14	3,20	2,00	2,90

4 Diskussion

Das vorgestellte Verfahren ist ein vielversprechender Ansatz für die schnelle Detektion nichtrigider Deformationen. Gegenüber dem Vergleichsalgorithmus kann durch lokale Interpolation des Deformationsvektorfeldes fast die ganze Rechenzeit für diesen Schritt eingespart werden. Andererseits werden mehr Matchings bei gleichzeitig niedrigerer Erfolgsrate durchgeführt.

Gegenwärtig werden Deformationen berücksichtigt, die durch Matching mit lokal-rigiden Templates erfassbar sind. Bei schnellen Deformationsänderungen, etwa im Darm, misslingt das Matching, weswegen dann keine Deformationen bestimmbar sind. Durchweg wurden mittlere Registrierungsungenauigkeiten im Subvoxelbereich erreicht. Allerdings führt das lokale Fehlen von Kontrollpunkten dazu, dass nicht alle Lageunterschiede ausreichend korrigiert werden.

FFD in Verbindung mit lokaler Interpolation eignet sich für die Beschreibung von Lageunterschieden. In Verbindung mit Template Matching entstehen zwar weitgehend gute Ergebnisse, das Potential des FFD-Modells wird jedoch nicht ausgeschöpft. Verbesserungen sind durch besseres Propagieren gefundener Translationen sowie weitere Methoden zur Translationsbestimmung erzielbar.

Literaturverzeichnis

1. Malsch U. An enhanced block matching algorithm for fast elastic registration in adaptive radiotherapy. Phys Med Biol. 2006;51(51):4789–4806.
2. Sederberg TW, Parry SR. Free-form deformation of solid geometric models. Computer Graph Procs. 1986; p. 151–160.
3. Söhn M, Birkner M, Chi Y, et al. Model-independent, multimodality deformable image registration by local matching of anatomical features and minimization of elastic energy. Med Phys. 2008;35:866 ff.
4. Bookstein F. Principal warps: Thin-plate splines and the decomposition of deformations. IEEE Trans Pattern Anal Mach Intell. 1998;11(11):567–585.
5. Lekien J F und Marsden. Tricubic interpolation in three dimensions. Int J Numer Methods Eng. 2005;63(63):455–471.

A Scale-Space Approach for Image Registration of Vessel Structures

Stefan Heldmann, Nils Papenberg

Institute of Mathematics, University of Lübeck
heldmann@math.uni-luebeck.de

Abstract. We present a multi-scale approach for non-rigid image registration of tubular tree-like structures such as vessels. Therefore, we consider a Gaussian and a combined morphological and Gaussian scale-space. Similar to a multi-level framework, we solve a sequence of registration problems on several scale-space levels using a standard variational approach for non-liner volumetric image registration. The overall idea is to avoid locally ambiguous mappings between parts of the images by removing morphological details but also finding a global optimal solution by spreading remaining local information using Gaussian scaling. We successfully tested our method on registration of 3D CT and ultrasound images of hepatic vessels.

1 Introduction

Image registration of tubular tree-like structures is a very difficult task. Our work is motivated by a project on Liver surgery. Here, image registration comes into play for the alignment of 3D images of liver where the target structures are vessels. Another example is the analysis of lungs where registration is used for the alignment of the respiratory system. The particular difficulty for image registration is that there are locally many ambiguous mappings between tree-like structures which makes it hard to find a globally optimal alignment.

State-of-the-art approaches rely on intelligent pre-processing. Typically, in a first step segmentation is used to extract vessels. Model-based approaches then try to identify few bifurcation points that are used as landmarks [1, 2] and/or to build a 3D model from the image data [3, 4, 5]. Other approaches use volumetric image registration techniques focusing on edges in the image data. However, all these approaches suffer from the local structure such that extensive user-interaction by an expert is required typically by identifying corresponding bifurcation points.

Our new approach uses ideas from scale-space. For the alignment of major structures we spread local information in the images and construct a Gaussian scale-space from the images and use it in a multi-level fashion. Furthermore, we extent the Gaussian scale-space by a second morphological scale that builds on the observation that anatomical tree-like structures become thinner as ramification becomes finer.

2 Material and methods

We use a standard variational approach for non-liner volumetric image registration [6]. Given two images R (reference) and T (template) we compute a deformation y of the template by minimizing a suitable cost-function $\mathcal{J}$ given by

$$\mathcal{J}(R,T,y) := \mathcal{D}(R,T(y)) + \mathcal{S}(y). \tag{1}$$

Here, $\mathcal{D}$ measures the distance between the reference R and the deformed template $T(y)$. The second building block $\mathcal{S}$ penalizes derivatives of the deformation and thus forces smoothness. We assume the images have been preprocessed by segmentation and therefore are binary images. Consequently, we choose the sum-of-squared-difference (SSD) distance measure. We will not discuss a particular regularizer here. Suitable choices include diffusive, elastic, or curvature regularization [6].

Instead of using the original images directly we construct a scale-space [7] from the images by successively smoothing the image data and removing details. Finally, we solve a sequence of registration problems. Starting on the coarsest scale (least detailed images) we compute a deformation and use the result as initial guess for the next finer scale.

We consider two strategies. First, we construct a Gaussian scale by smoothing the original image data and creating an image pyramid for its use in a multi-level framework. This procedure basically spreads local information. Second, we extend the pure Gaussian scale by a morphological axis to eliminate small vessels structures and thus to focus on the alignment of thick vessels. The second approach is a generalization of the first one. Therefore, we only describe the combined morphological and Gaussian approach in the following.

Addressing the problem of locally ambiguous mappings we introduce morphological scaling of the images. The leading idea is that major vessels are thicker than peripheral ones. For that reason, we use a morphological opening with a ball $\bar{B}_r := \{x : \|x\| \leq r\}$ of radius r. For binary images $R, T : \mathbb{R}^d \to \{0,1\}$ we set

$$R^r := (R \ominus \bar{B}_r) \oplus \bar{B}_r \quad \text{and} \quad T^r := (T \ominus \bar{B}_r) \oplus \bar{B}_r \tag{2}$$

where $(R \ominus \bar{B}_r)(x) := 1$ if $R = 1$ on $x + \bar{B}_r$ and 0 else denotes erosion and $(R \oplus \bar{B}_r)(x) := 1$ if $R \neq 0$ on $x + \bar{B}_r$ and 0 else is dilation. As a result, for $r = 0$

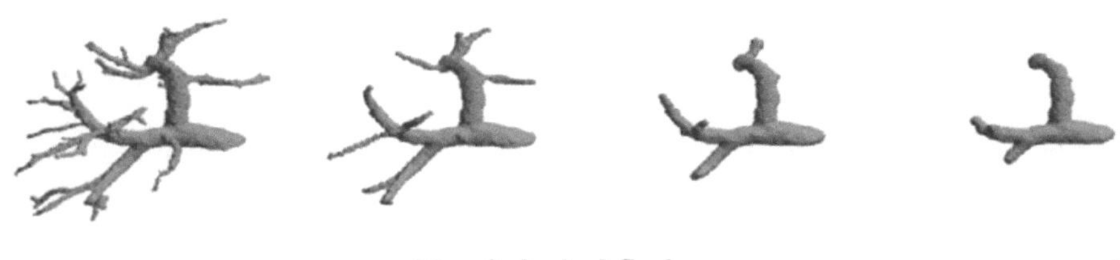

Fig. 1. Morphological scale-space of a 3D vessel system (increasing r left to right)

we have $R^0 = R$, $T^0 = T$ and for increasing scale-space parameter r we remove details from the images. An example is given in Figure 1.

Besides ambiguous mappings another problem is that structural information is very local, i.e., corresponding vessels do not initially overlap which makes registration difficult. To this end, we additionally use a Gaussian scale-space. We define

$$R^{r,\sigma} := R^r * K_\sigma \quad \text{and} \quad T^{r,\sigma} := T^r * K_\sigma$$

where $K_\sigma(x) = (2\pi\sigma^2)^{-\frac{d}{2}} \exp(-\frac{\|x\|^2}{2\sigma^2})$ is a Gaussian with standard deviation σ. Consequently, $R^{r,\sigma} \to R^r$, $T^{r,\sigma} \to T^r$ as $\sigma \to 0$ and with increasing σ more and more local information is dispersed. A 2D example for simulated data with combined morphological and Gaussian scale-space is shown in Figure 2.

Summarizing, we solve a sequence of registration problems for scale-space parameters $(r_1, \sigma_1), \ldots, (r_N, \sigma_N)$ with $r_1 \geq \ldots \geq r_N = 0$ and $\sigma_1 \geq \ldots \geq \sigma_N = 0$. Note that choosing $r_1 = \ldots = r_N = 0$ results a pure Gaussian scale space.

For our numerical method we first discretize the objective function (1) and use a Gauss-Newton optimization method.

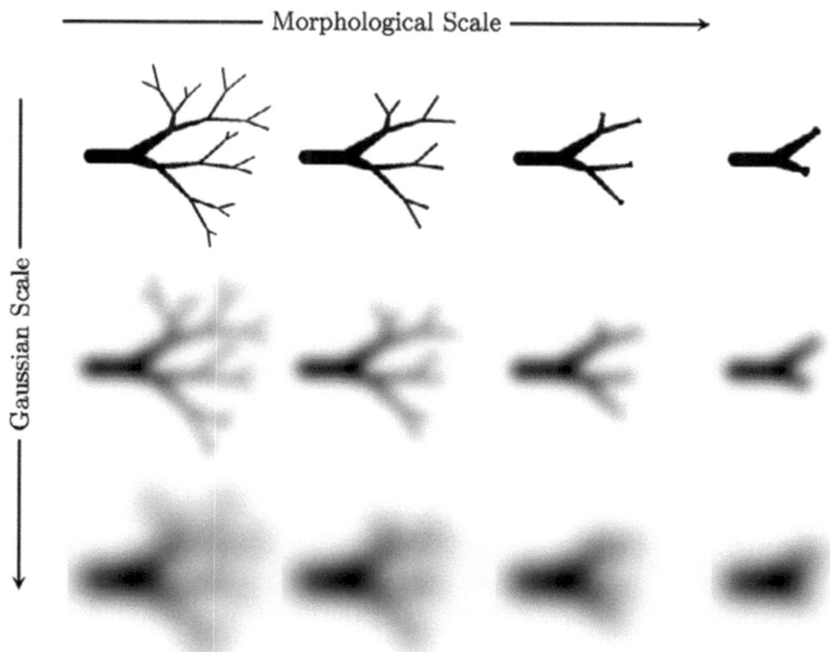

Fig. 2. 2D combined morphological and Gaussian scale

Table 1. SSD relative to pre-registered data after non-rigid registration on the finest-level, using the Gaussian scale-space, and using the combined morphological and Gaussian scale-space.

Strategy	Case 1	Case 2	Case 3	Case 4	Case 5	Case 6
Original	63.95%	36.27%	43.90%	52.71%	17.16%	34.75%
Gaussian	20.59%	23.46%	22.70%	27.52%	9.21%	24.15%
Morph.+Gauss.	19.45%	23.17%	23.49%	26.59%	8.31%	21.25%

3 Results

We tested our method on the registration of hepatic vessels obtained from 3D CT and ultrasound. We totally considered 6 cases. The size of the images was between 128^3 and 256^3 voxels and for each image we constructed 4 morphological and 4 Gaussian scales. The morphological scales were constructed by opening the images with balls of diameters $r = 1, 5, 11, 15$ voxels. For the Gaussian scales we used discrete convolution kernels based on the 1D stencil [0.25 0.5 0.25]. Higher order smoothing was achieved by repeated convolution. Therefore, here the smoothing parameter σ is a discrete number that denotes the number of subsequent convolutions. For our tests we generated 4 scales for $\sigma = 0, 4, 8, 16$.

We compared three different registration strategies. First, we used plain non-rigid registration on the finest level for $(r, \sigma) = (1, 0)$. Second, we used the Gaussian scale-space and performed 4 registrations by choosing (r, σ) as $(1, 16)$, $(1, 8)$, $(1, 4)$, and $(1, 0)$. The third strategy uses both, the morphological and Gaussian scale. Here, we chose the sequence of (r, σ) as $(15, 16)$, $(15, 8)$, $(11, 8)$, $(11, 4)$, $(5, 4)$, $(5, 0)$, and $(1, 0)$.

Furthermore, for each strategy we performed rigid pre-registration.

The results are summarized in Table 1 and a visual comparison for the 4th case is shown in Figure 3.

We found that both scale-space approaches produced good results and significantly outperformed only registration on the finest scale. Thereby, the combined morphological and Gaussian strategy produced the best results.

4 Discussion

We have presented a scale-space approach for the registration of tubular tree-like structures such as vessels. The key-feature is a combined two-dimensional morphological and Gaussian scale-space. The morphological axis allows for scaling the structural level and the Gaussian axis spreads local information to find a globally optimal deformation.

We tested our approach on real data and compared non-rigid registration of the initial images, using a pure Gaussian scale-space, and the combined two-dimensional scale-space. Our experiments showed that the registration significantly benefits from using scale-spaces. Although, the results of the combined

Fig. 3. Registration results for Case 4 (reference bright, template dark)

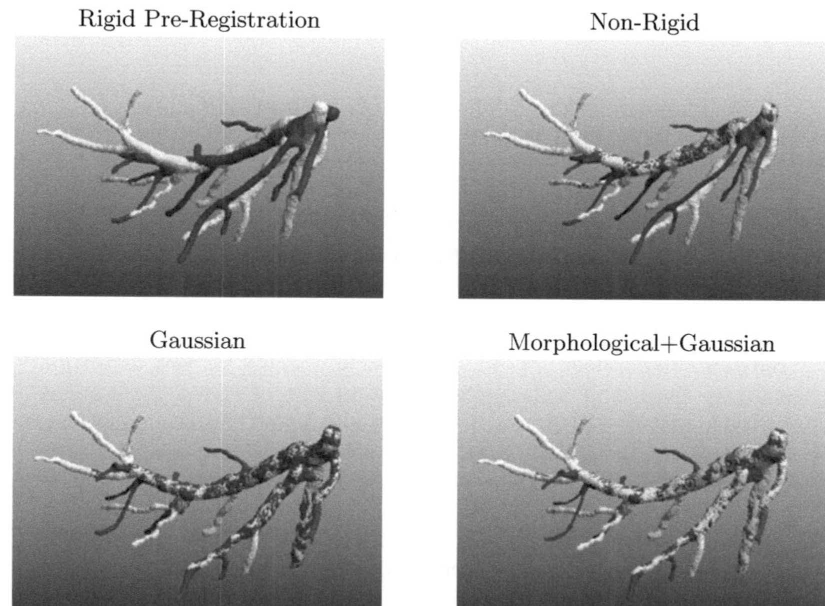

framework are best, to our surprise they are comparable to the pure Gaussian approach which needs further investigation in the future.

A practical benefit is that the method is easy to implement and due to the used scale-spaces it is robust with respect to noise and lack of data.

Summarizing, we conclude that using scale-spaces ideas is inevitable for successful registration of vessel structures.

References

1. Charnoz A, Agnus V, Malandain G, et al. Design of robust vascular tree matching: Validation on liver. LNCS. 2005;3566:443–455.
2. Reinertsen I, Descoteaux M, Siddiqi K, et al. Validation of vessel-based registration for correction of brain shift. Med Image Anal. 2007;11(4):374–388.
3. Aylward SR, Jomier J, Weeks S, et al. Registration and analysis of vascular images. Int J Computer Vis. 2003;55(2-3):123–138.
4. Bühler K, Felkel P, La Cruz A. Geometric methods for vessel visualization and quantification: A survey. In: Brunett G, Hamman B, Müller H, editors. Geometric Modelling for Scientific Visualization. Springer; 2003.
5. Lange T, Eulenstein S, Hünerbein M, et al. Vessel-based non-rigid registration of MR/CT and 3D ultrasound for navigation in liver surgery. Comput Aided Surg. 2003;8(5):228–240.
6. Modersitzki J. Numerical Methods for Image Registration. Numerical Mathematics and Scientific Computation. Oxford University Press; 2003.
7. Weickert J. Anisotropic Diffusion in Image Processing. Teubner; 1998.

Dynamic Distortion Correction for Endoscopy Systems with Exchangeable Optics

Thomas Stehle, Michael Hennes, Sebastian Gross,
Alexander Behrens, Jonas Wulff, Til Aach

Institute of Imaging & Computer Vision,
RWTH Aachen University, D-52056 Aachen, Germany
Thomas.Stehle@lfb.rwth-aachen.de

Abstract. Endoscopic images are strongly affected by lens distortion caused by the use of wide angle lenses. In case of endoscopy systems with exchangeable optics, e.g. in bladder endoscopy or sinus endoscopy, the camera sensor and the optics do not form a rigid system but they can be shifted and rotated with respect to each other during an examination. This flexibility has a major impact on the location of the distortion centre as it is moved along with the optics. In this paper, we describe an algorithm for the dynamic correction of lens distortion in cystoscopy which is based on a one time calibration. For the compensation, we combine a conventional static method for distortion correction with an algorithm to detect the position and the orientation of the elliptic field of view. This enables us to estimate the position of the distortion centre according to the relative movement of camera and optics. Therewith, a distortion correction for arbitrary rotation angles and shifts becomes possible without performing static calibrations for every possible combination of shifts and angles beforehand.

1 Introduction

For many image processing applications like mosaicing [1, 2] or 3D reconstruction [3] the pinhole camera model is assumed as underlying imaging model. In the case of endoscopy, however, this assumption does not hold as the use of wide angle lenses leads to severe lens distortion. Many algorithms are known to compensate for this distortion, e.g. [4, 5].

They rely on the assumption that the optical properties of the imaging system are invariant. Systems for bladder or sinus endoscopy, however, usually feature exchangeable optics so that this assumption does not hold. Because of special mounting adapters used in those systems, which connect the optics to the actual camera, both components can be rotated with respect to each other. As the adapters exhibit some mechanical slackness both components can also be shifted with respect to each other. For these reasons, the distortion centre's location also changes, which makes a successful distortion correction using solely a conventional static approach impossible (Fig. 1).

Fig. 1. Influence of movement of camera sensor and optics with respect to each other. Left: The elliptic field of view is located on the left of the image and its orientation marker is located at the bottom (indicated by circle). Right: The field of view is centred in the image and its orientation marker is located at the lower left. The different positions of the distortion centre in both images are indicated by the cross.

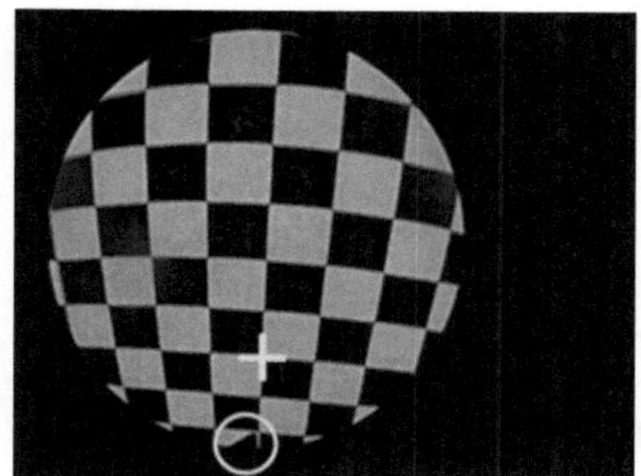

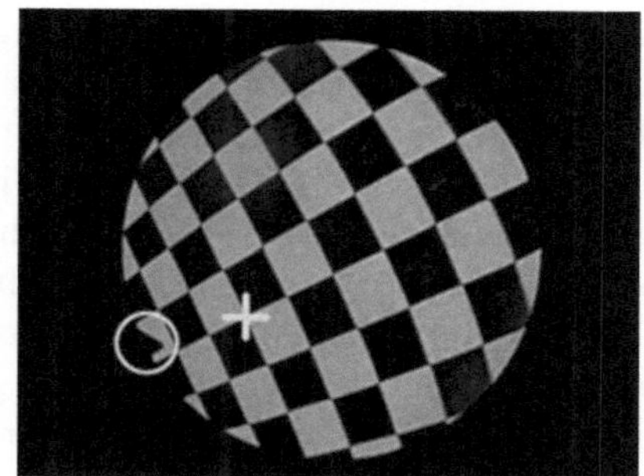

The remainder of this paper is organised as follows: We first present a method for *dynamic* lens distortion correction. To this end, we extend a conventional static distortion correction algorithm with the localisation and the orientation detection of the field of view in each image. Using this information, we estimate the distortion centre's new position. This, in turn, enables us to perform a distortion correction without an explicit calibration for the current rotation angle and shift. We then present a quantitative evaluation which was carried out on synthetically distorted data as well as on real calibration images acquired with an Olympus Excera II video endoscope.

2 Materials and methods

Our dynamic distortion correction algorithm combines the results of a static approach with the localisation and the orientation detection of the field of view (FOV, Fig. 1). The underlying assumption is that the distortion function itself does only change its position and orientation but not its actual shape when camera and optics are shifted and rotated with respect to each other.

For the initial static distortion correction, we use a planar checkerboard pattern as calibration object. The images of this pattern are analysed using Mühlich and Aach's feature extractor for high accuracy camera calibration [6]. As method for static distortion correction, we use Hartley and Kang's approach based on the fundamental matrix [5]. Since their algorithm assumes pure radial distortion, it suffices to estimate the distortion centre's new position and to shift the statically calibrated distortion function to this new location without a further change of the distortion function. However, if a distortion correction model, which also considers tangential distortion (i.e. a function which is not radially symmetric) is used, the distortion field also needs be rotated according to the FOV's rotation.

For FOV detection, we analyse grey value profiles from the image centre to the image border pixels [7]. The position of the FOV border pixels can then be determined by finding the maximum correlation value of a step edge model and the grey value profile. As next step, an ellipse model is robustly fitted to these detected border points using the RANdom SAmple Consensus (RANSAC) algorithm [8]. The RANSAC algorithm rejects border points which do not fit the ellipse model close enough so the parameter estimation becomes more stable. The centre of the ellipse is regarded as the position of the FOV.

As the orientation marker (indicated by a circle in Fig. 1) downsizes the FOV locally, the rejected point with the largest distance to the ellipse is chosen as initial guess for the position of the orientation marker. As the region around the initial position is not sampled densely enough by the grey value profiles to allow an accurate detection of the orientation marker, the region around this point is analysed more closely in order to refine the initial guess. To this end, the contour point is found which maximises the Euclidian distance from the ellipse to the marker contour.

Finally, a new coordinate system is introduced with one axis pointing from the ellipse centre to the orientation marker. The other axis is chosen to be perpendicular to the first one. The distortion centre coordinates are now transformed to this coordinate system, which is invariant with respect to the endoscope's shift and rotation.

In our first experiment, we evaluated the repeatability of the ellipse location detection. To this end, 200 images were taken in which the location of the FOV remained constant. Subsequently, the ellipse detection was carried out and the mean distance to the location as well as the respective standard deviation was calculated.

To verify the hypothesis that the distortion centre moves along with the shift and rotation of the lens, we carried out a second experiment in which the orientation of the FOV was also taken into account. The optic was rotated to eight different angles and 200 calibration images were taken at each orientation. For each position, the distortion centre was determined using Hartley and Kang's algorithm. One of these distortion centres was defined as reference and subsequently shifted and rotated to the remaining seven positions. Then, the distance between the computed and estimated positions was calculated.

A last experiment was carried out in order to assess the impact of a slightly displaced distortion centre on the accuracy of the distortion correction. To this end, the error introduced by a distortion centre, which was displaced by the mean error found in the second experiment, was calculated using a real endoscope's distortion function.

3 Results

In our first experiment, we found that the mean error in the detection of the ellipse position was 0.84 pixels with a standard deviation of 0.63 pixels. Fig. 2(a) shows the results of estimating the distortion centre position. The crosses cor-

Fig. 2. Evaluation of distortion centre estimation. (a) Position of calculated (crosses) and estimated (circles) distortion centres. (b) Mean distance between calculated and updated distortion centres with respective standard deviation.

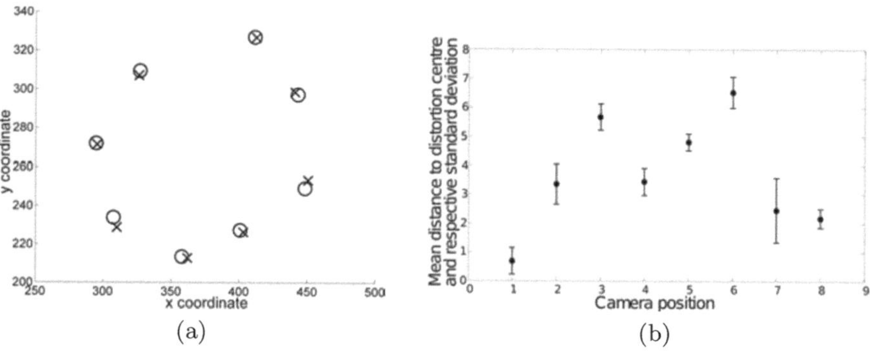

(a) (b)

respond to distortion centres computed with Hartley and Kang's method. The circles correspond to estimated distortion centres. The mean distance between the computed and the estimated distortion centres was 3.1 pixels. These results are quantitatively shown for all rotations in Fig. 2(b).

In Fig. 3, the error in distortion corrected images introduced by a displacement of 3.1 pixels is depicted. Fig. 3(a) shows the error inside of the circular field of view. In Fig. 3(b) a profile through the error function along the plane in Fig. 3(a) can be seen. It is evident that the error in a circular region with a diameter of 450 pixels centred at the estimated centre of distortion is one pixel or lower. The whole FOV has a diameter of about 500 pixels.

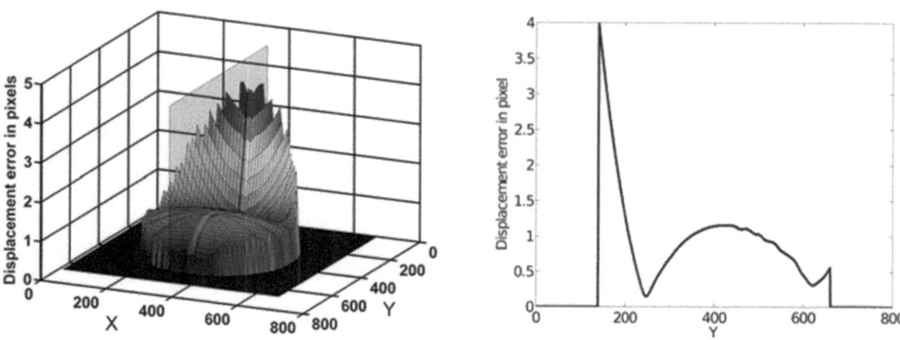

(a) 3D plot showing the error inside the field of view

(b) Profile through 3D error plot along plane indicated in (a)

Fig. 3. Errors introduced by a distortion centre displacement of 3.1 pixels

4 Conclusion

In this paper, we have identified a yet unaddressed topic in the calibration of endoscopes with exchangeable optics. These lenses cannot be fixed entirely to the camera to form a rigid object. Instead, the camera sensor and the optic can be shifted and rotated with respect to each other which has a major influence on the position of the distortion centre.

We have proposed a method to estimate the new position of the distortion centre after a rotation or a shift. Our method combines a classical approach for distortion correction with the detection of the FOV location and orientation. With our approach it becomes possible to carry out one single static calibration, and successfully compensate distortions with arbitrary rotation angle and shift of the optics with respect to the camera sensor.

In our experiments, we have shown that the proposed FOV detection method offers subpixel accuracy for the estimation of the FOV location. In a second experiment, we could verify our hypothesis that the distortion centre moves along with the FOV. In our third experiment, we have evaluated the impact of an imprecisely estimated distortion centre. As displacement we have chosen the mean error as calculated from the second experiment. We found that in a circular area around the estimated centre of distortion with 450 pixels diameter, an acceptable error of less than a pixel is present in the image.

In the future, we will investigate the sources of the remaining error. One possibility which has not yet been addressed is a tilt between camera and optics.

References

1. Konen W, Breiderhoff B, Scholz M. Real-time image mosaic for endoscopic video sequences. Proc BVM. 2007; p. 298–302.
2. Behrens A. Creating panoramic images for bladder fluorescence endoscopy. Acta Polytech: J Adv Eng. 2008;3:50–54.
3. Stehle T, Truhn D, Aach T, et al. Camera calibration for fish-eye lenses in endoscopy with an application to 3D reconstruction. Procs IEEE ISBI. 2007 April; p. 1176–1179.
4. Kannala J, Brandt SS. A generic camera model and calibration method for conventional, wide-angle, and fish-eye lenses. IEEE Trans PAMI. 2006;28(8):1335–1340.
5. Hartley R, Kang SB. Parameter-free radial distortion correction with center of distortion estimation. IEEE Trans PAMI. 2007;29(8):1309–1321.
6. Mühlich M, Aach T. High accuracy feature detection for camera calibration: A multi-steerable approach. LNCS. 2007;(4713):284–293.
7. Stache NC, Zimmer H, Gedicke J, et al. Robust high-speed melt pool measurements for laser welding with sputter detection capability. LNCS. 2007;4713:476–485.
8. Fischler MA, Bolles RC. Random sample consensus: A paradigm for model fitting with applications to image analysis and automated cartography. Commun ACM. 1981 June;24(6):381–395.

Evaluation Scheme for a Positron Emission Tomography System Used in Monitoring of Radiation Therapy

Georgy Shakirin[1], Fine Fiedler[1], Wolfgang Enghardt[1,2]

[1]Institute of Radiation Physics, Forschungszentrum Dresden-Rossendorf, Dresden
[2]OncoRay, Technische Universität Dresden
g.shakirin@fzd.de

Abstract. Positron emission tomography (PET) is used for independent monitoring of dose delivery in ion therapy. An in-beam PET scanner registers the annihilation γ-rays following the decay of β^+-radioactive nuclei produced via nuclear reactions between the ions of the therapeutic beam and the irradiated tissue. From a comparison of the reconstructed activity distributions with those predicted from the treatment plan, deviations between the prescribed and the applied dose can be detected. In-beam PET, therefore, allows to verify the physical beam model of the treatment planning, to detect patient dislocations and density changes in the irradiated tissue. Issues related to the image quality and evaluation of a whole PET imaging system are discussed in this paper.

1 Introduction

An in-beam PET scanner is used to measure β^+-activity distributions corresponding to the applied dose during therapeutic irradiation. The reconstructed β^+-activity image allows to evaluate the conformity and accuracy of the performed treatment. The main task of in-beam PET is to detect and interpret deviations from the prescribed and actually applied dose. The applied dose is characterized by the measured β^+-activity distribution. Representing different physical processes, dose and β^+-activity distribution cannot be compared directly. Therefore, an expected β^+-activity distribution based on the prescribed dose is simulated [1]. The quality assurance of the irradiation is then performed by a comparison of the expected (corresponding to the prescribed dose) and the measured (corresponding to the actually applied dose) β^+-activity distributions.

The in-beam PET scanner BASTEI (Fig. 1) is installed at the heavy ion therapy facility at the Gesellschaft für Schwerionenforschung (GSI), Darmstadt, Germany [1, 2]. Since 1997 irradiation of more than 400 patients have been monitored there by means of in-beam PET. A dedicated, limited angle configuration of the in-beam PET scanner (Fig. 1), a very low counting statistics, and requirement of fast (ideally, real time) availability of in-beam PET images for analysis make the imaging process a challenging task. Based on more than 10 year experience of the clinical exploitation of the in-beam PET technology specific quality criteria and an evaluation workflow for an in-beam PET imaging system have been developed.

2 Materials and methods

2.1 Quality criteria for in-beam PET

Three criteria are used for evaluation of imaging capabilities of an in-beam PET system: root mean square error (RMSE), contrast recovery value for NEMA-like phantom, and range modification trials [3]. RMSE (1) shows the average image noise and is not sensitive to particular image details.

$$RMSE = \sqrt{\sum_{j=1}^{N}(x_j - x_j^*)^2/N}, \tag{1}$$

where N is a number of elements (pixels for 2D or voxels for 3D) of the image, x_j is the reference value of activity, and x_j^* is the reconstructed activity value at element j. NEMA-like phantom (Fig. 2) specially adapted for counting statistics and size of irradiated volume of in-beam PET is used for the contrast recovery calculation (2):

$$LCRH = \frac{MH - MB}{3MB} \cdot 100\%; \quad LCRC = \frac{MB - MC}{MB} \cdot 100\%, \tag{2}$$

where $LCRH$ is local contrast recovery ratio for the high activity areas (four hot spheres), $LCRC$ is local contrast recovery ratio for the areas of no activity (two cold spheres and the central cylinder). MH, MB, and MC are median values for activity inside hot spheres, background, and cold areas, respectively. The median value for the background is calculated locally near each cold or hot

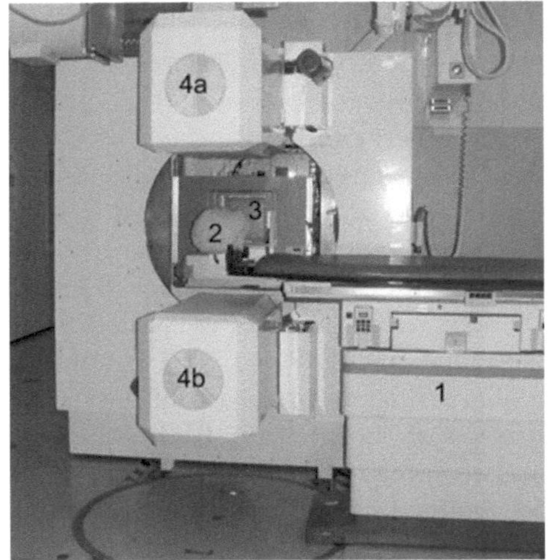

Fig. 1. In-beam PET scanner BASTEI installed at GSI. Positioning of a patient is performed with rotation, vertical, and horizontal movements of the couch (1). The individual patient immobilization mask (2) is fixed on the couch. The irradiation beam arrives through the window (3). The PET scanner consists of two heads (4a and 4b).

area. In the ideal case $MH = 4MB$, $MC = 0$ and $LCRH = LCRC = 100\%$. In the worst case $MH = MC = MB$ (hot area and cold areas are not recognized from the background) and $LCRH = LCRC = 0\%$.

For in-beam PET any deviations from norm, e.g. changes in the structure (density) of the irradiated tissue or mispositioning of the patient, usually cause a deviation in the maximum particle range. Therefore, the third image quality criterion is based on the light modification of the maximum particle range for real treatment plans and simulation of β^+-activity distributions [3] as shown in (Fig. 3). This quality criterion evaluates the most important imaging characteristics of in-beam PET - the sensitivity of the system to modification of irradiation range. However, it is the most time consuming and requires skills in visual analysis of in-beam PET images.

2.2 Scheme for quality evaluation

The integration of an in-beam PET system into particle therapy facility relies on the two main issues: i) choosing of an optimum form of the scanner which fulfills the requirements of the treatment room and provides acceptable imaging capabilities and ii) optimization of reconstruction algorithm for fast delivery of high quality images. The first problem can be solved using a dedicated software tool based on the OpenGL technology. The program receives the dimensions and degrees of freedom for objects (beam nozzle, patient couch, etc.) inside the treatment room as parameters. Then a collision free solution for the integrated in-beam PET scanner is manually generated. The program returns a lookup table with coordinates and position of all detectors of the PET scanner. ML-EM [4], RFS-EM [5], and dTOF [6] reconstruction algorithms can be applied for in-beam PET data. Each reconstruction algorithm has a number of parameters to optimize (number of iterations, size of the image element, etc.). A semiautomatic workflow has been developed in order to find an optimum solution concerning position and geometry of a PET scanner and the reconstruction algorithm (Fig. 4). The steps of the evaluation workflow are performed automatically except the range modification trial which requires experienced human observers. The rough selection of reconstruction parameters and a scanner is

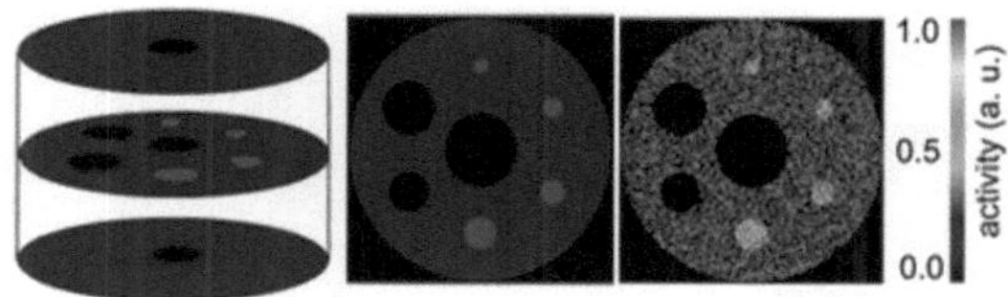

Fig. 2. Left: Schematic view of the NEMA phantom for in-beam PET (up, middle and bottom slices). Central slices of the ideal (center) and simulated (right) NEMA phantoms. The simulated phantom consists of annihilation points distributed according to the predefined concentrations(4 : 1 : 0 for hot, background, and cold areas, respectively).

done using only two image quality criteria - RMSE and the contrast recovery. Finally, a whole imaging system with the selected parameters must be proven by means of the range modification trial.

3 Results

The discussed evaluation workflow and the image quality criteria have been used to find an optimum solution for in-beam PET system. Different reconstruction algorithms (ML-EM [4], RFS-EM [5], and dTOF [6]) have been tested. The dTOF algorithm showed the best image quality. It reconstructed images in real time. However, the detectors required for it are not yet commercially available. More than 50 different schemes for the iterative ML-EM and RFS-EM algorithms have been automatically tested using RMSE and the contrast recovery criteria. The optimum scheme with only 4 iterations through the whole dataset (only 20-120 s of reconstruction time depending on the image size and the counting statistics) has been found and finally tested with the range modification trial. It was possible to recognize the range modification equivalent to 6 mm in water for the most typical patient cases. These results allowed to substitue the standard ML-EM algorithm (5-10 min of reconstruction time) with the fast RFS-EM algortihm (20-120 s of reconstruction time) without reducing the sensitivity of the in-beam PET method to the range modifications.

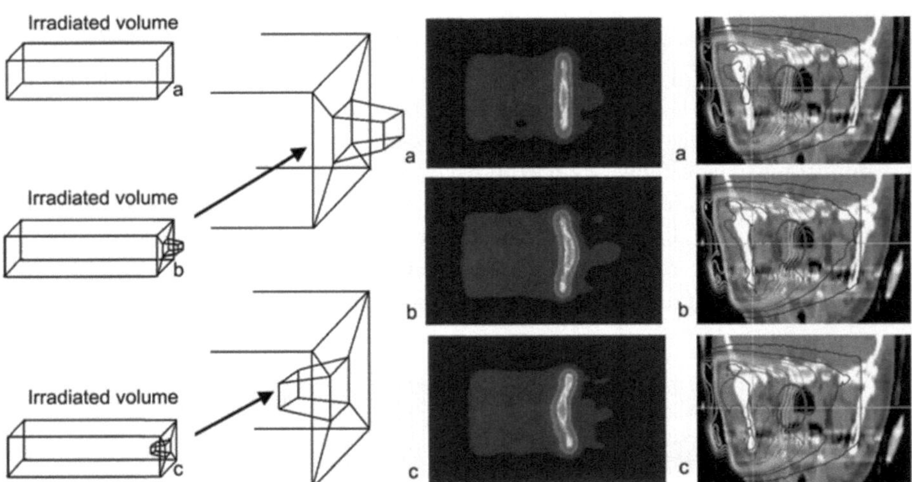

Fig. 3. Schematic view of the range modification (left). Simulations of the β^+-activity distribution in PMMA phantom (centre) and based of the patient plans (right). (a) corresponds to unmodified range, (b) - to enlarged range, and (c) - to reduced range.

4 Discussion

The dedicated image quality criteria for evaluation of an in-beam PET imaging system have been developed. It is suggested to apply the two numeric criteria - RMSE and the contrast recovery - first in order to exclude the low image quality cases. Finally, the range modification trial must be performed using data of several patients. This test has to be accomplished by the experienced human observers using representative set of the real patient treatment plans. The sequential way of the image quality evaluation allows to save a lot of time because most of non-optimal parameters can be rejected during the fast automated analysis. The evaluation workflow (Fig. 4) allows to select and evaluate the geometry and a position of the PET scanner in 3D taking into account position and degrees of freedom of other equipment of the treatment room using a dedicated software tool based on the OpenGL technology. Only simulated data are required for this workflow. Therefore, it is possible to perform a fully virtual analysis of imaging capabilities of an in-beam PET system before any prototype is built.

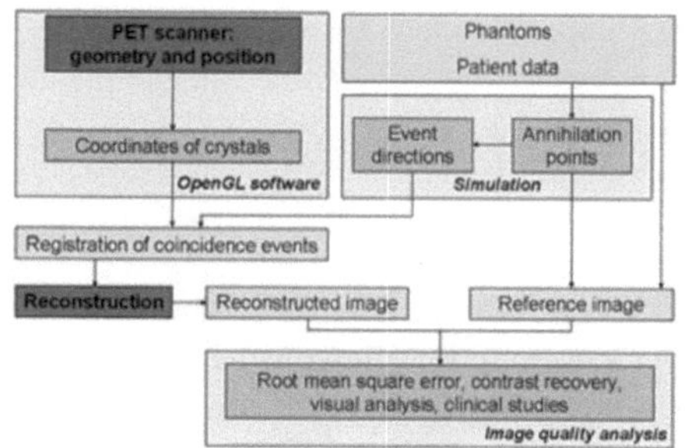

Fig. 4. Evaluation workflow for a PET scanner and reconstruction algorithm. The position and geometery of a PET scanner and a reconstruction algorithm are evaluated using simulated phantoms and patient data. The evaluation is performed using the image quality criteria: RMSE, contrast recovery, visual analysis, and the range modification trial (clinical srudies).

References

1. Enghardt W, Parodi K, Crespo P, et al. Dose quantification from in-beam positron emission tomography. Radiother Oncol. 2004;73:96–98.
2. Enghardt W, Crespo P, Fiedler F, et al. Charged hadron tumour therapy monitoring by means of PET. Nucl Instrum Methods Phys Res. 2004;525:284–288.
3. Fiedler F, Shakirin G, Crespo P, et al. On the efficiency of ion range determination from in-beam PET data. Radiother Oncol. submitted.
4. Pönisch F, Enghardt W, Lauckner K. Attenuation and scatter correction for in-beam positron emission tomography monitoring of tumour irradiations with heavy ions. Phys Med Biol. 2003;48:2419–2436.
5. Shakirin G, Crespo P, Enghardt W. A method for system matrix construction and processing for reconstruction of in-beam PET data. IEEE Trans Nucl Sci. 2007;54:1710–1716.
6. Crespo P, Shakirin G, Fiedler F, et al. Direct time-of-flight for quantitative, real-time in-beam PET: A concept and feasibility study. phys. med. biol., 52: pp. 6795-6811, 2007. Phys Med Biol. 2007;52:6795–6811.

Super-Resolution für mobile C-Bogen-Systeme

C. Bodensteiner[1], C. Darolti, A. Schweikard[1]

[1]Institut für Robotik und Kognitive Systeme, Uni Lübeck
bodensteiner@rob.uni-luebeck.de

Kurzfassung. Unter dem Begriff der Superresolution versteht man Algorithmen aus der Bildverarbeitung zur Auflösungssteigerung mittels niedrig aufgelöster Bilddaten. Die Roboterisierung eines mobilen C-Bogens bietet nun die Möglichkeit die physikalische Auflösung des Aufnahmesystems mittels dieser Techniken zu erhöhen. Anhand eines synthetischen CT-Phantoms wurden hierbei gängige Super-Resolution Verfahren evaluiert. Daneben werden Details zur Daten-Akquise und Fehler-Kompensation erläutert. Mittels eines prototypischen C-Bogen Systems konnten 3-4 fache Auflösungssteigerungen erreicht werden. Hierbei wurden Strukturen sichtbar, welche in den ursprünglichen Daten nicht erkennbar waren.

1 Einleitung

Unter dem Begriff der Superresolution (SR) versteht man Algorithmen aus der Bildverarbeitung zur Errechnung hoch aufgelösten (HR) Bildmaterials aus einer Sequenz von Bilddaten, die jedoch nur in einer niedrigen Auflösung (LR) vorliegen. Hierbei sind im Allg. zwei eng gekoppelte Probleme zu lösen. Einerseits gilt es die Bewegung zwischen den gemessenen LR-Daten zu bestimmen, andererseits muss ein Rekonstruktionsproblem gelöst werden um die HR-Daten aus den LR-Daten unter der Modellierung des Bildaufnahmenprozesses zu errechnen. Super-Resolution ist seit über 30 Jahren ein äußerst aktives Forschungsgebiet der Bildverarbeitung. Jedoch werden diese Techniken erst seit kurzem erfolgreich im Bereich der medizinischen Bildgebung verwendet [1]. Einen guten Überblick über gängige SR-Methoden bieten hierbei die Arbeiten von Farsiu et al. [2]. Frühere Ansätze in diesem Feld arbeiteten meist im Frequenzraum. Neuere Verfahren arbeiten meist im Ortsraum, da hier komplexere Bewegungsmodelle eingesetzt werden können. Sie zielen vor allem auf die gekoppelte Lösung der Bewegungs- und Rekonstruktionsparameter [3] ab. Im Bereich der Röntgenbildgebung finden sich erstaunlicherweise nur wenige Arbeiten. Bernhardt et al. [4] schlagen vor Super-Resolution Algorithmen in der pädiatrischen Radiologie zu verwenden, jedoch werden weder Details über benutzte Verfahren noch detaillierte Ergebnisse präsentiert. Mögliche medizinische Applikationen könnten sich dabei bei der frühzeitigen Diagnose von Osteoporose oder der Detektion von Calcifikationen ergeben.

2 Material und Methoden

Die Aufnahme der Bildsequenzen erfolgte mit zwei verschiedenen Aquisitionsprofilen. Generell besteht bei der SR-Röntgen-Bildgebung das Problem der Parallaxe, welche beispielsweise bei der Translation der Röntgenquelle zu unterschiedlichen Strahlverläufen und damit zu Inkonsistenzen in der Rekonstruktion führt. Vorerst wurden folgende Aquisitionsstrategien verwendet:

2.1 Rotation um die Strahlenquelle

Die allgemeine projektive Abbildung zwischen den einzelnen Projektionsdaten lässt sich hierbei folgendermaßen formalisieren: Ohne Beschränkung der Allgemeinheit wird das Weltkoordinatensystem in das erste Kamarakoordinatensystem gelegt. Jedes Projektionsbild $I_i, i \in 1,..,m$ muss dabei von einer leicht veränderten Kameraposition akquiriert werden, die mittels der Transformation T_i erreicht wird. Die Transformation kann dabei in einen $3x3$ Rotationsanteil R_i und einen Translationsanteil t_i zerlegt werden. Die Abbildung durch das Röntgensystem wird mittels einer einfachen Lochkamera mit Projektionsmatrix K (intrinsische Parameter) modelliert. Dies führt zu folgender Beziehung zwischen einem Punkt p und seinen zwei-dimensionalen Projektionen p_i in homogenen Koordinaten:

$$\boldsymbol{p_i} = K(R_i\boldsymbol{p} + \boldsymbol{t_i}). \tag{1}$$

Durch Einbeziehung der projektiven Tiefe z bzw. z' des Punktes $\boldsymbol{p} = (x, y, z)^T$ gelten folgende Gleichungen:

$$p = zK^{-1}\boldsymbol{p_0}, R_i\boldsymbol{p} + \boldsymbol{t} = z'K^{-1}\boldsymbol{p_i} \tag{2}$$

Eine alleinige Rotation um die Strahlenquelle führt dabei zu der bekannten projektiven Transformation H_i:

$$z'K^{-1}\boldsymbol{p_i} = zR_iK^{-1}\boldsymbol{p_0}, \boldsymbol{p_i} = \frac{z}{z'}KR_iK^{-1}\boldsymbol{p_0} \tag{3}$$

Diese Homography $H_i = KR_iK^{-1}$ (konjugierte Rotation) ist dabei unabhängig von der aufgenommen 3D Struktur und gilt für alle Punkte p. Abhängig von der Zielauflösung wird nun das HR-Gitter mit dem C-Bogensystem abgefahren (Versätze ensprechen den Pixelabständen im HR-Bild).

2.2 Planare Translation

Bei einer Translation der Röntgenkamera können nur koplanare Punkte mittels einer Homographie ([5]) zueinander in Beziehung gesetzt werden. Aus diesem Grund können keine guten SR-Ergebnisse erwartet werden, wenn das Objekt eine große Ausdehnung in Richtung der Kamerahauptachse besitzt. Durch die Roboterisierung lassen sich jedoch äußerst kleine Translationen realisieren was

Tabelle 1. Rekonstruktionsergebnisse mit verrauschten Eingabedaten. 4-fache Auflösungserhöhung. Alle Angaben geben die L_2-Norm des Differenzvektors wieder.

	Anzahl Bilder								
Algorithmus	15	16	17	18	19	20	21	22	23
Interpolation	2465	2593	2565	2666	2485	2522	2545	2519	2524
N. Convol.	1764	1782	1663	1702	1623	1663	1626	1646	1611
Papoulis G.	24203	30000	26157	22372	18586	18602	18620	14823	14841
POCS	2831	2904	2903	2957	3032	3038	3045	3150	3157
Zomet	6016	5770	5602	5541	5609	5564	5542	5470	5524

in der Praxis dennoch gute Ergebnisse zur Folge hatte. Analog zur Rotationsaufnahme wurde hierbei das HR-Gitter durch Translationen in der Bildebene des C-Bogens abgefahren.

Es ist allgemein bekannt, dass SR-Algorithmen in der Praxis durch die Genauigkeit der Bestimmung der stattgefundenen Bewegung limitiert sind. Um etwaige Positionierungs- und Aufnahmefehler des robotischen Röntgen-Systems auszugleichen, konnte nicht auf eine 2D-Registrierung der einzelnen LR-Daten verzichtet werden. Hierbei kam die Methode nach [6] zum Einsatz. Zur Evaluation gängiger SR-Algorithmen wurde ein synthetischer CT-Datensatz entworfen (Fig. 1). Er setzt sich aus fünf kreisförmigen Objekten zusammen welche wiederum aus dreidimensionalen Gittern (Gitterdicke 0,3 mm) mit ansteigenden Abständen (0,3 mm, ..., 1,8 mm) bestehen. Basierend auf diesem CT-Datensatz wurden nun simulierte Röntgenbilder (DRR's) in vier unterschiedlichen Auflösungen generiert ($568^2, ..., 2272^2$). Die intrinsischen Parameter wurden dabei analog zum bestehenden prototypischen C-Bogen gewählt: focal length: 960mm, pixel scale 0.40mm/px). Anschließend wurden aus einer Menge (Anzahl abhängig von der jeweiligen Auflösungsstufe) von niedrig aufgelösten Projektionsdaten eine Projektion in hoher Auflösung rekonstruiert (mit Verwendung der 2D-Registrierung für die Bewegungsschätzung) und mit der vorher exakt berechneten hochaufgelösten Projektion verglichen. Echte Projektionsdaten wurden mittels eines experimentellen roboterisierten C-Bogen aufgenommen. Als Rekonstruktionsverfahren kamen dabei die folgenden Verfahren zum Einsatz: Bi-Cubische Interpolation [7], Projection on Convex Sets (POCS) [6], Normalized Convolution (NC) [8], Papoulis Gerchberg (PG) [9], Robust Super-Resolution nach Zomet [10]. Für eine detaillerte Beschreibung verweisen wir auf die entsprechende Literatur. Als Rekonstruktionsverfahren kamen dabei die Folgenden Verfahren zum Einsatz: Bi-cubische Interpolation der Daten am HR-Gitter, Normalized Convolution, Projection on Convex Sets (POCS), Verfahren nach Papoulis Gerchberg und Verfahren nach Zomet. Für eine detaillerte Beschreibung der einzelnen Verfahren verweisen wir auf die entsprechende Literatur.

Abb. 1. Synthetischer CT-Datensatz zur Evaluation (links). Eingabebild mit künstlichem Rauschen. Rekonstruierte Projektion aus 16 Eingabebildern mittels NC.

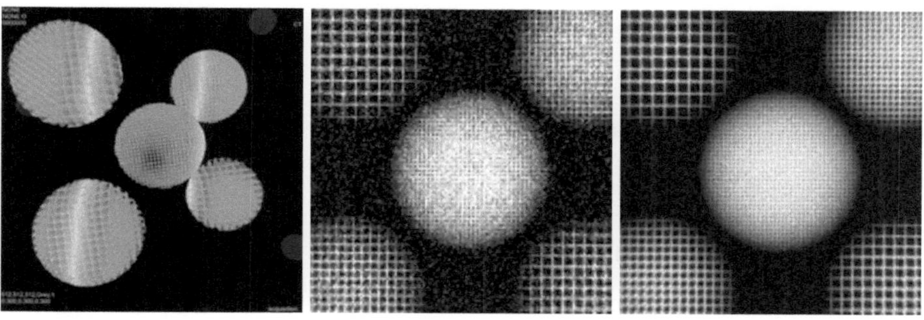

Abb. 2. Implementierte Super-Resolution Software Umgebung (links). Durch die Automatisierung des Bildgebungssytems erfolgt eine adaptive Akquisition. Visualisierung der Auflösungsverbesserung von realen Daten: Ausschnitt einer Projektion in Originalauflösung (mitte). Rechts: Gleicher Ausschnitt mit 4-facher Auflösungserhöhung.

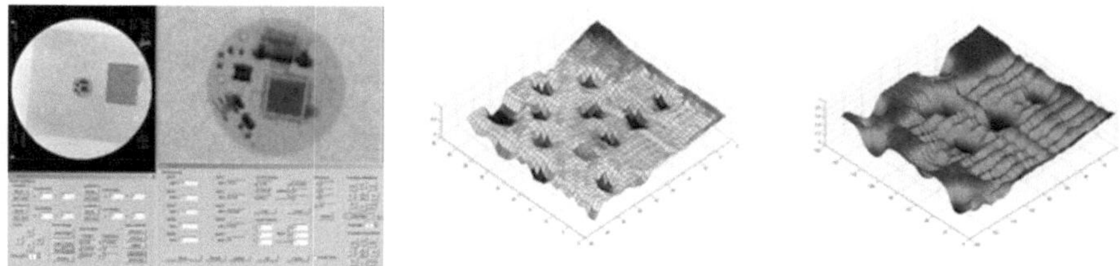

3 Ergebnisse

Bei den simulierten Projektionsdaten ergaben sich die in Tab. 1 dargestellten Ergebnisse. Eine beispielhafte Rekonstruktion ist in Fig. 1 abgebildet.

4 Diskussion

Obwohl die mathematischen Grundlagen der Super-Resolution weitgehendst untersucht wurden [2], gibt es unserer Kenntnis nach im Bereich der Röntgenbildgebung mittels mobiler C-Bögen keine detaillierte Literatur zur Anwendung dieser Techniken. Hierbei bietet die Roboterisierung eines C-Bogen Systems eine elegante Möglichkeit zur adaptiven Steigerung der Auflösung. Bei der Evaluation erwies sich dabei das Normalized Convolution Verfahren meist als überlegen. In diesem Beitrag wurden dabei Details erläutert, um diese Techniken praktisch umzusetzen. Darüber hinaus wurde neben einer Evaluation gängiger Verfahren auch eine erste prototypische Implementierung mit einem robotischen C-Bogen System präsentiert. Hierbei konnten 3-4 fache Auflösungssteigerungen erzielt werden. Zukünftige Arbeiten zielen vor allem auf die weitere Optimierung der Rekonstruktions- und Positionskorrektur-Verfahren.

Abb. 3. a) Beispiel eines Eingabebildes. Ergebnisse: b) Zomet. c) Bi-cub. Interp d) POCS e) NC f) NC mit Polynombasis 3.Grades.

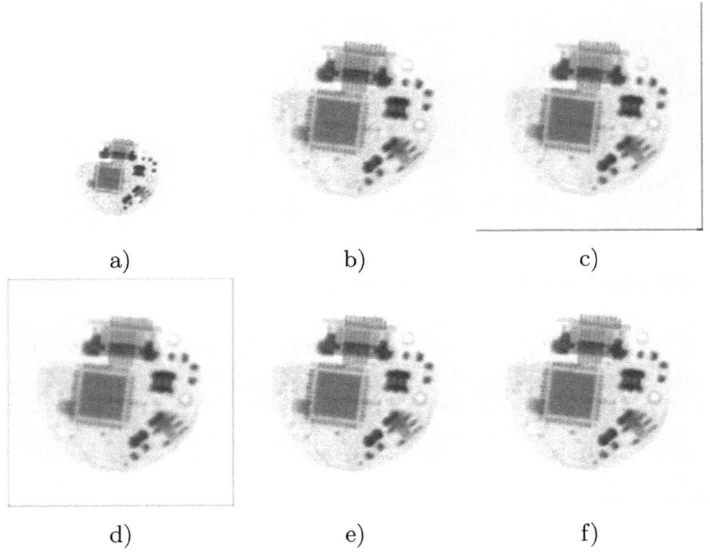

Literaturverzeichnis

1. Greenspan H. Super-resolution in medical imaging. The Computer Journal Advance Access. 2008.
2. Farsiu S, Robinson D, Elad M, et al. Advances and challenges in super-resolution. Int J Imag Sys Tech. 2004;14:47–57.
3. Chung J, Haber E, Nagy J. Numerical methods for coupled super-resolution. Inverse Problems. 2006;22:1261–1272.
4. Bernhardt P, Lendl M, Deinzer F. New technologies to reduce pediatric radiation doses. Pediatr Radiol. 2006;36:212–215.
5. Yaniv Z, Joskowicz L. Long bone panoramas from fluoroscopic x-ray images. IEEE Trans Med Imaging. 2004;23:26–35.
6. Vandewalle P. Super Resolution from unregistered aliased images. EPF Lausanne; 2006.
7. Kim SP, Bose NK, Valenzuela HM. Recursive reconstruction of high resolution image from noisy undersampled multiframes. IEEE Trans Acoust Speech. 1990;38:1013–1027.
8. Pham TQ, van Vliet LJ, Schutte K. Robust fusion of irregularly sampled data using adaptive normalized convolution. EURASIP J Appl Signal Process. 2006; p. 12.
9. Marques M, Neves A, Marques JS, et al. The Papoulis-Gerchberg algorithm with unknown signal bandwidth. In: Image Analysis and Recognition. Springer, Berlin; 2006.
10. Zomet A, Rav-acha A, Peleg S. Robust super resolution. In: Proc IEEE Workshop on Applications of Computer Vision; 2001. p. 645–650.

Echtzeit-Ultraschallsimulation auf Grafik-Prozessoren mit CUDA

Tobias Reichl[1,2], Josh Passenger[2], Oscar Acosta[2], Olivier Salvado[2]

[1] Computer-Aided Medical Procedures (CAMP), TUM, München
[2] CSIRO, ICTC, The Australian e-Health Research Centre – Biomedical Imaging, Royal Brisbane and Women's Hospital, Herston, Australien
reichl@in.tum.de

Kurzfassung. Trotz der zunehmenden Verbreitung jüngerer bildgebender Verfahren bleibt medizinischer Ultraschall (US) weiterhin ein wichtiges Hilfsmittel bei chirurgischen Eingriffen und der klinischen Diagnose. Viele US-gestützte medizinische Prozeduren erfordern allerdings ausgiebiges Training, so dass es wünschenswert ist, eine realistische Simulation von US-Bildern zur Verfügung zu stellen. Im Gegensatz zu früheren Ansätzen simulieren wir solche Bilder auf der „Graphics Processing Unit". Wir erweitern hierzu eine Methode, die von Wein et al. für die Abschätzung von US-Reflexionen aus Daten der Computertomographie (CT) vorgeschlagen wurde, zu einer leichter zu berechnenden Form. Zusätzlich schätzen wir die US-Absorption aus den CT-Daten ab. Mit Hilfe von NVIDIAs „Compute Unified Device Architecture" (CUDA) simulieren wir Reflexion, Verschattung, Rauschen und radiale Unschärfe, ausgehend von unbearbeiteten CT-Daten in Echtzeit und ohne Vorausberechnung.

1 Einleitung

Für bereits existierende Ansätze zur Simulation von US-Bildern sind die verfügbaren Rechnerkapazitäten üblicherweise begrenzt durch Echtzeit-Anforderungen. Aktuelle Veröffentlichungen [1, 2, 3, 4] zeigen teils viel versprechende Ergebnisse, sind aber wegen oftmals fehlender Angaben zum Umfang bzw. der erreichbaren Bildgröße der Simulation meist nicht direkt vergleichbar.

Es wurden bereits Ansätze vorgestellt, die Rechenleistung moderner Grafikkarten für diese Zwecke zu nutzen, diese nutzen die „Graphics Processing Unit" (GPU) allerdings entweder nicht durchgängig [5] oder nur z.B. zur nachträglichen Simulation von radialer Unschärfe [2]. Wir stellen nun das Konzept einer Implementierung mittels NVIDIAs „Compute Unified Device Architecture" (CUDA) vor, bei der die US-Simulation durchgehend auf der Grafikkarte stattfindet.

2 Materialien und Methoden

Die einzelnen Berechnungsschritte unserer Simulation sind in Abbildung 1 zusammengefasst: in Abhängigkeit von der aktuellen Position und Orientierung

Abb. 1. Aus 3-D CT-Daten, 3-D Rauschen, Position und Einstellungen der virtuellen Sonde wird ein Ultraschallbild simuliert.

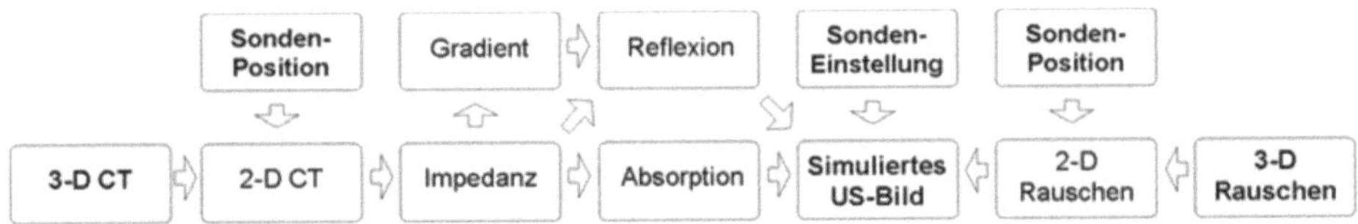

der virtuellen US-Sonde wird ein 2-D Bild aus einem 3-D CT-Datensatz ausgeschnitten. Anschließend werden die physikalischen Eigenschaften des Gewebes, d.h. akustische Impedanz, Reflexion und Absorption anhand von Gewebedichte und -grenzen abgeschätzt. Schließlich werden in einem weiteren Schritt künstlich US-typisches Rauschen und radiale Unschärfe eingefügt. Das entstandene Bild (vgl. Abbildung 2) kann in Echtzeit und entsprechend den vom Benutzer gewählten Parametern aktualisiert werden.

Die akustische Impedanz schätzen wir hierbei anhand der bekannten Werte für Luft, Wasser und eines geschätzten Wertes für Knochengewebe ($Z = 7$ Mrayl und $\mu = 1000$ HU) aus den ursprünglichen CT-Daten ab. Wie in der Optik lässt sich zeigen, dass das Snelliussche Brechungsgesetz auch für US gilt, und dass der Anteil I_r/I_i der an einer spekularen Grenzfläche reflektierten Intensität berechnet werden kann als

$$\frac{I_r}{I_i} = \left(\frac{Z_2 \cdot \cos\theta_i - Z_1 \cdot \cos\theta_t}{Z_2 \cdot \cos\theta_i + Z_1 \cdot \cos\theta_t}\right)^2 \overset{\theta \approx 0}{\approx} \left(\frac{Z2 - Z1}{Z2 + Z1}\right)^2 \tag{1}$$

wobei Z_1 und Z_2 die akustischen Impedanzen der beiden Gewebearten und θ_i und θ_t die Einfalls- bzw. Ausfallswinkel sind. Diese Gleichung wird üblicherweise zum

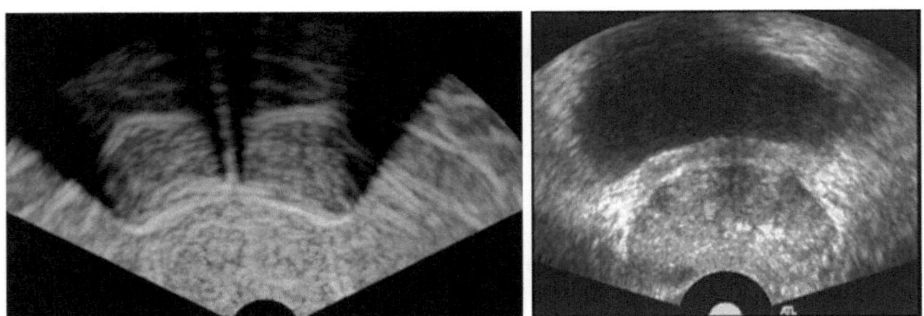

Abb. 2. Screenshot der Ultraschallsimulation, konfiguriert wie eine transrektale Sonde (links, Abbildung aus [6]), zusammen mit einem ähnlichen Bild aus einer realen transrektalen Ultraschalluntersuchung (rechts, Bild mit freundlicher Genehmigung von Robarts Research Institute). Zur besseren Darstellung wurden beide Bilder identisch aufgehellt. Die ausgeprägten Verschattungen im simulierten Bild entstehen durch Reflexion und Absorption an Grenzflächen und sind in diesem Fall deutlich stärker als im Vergleichsbild.

Fall des senkrechten Einfalls $\theta = 0$ vereinfacht, falls keine oder nur unzuverlässige Informationen über die lokalen Normalen vorhanden sind.

Nachdem wir nur Intensität betrachten, die direkt zur Sonde zurück reflektiert wird, müssen wir im allgemeinen Fall diffuse statt spekulare Reflexion berücksichtigen. Bei ideal diffuser Reflexion wird die eintreffende Intensität gleichförmig in alle Raumrichtungen reflektiert. Ein Modell für diffuse Reflexion ist das Lambertsche Gesetz $I_r/I_i = \cos(\alpha)$, wobei α der Winkel zwischen der Richtung des eintreffenden Strahls und der Oberflächennormalen ist.

Üblicherweise wird durch die Verwendung von $I_r/I_i = \cos(\alpha)^n$ eine Kombination aus diffuser und spekularer Reflexion angenähert, wobei $n = 1$ der ideal diffusen Reflexion entspricht. Spekulare Reflexion tritt in US-Aufnahmen tatsächlich auf, z.B. an Grenzflächen zu Knochengewebe, aber die Größenordnung der für US-Reflexion relevanten Unregelmäßigkeiten in den Grenzschichten (US-Wellenlänge rund 0,6 bis 0,15 mm) ist deutlich unterhalb der üblichen Auflösung für CT-Aufnahmen des Bauchraums (z.B. 0,88 mm), so dass wir $n = 2$ annehmen, da es die weitere Berechnung vereinfacht.

Wir kombinieren $\cos(\alpha)^2$ mit Gleichung 1, wie ähnlich von Wein et al. vorgeschlagen. Wir ersetzen den Cosinus durch das Skalarprodukt eines Einheitsvektors d in Strahlrichtung mit dem normierten Gradientenvektor und erhalten

$$\frac{I_r}{I_i}(x) \approx \left(d^T \cdot \frac{\nabla Z(x)}{\|\nabla Z(x)\|}\right)^2 \left(\frac{\|\nabla Z(x)\|}{2 \cdot Z(x)}\right)^2 = \left(\frac{d^T \cdot \nabla Z(x)}{2 \cdot Z(x)}\right)^2 \tag{2}$$

wobei $d^T \cdot \nabla Z(x)$ dem Betrag des Gradientenvektors in Strahlrichtung entspricht, was innerhalb der simulierten US-Ebene leicht berechnet werden kann. Für die Berechnung sind keine weiteren Information über das ursprüngliche 3-D Bild notwendig und sie somit kann komplett in 2-D durchgeführt werden.

Absorption, d.h. der Energieverlust durch eine lokale Erwärmung des Gewebes, macht fast die gesamte Abschwächung von US-Wellen in weichem Gewebe aus, mindestens 95% laut Lyons et al. [7]. Sie kann durch ein exponentielles Gesetz $I/I_0 = e^{-\beta x}$ charakterisiert werden, ähnlich Röntgenstrahlen. Dies wird üblicherweise auf Einheitslänge normiert $\alpha = -10 \cdot \log_{10}(I/I_0)$, wobei α der Absoptionskoeffizient in Dezibel pro Einheitslänge ist. Zwischen α und der US-Frequenz besteht ein annähernd linearer Zusammenhang über den Bereich von 200 kHz bis 100 MHz.[8] Koeffizienten für verschiedene Gewebearten reichen üblicherweise von 0,6 bis 1,2 dB/cm bei 1 MHz, bei Knochen bis zu 20 dB/cm. Wir schätzen die Koeffizienten durch eine Interpolation aus bekannten Werten von Luft, Wasser und Knochen ab, und somit kann der Anteil an absorbierter Intensität entlang einer bekannten Wegstrecke d berechnet werden als $I/I_0 = 10^{-\alpha \cdot d \cdot f/10}$, wobei f die gerade verwendete US-Frequenz darstellt.

Um nun ein US-Bild zu simulieren, verfolgen wir US-Wellen durch das Gewebe. Dies ist der einzige Schritt, der nicht für jeden Pixel unabhängig berechnet werden kann. Wir initialisieren die ursprüngliche Intensität an der Position der virtuellen Sonde, und anschließend berechnen wir für jeden Pixel entlang einer Spalte die Intensität, die diesen Pixel erreicht und reflektiert bzw. absorbiert wird oder weiter ins Gewebe eindringt. Auf diese Weise können die Abschät-

Tabelle 1. Laufzeit-Informationen für die Ultraschall-Simulation (links) und Aufschlüsselung der Teilschritte auf GPU (rechts).

2-D Schnitt	0,300 ms
Daten-Transfers	4,076 ms
Berechnung auf GPU	8,690 ms
3-D Anzeige	0,208 ms

Synthese	2,325 ms
Verwischen	4,157 ms
Kompression	1,060 ms
Sonstige	0,968 ms

zungen für Reflexion, Transmission und Absorption kombiniert werden, um die reflektierte Intensität für jede Tiefe x entlang der Strahlrichtung zu berechnen:

$$I(x) \approx I_0 \cdot \left(\prod_{0 \le k < x} \underbrace{\left[\frac{I_t}{I_i}(k) \right]}_{\text{Transmission}} \underbrace{\left[1 - \frac{I_a}{I_i}(k,d) \right]}_{\text{Absorption}} \right)^2 \cdot \underbrace{R(x)}_{\text{Reflexion}} \tag{3}$$

In unserer Implementierung verwenden wir in CUDA je einen Thread pro Spalte und die aktuell verbleibende Intensität pro Spalte wird in gemeinsam genutztem Speicher auf der GPU verwaltet. Alle Threads werden vor und nach dem Zugriff auf diese Werte synchronisiert, da im allgemeinen Fall die Intensität aus zwei Werten in der darüber liegenden Reihe interpoliert werden muss. In einem Nachbearbeitungsschritt fügen wir noch US-typische Artefakte wie Rauschen und Unschärfe ein.

3 Ergebnisse

Wir haben die Laufzeit unserer Simulation für ein US-Bild der Größe 512×384 Pixel (Seitenverhältnis 3:4) aus einem CT-Datensatz der Größe $512 \times 512 \times 148$ Voxel auf einem Rechner mit GeForce 8800 GTX, Dual Intel Xeon 3 GHz und 2 GB RAM gemessen. Der größte Anteil der Berechnungsschritte erfolgt in CUDA auf der GPU und benötigt rund 8,7 ms. Eine genaue Aufschlüsselung der anderen Schritte und der Teilschritte auf der GPU sind in Tabelle 1 verfügbar.

Anzumerken ist, dass Transfers zwischen CPU und GPU rund 4,1 ms ausmachen, weil mit CUDA 1.1 Transfers zwischen OpenGL und CUDA noch über den Arbeitsspeicher laufen. Insgesamt übertreffen wir aber die Anforderungen an eine Echtzeit-Darstellung mit rund 30 Bildern pro Sekunde.

4 Diskussion

Wir haben einen bereits existierenden und physikalisch plausiblen Ansatz zur Simulation von US-Bildern dahin gehend erweitert, dass die Berechnung nun komplett innerhalb der US-Bildebene möglich ist, d.h. nur mit einem 2-D Ausschnitt der ursprünglich 3-D CT-Daten. Wir stellen das Design einer Implementierung in CUDA vor, die im Vergleich zu existierenden CPU-basierten Ansätzen einen deutlichen Geschwindigkeitsgewinn liefert. Es ist keine manuelle Aufbereitung der Eingangsdaten notwendig und wir erfüllen deutlich die Anforderungen an eine Echtzeit-Simulation.

Artefakte wie Reflexion, Abschwächung, Verschattung, Rauschen und radiale Unschärfe werden reproduziert. Insbesondere zur Absorption wurden bislang noch keine Ansätze vorgestellt, die über ein Zählen von „Knochenpixeln" hinaus gehen, wie z.B. implementiert von Zhu et al. [2]. Noch nicht berücksichtigt ist die Beugung von Ultraschallwellen an Grenzflächen, unserer Erfahrung nach sind aber insbesondere beim CT-üblichen Auflösungsvermögen die dafür benötigten genauen Informationen über die örtlichen Oberflächennormalen nicht rekonstruierbar bzw. zu stark verrauscht.

Wie bei einer realen US-Sonde können alle Einstellungen unserer Simulation interaktiv angepasst werden, darunter die US-Frequenz und -Intensität, „time gain compensation" und die Feld-Geometrie, sowie Rauschanteil und Ausmaß der radialen Unschärfe. Ein breites Spektrum an Sonden-Typen kann simuliert werden und unser Konzept ist allgemein anwendbar für das Training verschiedener US-Untersuchungen oder US-gestützter chirurgischer Eingriffe.

Literaturverzeichnis

1. Hostettler A, Forest C, Forgione A, et al. Real-Time Ultrasonography Simulator Based on 3D CT-Scan Images. Medicine Meets Virtual Reality 13. 2005;111:191–193.
2. Zhu Y, Magee D, Ratnalingam R, et al. A virtual ultrasound imaging system for the simulation of ultrasound-guided needle insertion procedures. In: Procs Med Image Underst Anal; 2006.
3. Wein W, Brunke S, Khamene A, et al. Automatic CT-ultrasound registration for diagnostic imaging and image-guided intervention. Med Image Anal. 2008;12:577–585.
4. Shams R, Hartley R, Navab N. Real-time simulation of medical ultrasound from CT images. Procs MICCAI. 2008.
5. Vidal FP, John NW, Healey AE, et al. Simulation of ultrasound guided needle puncture using patient specific data with 3D textures and volume haptics. Computer Animation Virtual Worlds. 2008;19(2):111–127.
6. Reichl T, Passenger J, Acosta O, et al. Ultrasound goes GPU: Real-time simulation using CUDA. Procs SPIE. 2008;To appear.
7. Lyons ME, Chivers RC, Parker KJ. Absorption Dominates Attenuation in Soft Tissues. In: Procs IEEE 1986 Ultrasonics Symposium; 1986. p. 871–874.
8. Dowsett DJ, Kenny PA, Johnston RE. The Physics of Diagnostic Imaging. Chapman & Hall Medical; 1998.

3D Segmentation and Quantification of the Aortic Arch for Endovascular Aortic Repair

Stefan Wörz[1], Hendrik von Tengg-Kobligk[2], Verena Henninger[2], Dittmar Böckler[3], Hans-Ulrich Kauczor[4], Karl Rohr[1]

[1]University of Heidelberg, BIOQUANT, IPMB, and DKFZ Heidelberg, Dept. Bioinformatics and Functional Genomics, Biomedical Computer Vision Group
[2]German Cancer Research Center (DKFZ) Heidelberg, Dept. Radiology
[3]University of Heidelberg, Dept. Vascular and Endovascular Surgery
[4]University of Heidelberg, Dept. Diagnostic Radiology
s.woerz@dkfz.de

Abstract. We introduce a novel model-based approach for the segmentation and quantification of the aortic arch morphology in 3D CTA images for endovascular aortic repair. The approach is based on a 3D analytic intensity model for thick vessels, which is directly fitted to the image. Based on the fitting results we compute the (local) 3D vessel curvature and torsion as well as the relevant lengths not only along the 3D centerline but particularly along the inner and outer contour. These measurements are important for pre-operative planning. We have successfully applied our approach using 3D CTA images and have compared the results with ground truth obtained by a radiologist. It turned out that our approach yields accurate estimation results.

1 Introduction

Aortic arch repair (AAR) poses a major challenge for cardiac and vascular surgeons as well as radiologists due to its tortuous anatomy (Fig. 1a). Since patients often have many comorbidities, more and more aortic arch pathologies are treated by minimal-invasive therapy using an endovascular graft (EVG, Fig. 1b). Endovascular aortic repair (EVAR) was initially used for the abdominal aorta but is currently also being explored for the thoracic aorta comprising the aortic arch (e.g., [1]). However, the EVGs currently used for AAR were designed for the abdominal aorta or are not yet optimized for the curved aortic arch. Therefore, these grafts fail to represent the tortuous anatomy of the arch, so misalignment of the EVG is often the case (Figs. 1c,d).

Since EVAR does not require opening the whole chest, pre-operative imaging is crucial to assess the vascular anatomy, for example, using 3D CT angiography (CTA). To choose the type of EVG for EVAR, morphological parameters need to be known such as aortic diameters, length of pathology along the centerline, and tortuosity of the aorta. In addition, we propose to choose an EVG also based on the relevant lengths along the outer and inner contours of the aortic arch. These measurements are important, for example, for planning the landing zone of the EVG, in particular, in case the landing zone is between two supra aortic branches. However, whereas in clinical practice the vessel diameters and lengths along the vessel centerline can be measured using commercial tools (e.g., [2]), the lengths along the inner and outer contour of the curved aortic arch as well as the (local) curvature and torsion are often not quantified at all, or only manually determined. Note that for the curved arch the lengths along the contour, in general, significantly deviate from the corresponding length along the centerline.

Previous work on the segmentation of the aorta from 3D images is often based on deformable models (e.g., [3, 4]). These approaches typically exploit contour information of vessel structures. Alternatively, deformable parametric intensity models have been suggested (e.g., [5, 6]). In comparison to contour-based models more image information is taken into account to improve the robustness and accuracy of the segmentation result. Concerning the segmentation of the abdominal aorta, i.e., the lower part of the aorta, contour-based approaches have been proposed (e.g., [3, 4, 7]). However, we are not aware of an intensity model-based approach which has been used to quantify the morphology of the aortic arch, i.e., the curved part of the aorta, for pre-operative planning of EVAR using grafts.

In this contribution, we introduce an approach based on a new intensity model for the quantification of the aortic arch morphology in 3D CTA images for EVAR. In contrast to previous work we quantify the (local) 3D vessel curvature and torsion as well as the relevant lengths not only along the 3D centerline but particularly along the inner and outer contour. Moreover, in contrast to previous approaches based on intensity models, our model is particularly suited for vessels of large widths such as the aorta, which is in contrast to, e.g., [5].

2 Materials and Methods

To quantify the aortic arch morphology, we have developed a 3D analytic intensity model, which represents the shape as well as the image intensities of the aortic arch within a 3D ROI. The parametric model is an ideal sharp 3D cylinder

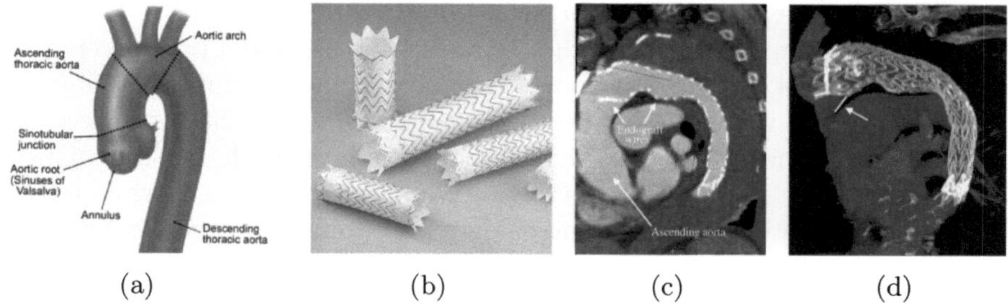

Fig. 1. Anatomy of the thoracic aorta (a), examples of endovascular grafts (b), as well as a 2D section (c) and a maximum intensity projection (d) of a 3D CTA of a patient after implantation of an EVG into the aortic arch. The EVG shows a significant misalignment w.r.t. the inner contour of the proximal aortic arch (see the arrow, (d)).

of radius R convolved with a 3D Gaussian (standard deviation σ) to incorporate the blurring effect of the image formation process. In particular, this model allows to represent the plateau-like intensity structure of thick vessels such as the aorta. Unfortunately, the exact solution of a Gaussian smoothed cylinder cannot be expressed analytically. In [6], an approximation of a Gaussian smoothed cylinder has been introduced, which uses two different approximations based on a Gaussian function and a Gaussian error function, and which employs blending functions to switch between both approximations. However, the application here concerns the segmentation of the aorta, which has a large width. Therefore, we here use a different approximation which is particularly suited for thick cylinders and which is computationally more efficient than the one in [6]. This 3D approximation is based on a 2D approximation of a Gaussian smoothed large disk using the Gaussian error function $\Phi(x) = \int_{-\infty}^{x} (2\pi)^{-1/2} e^{-\xi^2/2} d\xi$, and is defined as

$$g_{\text{Cylinder}'}(\mathbf{x}, R, \sigma) = \Phi(\rho_{\text{radial}}(r, R, \sigma)) \quad (1)$$

with $\mathbf{x} = (x, y, z)$ and $r = \sqrt{x^2 + y^2}$. Based on (1), the complete 3D intensity model is constructed by incorporating intensity levels a_0 (surrounding tissue) and a_1 (vessel) as well as a 3D rigid transform $\mathcal{R}$ with rotation parameters $\boldsymbol{\alpha} = (\alpha, \beta, \gamma)$ and translation parameters $\mathbf{x}_0 = (x_0, y_0, z_0)$. This results in the 3D intensity model $g_{M,\text{Cylinder}}(\mathbf{x}, \mathbf{p}) = a_0 + (a_1 - a_0)\ g_{\text{Cylinder}'}(\mathcal{R}(\mathbf{x}, \boldsymbol{\alpha}, \mathbf{x}_0), R, \sigma)$.

To segment the aortic arch we utilize an incremental process which starts from a given point D at the descending aorta and proceeds along the aorta until it reaches a given point A at the ascending aorta (Fig. 2a). In each increment, the parameters of a cylinder segment are determined by fitting the model $g_{M,Cylinder}$ to the image intensities $g(\mathbf{x})$ within a 3D ROI. Initial parameters for the fitting process are determined from the estimated parameters of the previous segment using a Kalman filter. To increase the robustness and accuracy of model fitting, we here apply a two-step refinement procedure. In the first step, we segment the aorta as described above using a larger size of the 3D ROI, i.e., we include more image information to robustly estimate the position $\mathbf{x}_0$ and orientation $\boldsymbol{\alpha}$ defining the centerline. In the second step, the remaining parameters such as the radius are refined by applying the model again but using a smaller size of the ROI in the direction of the centerline to increase the accuracy.

Applying our approach, we obtain estimates of the model parameters $\mathbf{p}$ for each vessel segment. In particular, based on the estimated radius R, position $\mathbf{x}_0$, and orientation $\boldsymbol{\alpha}$, we yield a 3D description of the shape of the aortic arch. For example, Fig. 2b shows the computed 3D shape overlayed with the original image data. To compute the (local) 3D curvature and torsion of the aortic arch, we apply a least-squares approach using cubic polynomials, which are locally fitted to a range of centerline positions. To visualize the results and to compute the lengths along the inner and outer contour of the curved aortic arch, we project the segmentation results onto a plane. This plane is specified by the centerline points A and D as well as the most anterior point along the centerline. For example, Fig. 2c shows the projected plane with the centerline (dashed), the inner and outer boundary (white), as well as the points A, 1, 2, 3, and D where the points 1, 2, and 3 are distal to the three supra aortic branches.

3 Results

We have applied our approach to quantify the morphology of the aortic arch in ten 3D CTA images. The images consist of about $512 \times 512 \times 700$ voxels with a slice spacing of 0.8 mm and a within-slice resolution between 0.512 mm and 0.625 mm. In all ten 3D images the automatic segmentation and quantification of the aortic arch was successful. As an example, Fig. 2b shows the computed 3D shape for one 3D image and Fig. 2c shows the 2D projection of the segmentation result. To illustrate the application for pre-operative planning of EVAR, Fig. 2d shows a picture of a real graft, which has been (interactively) aligned in accordance with the segmented shape of the aortic arch.

To validate our approach, we compared the results with ground truth, which was manually obtained by a radiologist. In addition, we compared the results with results obtained using a workstation with a commercial vascular analysis software. Fig. 2e shows the estimated radius in *mm* along the aortic arch for the new approach (bold) and the segmentation results of the radiologist (small grey squares and grey line) as well as for the commercial software (dashed). It turns out that our approach yields a much better result w.r.t. the ground truth than the commercial software. The maximal difference of the estimated radius

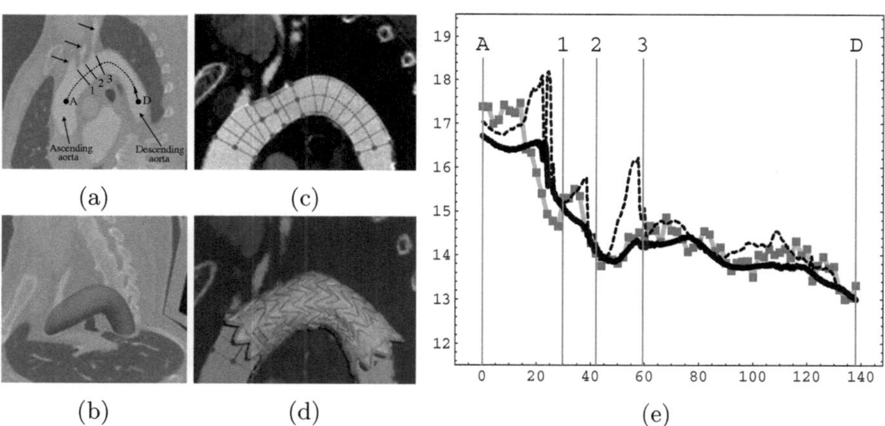

Fig. 2. 2D section of a 3D CTA showing the aortic arch (a), 3D segmentation result overlayed with two 2D sections of the 3D CTA image (b), a projected plane displaying the aortic arch and the segmentation result (centerline (dashed), inner and outer boundary (white), and several diameters) (c), as well as a picture (d) of a graft which has been aligned in accordance with the segmented shape shown in (c). The diagram (e) shows the estimated radius in *mm* along the arch for our approach (bold), the segmentation results of a radiologist (grey), and the result of the commercial software (dashed).

between our approach (bold) and that of the radiologist (grey) is 1.02 mm for all 70 measured radii, and the mean error is 0.34 mm. In contrast, the commercial software (dashed) yields a maximal error of 3.26 mm and a mean error of 0.44 mm. Moreover, for all ten 3D images we have compared the estimated radius of the aorta using our approach with the radius determined by the radiologist at the 3D points *A*, *1*, *2*, *3*, and *D*. It turned out that the results of our approach well agree with the ground truth with a maximal error over all points in all 3D images of 1.31 mm and a mean error of 0.38 mm.

4 Discussion

We introduced a new model-based approach for the segmentation and quantification of the aortic arch morphology in 3D CTA images for endovascular aortic repair (EVAR). The approach is based on a 3D analytic intensity model which is particularly suited for vessels of large widths. To increase the robustness and accuracy of model fitting we suggested a two-step refinement procedure. Based on the fitting results we directly compute the (local) 3D vessel curvature and torsion as well as the relevant lengths along the 3D centerline and along the inner and outer contour, which are important parameters for pre-operative planning in EVAR applications. We have successfully applied our approach to segment and quantify the aortic arch morphology using ten 3D CTA images.

Acknowledgement. Support of the Deutsche Forschungsgemeinschaft (DFG) within the project QuantVessel (RO 2471/6) is gratefully acknowledged. The work has partly been supported by the "Research training group 1126: Intelligent Surgery" funded by the DFG. We thank Heiko Heckmann for implementing the user-interface.

References

1. Schumacher H, Böckler D, von Tengg-Kobligk H, et al. Acute traumatic aortic tear: Open versus stent-graft repair. Semin Vasc Surg. 2006;19(1):48–59.
2. Lell MM, Anders K, Uder M, et al. New techniques in CT angiography. RadioGraphics. 2006;26:45–62.
3. de Bruijne M, van Ginneken B, Viergever MA, et al. Interactive segmentation of abdominal aortic aneurysms in CTA images. Med Image Anal. 2004;8:127–38.
4. Olabarriaga SD, Rouet JM, Fradkin M, et al. Segmentation of thrombus in abdominal aortic aneurysms from CTA with nonparametric statistical grey level appearance modeling. IEEE Trans Med Imaging. 2005;24(4):477–485.
5. Noordmans HJ, Smeulders AWM. High accuracy tracking of 2D/3D curved line structures by consecutive cross-section matching. Pattern Recognit Lett. 1998;19(1):97–111.
6. Wörz S, Rohr K. Segmentation and quantification of human vessels using a 3-D cylindrical intensity model. IEEE Trans Image Proc. 2007;16(8):1994–2004.
7. Egger J, Großkopf S, Freisleben B. Präoperative Simulation von Rohrprothesen und Y-Stens zur endovaskulären Behandlung von Stenosen und Aneurysmen. Proc BVM. 2007; p. 182–186.

Level-Set-Segmentierung von Rattenhirn MRTs

Björn Eiben[1,2], Dietmar Kunz[2], Uwe Pietrzyk[1,3] und Christoph Palm[1,3]

[1]Institut für Neurowissenschaften und Biophysik, Jülich Forschungszentrum
[2]Institut für Medien- und Phototechnik, Fachhochschule Köln
[3]Fachgruppe Physik, Bergische Universität Wuppertal
ch.palm@fz-juelich.de

Kurzfassung. In dieser Arbeit wird die Segmentierung von Gehirngewebe aus Kopfaufnahmen von Ratten mittels Level-Set-Methoden vorgeschlagen. Dazu wird ein zweidimensionaler, kontrastbasierter Ansatz zu einem dreidimensionalen, lokal an die Bildintensität adaptierten Segmentierer erweitert. Es wird gezeigt, dass mit diesem echten 3D-Ansatz die lokalen Bildstrukturen besser berücksichtigt werden können. Insbesondere Magnet-Resonanz-Tomographien (MRTs) mit globalen Helligkeitsgradienten, beispielsweise bedingt durch Oberflächenspulen, können auf diese Weise zuverlässiger und ohne weitere Vorverarbeitungsschritte segmentiert werden. Die Leistungsfähigkeit des Algorithmus wird experimentell an Hand dreier Rattenhirn-MRTs demonstriert.

1 Einleitung

Die Segmentierung von Gehirngewebe aus Kopfaufnahmen unterschiedlicher Modalitäten wird unter dem Begriff *Skull-Stripping* zusammengefasst. Dieses stellt einen wichtigen Vorverarbeitungsschritt für quantitative morphometrische Untersuchungen dar oder kann in vivo Konturinformationen für die Registrierung von Schnittmodalitäten bereitstellen. Im Rahmen dieser Arbeit werden MRTs von Rattenhirnen für die Evaluation des vorgeschlagenen Algorithmus verwendet.

Für die Segmentierung dreidimensionaler Daten sind leistungsstarke, flexible Modelle von hoher Bedeutung. Eine besondere Stellung nehmen hier aktive Konturmodelle ein, welche durch die Level-Set-Formulierung eine implizite Oberflächendarstellung und -entwicklung erlauben. Sie weisen insbesondere bei numerischen Berechnungen gutmütige Eigenschaften auf [1, 2].

Ein weit verbreitetes Werkzeug zum Skull-Stripping von Kopf-MRTs des Menschen ist das Brain-Extraction-Tool (BET), welches am FMRIB-Center der University of Oxford entwickelt wurde. Es basiert auf einem deformierbaren Netz, an dessen Knoten Formkräfte angreifen [3]. Zhuang et al. [4] haben diese Formkräfte in die Geschwindigkeitsfunktion der Level-Set-Methoden überführt und dabei einen zweidimensionalen Ansatz gewählt, welcher durch Konturpropagation auf benachbarte Schichten für dreidimensionale Daten einsetzbar ist. In dieser Arbeit wird ein echt-dreidimensionales Level-Set-basiertes Skull-Stripping auf Rattenhirn-MRTs vorgestellt und damit ein in allen Raumrichtungen konsistentes Segmentierungsergebnis ermöglicht.

2 Material und Methoden

Für die Segmentierungsaufgabe wird auf die Level-Set-Methoden nach [2] zurückgegriffen. Level-Sets sind Höhenlinien einer Funktion $\phi(\boldsymbol{x}) : \boldsymbol{x} \in \mathbb{R}^n \mapsto \mathbb{R}$ mit der Bilddimension n. Die zu beschreibende Kontur $\partial\Omega$ wird implizit durch den Nulldurchgang der Funktion ϕ beschrieben, das so genannte Zero-Levelset: $\partial\Omega = \{\boldsymbol{x} \mid \phi(\boldsymbol{x}) = 0\}$. Eine auf diese Weise definierte Startkontur, welche komplett innerhalb des zu segmentierenden Objektes liegt, wird durch eine partielle Differentialgleichung zeitlich deformiert und führt zu den Level-Set-Methoden:

$$\frac{\partial\phi}{\partial t} + \beta S(\boldsymbol{x}, \phi(\boldsymbol{x}, t))|\nabla\phi| = \gamma\kappa|\nabla\phi| \tag{1}$$

Hierbei bezeichnet t die Zeit, $S(\boldsymbol{x}, \phi(\boldsymbol{x}, t))$ die Geschwindigkeitsfunktion in Normalenrichtung $\nabla\phi$ der Kontur und κ die Krümmung der Kontur. Damit ist die Geschwindigkeitsfunktion bestimmend für den Segmentierungsprozess, wobei sich die Minimierung der Krümmung glättend auf die Kontur auswirkt. β und γ sind skalare Gewichtungsfaktoren.

Die Geschwindigkeitsfunktion wird, wie schon in [4], örtlich und zeitlich adaptiv berechnet. Hierzu wird entlang der nach innen zeigenden Konturnormalen das Intensitätsminimum und -maximum bestimmt. Der hieraus ermittelte Kontrast definiert, wie schnell die Kontur orthogonal zu sich selbst deformiert wird. Vor der Segmentierung wird eine Histogrammauswertung innerhalb der Startkontur vorgenommen. Das ermittelte Minimum darf nicht größer und das Maximum nicht kleiner werden als der Median des Histogramms. Dieses Prinzip findet auch beim BET Anwendung [3]. Globale Helligkeitsgradienten im Bild führen daher zu frühzeitigen Segmentierungsabbrüchen (Abb. 1, helle Kurve).

Zur Steigerung der Robustheit bei Helligkeitsgradienten im Bild wird im ersten Versuch auf den globalen Median verzichtet und stattdessen auf den lokalen Kontrast an der Objektgrenze abgehoben:

$$S(\boldsymbol{x}, \phi(\boldsymbol{x}, t)) = \frac{I_m(\boldsymbol{x}, \phi(\boldsymbol{x}, t), d_m)}{I_M(\boldsymbol{x}, \phi(\boldsymbol{x}, t), d_M)} - T, \tag{2}$$

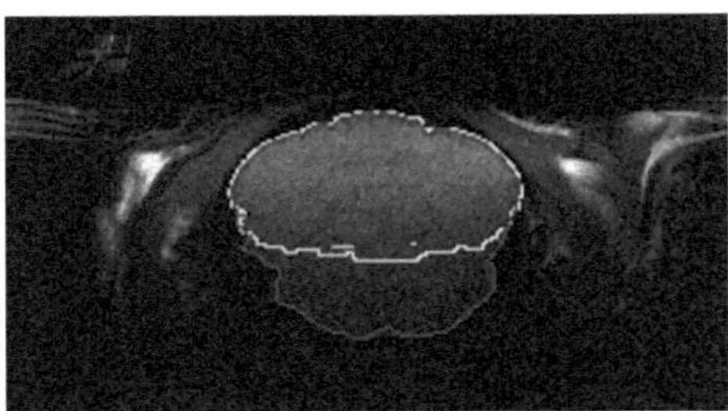

Abb. 1. Vergleich des Segmentierungsergebnisses an der sagittalen Schicht 140 zwischen dem 2D- (hell) und dem 3D-Segmentierer (dunkel). Der 2D-Ansatz führt zu einem frühzeitigen Abbruch der Segmentierung.

wobei I_m das Minimum auf der Normalen $\boldsymbol{N} = \frac{\nabla\phi}{|\phi|}$ in einem einstellbaren, maximalen Abstand d_m zur Kontur und I_M das entsprechende Maximum mit dem maximalen Abstand d_M darstellt. T bezeichnet den erwarteten Konturkontrast.

In einem zweiten Ansatz wird I zusätzlich lokal kontrastverstärkt:

$$I' = \mathrm{Median}(I, \boldsymbol{x}, \boldsymbol{N}) + w \frac{\mathrm{Var_i}(I, \boldsymbol{x}, \boldsymbol{N}) - \mathrm{Var_o}(\mathrm{I}, \boldsymbol{x}, \boldsymbol{N})}{\mathrm{Median}(I, \boldsymbol{x}, \boldsymbol{N})} \tag{3}$$

Die Differenz zwischen den auf $\boldsymbol{N}$ gleitenden, nach außen und nach innen gerichteten Varianzen $\mathrm{Var_i}$ und $\mathrm{Var_o}$ ruft eine Kontrastverstärkung hervor, welche insbesondere in schwachkontrastigen Bereichen bedingt durch die Normierung auf den gleitenden Median stärker wirkt. w gewichtet diese Signalaufsteilung. Die korrespondierende Geschwindigkeitsfunktion ergibt sich analog zu (2). Abbildung 2 zeigt die Wirkung der Signaladaption exemplarisch an einer Scanline in einem schwachkontrastigen Bereich. Nulldurchgänge bedingen einen Richtungswechsel der Konturpropagation (positive Werte bedeuten Expansion).

Beim Übergang von einer 2D-Konturpropagation mit globalem Median [4] zu einer 3D-Segmentierung mit lokaler Auswertung der Kontrastverhältnisse und späterer Erweiterung mit Signaladaption besteht die Hypothese, dass im Hinblick auf Leakage bzw. vorzeitigen Abbruch robustere und an problematischen Stellen genauere Ergebnisse resultieren.

Die Implementation wurde mit dem Insight Segmentation and Registration Toolkit (ITK) vorgenommen, welches für die Level-Set-Methoden jedoch isotrope Daten voraussetzt. Zur Generierung isotroper Daten wurde eine registrierungsbasierte Interpolation nach Penney verwendet [5].

3 Ergebnisse

Drei Datensätze eines 9,4 T Kleintier MRI-Scanners (21 cm Innendurchmesser, Oberflächenspule, Gradientenfeld: 270 mT/m, UnityInova Konsole (Varian, Palo Alto, USA)) standen zur Verfügung. Das T2 gewichtete Echo (TE = 24 ms)

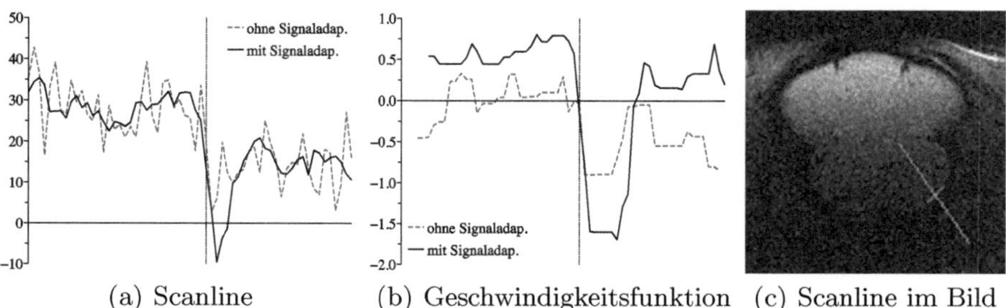

(a) Scanline (b) Geschwindigkeitsfunktion (c) Scanline im Bild

Abb. 2. Signal (hell gestrichelt) und adaptiertes Signal (durchgezogen) der Scanline (von innen nach außen) mit den zugehörigen Geschwindigkeitsfunktionen und der Scanline im Bild. Nulldurchgänge bewirken einen Richtungswechsel der Konturpropagation.

Tabelle 1. Die Dice-Koeffizienten gemäß (4) für drei Datensätze, wobei der erste Datensatz einen deutlichen Helligkeitsgradienten aufweist.

Datensatz	D_{2D}	D_{3D}	$D_{3D,SA}$
1	0.939	0.964	**0.966**
2	0.938	**0.945**	0.938
3	0.939	**0.942**	0.931

ergab 40 Schichtbilder mit einer Auflösung von 256 × 256 Bildpunkten und einer Ortsauflösung von 0,117 × 0,117 × 0,5 mm.

Die rekonstruierten 3D-Daten wurden einmal mit dem in [4] vorgestellten Algorithmus 2D schichtweise segmentiert und einmal 3D ohne und mit Signaladaption. Als Referenz zur Qualitätsbestimmung der Segmentierungsergebnisse wurden die Daten manuell segmentiert. Als Qualitätsmaß dient der Dice-Koeffizient:

$$D = \frac{2|X \cap Y|}{|X| + |Y|} \tag{4}$$

Dabei sind X und Y die Mengen der Bildpunkte, welche zum Referenz- bzw. segmentierten Volumen gehören. Die Dice-Koeffizienten für drei Datensätze sind

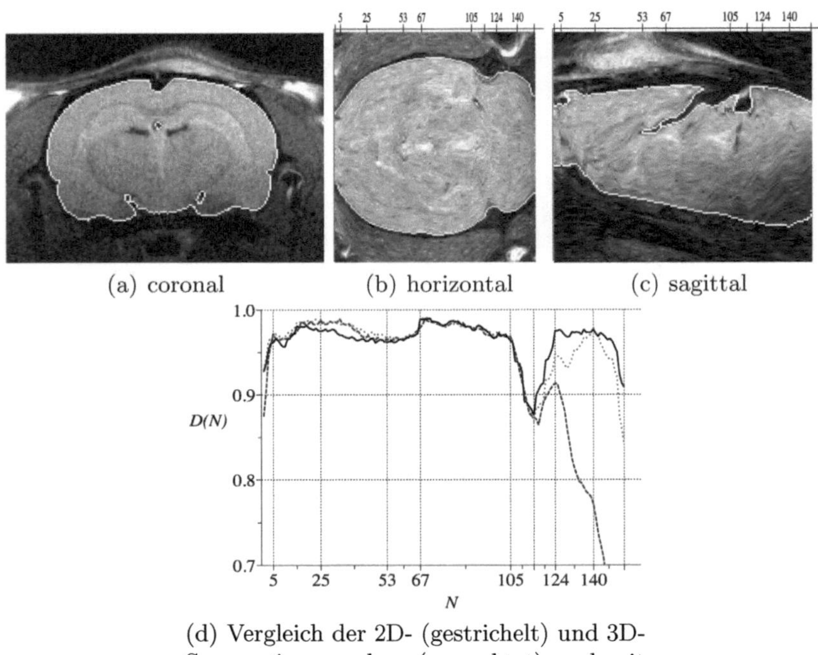

(a) coronal (b) horizontal (c) sagittal

(d) Vergleich der 2D- (gestrichelt) und 3D-Segmentierung ohne (gepunktet) und mit Signaladaption (durchgezogen)

Abb. 3. Darstellung des Segmentierungsergebnisses zu Datensatz 1 in zueinander orthogonalen Schnitten.

in Tabelle 1 dargestellt. Für alle Tests schneidet ein 3D-Ansatz besser ab. Besonders deutlich ist mit 0.966 zu 0.939 der Unterschied für den ersten Datensatz. Dieser weist, bedingt durch eine Oberflächenspule, einen deutlichen Helligkeitsgradienten auf. Bei den übrigen Daten ist diese Eigenschaft weniger ausgeprägt.

Abbildung 3(d) zeigt D aufgetragen über die Schichten N des ersten Datensatzes, aus welchem zueinander orthogonale Schnitte in Abbildung 3(a)-3(c) dargestellt sind. Die gestrichelte Kurve zeigt das Ergebnis der zweidimensionalen, die gepunktete das der dreidimensionalen, lokal modifizierten Segmentierung und die durchgezogene Kurve das Segmentierungsergebnis mit Signaladaption.

4 Diskussion

Die gewählte Kombination aus 3D-Datenverwertung und einer lokalen Signaladaption bei der Level-Set-Segmentierung liefert insbesondere bei Datensätzen mit einem ausgeprägten, globalen Helligkeitsgradienten eine deutliche Verbesserung des Segmentierungsergebnisses. Eine Vorverarbeitung zur globalen Helligkeitsangleichung ist damit für den Segmentierungsprozess nicht erforderlich. Bei Daten ohne ausgeprägten Helligkeitsgradienten konnte das Qualitätsniveau mindestens gehalten oder sogar leicht verbessert werden (siehe Tab. 1, Zeile 2 und 3). Die Erwartung, dass eine 3D-Verarbeitung an stark gekrümmten Strukturen zu stark glätten könnte, wurde nicht bestätigt. Der 3D-Ansatz ist demnach der 2D-Segmentierung vorzuziehen.

Die Signaladaption verbessert die Segmentierung in Bereichen mit schwachem Signal-zu-Rausch-Verhältnis beispielsweise im Bereich des Cerebellums. In den Schichten 25-40 zeigen sich jedoch leichte Schwächen durch Leakage.

In weiteren Studien werden die Einbindung von Formmodellen in Anlehnung an Leventon [6] beabsichtigt, um die Robustheit weiter zu erhöhen. Darüber hinaus wird die Übertragbarkeit der Ergebnisse auf Menschen-MRs untersucht.

Literaturverzeichnis

1. Sethian JA. Level Set Methods and Fast Marching Methods. Cambridge: Cambridge University Press; 1999.
2. Osher S, Fedkiw R. Level Set Methods and Dynamic Implicit Surfaces. Berlin: Springer; 2002.
3. Smith SM. BET: Brain Extraction Tool. Oxford: FMRIB; 2002.
4. Zhuang AH, Valentino DJ, Toga AW. Skull-stripping magnetic resonance brain images using a model-based level set. NeuroImage. 2006;32:79–92.
5. Penney GP, Schnabel JA, Rueckert D, et al. Registration-based interpolation. IEEE Trans Med Imaging. 2004;23:922–926.
6. Leventon ME, Grimson WEL, Faugeras O. Statistical shape influence in geodesic active contours. Proc CVPR. 2000;01:316–323.

Atlasbasierte 3D-Segmentierung medizinischer Bilddaten mit Fast-Marching-Methoden

Michael Schwenke[1,2], Matthias Färber[1], Jan Ehrhardt[1], Andreas Plaß[2], Heinz Handels[1]

[1]Institut für Medizinische Informatik, Universitätsklinikum Hamburg-Eppendorf
[2]Hochschule für Angewandte Wissenschaften Hamburg
michaelschwenke@web.de

Kurzfassung. In diesem Beitrag wird ein automatisches atlasbasiertes 3D-Segmentierungsverfahren unter Verwendung von *Fast-Marching*-Verfahren vorgestellt. Nach einer affinen Registrierung des Atlas- auf den Patientendatensatz werden ausgewählte Punkte der Oberfläche der Atlassegmentierung mittels Korrelationsverfahren auf den Patientendatensatz übertragen. Ausgehend von dieser Punktwolke wird in einem zweistufigen *Fast-Marching*-Verfahren die Objektoberfläche berechnet. Zentraler Punkt des Verfahrens ist eine aus dem Patientenbild abgeleitete Kostenmetrik, die Konturpunkten geringe, anderen Bildpunkten hohe Kostenwerte zuweist. Die Kostenfunktion kann flexibel auf unterschiedliche Kanten justiert werden, um zu gewährleisten, dass das Verfahren für unterschiedliche medizinische Strukturen verwendet werden kann. Das Verfahren wird in diesem Beitrag beispielhaft zur automatischen Nierensegmentierung in 3D-CT-Datensätzen angewendet.

1 Einleitung

Die Bandbreite von Segmentierungsverfahren reicht von vollständig manuellen über semiautomatische bis hin zu vollautomatischen Verfahren. Probleme manueller Segmentierung sind der hohe Aufwand und große Inter-Observer-Variabilitäten. Automatische Segmentierungsverfahren führen in medizinischen Bilddaten oft zu nicht ausreichender Genauigkeit der Segmentierung.

Um eine robuste automatische Segmentierung zu ermöglichen muss Wissen über die zu segmentierende Struktur in das Verfahren eingebracht werden. Man unterscheidet zwei generelle Ansätze: Statistische Modelle sowie atlasbasierte Methoden [1]. Bei Ersteren wird durch statistische Auswertung einer Menge von Observationen ein mittleres Modell und Eigenmoden berechnet. Das Modell wird unter Verwendung der Eigenmoden deformiert und auf den Patientendatensatz angepasst. Dieser Ansatz ist flexibel, hat aber den Nachteil, dass zur Erstellung des Modells eine große Zahl bereits segmentierter Daten vorliegen muss. Bei der Segmentierung mit Hilfe von Atlanten wird von einem segmentierten Referenzdatensatz, dem Atlas, die Segmentierung auf den Patientendatensatz übertragen. Eine Möglichkeit hierfür bilden nicht-lineare Registrierungsverfahren [1]. Färber et al. stellen in [2] ein Verfahren auf Basis des Live-Wire-Verfahrens [3] vor, bei dem nach affiner Registrierung einzelne Konturpunkte der Atlassegmentierung auf den Patientendatensatz übertragen werden. Zwischen den Punkten werden geschlossene Konturen berechnet. Lokale Formunterschiede werden somit anhand der Bilddaten ausgeglichen. Problematisch ist allerdings die schichtweise Betrachtung des Problems durch Verwendung des Live-Wire-Verfahrens. Fast-Marching-basierte Segmentierungsverfahren, wie vorgestellt in [4], ermöglichen hingegen die Berechnung von 3D-Oberflächen in Bilddaten.

Wesentlicher Fortschritt des vorgestellten Verfahrens liegt in der Automatisierung des Segmentierungsverfahrens aus [4] durch die automatische Übertragung ausgewählter Oberflächenpunkte vom Atlas- auf den Patientendatensatz. Dies ersetzt die im Allgemeinen aufwändige manuelle Initialisierung, wie sie in [4] vorgesehen ist.

2 Material und Methoden

2.1 Minimal-Pfad-basierte Berechnung von Oberflächen

Das Verfahren zur Berechnung der Oberflächen aus [4] baut auf dem Verfahren zur Berechnung minimaler Pfade aus [5] auf, bei dem minimale Pfade auf der Objektoberfläche über die Berechnung einer metrischen Distanzfunktion von einem Startpunkt und nachfolgendem Gradientenabstieg vom Endpunkt des Pfads zum Startpunkt bestimmt werden.

Sei $I : \Omega \to \mathbb{R}$ ein kontinuierlich definiertes Grauwertbild und $f : \Omega \to \mathbb{R}^+$ eine von I abgeleitete Kostenfunktion. Der kostenminimale Pfad zwischen $p_1, p_2 \in \Omega$, ist der Pfad γ aus der Menge A_{p_1,p_2} aller Verbindungspfade, der das Funktional

$$E : A_{p_1,p_2} \to \mathbb{R}^+,\ E(\gamma) = \int_\gamma f(\ \gamma(s) + w\ )\mathrm{d}s = \int_\gamma \tilde{f}(\ \gamma(s)\ )\mathrm{d}s, \tag{1}$$

mit dem Pfadlängenparameter s, einem Regularisierungsterm $w > 0$ zur Glättung der Pfade und $\tilde{f} = (f + w)$ global minimiert. Die Lösung dieses Minimierungsproblems wird durch Berechnung einer metrischen Distanzfunktion $U : \overline{\Omega} \to \mathbb{R}^+$ erreicht. Diese Funktion ist für einen der beiden Endpunkte, hier p_1, definiert durch:

$$\forall\ p \in \Omega,\ U_{p_1}(p)\ =\ \min_{\gamma \in A_{p_1,p}}\ \{E(\gamma)\}\ . \tag{2}$$

Die Funktion gibt folglich für jeden Punkt p des Bildes die integrierten Kosten entlang des minimalen Pfades vom Quellpunkt p_1 zum Punkt p an und erfüllt die Eikonalgleichung

$$\|\nabla U_{p_1}(p)\| = \tilde{f}(p)\ ,\ p \in \Omega \quad \text{und} \quad U_{p_1}(p_1) = 0\ . \tag{3}$$

Die Segmentierung geschlossener Objekte erfolgt, indem die Berechnung der Distanzfunktion auf ein Band um die Oberfläche des Objekts beschränkt wird.

Die Distanzwerte werden ausgehend von mehreren Saatpunkten auf der Oberfläche des Objekts berechnet, bis die besuchte Region $\overline{\Omega}_F$ den Bilddefinitionsbereich $\overline{\Omega}$ global in das Innere des Objekts und den Bildhintergrund trennt. Es erfolgt anschließend die Berechnung einer implizierten Oberfläche nach einem Verfahren aus [6]. Die Oberfläche wird als Zero-Level-Set einer Funktion $\Psi : \Omega \to \mathbb{R}$ bestimmt, die durch Lösung des Anfangswertproblems

$$\begin{cases} \nabla\Psi(p)\cdot\nabla U \;+ G\circ\Psi(p) \;=\; 0 & \text{falls } p\in int(\overline{\Omega}_F), \\ \Psi(p) \;=+k & \text{falls } p\in\partial\overline{\Omega}_F^{\text{Innen}}, \\ \Psi(p) \;=-k & \text{falls } p\in\partial\overline{\Omega}_F^{\text{Außen}}, \end{cases} \tag{4}$$

berechnet wird [4]. Die als konstant gesetzten Anfangswerte ($\pm k$) auf der inneren und äußeren Hülle der besuchten Region ($\partial\overline{\Omega}_F^{\text{Innen}}$ und $\partial\overline{\Omega}_F^{\text{Außen}}$) werden entlang des Gradienten der Distanzfunktion ∇U propagiert und die unterschiedlichen Vorzeichen kollidieren auf der gesuchten Oberfläche des Objekts, die somit als Nullschnitt extrahiert werden kann.

2.2 Die Kostenfunktion

In dieser Arbeit wird die Kostenfunktion aus vier Bildmerkmalen gebildet: dem Betrag des Sobel-Gradienten f_{G}, dem Deriche-Kantenmerkmal f_{D}, einem Laplace-Zero-Crossing f_{L} und einem Grauwert-Merkmal f_{Gw}. Die Merkmale werden nach Fensterung und Glättung auf den Wertebereich $[0,1]$ normiert und bis auf das Grauwert-Merkmal invertiert. Die Wertebereiche des Sobel-Gradientenbetrags und des Grauwert-Merkmals werden Gauß-gewichtet, so dass die Kostenfunktion auf bestimmte Merkmalswertebereiche justiert werden kann. Mittelwert und Standard-Abweichung der Gaußfunktion für jedes Merkmal werden auf Basis der Merkmalswerte an den Saatpunkten im Patientenbild geschätzt. Die Kostenfunktion weist jedem Bildpunkt $p \in \overline{\Omega}$ unter Verwendung der Bewertungsfunktionen G_{Gw} für das Grauwert-Merkmal und G_{G} für das Gradienten-Merkmal und der Gewichte für jedes Merkmal (w_{G}, w_{D}, w_{L} w_{Gw}) den Kostenwert zu:

$$f(p) = w_{\text{Gw}}\cdot G_{\text{Gw}}\left(f_{\text{Gw}}(p)\right) + w_{\text{G}}\cdot G_{\text{G}}\left(f_{\text{G}}(p)\right) + w_{\text{L}}\cdot f_{\text{L}}(p) + w_{\text{D}}\cdot f_{\text{D}}(p)\ . \tag{5}$$

2.3 Beschränkung auf eine konvexe Region-Of-Interest

Zur Verhinderung des Überlaufens des Verfahrens auf benachbarte Strukturen und zur Verringerung des Rechenaufwands wird in dieser Arbeit das Verfahren mittels konvexer Region-Of-Interest beschränkt, die automatisch auf Basis der Saatpunktwolke bestimmt wird. Es wird dabei die konvexe Hülle der Wolke berechnet, die mit Bezug auf den Schwerpunkt der Wolke mit $\alpha > 1$ skaliert und als Region-Of-Interest verwendet wird.

2.4 Atlasbasierter Segmentierungsansatz

Das Verfahren gliedert sich in folgende Phasen: 1. Patienten- und Atlasdatensatz werden derselben Vorverarbeitung unterzogen. Der Atlasdatensatz wird affin auf den Patientendatensatz registriert; 2. Es werden einzelne äquidistante Konturpunkte der Atlassegmentierung ausgewählt; 3. Die Konturpunkte werden mittels Korrelationsverfahren auf den Patientendatensatz übertragen; 4. Das Kostenbild des Patientendatensatz wird berechnet; 5. Ausgehend von den übertragenen Saatpunkten wird das Segmentierungsverfahren durchgeführt.

2.5 Evaluation

In CT-Datensätzen wurden die Nieren durch einen medizinischen Experten semiautomatisch segmentiert. Diese Segmentierungen stellen den Goldstandard für die Bewertung der Güte des Verfahrens dar. Die Evaluation des Verfahrens zur automatischen atlasbasierten Segmentierung erfolgt durch drei Versuche: 1. *Test-Transfer*: Ein CT-Nierendatensatz wird durch Transformation und Hinzufügen von Rauschen verändert und dient als Atlas für den untransformierten Datensatz; 2. *Intrapatient-Transfer*: Es wird innerhalb eines Patienten die Segmentierung einer gespiegelten Niere auf die andere Niere übertragen; 3. *Interpatient-Transfer*: Es wird von einem Patientendatensatz die Segmentierung einer Niere auf einen anderen Patientdatensatz übertragen.

3 Ergebnisse

Tab. 1 stellt die Ergebnisse der Evaluation dar. In allen Versuchen wurden 50-70 Saatpunkte übertragen, die bis auf einige Outlier nur geringen Abstand zur Goldstandard-Segmentierung aufweisen. Der Vergleich der berechneten Segmentierungen mit dem Goldstandard zeigt in allen Versuchen Jaccard-Index-Werte ≥ 0.923, mittlere Konturabstände ≤ 0.576 und Hausdorff-Distanzen ≤ 9.28. Abb. 1 visualisiert die Segmentierungen in 3D.

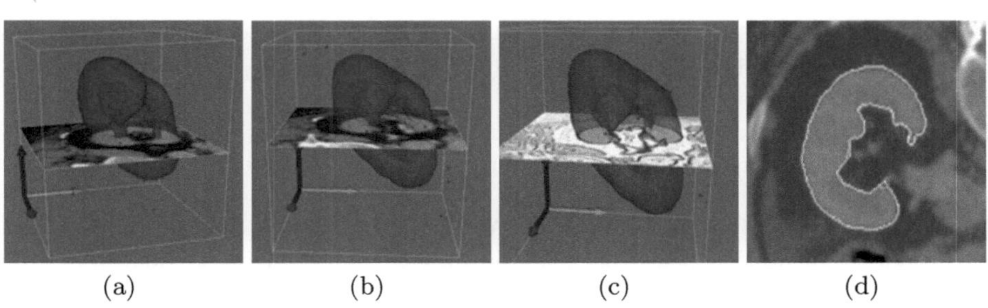

(a) (b) (c) (d)

Abb. 1. Ergebnisse der automatischen atlasbasierten Segmentierung. a) Test-Transfer; b) Intrapatient-Transfer; c) Interpatient-Transfer mit Schnitt durch das Kostenbild; d) Patientenbild mit Segmentierungskonturen: Goldstandard (weiß), Test-Transfer (blau), Intrapatient-Transfer (gelb) und Interpatient-Transfer (grün).

Tabelle 1. Ergebnisse: Atlasbasierte Saatpunktübertragung und Vergleich der Segmentierung mit dem Goldstandard. Güte des Saatpunktetransfers: Abstände der Saatpunkte zur Goldstandard-Kontur (Mittelwert $\overline{d}$, Minimum d_{Min} und Maximum d_{Max}. Güte der Segmentierung: Jaccard Index $J(S,G)$, mittlerer Konturabstand $\overline{d}(S,G)$ und Hausdorff-Distanz $H(S,G)$ von Segmentierung S zum Goldstandard G.

Versuch	Anzahl Punkte	Distanzmaße $\overline{d}$ [mm]	d_{Max} [mm]	Anzahl Outlier	$J(S,G)$	$\overline{d}(S,G)$ [mm]	$H(S,G)$ [mm]
Test-Transfer	68	2.02	25.57	1	0.923	0.576	7.810
Intrapatient-Transfer	57	3.15	29.19	5	0.938	0.535	8.943
Interpatient-Transfer	51	2.20	13.42	1	0.955	0.415	9.276

4 Diskussion

Die Übertragung der Saatpunkte des affin auf den Patienten registrierten Atlasdatensatzes ist in der Regel erfolgreich gewesen. Dies zeigen die geringen mittleren Abstände zur Goldstandard-Segmentierung. Einige Ausreißer zeigt der maximale Abstand an. Diese wurden jedoch in allen Fällen, da sie weit von der Objektoberfläche entfernt detektiert wurden, vom Verfahren implizit verworfen: Sie waren nicht Teil der beiden Grenzkomponenten der besuchten Region und wurden nicht in die Berechnung der Oberfläche einbezogen. Die Güte der Segmentierung ist in allen Versuchen als sehr gut einzustufen. Das Verfahren zur atlasbasierten Segmentierung hat sich zur Segmentierung von Nieren als gut geeignet erwiesen und wird in weiteren Untersuchungen an weiteren Strukturen getestet.

Literaturverzeichnis

1. Ehrhardt J, Handels H, Plötz W, et al. Atlas-based recognition of anatomical structures and landmarks and the automatic computation of orthopedic parameters to support the virtual planning of hip operations. Methods Inf Med. 2004;43:391–397.
2. Färber M, Ehrhardt J, Handels H. Live-wire based segmentation using similarities between corresponding image structures. Comput Med Imaging Graph. 2007;31:549–560.
3. Mortensen E, Morse B, Barrett W, et al. Adaptive boundary detection using live-wire two-dimensional dynamic programming. IEEE Computers Cardiol. 1992; p. 635–638.
4. Benmansour F, Bonneau S, Cohen L. An implicit approach to closed surface and contour segmentation based on geodesic meshing and transport equation. Proc RFIA. 2008.
5. Cohen L, Kimmel R. Global minimum for active contour models: a minimal path approach. Proc CVPR. 1996; p. 666–673.
6. Ardon R, Cohen L, Yezzi A. Fast surface segmentation guided by user input using implicit extension of minimal paths. J Math Imaging Vis. 2006;25:289–305.

Evaluation of the Twofold Gaussian Mixture Model Applied to Clinical Volume Datasets

Jan Bruijns

Philips Research Eindhoven, The Netherlands
jan.bruijns@philips.com

Abstract. Volume representations of blood vessels acquired by 3D rotational angiography are very suitable for diagnosing a stenosis or an aneurysm. For optimal treatment, physicians need to know the shape of the diseased vessel parts. Binary segmentation by thresholding is the first step in our shape extraction procedure. Assuming a twofold Gaussian mixture model (GMM), the model parameters (and thus the threshold for binary segmentation) can be extracted by the Expectation-Maximization (EM) algorithm. The question is whether this GMM threshold gives a good segmentation. Therefore we compared segmentations induced by the GMM threshold with segmentations induced by thresholds derived in a different way. It appeared that a twofold Gaussian mixture model is not always a correct assumption for the distribution of the gray values.

1 Introduction

Volume representations of blood vessels acquired by 3D rotational angiography after injection with a contrast agent [1] have a clear distinction in gray values between tissue and vessel voxels. Therefore, these volume representations are very suitable for diagnosing a stenosis, a local narrowing of a vessel caused for example by cholesterol, or an aneurysm, a local widening of a vessel caused by a weak vessel wall.

For optimal treatment of a stenosis or an aneurysm, physicians need to know the cross-sectional shape parameters in the neighborhood of the diseased vessel parts. The starting point for many shape extraction methods is a segmented volume. Such a segmented volume can be created by thresholding (given further detail in Section 2.3).

To eliminate inter- and intra-operator variations this threshold should be extracted automatically from the data. Starting point for automatic threshold extraction can be a twofold Gaussian mixture model [2, 3, 4]. The question is whether the threshold derived from such a model results in a good segmentation. If the threshold is too low, many noise bulges arise; if the threshold is too high, an undersized vessel surface results.

1.1 Related work

Gan et al. introduced a method for vascular segmentation of 3D rotational angiography volumes based on MIP images [3]. Applying the Expectation-

Maximization (EM) algorithm for a twofold Gaussian mixture model, they estimate a threshold from a MIP image because the standard deviation of the individual classes in a MIP image is smaller. This threshold is used to classify the voxels belonging to this MIP image (i.e. the voxels with the maximum gray value in the projection direction). After the resulting vessel voxels are labelled in a corresponding binary volume, their gray values in the original volume is set to zero, and the procedure is repeated until over fitting of the non-vessel class is detected. This iterative algorithm is applied in the three axis directions and the resulting segmentations are combined by minimizing an energy functional for a spatially smooth result.

1.2 What is new

Since segmentations of our clinical volume datasets by one or more experienced radiologist were not available, we developed a new method to quantify segmentations on the basis of the gradient information of the gray value volumes (given further detail in Section 2.4).

Since we apply this method to quantify not only segmentations induced by the GMM threshold but also segmentations induced by thresholds derived in a different way (given further detail in Section 2.2), we can assess the segmentations and thus the GMM threshold.

2 Method

2.1 EM algorithm

Since the Expectation-Maximization (EM) algorithm [5, 6] requires a number of iterations through the observations (e.g. the gray values), and because of the large number of observations (e.g. 512x512x512 volumes), the EM algorithm is very time-consuming. To accelerate the extraction of the parameters of a twofold Gaussian mixture model (GMM) by the EM algorithm, we use the variant developed by Bruijns [4]. He applies the EM algorithm on to the histogram of the observations, requiring a single pass through the volume and a number of iterations through the much smaller histogram. After the parameters of the Gaussian mixture model are extracted, the GMM threshold is given by the intersection point of the two Gaussian components.

2.2 Bench mark thresholds

As already told in Section 1.2, we have not only used the GMM threshold for binary segmentation but also thresholds extracted in a different way from the gray value volumes. We have used the threshold proposed in [7] (indicated by "OT"), the threshold proposed in [2] (indicated by "KI"), the threshold proposed in [8] (indicated by "RF") and the threshold proposed in [9] (indicated by "GR").

2.3 Segmentation

As explained in Section 2.1 of [9], binary segmentation of a gray value volume with a single threshold gives too much noise. To remove this noise, the gray value volume is transformed to a segmented volume by a region growing algorithm with two thresholds [10].

Voxels with a gray value below the lower threshold are classified as tissue voxels. Voxels with a gray value above the upper threshold are classified as vessel voxels. Voxels with a gray value between the two thresholds are classified as potential vessel voxels. A potential vessel voxel is classified as vessel voxel if it is face connected to a vessel voxel, possibly via a chain of face connected potential vessel voxels.

The GMM threshold and the bench mark thresholds (Sec. 2.2) are used as lower threshold. The upper thresholds are derived from the lower thresholds and the gray value volume similar as in Section 2.2 of [9].

2.4 Evaluation

The true boundary between vessels and tissue is located at (a subset of) the positions $\{\mathbf{p}_{max}\}$ of the maxima of the gradient magnitude $||\mathbf{g}(\mathbf{p})||$ in the direction of the gradient vector $\mathbf{n}(\mathbf{p})$. These positions are given by the following relation:

$$||\mathbf{g}(\mathbf{p}_{max} + \mathbf{n}(\mathbf{p}_{max}) * dt)|| < ||\mathbf{g}(\mathbf{p}_{max})|| \tag{1}$$

Since the high gray value gradient ridge voxels (Section 2.3.2 of [9]) are located close to the maxima of the gradient magnitude, these voxels are used as reference boundary for a quantitative evaluation of the segmentations.

Since the Manhattan distance transform [11] with regard to the high gray value gradient ridge voxels gives the Manhattan distance between every voxel and its closest high gray value ridge voxel, and since the Manhattan distance transform is faster to compute than the Euclidian distance transform, we have used these Manhattan distances to indicate the segmentation performance. We have computed per volume the following characteristic numbers from the Manhattan distances of the border vessel voxels (i.e. vessel voxels with a tissue voxel as neighbor):

1. The fraction of border vessel voxels with a Manhattan distance greater than zero (i.e. the border vessel voxels not located on the high gray value ridges). This fraction is indicated by "border_off_ridges".
2. The average Manhattan distance of the border vessel voxels (indicated by "avg_dist2ridges").
3. The maximum Manhattan distance of the border vessel voxels (indicated by "max_dist2ridges").

Table 1. Median MD, mean MN and maximum MX of the three characteristic numbers.

	"border_on_ridges"			"avg_dist2ridges"			"max_dist2ridges"		
	MD	MN	MX	MD	MN	MX	MD	MN	MX
GMM	0.3839	0.4253	0.9854	0.4345	1.0924	20.9937	7	12.1938	93
OT	0.3394	0.3522	0.8499	0.3516	0.6760	19.6738	4	7.3718	91
KI	0.3692	0.3887	0.8875	0.4022	0.4501	1.8899	6	8.1125	35
RF	0.3770	0.3988	0.9352	0.4016	0.4738	2.1754	6	9.6296	46
GR	0.3176	0.3274	0.6537	0.3479	0.3707	1.7681	4	5.5988	33

2.5 Remarks

1. When the gradient ridges are used for extraction of the lower threshold (Section 2.3.3 of [9]), faultless detecting of all gradient ridge voxels at all vessel-tissue boundaries is not required. Better a number of gradient ridge voxels at the vessel-tissue boundaries ruled out than a number of voxels at possible artefacts included. But, when the gradient ridges are used for quantitative evaluation of segmentations, it is better that a number of voxels at possible artefacts are included, than that a number of gradient ridge voxels at the vessel-tissue boundaries are ruled out. Indeed, a significant loss of gradient ridge voxels at the vessel-tissue boundaries result in overestimated characteristic numbers.
2. In case of a "perfect segmentation" the vessel boundary is coincident with the high gray value gradient ridges. In this case all border vessel voxels are located on the high gray value gradient ridges. So "border_on_ridges" closer to 0.0 is better, "avg_dist2ridges" closer to 0.0 is better, and "max_dist2ridges" closer to 0.0 is better.

3 Results and discussion

We have applied the variants for extraction of the thresholds to 81 clinical volume datasets (24 of them with a resolution of 256x256x256 voxels, the rest 128x128x128 voxels), acquired with the 3D Integris system [12]. The voxel size varies between 0.2 and 1.2 millimeter.

The median MD, mean MN and maximum MX of the three characteristic numbers (Sec. 2.4) of the 81 clinical volume datasets are given in Table 1.

The following conclusions can be drawn from the results and the experience gained:

1. Since the GR threshold is derived from the gray values of the gradient ridge voxels, the GR threshold gives the best (i.e. lowest) results. But, since the GR threshold is a global threshold (as all thresholds used for segmentation of the 81 clinical volume datasets) and since the gray values of the gradient ridge voxels vary considerably (Fig. 5 of [9]), the median, mean and maximum are

still not close to zero. So, a better segmentation is probably only possible by local thresholds.

2. The OT threshold gives compared to the GMM, KI and RF thresholds good results except for the maximum (MX) of the characteristic numbers "avg_dist2ridges" and "max_dist2ridges". However, it was not possible to extract an OT threshold for three of the 81 clinical volume datasets.
3. The KI threshold and the RF threshold give more or less the same results. However, it was not possible to extract an KI threshold for one of the 81 clinical volume datasets.
4. The GMM threshold gives the worst results, especially for the mean (MN) and the maximum (MX) of the characteristic numbers "avg_dist2ridges" and "max_dist2ridges". This indicates that a twofold Gaussian mixture model is not always a correct assumption for the distribution of the gray values.

References

1. Moret J, Kemkers R, de Beek JO, et al. 3D rotational angiography: Clinical value in endovascular treatment. Medicamundi. 1998;42(3):8–14.
2. Kittler J, Illingworth J. Minimum error thresholding. Pattern Recognit. 1986;19(1):41–47.
3. Gan R, Wong WCK, Chung ACS. Statistical cerebrovascular segmentation in three-dimensional rotational angiography based on maximum intensity projections. Med Phys. 2005;32(9):3017–3028.
4. Bruijns J. The expectation-maximization algorithm for a twofold Gaussian mixture model applied to the histogram of the observations. Proc CAR. 2008; p. S392–S393.
5. Bilmes J. A Gentle Tutorial on the EM Algorithm and its Application to Parameter Estimation for Gaussian Mixture and Hidden Markov Models. Berkeley, CA, USA: University of Berkeley; 1997. ICSI-TR-97-021.
6. Dempster AP, Laird NM, Rubin DB. Maximum likelihood from incomplete data via the EM algorithm. J Royal Statist Soc B. 1977;39(1):1–38.
7. Otsu N. A threshold selection method from gray level histograms. IEEE Trans Sys Man Cybern. 1979;9(1):62–66.
8. Bruijns J. Verification of the self-adjusting probe: Shape extraction from cerebral vasculature. Proc VMV. 2003; p. 159–166.
9. Bruijns J. Segmentation of vessel voxel structures using gradient ridges. Proc VMV. 2003; p. 391–398.
10. Canny J. A Computational approach to edge detection. IEEE Trans Pattern Anal Machine Intell. 1986;8(6):679–698.
11. Borgefors G. Distance transformations in arbitrary dimensions. Computer Vis Graph Image Process. 1984;27(3):321–345.
12. Philips-Medical-Systems-Nederland. INTEGRIS 3D-RA. Instructions for use. Release 2.2. Best, The Netherlands: Philips Medical Systems Nederland; 2001. 9896 001 32943.

Integrierte Segmentierung und Trajektorienberechnung mittels diffeomorpher Registrierung in räumlich-zeitlichen CT-Bildfolgen

Alexander Schmidt-Richberg, Jan Ehrhardt, René Werner, Heinz Handels

Institut für Medizinische Informatik, Universitätsklinikum Hamburg-Eppendorf
a.schmidt-richberg@uke.uni-hamburg.de

Kurzfassung. Verfahren zur integrierten Segmentierung und Registrierung von 4D-Bilddaten ermöglichen die Berücksichtigung der gegenseitigen Abhängigkeiten beider Komponenten. Bestehende Ansätze konzentrieren sich dabei meist auf die Betrachtung zweier 3D-Bilder und lassen sich nicht direkt auf vollständige Bildfolgen übertragen. In dieser Arbeit wird ein Verfahren vorgestellt, in dem ein diffeomorpher Registrierungsansatz verwendet wird, um eine integrierte Berechnung von Segmentierungen und 3D-Voxeltrajektorien in 4D-Daten zu ermöglichen.

1 Einleitung

Die Berechnung von 3D-Voxeltrajektorien anhand räumlich-zeitlicher Bilddaten sowie die Segmentierung relevanter Strukturen sind Voraussetzung vieler Diagnose- und Therapieverfahren der medizinischen Praxis. Sie stellen beispielsweise in der Strahlentherapie zur Behandlung thorakaler Tumoren die Grundlage zur Erstellung zeitlich modellierter Bestrahlungspläne und zur Akkumulation von Dosisverteilungen dar [1].

In Vorarbeiten konnte gezeigt werden, dass durch die Integrierung von Segmentierung und Registrierung die Ergebnisse beider Verfahren verbessert werden können [2]. Dabei wurden zunächst zwei 3D-Bilder des 4D-Bilddatensatzes betrachtet. Grundlegende Idee ist es, die als bekannt vorausgesetzte Segmentierung eines Bildes (Referenzbild) mithilfe nichtlinearer Registrierung in den Bildraum des anderen Bildes (Zielbild) zu überführen. Die transformierte Referenzsegmentierung dient einerseits als *a priori*-Information zur Verbesserung der Segmentierung des Zielbildes, andererseits wird sie zur Verbesserung der Registrierung genutzt, indem gefordert wird, dass sie eine valide Segmentierung des Zielbildes darstellt.

Ziel der vorgestellten Arbeit ist die Erweiterung des Verfahrens für die Betrachtung von 4D-Datensätzen, d.h. einer Folge $I_0(\boldsymbol{x}), I_1(\boldsymbol{x}), \ldots, I_{n-1}(\boldsymbol{x})$ von 3D-Bilddaten zu n Zeitpunkten. Dabei wird ein Zeitpunkt als festes Referenzbild gewählt, z.B. $I_{\text{Ref}} := I_0$. Gesucht ist zum einen die Registrierung der Zielbilder $I_i(\boldsymbol{x}), i \in \{1, \ldots, n-1\}$ mit dem Referenzbild, zum anderen die Segmentierungen $\phi_i(x)$ der Zielbilder.

Eine Adaption auf Bildfolgen des in [2] vorgeschlagenen Verfahrens und anderer in der Literatur zu findenden Ansätze (z.B. [3, 4, 5, 6]) ist nicht ohne weiteres möglich, da in diesen die Segmentierung für das zu transformierende Bild gegeben ist. Auf die Aufgabenstellung übertragen hieße das, dass die Verschiebungsfelder über den Zielbildern $I_1, \ldots, I_{n-1}$ definiert sind, da für dieses die Segmentierung gesucht ist. Jedoch ist es zur Berechnung von Voxeltrajektorien $\boldsymbol{T}(\boldsymbol{x}) := \big(\boldsymbol{x}, \boldsymbol{x}+\boldsymbol{u}_1(\boldsymbol{x}), \ldots, \boldsymbol{x}+\boldsymbol{u}_{n-1}(\boldsymbol{x})\big)$ erforderlich, dass die Verschiebungsfelder über dem Bildraum eines fest gewählten Referenzbildes definiert sind. Dies ist weiterhin notwendig, um die Registrierung der Bilder I_0 mit I_i sukzessive mit dem Ergebnis des vorherigen Schrittes $\boldsymbol{u}_{i-1}$ zu initialisieren. Die Übertragung der Referenzsegmentierung in den Zielbildraum ist in diesem Fall jedoch nur unter Kenntnis des inversen Verschiebungsfeldes $\boldsymbol{u}_i^{-1}$ möglich.

Aus diesen Gründen wird der Ansatz um eine diffeomorphe Registrierung erweitert, durch die zum einen die Invertierbarkeit des Verschiebungsfeldes garantiert ist, zum anderen das inverse Verschiebungsfeld effizient berechnet werden kann.

2 Material und Methoden

Das in dieser Arbeit vorgestellte Verfahren zur integrierten Berechnung von Segmentierung und Registrierung besteht aus zwei Teilen:

- Registrierung der Bilder I_i mit dem Referenzbild I_{Ref} unter Berücksichtigung der transformierten Segmentierung $\phi_i(\boldsymbol{x} + \boldsymbol{u}_i(\boldsymbol{x}))$
- Segmentierung der Zielbilder I_i unter Berücksichtigung der transformierten Referenzsegmentierung $\phi_{\mathrm{Ref}}(\boldsymbol{x} + \boldsymbol{u}_i^{-1}(\boldsymbol{x}))$

Im Folgenden wird zunächst näher auf den verwendeten Registrierungsansatz eingegangen (Abschnitt 2.1) und anschließend ein variationelles Modell für die integrierte Segmentierung und Registrierung vorgestellt (2.2).

2.1 Diffeomorphe Registrierung

Ziel der Registrierung ist die Bestimmung einer Abbildung $\varphi_i(\boldsymbol{x}) := \boldsymbol{x} + \boldsymbol{u}_i(\boldsymbol{x})$, so dass die Distanz $\mathcal{D}$ zwischen $I_i \circ \varphi_i(\boldsymbol{x})$ und $I_{\mathrm{Ref}}(\boldsymbol{x})$ unter Berücksichtigung einer Glattheitsbedingung $\mathcal{S}$ minimiert wird:

$$\mathcal{J}_{\mathrm{Reg}}[\boldsymbol{u}_i] := \mathcal{D}[I_{\mathrm{Ref}}, I_i; \boldsymbol{u}_i] \;+\; \mathcal{S}[\boldsymbol{u}_i] = \min! \tag{1}$$

Die Minimierung lässt sich z.B. mithilfe des semi-impliziten Iterationsschemas

$$\big(\mathrm{Id} - \tau \boldsymbol{A}\big)\boldsymbol{u}_i^{(k+1)} = \boldsymbol{u}_i^{(k)} + \tau \boldsymbol{f}_{\mathrm{Reg}}(\boldsymbol{u}_i^{(k)}) \tag{2}$$

schrittweise lösen, wobei Id die identische Abbildung und τ die Schrittweite angibt. In diesem Beitrag wird eine diffusive Regularisierung gewählt, d.h. $\boldsymbol{A} = \Delta$. Der verwendete Kraftterm

$$\boldsymbol{f}_{\mathrm{Reg}} := \boldsymbol{f}_{\mathcal{D}}(\boldsymbol{x}) = \frac{I_{\mathrm{Ref}}(\boldsymbol{x}) - I_i(\boldsymbol{x} + \boldsymbol{u}_i(\boldsymbol{x}))}{\|\nabla I_i(\boldsymbol{x} + \boldsymbol{u}_i(\boldsymbol{x}))\| + \kappa} \nabla I_i(\boldsymbol{x} + \boldsymbol{u}_i(\boldsymbol{x}))$$

ist zu Thirions *Demons* verwandt und zeichnet sich im Vergleich zum SSD-Maß durch größere Kräfte an schwachen Kanten aus, wodurch kontrastarme Objekte besser registriert werden. Gleichung (2) lässt sich mithilfe von *Additiv Operator Splitting* effizient lösen [7].

Wie eingangs beschrieben, sollen diffeomorphe, d.h. invertierbare und in beide Richtungen differenzierbare Abbildungen erzielt werden. In diesem Beitrag werden diffeomorphe Abbildungen betrachtet, die durch stationäre Vektorfelder beschrieben werden können: $d\varphi_i(\boldsymbol{x},t)/dt = \boldsymbol{v}_i(\varphi_i(\boldsymbol{x},t))$ [8]. Dabei bezeichnet $\varphi_i(\boldsymbol{x},t)$ den Fluss der Transformation zum Zeitpunkt t, $\boldsymbol{v}_i$ lässt sich als Geschwindigkeitsfeld interpretieren. Die gesuchte Transformation ist gegeben durch $\varphi_i(\boldsymbol{x}) = \varphi_i(\boldsymbol{x},1) = \exp(\boldsymbol{v}_i(\boldsymbol{x}))$, wobei eine effiziente Berechnung der *Exponential Map* aufgrund der Gruppenstruktur der Diffeomorphismen möglich ist.

Das oben formulierte Iterationsschema (2) wird hiermit zu

$$\exp\left((\mathrm{Id} - \tau \boldsymbol{A})\boldsymbol{v}_i^{(k+1)}\right) = \exp\left(\boldsymbol{v}_i^{(k)}\right) \circ \exp\left(\boldsymbol{f}_{\mathrm{Reg}}(\boldsymbol{u}_i^{(k)})\right) . \tag{3}$$

Die rechte Seite der Gleichung wird mithilfe der *Baker-Campbell-Hausdorff*-Formel approximiert [9]. Im Gegensatz zu (2) wird im diffeomorphen Ansatz das Geschwindigkeitsfeld und nicht das Verschiebungsfeld geglättet.

2.2 Integrierte Level-Set-Segmentierung

Die Segmentierung der Zielbilder mittels Level-Set-Verfahren lässt sich als Minimierung des Funktionals

$$\mathcal{J}_{\mathrm{Seg}}[\phi_i] := \mathcal{I}[\phi_i] \; + \; \mathcal{E}[I_i;\phi_i] = \min! \tag{4}$$

formulieren, wobei $\mathcal{I}$ die interne Energie und $\mathcal{E}$ eine regionenbasierte externe Energie bezeichnen [10]. Die optimale Level-Set-Funktion ϕ_i wird iterativ durch

$$\phi_i^{(k+1)} = \phi_i^{(k)} - \delta(\phi_i^{(k)}) \left(\nabla \frac{\nabla \phi_i^{(k)}}{\|\nabla \phi_i^{(k)}\|} + f_{\mathrm{Seg}}(\phi_i^{(k)}, I_i) \right) \tag{5}$$

berechnet, wobei $f_{\mathrm{Seg}} := f_{\mathcal{E}}$ ein aus der externen Energie resultierender Kraftterm ist [2, 10] und $\delta(x)$ die Dirac-Distribution bezeichnet.

Die Segmentierung wird mit der Registrierung gekoppelt, indem zusätzlich gefordert wird, dass ϕ_{Ref} und ϕ_i korrespondierende Segmentierungen darstellen, im Fall der Segmentierung also der Abstand der ins Zielbild transformierten Referenzsegmentierung $\phi_{\mathrm{Ref}}(\boldsymbol{x} + \boldsymbol{u}_i^{-1}(\boldsymbol{x}))$ zur Oberfläche von $\phi_i(\boldsymbol{x})$ gering ist. Der Kraftterm wird demnach erweitert zu

$$f_{\mathrm{Seg}} := f_{\mathcal{E}} + \left(\phi_i(\boldsymbol{x}) - \phi_{\mathrm{Ref}}(\boldsymbol{x} + \boldsymbol{u}_i^{-1}(\boldsymbol{x}))\right) ,$$

d.h. ϕ_i wird in Richtung der transformierten Referenzsegmentierung gelenkt.

Gleichzeitig wird an die Registrierung die zusätzliche Forderung gestellt, dass die Referenzsegmentierung möglichst nahe der transformierten Segmentierung des Zielbildes liegen soll. Es resultiert eine Kraft

$$\boldsymbol{f}_{\mathrm{Reg}} := \boldsymbol{f}_{\mathcal{D}} + \delta(\phi_{\mathrm{Ref}}(\boldsymbol{x})) \; \left(\phi_{\mathrm{Ref}}(\boldsymbol{x}) - \phi_i(\boldsymbol{x} + \boldsymbol{u}_i(\boldsymbol{x}))\right) \nabla \phi_i(\boldsymbol{x} + \boldsymbol{u}_i(\boldsymbol{x})) ,$$

die an der Objektoberfläche von ϕ_{Ref} in Richtung der Segmentierung ϕ_i wirkt.

Optimiert werden ϕ_i und $\boldsymbol{u}_i$ alternierend nach Gleichungen (3) und (5). Es ist zu beachten, dass die Kraftterme von Segmentierung und Registrierung über unterschiedlichen Bildräumen definiert sind und Kräfte an unterschiedlichen Stellen auftreten, bei der Segmentierung an der Oberfläche von ϕ_i, bei der Registrierung am Rand von ϕ_{Ref}.

2.3 Methodik der Evaluation

Für die Evaluation standen 4D-CT-Daten von 7 Patienten zur Verfügung, die jeweils 8 Zeitpunkte der Einatmung von max. Exhalation zu max. Inhalation abbilden. Als Referenzbild wurde I_0 (max. Exhalation) gewählt. Die Integrierung der Segmentierung wurde am Beispiel der Leber evaluiert.

Es wurden die Ergebnisse einer einfachen diffeomorphen Registrierung (Abschn. 2.1) denen des vorgeschlagenen integrierten Verfahrens gegenübergestellt (jeweils bei Registrierung mit max. Inhalation I_7) und somit der Qualitätsgewinn durch die vereinigte Segmentierung und Registrierung untersucht.

Weiterhin wurde der Nutzen einer sukzessiven Initialisierung untersucht. Dabei wurden einerseits die Verfahren unabhängig mit den Zielbildern $I_1(\boldsymbol{x}), \ldots, I_7(\boldsymbol{x})$ ausgeführt, andererseits wurde die Anwendung für jeden Schritt i mit $\boldsymbol{v}_{i-1}$ initialisiert. Die Ergebnisse wurden im Hinblick auf Registrierungsgüte (MSD, *Mean Squared Differences* zwischen Referenz- und transformiertem Zielbild) evaluiert und der Einfluss einer Multi-Resulution-Strategie untersucht.

3 Ergebnisse

Durch Integrierung von Segmentierung und Registrierung konnte der MSD-Abstand bei sieben Patienten um durchschnittlich 21% verringert werden, es ist eine signifikante Verbesserung der Ergebnisse zu beobachten ($p < 0,01$, gepaarter

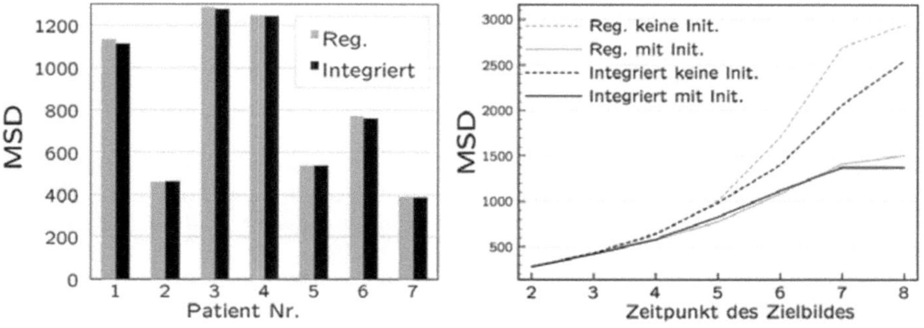

Abb. 1. *Links:* Vergleich des MSD der einfachen Registrierung mit dem vorgeschlagenen Verfahren (3 Level Multi-Resolution). *Rechts:* Verbesserung der Verfahren durch sukzessive Initialisierung mit $\boldsymbol{v}_{i-1}$ (kein Multi-Resolution).

t-Test). Bei Verwendung einer Multi-Resolution-Strategie verliert die Verbesserung jedoch an Signifikanz und sinkt auf durchschnittlich 2,6% bei zwei Levels, bzw. 0,9% bei 3 Levels (jeweils $p < 0,1$). Weiterhin konnte gezeigt werden, dass eine sukzessive Initialisierung, wie sie durch den vorgeschlagenen Ansatz ermöglicht wird, zu einer deutlichen Verbesserung der Ergebnisse führt (Abb. 1).

4 Diskussion

Es wurde gezeigt, dass die Integrierung von Segmentierung und Registrierung zu einer Verbesserung der Bewegungsfeldschätzung führt. Dabei erlaubt die Verwendung einer diffeomorphen Registrierung die Betrachtung räumlich-zeitlicher Sequenzen und die Berechnung von 3D-Trajektorien. Zudem ist die Kenntnis der Inversen Voraussetzung für diverse Applikationen [11].

Die quantitativ geringe Verbesserung des MSD-Maßes ist v.a. darauf zurückzuführen, dass bereits die einfache diffeomorphe Registrierung sehr gute Ergebnisse liefert, was in der Wahl des Distanzmaßes (Thirion statt SSD) und der Verwendung einer Multi-Resulution-Strategie begründet ist.

Weiterhin zeigen die Ergebnisse, dass eine sukzessiven Initialisierung zur Verbesserung der Ergebnisse führt, da auf diese Weise große Bewegungen präziser abgebildet werden. Dies ist besonders dann von Bedeutung, wenn keine Multi-Resolution-Strategie verwendet wird und große Bewegungsamplituden im Verhältnis zur Objektgröße auftreten.

Literaturverzeichnis

1. Sarrut D. Deformable registration for image-guided radiation therapy. Z Med Phys. 2006; p. 1–38.
2. Schmidt-Richberg A, et al. Variationeller Ansatz fur eine integrierte Segmentierung und nicht-lineare Registrierung. Proc BVM. 2008; p. 26–20.
3. Yezzi A, Zollei L, Kapur T. A variational framework for integrating segmentation and registration through active contours. Med Image Anal. 2003;7(2):171–185.
4. Paragios N, Rousson M, Ramesh V. Knowledge-based registration and segmentation of the left ventricle: A level set approach. IEEE Comput Graph Appl. 2002; p. 37–42.
5. An J, Chen Y, Huang F, et al. A variational PDE based level set method for a simultaneous segmentation and non-rigid registration. Procs MICCAI. 2005; p. 286–293.
6. Ashburner J, Friston KJ. Unified segmentation. NeuroImage. 2005;26(3):839–851.
7. Modersitzki J. Numerical Methods for Image Registration. Oxford Univ; 2004.
8. Arsigny V, Commowick O, Pennec X, et al. A log-euclidean framework for statistics on diffeomorphisms. Proc MICCAI. 2006; p. 754–761.
9. Vercauteren T, Pennec X, Perchant A, et al. Symmetric log-domain diffeomorphic registration: A demons-based approach. Proc MICCAI. 2008; p. 924–931.
10. Chan TF, Vese LA. Active contours without edges. IEEE Trans Image Process. 2001;10(2):266–277.
11. Ehrhardt J, Werner R, Schmidt-Richberg A, et al. Generation of a mean motion model of the lung using 4D-CT image data. Proc VCBM. 2008; p. 69–76.

Verbesserung der Symmetrie von Hirnaufnahmen entlang der Sagittalebene

Konstantin Ens[1,2], Fabian Wenzel[2], Bernd Fischer[1]

[1]Universität zu Lübeck, Institut für Mathematik, Wallstraße 40, 23560 Lübeck
[2]Philips Research Hamburg, Röntgenstraße 24–26, 22335 Hamburg
ens@math.uni-luebeck.de

Kurzfassung. Die lokale Symmetrie von Hirnscans entlang der Sagittalebene zu ermitteln und zu modifizieren, ist für eine Reihe neurologischer Anwendungen interessant. Beispielsweise kann der voxelweise Vergleich von rechter und linker Hirnhälfte nur dann Aufschluss über die Lokalisierung von Läsionen geben, wenn durch Transformation ein Hirnscan eine möglichst hohe Symmetrie aufweist. Ein weiteres Anwendungsgebiet ist die Visualisierung von medialen Hirnschnitten, für die die Trennfläche beider Hirnhälfte möglichst eben sein sollte. Diese Arbeit stellt die Entwicklung eines Verfahrens vor, mit dessen Hilfe die Symmetrie von Hirnaufnahmen entlang der Sagittalebene verbessert werden kann. Dies geschieht unter Verwendung von aktiven Konturen, die mit Hilfe einer neuartigen Kostenfunktion gesteuert werden. Experimente am Ende der Arbeit mit strukturellen Kernspinaufnahmen demonstrieren die Leistungsfähigkeit des Verfahrens.

1 Einleitung

Die Tatsache, dass jede Hirnaufnahme durch eine Ebene in zwei Hirnhälften geteilt werden kann, ist prinzipiell falsch. In aller Regel ist das menschliche Gehirn bezüglich der sagittalen Ebene nicht symmetrisch [1]. Es existieren jedoch eine Reihe von Anwendungen, für die ein entlang der Sagittalebene symmetrisches Gehirn von Vorteil wäre, beispielsweise die Visualisierung eines medialen Hirnschnitts, die Verwendung von symmetrischen Hirnatlanten oder die voxelweise Symmetrieanalyse beider Hirnhälften, die man durch üblicherweise durch Spiegelung der Aufnahme erreicht [2]. Derzeit wird die fehlende Symmetrie bei Atlanten nicht berücksichtigt [3] oder vernachlässigt [4]. Beispielsweise führt kein Registrierverfahren für Hirnscans einen Ausgleichsschritt durch, der die Trennfläche beider Hirnhälften auf eine Ebene transformiert. So sind Symmetriemaße medial fehlerbehaftet. Schließlich ist auch für die Erstellung von Hirnatlanten aus individuellen Aufnahmen eine in diesem Artikel beschriebene Verarbeitung wünschenswert. Im Folgenden wird ein Konzept vorgestellt, mit dem die Symmetrie der Hirnhälf- ten entlang der Sagittalebene verbessert werden kann. Im Rahmen dieser Arbeit wird eine Möglichkeit vorgestellt, wie mit Hilfe einer speziellen Kostenfunktion eine sagittale Trennfläche zwischen den Hirnhälften ermittelt wird, die anschließend auf eine Ebene transformiert werden kann.

2 Material und Methoden

Die Ermittlung der Trennfläche beider Hirnhälften, die hinterher auf eine Ebene abgebildet werden soll, ist nicht trivial, denn sie verläuft zwar zwischen den Kortexoberflächen beider Hirnhälften, aber sie schneidet Strukturen im Klein- und Mittelhirn. Einfache, schwellwertbasierte Methoden zur Segmentierung der beiden Hirnhälften sind deshalb nicht anwendbar. Ein komplexes, modellbasiertes Verfahren wäre hingegen wegen der großen individuellen Variabilität von Hirnstrukturen nur mit großem Aufwand zu entwickeln. In dieser Arbeit wird deshalb lediglich die Trennfläche beider Hirnhälften modelliert und durch aktive Konture detektiert. Das vorliegende Problem kann mathematisch als Minimierungsaufgabe formuliert werden. Gegeben sei ein Bild $\mathbf{I}(x, y, z) \in \mathbb{R}$ auf dem Einheitswürfel $\Omega = [0, 1]^3$, gesucht sei eine über der (y, z)-Ebene parametrisierte Fläche $\mathbf{P} : \mathbb{R}^2 \rightarrow \mathbb{R}, x = \mathbf{P}(y, z)$, die erstens in der Mitte zwischen den beiden Hirnhälften verläuft und zweitens möglichst glatt ist. Beide Bedingungen lassen sich in einem zu minimierendem Funktional

$$J(\mathbf{P}; \mathbf{I}) = C(\mathbf{P}; \mathbf{I}) + S(\mathbf{P}) \tag{1}$$

kombinieren, wobei C eine spezielle Kostenfunktion ist, die die Position der Trennfläche beschreibt. Durch den Regularisierer S wird die Glattheit der geforderten Fläche beschrieben. Als interne Energie für die Regularisierung dient die 1987 von Kass, Withkin und Terzopolous [5] vorgeschlagene Komponente

$$S(\mathbf{P}) := \frac{1}{2} \int_0^1 \int_0^1 |\mathbf{P}'(y, z)|^2 + |\mathbf{P}''(y, z)|^2 dy\, dz, \tag{2}$$

durch die sowohl eine starke Krümmung als auch die Bildung von Löchern der Fläche vermeidet. Die Kostenfunktion C soll berücksichtigen, dass die zu berechnende Fläche das Bild in zwei Teilen mit möglichst symmetrischem Inhalt aufteilt. Idealerweise sollten also zu beiden Seiten der Fläche die entsprechenden Grauwerte gleich sein. Dies ist der Fall, wenn das folgende Funktional den Wert Null hat

$$C(\mathbf{P}; \mathbf{I}) := \frac{1}{2} \int_0^1 \int_0^1 \int_0^{\Delta x} |\mathbf{I}(\mathbf{P}(y, z) + s, y, z) - \mathbf{I}(\mathbf{P}(y, z) - s, y, z))|^2 ds\, dy\, dz. \tag{3}$$

Für die Berechnung eines Minimums von (1) lässt sich mit Hilfe der Variationsrechnung eine notwendige Bedingung erster Ordnung angeben, die mit finiten Differenzen diskretisiert und schließlich über eine Fixpunktiteration gelöst werden kann. Als Startposition der Trennfläche bietet sich die (y, z)-Ebene in der Mitte des Volumens an, wenn durch einen vorgeschalteten Registrierschritt, z.B. [6], der Hirnscan in etwa mittig im Volumen liegt. Gängige Koordinatensysteme für Atlasscans (MNI, Talairach) haben diese Eigenschaft [7, 8]. Im letzten Schritt soll nun basierend auf der berechneten Symmetriefläche eine Symmetrieebene in der Mitte des Volumens erzeugt werden. Hinzu wird das gesamte Volumen entsprechend zeilenweise entlang der x-Achse linear interpoliert.

Tabelle 1. C_0: Mittelwert des Symmetriemaßes vor der Anwendung des Verfahrens. C_{end}: Mittelwert des Symmetriemaßes nach der Anwendung des Verfahrens, $\frac{C_0}{C_{\text{end}}} \cdot 100\%$: Verbesserung des Symmetriemaßes in %, std(C_{end}): Standardabweichung der Verbesserung. I_0: Mittelwert des Intensitätsmaßes vor der Anwendung des Verfahrens. I_{end}: Mittelwert des Intensitätsmaßes nach der Anwendung des Verfahrens, $\frac{I_0}{I_{\text{end}}} \cdot 100\%$: Veränderung des Intensitätsmaßes in %, std(I_{end}): Standardabweichung der Veränderung.

C_0	C_{end}	$\frac{C_0}{C_{\text{end}}} \cdot 100\%$	std(C_{end})	I_0	I_{end}	$\frac{I_0}{I_{\text{end}}} \cdot 100\%$	std(I_{end})
2255	1524	67.6	4.86	8394	7970	95	1.03

3 Ergebnisse

Dieser Abschnitt beschreibt die Anwendung der vorgestellte Methode in zwei Szenarien: (i) Visualisierung eines medial geschnittenen, T1-gewichteten MR-Hirnscans, (ii) Symmetrieanalyse. Für die Visualisierungsaufgabe wurde der vom *International Consortium for Brain Mapping* (ICBM) [3] zur Verfügung gestellte MR Atlas verwendet, der sich im MNI-Raum befindet. Die Ausschnitte des Atlasses vor und nach der Erstellung der Symmetrie sind in Abbildung 1 zu sehen. Rote Pfeile in Abbildung 1(a) markieren Regionen, die deutlich von der Symmetrieebene abweichen. Nach der Anwendung der vorgestellten Methode auf den ICBM-Atlas erhalten wir die in Abbildung 1(b) illustrierte Trennfläche. Abbildung 2 zeigt exemplarisch einige Transversalschnitte mit detektierter Trennfläche. Die entprechenden Bilder nach der Interpolation sind in Abbildung 3 und 1(c) dargestellt. Es ist leicht zu erkennen, dass die Trennfläche jetzt eben zwischen den Hirnhälften verläuft. Die visuell festgestellte Verbesserung lässt sich quantitativ durch Symmetrieanalyse bestätigen. Es wurden zwei Qualitätsmaße ausgewertet: das Symmetriemaß $C(\mathbf{P}; \mathbf{I})$ aus (3) und die Summe I der Grauwerte

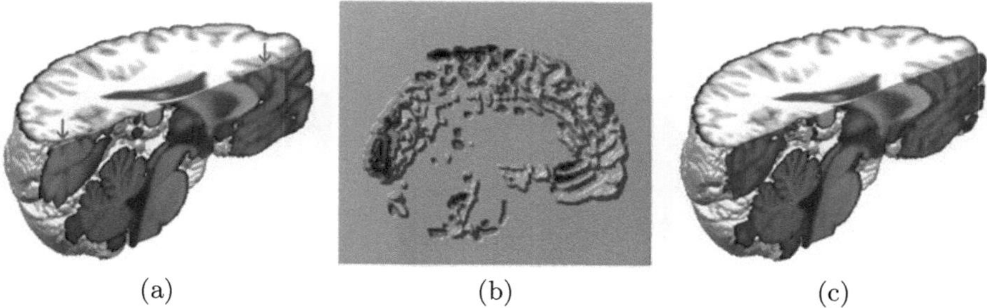

(a) (b) (c)

Abb. 1. (a) Ein Ausschnitt aus dem 3D MR Volumen. Die Schnittebene verläuft zwar in der Mitte der beiden Hirnhälften, trotzdem wurden lokal Kortexstrukturen geschnitten (rote Pfeile). (b) Die berechnete Abweichung der detektierten Trennfläche von einer Ebene. Die Farbgebung entspricht einer Abweichung von -3 (dunkelblau) über 0 (Hintergrundfarbe) bis +6 Voxeln (dunkelrot). (c) Ein Ausschnitt aus dem transformiertem 3D Volumen. Die transformierte Trennfläche beider Hirnhälften entspricht der Schnittebene.

auf der sagittalen Ebene vor und nach Transformation des Volumens. Motivation für I ist die Tatsache, dass T1-Intensitätswerte im Gewebe höher sind als in der Hirnflüssigkeit. Eine optimale Trennfläche beider Hirnhälften sollte also eine minimale Summe der auf ihr enthaltenen Intensitätswerte zeigen. Die Symmetrieanalyse fand auf 53 Datensätzen aus der ADNI-Datenbank [9] statt. Die Scans wurden vorher mit einem Registrierverfahren und einem entsprechendem Referenzbild mit $181 \times 217 \times 181$ Voxeln in den MNI Raum transformiert [7].

Die Ergebnisse in Tabelle 1 zeigen eine mittlere Verbesserung des Symmetriemaßes von 67.6 % (min: 57 %, max: 82 %). Die mittlere Intensitätssumme I auf der Trennebene könnte um 5% verringert werden. Beide Maße haben geringe Streuung, sind also als robust einzuschätzen. Für die Berechnungen und die gegebene Bildgröße wurde als Grenze des Vertrauensintervalls $\Delta x = 5$ gewählt. Die Berechnungen erfolgten in Matlab 7.6.0 auf einem Pentium Centrino mit 2 GHz und 2 GB Arbeitsspeicher. Das Verfahren brauchte für die Berechungen ca. 5 Sekunden je Datensatz. Für Anwendungen mit speziellen Anforderungen hinsichtlich der Rechenzeit sei erwähnt, dass das Verfahren durch Modifikationen, wie z.B. der Integration eines Multi-Level-Ansatzes, beschleunigt werden kann.

4 Diskussion

In dieser Arbeit wurde ein Verfahren zur Verbesserung der Symmetrie von Kopfaufnahmen entlang der Sagittalebene vorgestellt. Die Methode nutzt aktive Konturen mit einer neu entwickelten Kostenfunktion zur Detektion der Trennfläche. Die Transformation der Trennfläche auf eine Ebene erfolgt mit einer eindimensionalen linearen Interpolation. Das Verfahren wurde mit 53 Scans und zwei Qualitätsmaße getestet. Die Ergebnisse haben gezeigt, dass die Symmetrie konsistent verbessern werden konnte. In der Zukunft planen wir unsere Methode in folgenden Punkten zu verbessern. Die Δx muss noch manuell gefunden werden, dieses Schritt lässt sich aber automatisieren. Die eindimensionale lineare Interpolation sollte durch ein intelligenteres Verfahren zur Deformation des Scans ersetzt

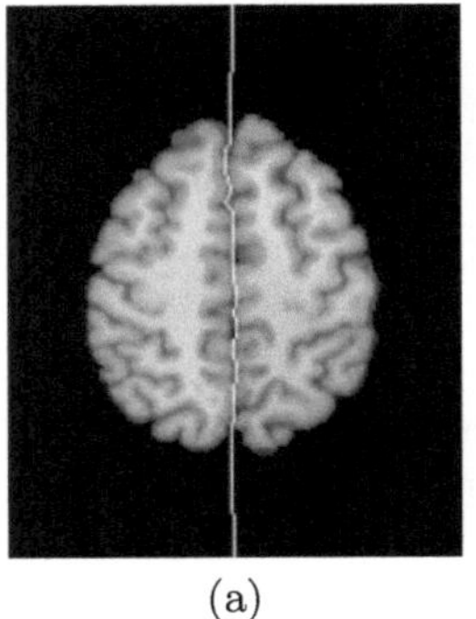

(a)

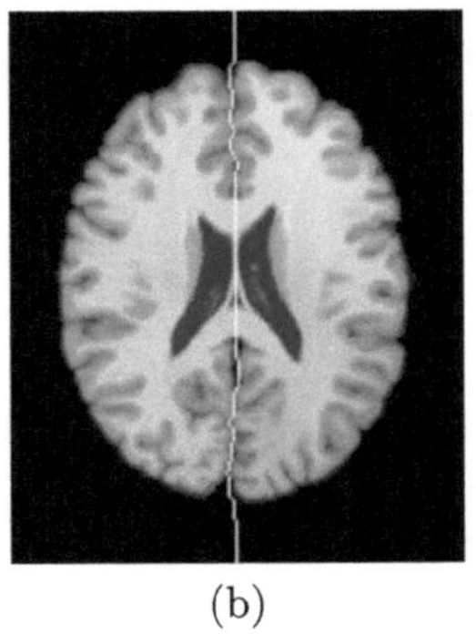

(b)

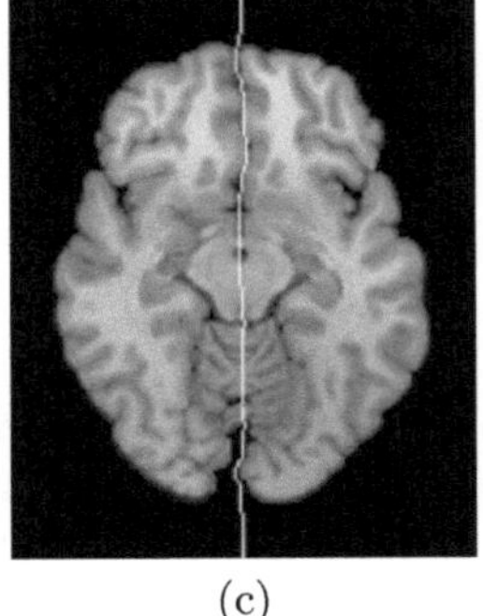

(c)

Abb. 2. Drei Schnitte aus dem ICBM Atlas entlang der Transversalebene. Die in diesem Schnitt ermittelte Trennlinie beider Hirnhälften ist in der Mitte des Volumens zu sehen.

Abb. 3. Drei Schnitte aus dem ICBM Atlas nach Verbesserung der Symmetrie entlang der Sagittalebene.

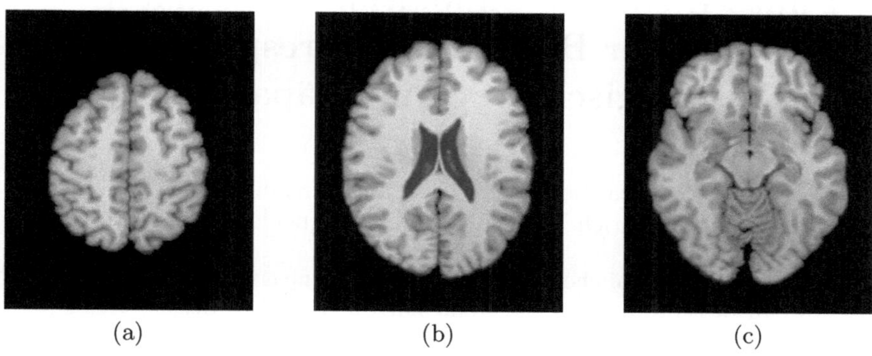

(a) (b) (c)

werden. Die Randbedingungen der Interpolation sollen besser an die Problemstellung angepasst werden. Die Segmentierung durch Trennfläche kann mit dem in [10] beschriebenem Verfahren verglichen werden.

Danksagung. Wir danken Steffen Renisch und Stewart Young von Philips Research Hamburg und Ralph Buchert von Universitätsklinikum Hamburg-Eppendorf für die fachliche Unterstützung.

Literaturverzeichnis

1. Kimura D. The asymmetry of the human brain. Sci Am. 1973;228(3):8–70.
2. Oostenveld R, et al. Brain symmetry and topographic analysis of lateralized event-related potentials. Clin Neurophys. 2003;114:1194–1202.
3. Abbott A. A new atlas of the brain. Nature. 2003; p. 249–250.
4. Apostolova I, et al. Detection of a possible epilepsy focus in the residual mesial temporal lobe in a patient operated on a ganglioglioma by ictal and interictal perfusion SPECT only after computer-aided sub-traction analysis. Nuklearmedizin. 2008;47:N65–N68.
5. Kass M, et al. Snakes: Active contour models. IJCV. 1987;1(4):321–331.
6. Maurer CR, Fitzpatrick JM. A review of medical image registration. Interactive Image-Guided Neurosurgery. 1993; p. 17–44.
7. Chau W, McIntosh AR. The Talairach coordinate of a point in the MNI space: How to interpret it. NeuroImage. 2005;25(2):408–416.
8. Talairach J, Tournoux P. Co-planar stereotaxic atlas of the human brain: 3-Dimensional proportional system - an approach to cerebral imaging. Thieme Medical Publishers, New York, NY. 1988.
9. ADNI. http://www.loni.ucla.edu/ADNI.
10. Zhao L, et al. Accurate 3D left-right brain hemisphere segmentation in MR images based on shape bottlenecks and partial volume estimation. Proc SCIA. 2007; p. 581–590.

Netzgenerierung und Finite-Elemente-Simulation muskulärer Strukturen unter Beachtung korrespondierender histologischer Schnittpräparate

Frank Weichert[1], Andreas Schröder[2], Constantin Landes[3], Lars Walczak[1], Heinrich Müller[1], Mathias Wagner[4]

[1]Lehrstuhl für Graphische Systeme, Technische Universität Dortmund
[2]Institut für Mathematik, Humboldt Universität zu Berlin
[3]Kiefer- und Plastische Gesichtschirurgie, Universitätsklinikum Frankfurt
[4]Institut für Allgemeine und Spezielle Pathologie, Universität des Saarlandes
frank.weichert@tu-dortmund.de

Kurzfassung. In dieser Arbeit wird ein Verfahren zur Netzgenerierung und Finite-Elemente-Simulation muskulärer Strukturen vorgestellt. Eine Herausforderung liegt dabei in der Fusion der Simulationsergebnisse mit den Daten histologischer Schnittpräparate. Basierend auf segmentierten histologischen Daten wird eine Rekonstruktion der relevanten muskulären Strukturen mittels eines BCC-Tetraedernetzes initiiert. Dieses wird getriggert über einen Level-Set-Ansatz. Die Deformation des Muskels wird dann mittels eines hyperelastischen Materialgesetzes modelliert und mithilfe der Finite-Elemente-Methode simuliert. Anschließend erfolgt eine Projektion der Ergebnisse der Simulation auf die histologischen Schnittpräparate. Als Anwendungsfall wurden Daten abortiver Feten mit einer Spaltbildung im Bereich der Lippen-, Kiefer- und Gaumenregion herangezogen.

1 Einleitung

Das Ziel gegenwärtiger rechnergestützter biologischer Simulationen besteht darin, anatomische Detailinformationen, dreidimensionale Rekonstruktionen der relevanten Regionen und mathematische Simulationen des Deformationsverhaltens zu vereinheitlichen. Aufgrund der Komplexität anatomischer und physiologischer Verhältnisse biologischer Objekte zum Beispiel im Viscerocranium sind hierzu Finite-Elemente-Methoden (FE-Methoden) aufgrund ihrer hohen Flexibilität in besonderem Maße als Simulationsverfahren geeignet [1]. Bei mesenchymalem Weichgewebe sind die Randflächen bisweilen durch feingliedrige Ausfransungen oder spitz zulaufende Geometrien relativ kompliziert, sodass Algorithmen zur Generierung von FE-Netzen gegenwärtig eine große Herausforderung bilden.

Der vorgestellte Ansatz unterscheidet sich insofern von anderen Arbeiten, dass der komplette Approximationsvorgang direkt am Volumennetz erfolgt, der gewünschten anatomischen Detailgrad berücksichtigt wird und den Vorgaben der FE-Methode genügt [2]. Eigene Studien deuten daraufhin, dass bestehende Verfahren diese Vorgabe nicht geeignet beachten [3]. Auch sind Möglichkeiten einer graphischen Rückführung der Ergebnisse einer FE-Simulation auf die komplexen und hoch detaillierten histologischen Strukturen noch wenig untersucht. Daher wird ergänzend eine Projektion der FE-Simulationsergebnisse auf die histologischen Daten vollzogen.

Ein hochrelevantes Anwendungsgebiet für die oben genannte Problemstellung ist die Therapie von Neugeborenen oder Kindern, bei denen krankhafte angeborene Spaltbildungen im Bereich der Lippen-, Kiefer- und Gaumenregion (LKG) vorliegen. Die derzeit üblichen Operationsmethoden zur Linderung der Erkrankung sind in mancherlei Hinsicht noch nicht vollständig ausgereift, sodass Langzeitergebnisse bisweilen leider noch unbefriedigend sind [4].

2 Material und Methoden

Initial wird zur Simulation der viscerocranialen Skelettmuskelaktivität ein Finite-Elemente konformes Tetraedernetz aus den Segmentierungsdaten digitalisierter histologischer Großflächenschnittpräparate generiert [3].

2.1 Mesh-Generierung

Realisiert wird die Bereitstellung eines FE-konformen Tetraedernetzes auf Basis einer Polygonzug-Segmentierung über einen Level-Set Ansatz, der eine implizite Oberfläche auf einem kartesischen Gitter erstellt [5]. Diese wird über die zeitliche Evolution einer initialen Schätzung der Oberfläche mit einem physikalisch motivierten Konvektionsmodell bestimmt, welches über die Level-Set Gleichung $\frac{\partial \phi}{\partial t} = \nabla d(\boldsymbol{x}) \cdot \nabla \phi$ modelliert wird. Dabei ist $\phi : \mathbb{R}^3 \mapsto \mathbb{R}$ eine vorzeichenbehaftete Distanzfunktion, dessen Nullmenge den Verlauf der gesuchten Kontur angibt. $d(\boldsymbol{x})$ ist eine zuvor aus dem Polygonzug-Datensatz berechnete vorzeichenlose Distanzfunktion, die als Potentialfeld dient, um die Kontur anzuziehen. Die Oberfläche wird im Folgenden genutzt, um eine Octree-Struktur durch mehrere Iterationen adaptiv zu verfeinern, wobei die Octree-Zellen aus sogenannten BCC-Tetraedern bestehen, die günstige Eigenschaften wie beispielsweise Unterteilungsinvarianz aufweisen und in ihren Qualitätsmaßen gleichschenkligen Tetraedern ähneln [2]. Zur Approximationsverbesserung wird das entsprechend generierte Netz über eine Masse-Feder-Simulation noch in Richtung der Null-Isokontur $\phi(\boldsymbol{x}) = 0$ des Level-Sets deformiert. Nach erfolgtem Abschluss der Netzgenerierung liegt die Rekonstruktion des ausgewählten Muskels der Lippen-, Kiefer- und Gaumenregion als Tetraedernetz vor. Basierend auf diesem Netz kann nachfolgend eine FE-Simulation erfolgen, die das Deformationsverhalten eines kontrahierenden Muskels unter Verwendung einer Volumenkraft geeignet nachzubilden versucht.

2.2 Modellierung der Muskeldeformation und FE-Simulation

Die Deformation des Muskels wird mithilfe eines hyperelastischen Materialgesetzes nach Mooney-Rivlin für isotropes und nahezu inkompressibles Materialverhalten modelliert. Dieses Materialgesetz bietet einen physikalisch begründbaren Rahmen zur Modellierung von Weich- und Muskelgewebe [6]. Zur Beschreibung von Anisotropien, die durch das Vorhandensein von Muskelfasern bedingt sind, kann das Materialgesetz zudem mit transvers-isotropen Modellanteilen erweitert werden [1]. Sofern von Isotropie ausgegangen wird, hat das Formänderungsenergiefunktional die Gestalt $W = \kappa W_{\text{vol}} + W_{\text{iso}}(\tilde{I}_1, \tilde{I}_2)$ mit den Hauptinvarianten $\tilde{I}_1 := \text{tr}(\tilde{C}) = \tilde{C}_{ii}$ und $\tilde{I}_2 := \frac{1}{2}(\tilde{I}_1^2 - \text{tr}(\tilde{C}^2))$ des volumetrisch-isochor entkoppelten Cauchy-Green-Tensors $\tilde{C}$. Das Materialgesetz wird durch die Angabe des isochoren Anteils W_{iso} spezifiziert. Beim Ansatz nach Mooney-Rivlin hat dieser die Form $W_{\text{iso}}(\tilde{I}_1, \tilde{I}_2) := c_1(\tilde{I}_1 - 3) + c_2(\tilde{I}_2 - 3)$ mit den Materialparametern c_1 und c_2. Durch Verwenden eines geeigneten volumetrischen Anteils W_{vol} und eines hinreichend großen Kompressibilitätsmoduls κ kann die Inkompressibilität des Weichgewebes wiedergegeben werden. Die für eine medizinische Bewertung aufschlussreiche Verteilung der Spannungsverhältnisse innerhalb des Muskels wird zu einer vorgegebenen Volumenkraft [1] mithilfe der Hauptspannungswerte ermittelt. Diese ergeben sich als die drei reellen Eigenwerte des symmetrischen Cauchyschen Spannungstensors (Abb. 1(d)). Zur numerischen Berechnung der Deformation sowie der Hauptspannungswerte wird ein verschiebungsbasierter, stückweise linearer FE-Ansatz verwendet, der auf einer nichtlinearen variationellen Formulierung des Modells basiert. Das hierbei entstehende nichtlineare Gleichungssystem wird mithilfe eines Newton-Raphson-Verfahrens gelöst.

Zur initialen Verifikation wurden der Prozess der Netzgenerierung und dessen nachgeschaltete FE-Simulation zunächst an synthetischen Daten analysiert. Bezogen auf den realen Muskel im dreidimensionalen Modell (Abb. 1(d)), repräsentieren die Farbwerte Bereiche hoher Spannungskonzentrationen, die durch die Kontraktion des Muskelgewebes hervorgerufen werden. Angemerkt sei, dass eine Validierung der Spannungen nicht im Fokus dieses Aufsatzes liegt. Als Ergebnis der FE-Simulation steht somit eine dreidimensionale Repräsentation zur Verfü-

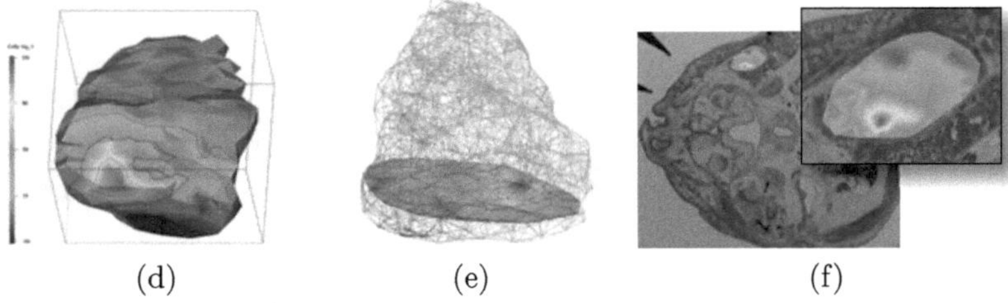

Abb. 1. (a) Visualisierung der Muskeldeformation (Spannungen) innerhalb eines FE-konformen Volumennetzes durch die Farbverteilung. (b) Visualisierung der Muskeldeformation bezogen auf eine ausgezeichnete Ebene innerhalb der 3D-Konformation und (c) Projektion der FE-Simulationsmerkmale auf das histologische Schnittpräparat.

gung, welche neben der deformierten Geometrie auch die Spannungswerte pro Tetraeder enthält. Da über eine konventionelle Darstellung die Simulationsergebnisse dem durchschnittlichen histologisch geschulten Untersucher mitunter nur schwer zu vermitteln sind, wird eine integrierte Visualisierung beider Informationskompartimente durch Projektion der FE-Simulation auf histologische Daten bereitgestellt. Zur Realisierung dieser Anforderung ist ein Schnitt des Volumennetzes mit einer achsenparallelen Ebene auf Höhe des betreffenden histologischen Schnittpräparats zu ermitteln und diese Ebene trianguliert bereitzustellen. Mittels linearer Interpolation innerhalb der entstandenen Dreiecke wird eine (farbliche) Textur generiert, die zusammen mit dem histologischen Schnittpräparat visualisiert werden kann (Abb. 1(f)).

3 Ergebnisse

Zur Verifikation des vorgestellten Verfahrens werden innerhalb der Abbildung 2(a) zuerst die Abstände der äußeren Volumennetzknoten zum Null-Level-Set $\phi = 0$ bewertet. Circa ein Viertel der gegebenen 4860 Oberflächenknoten liegt zu Beginn der physikbasierten Deformation zehn Pixel (60 Mikrometer pro Pixel) oder weiter vom Nullniveau entfernt. Mit fortschreitender Kompression verschiebt sich das Gros in Richtung der Null. Zudem dringen sehr wenige Knoten ($< 10\%$) in das Innere der impliziten Oberfläche ein. Bei der zehnten Iteration schließlich liegt der Mittelwert der Abstände (RMS) bei ungefähr 3.1 Pixel. Mit dem Verhalten der Konditionszahlen liegt ein weiteres Indiz zur Beurteilung der Netzqualität vor (Abb. 2(b)). Aus dem Kurvenverlauf der Konditionszahlen im Verhältnis zur fortschreitenden Annäherung an die Oberfläche ϕ lässt sich ableiten, dass nach Iteration vier jede weitere Annäherung die Kondition negativ beeinflusst – der optimale Zeitpunkt des Deformationsendes läge somit zwischen Iteration vier und acht. Die benötigte Zeit zur Erstellung eines Tetraedernetzes für die vorliegenden muskulären Strukturen beträgt auf einem aktuellen Intel Core2 Duo durchschnittlich fünf Minuten bei einem 200^3 Level-Set Gitter mit vier Verfeinerungsstufen sowie zehn Iterationen der physikbasierten Deformation.

Ausgehend von der Qualität des Netzes wird anhand der Abbildung 2(c) die Verteilung der Hauptspannungen entlang der z-Achse vermittelt. Es wird deut-

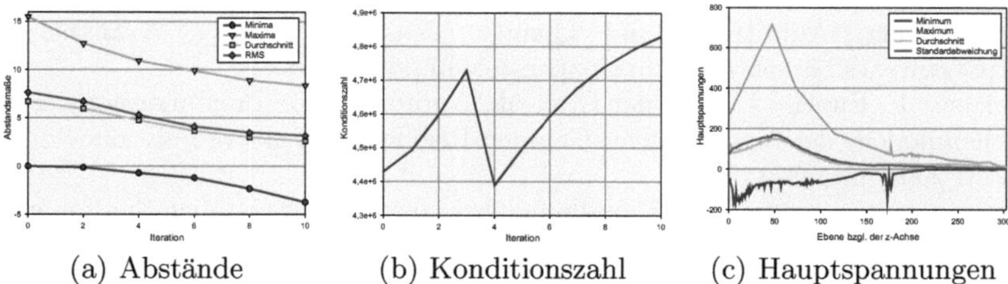

(a) Abstände (b) Konditionszahl (c) Hauptspannungen

Abb. 2. (a)-(b) Statistische Merkmale zur Beurteilung des FE-konformen Tetraedernetzes über Iterationen der Approximation und (c) zu den Hauptspannungen des Cauchyschen Spannungstensors über den Verlauf der Ebenen (bzgl. der z-Achse).

lich, dass in der Nähe der festgehaltenen Fläche (z-Wert = 0) hohe Spannungen im simulierten, lang gezogenen Muskel auftreten, die mit größerer Entfernung (nicht linear) abnehmen. Innerhalb der Abbildung 1(e) wird die Ebene mit dem Maximalausschlag visualisiert ($z \approx 50$). Erkennbar ist eine isolierte Region mit hohen Spannungswerten (rote Farbe), welches ein Indiz für eine (zu) starke Beanspruchung des Muskels in diesem Bereich sein könnte. In der dreidimensionalen Konformation (Abb. 1(d)) treten im oberen Bereich des Muskels derartige Regionen hingegen nicht auf.

4 Diskussion

Mit dem Ziel, neue Erkenntnisse für Operationsmethoden zu gewinnen, wurde eine FE-Simulation von Skelettmuskeln basierend auf einem Level-Set-Ansatz etabliert, die initial durch ein Tetraedernetz approximiert wurden. Insbesondere die integrierte Visualisierung von histologischen Strukturen und den Ergebnissen der FE-Simulation vermittelt einen ersten Eindruck der Spannungsverteilung in einem Muskel und liefert so mögliche erste Hinweise für nachfolgende Operationen. Über eine medizinische Gültigkeit der Ergebnisse kann in diesem Stadium noch keine Aussage getroffen werden. Trotz der subjektiv recht guten Ergebnisse besteht die Notwendigkeit, das vorliegende Verfahren weiter zu optimieren. Erste Hinweise liefert der sich teilweise ausprägende RMS-Abstand innerhalb der Abbildung 2(a). Dieses könnte darauf hindeuten, dass ab einem gewissen Zeitpunkt die im Masse-Feder-System vorherrschenden inneren Kräfte die weitere Deformation behindern. Eine Ursache könnte aus dem Sachverhalt resultieren, dass die Anzahl der Tetraeder mit geringem Volumen steigt, die Geometrie der kleinen Tetraeder aber insgesamt nicht entartet [2]. Eine genaue Analyse der Kondition des FE-Systems in Verbindung mit der Tetraederbeschaffenheit ist für die Zukunft geplant.

Literaturverzeichnis

1. Weiss JA, Maker BN, Govindjee S. Finite element implementation of incompressible, transversely isotropic hyperelasticity. Comput Methods Appl Mech Eng. 1996;135(1–2):107–128.
2. Shewchuk J. What Is a Good Linear Finite Element? Interpolation, Conditioning, Anisotropy, and Quality Measures; 2002. Available from: http://www.cs.berkeley.edu/ jrs/papers/elemj.pdf.
3. Weichert F, Ewerlin C, Büttner C, et al. Approximation dreidimensionaler Oberflächenmodelle der Lippen-Kiefer-Gaumen-Region durch aktive Polygonnetze. Proc BVM. 2008; p. 338–342.
4. Bitter K. Chirurgische Erstbehandlung der Lippen-Kiefer-Gaumen-Spalten im Jahr 2000. Mund Kiefer Gesichtschir. 2000;4(7):49–60.
5. Zhao HK, Osher S, Fedkiw R. Fast surface reconstruction using the level set method. Proc IEEE Workshop on Variational and Level Set Methods. 2001; p. 194.
6. Crisfield M. Non-linear Finite Element Analysis of Solids and Structures: Advanced Topics. John Wiley & Sons, Inc.; 1997.

Tumor-Wachstumsmodellierung als parametrisches Bildregistrierproblem

Stefan Becker, Jan Ole Jungmann, Andreas Mang, Thorsten M. Buzug

Institut für Medizintechnik, Universität zu Lübeck
buzug@imt.uni-luebeck.de

Kurzfassung. In der vorliegenden Arbeit stellen wir ein neues Modell zur Kopplung des Tumormasseeffektes an die, der Wachstumsmodellierung unterliegende, anisotrope Reaktionsdiffusionsgleichung vor. Die Gleichung wird auf einem hochaufgelösten Voxelgitter diskretisiert. Eine Modellierung der Anisotropie des Diffusionsprozesses ermöglicht die Integration von Diffusions-Tensor-Bildgebungsdaten. Die raumfordernde Wirkung des Tumors wird als parametrisches Bildregistrierproblem aufgefasst. Hierbei wird die resultierende Verteilung der Tumorzellkonzentration in die zu optimierende Zielfunktion integriert. Erste qualitative Ergebnisse zeigen, dass eine Minimierung der aufgestellten Zielfunktion zu einer plausiblen Modellierung des Masseeffektes führt.

1 Einleitung

Die Progression von primären Hirntumoren bleibt bis dato weitestgehend ungeklärt. Es gibt derzeit noch keine quantitativen Verfahren, die es erlauben, die räumlich heterogenen Muster der Tumorprogression, die Affinität von Gewebe zur Infiltration oder die Bildung eines Rezidives abzubilden.

Die aggressivste Manifestation primärer Hirntumoren, das *Glioblastom multiforme* (GBM), weißt, auch bei Einsatz modernster Therapieverfahren, eine sehr schlechte Prognose auf. Die Progression des GBM basiert auf drei Prozessen: (*i*) der Proliferation, (*ii*) der malignen Transformation und (*iii*) der Migration von kanzerösen Zellen in gesundes Gewebe. Vor allem der diffuse Charakter des GBM stellt ein fundamentales Problem für die Therapie dar, da die Konzentration von migrierten Tumorzellen meist unterhalb des Detektionsschwellwertes moderner bildgebender Verfahren liegt. Diese Eigenschaft ist insbesondere problematisch, falls Tumorzellen natürliche Pfade höherer Diffusivität finden.

Mit der mathematischen in-silico Modellierung der Progression von Tumoren steht uns ein vielseitiges Werkzeug zur Verfügung, welches das Verständnis des Einflusses unterschiedlicher Parameter auf den Krankheitsverlauf potenziell verbessern kann [1]. Ein zuverlässiges Modell würde unter anderem Aussagen über die raum-zeitliche Progression des Tumors zulassen, die Schätzung der Migration von kanzerösen Zellen ermöglichen und die Planung von räumlich variierenden Therapieverfahren erlauben.

2 Stand der Forschung und wesentlicher Beitrag

Die mathematische Beschreibung von Tumorwachstum kann prinzipiell in zwei Gruppen unterteilt werden: diskrete Modelle [2] und auf einer partiellen Differentialgleichung (DGL) basierende, kontinuierliche Modelle [3, 4, 5]. Aktuelle diffusionsbasierte Verfahren verwenden entweder isotrope Diffusionskoeffizienten für die weiße und graue Hirnmasse [5, 6] oder anisotrope Tensoren innerhalb der weißen Hirnmasse [4, 7]. Die mechanische Kopplung der Elastizität des neuronalen Gewebes an den Diffusionsterm erfolgt typischerweise über ein lokales Druckfeld, welches als eine parametrisierte Funktion der Zelldichte aufgefasst werden kann [4, 5], oder wird völlig vernachlässigt [3]. Neuere Arbeiten basieren auf simpleren Wachstumsmodellen und stellen den Masseeffekt in den Vordergrund [8]. Diese Vereinfachung ist dadurch motiviert, dass die Modellierung in ein Framework zur räumlichen Normalisierung von pathologischen Daten integriert wird [9]. In einer aktuellen Arbeit [5] werden die Modellparameter einer vereinfachten isotropen Reaktionsdiffusionsgleichung aus patientenindividuellen, longitudinalen Bilddaten bestimmt. Das entstehende inverse Optimierungsproblem verwendet als Randbedingung die das Modell beschreibenden partiellen DGLs.

Der wesentliche Beitrag der vorgestellten Arbeit ist (i) die Lösung der anisotropen Reaktionsdiffusionsgleichung auf einem hochaufgelöstem Voxelgitter und (ii) die Einbettung der Zellkonzentration in die Zielfunktion eines parametrischen Bildregistriermodells. Dieser Ansatz ermöglicht die Approximation der raumfordernden Wirkung von nicht-konvexen, multifokalen Tumoren basierend auf einer exakt modellierten Reaktionsdiffusionsgleichung.

3 Material und Methoden

3.1 Wachstumsmodell

Sei die Dimension $d \in \mathbb{N}$, die Domäne $\Omega =]0,1[^d \subset \mathbb{R}^d$, der Lösungsraum $\Psi = \Omega_T \times [0,\tau]$, $\Omega_T \subset \Omega$ und der Wertebereich $\Xi \in \mathbb{R}$ gegeben, dann beschreibt die skalare Funktion $c: \Psi \rightarrow \Xi$, $(\boldsymbol{x},t) \mapsto c(\boldsymbol{x},t), c \in [0,1]$ die relative Konzentration von Tumorzellen an der Position $\boldsymbol{x}$ zum Zeitpunkt $t \in [0,\tau]$. Hiermit ergibt sich die zu lösende partielle DGL zu

$$\partial_t c(\boldsymbol{x},t) = \mathcal{D}(c(\boldsymbol{x},t)) + \mathcal{P}(c(\boldsymbol{x},t)) = \nabla\left(\underline{\boldsymbol{D}}\nabla c(\boldsymbol{x},t)\right) + \rho c(\boldsymbol{x},t) \quad \text{in } \Psi. \tag{1}$$

$\mathcal{D}(c(\boldsymbol{x},t))$ beschreibt die Diffusion und $\mathcal{P}(c(\boldsymbol{x},t))$ die exponentielle Zunahme der Zellkonzentration (Proliferation). Entsprechend ist die Lösung der Reaktionsdiffusionsgleichung (1) auf einen hochaufgelösten d-dimensionalen Subraum $\Omega_T \subset \Omega_B$ innerhalb des Gehirns Ω_B beschränkt. Über die Proliferationsrate ρ und den Diffusionstensor $\underline{\boldsymbol{D}}$ lässt sich der Grad des Tumors modifizieren [6].

Um einer Ausbreitung der Tumorzellen außerhalb des Gehirnes vorzubeugen, führen wir die Randbedingung $\partial_t c(\boldsymbol{x},t) = 0$ für alle $\boldsymbol{x} \in \partial\Omega_B$ ein. Weiter initialisieren wir c mit dem Startwert $c(\boldsymbol{x}_S,0) = c_0$ in $\Omega_B \times [0,\tau]$. Die Werte für

$\underline{\boldsymbol{D}}$ variieren zwischen grauer ($\Omega_g \subset \Omega_B$) und weißer ($\Omega_w \subset \Omega_B$) Hirnmasse wie folgt [4]:

$$\underline{\boldsymbol{D}} = \begin{cases} \alpha \underline{\boldsymbol{D}} & \forall\, \boldsymbol{x} \in \Omega_w \text{ (anisotrop)} \\ \beta \max(\underline{\boldsymbol{D}}) & \forall\, \boldsymbol{x} \in \Omega_g \text{ (isotrop)} \\ 0 & \text{sonst.} \end{cases} \tag{2}$$

3.2 Parametrisches Deformationsmodell und Kopplung

In der vorliegenden Arbeit verzichten wir bewusst auf die Verwendung eines rechenaufwändigen, physikalischen Modells und approximieren die Deformation über eine Linearkombination von 1D kubischen B-Splines $\beta_s, s \in [0, 1, 2, 3]$ [10]. Die Grundidee der sog. Free-Form Deformation (FFD) ist es, den Lösungsraum über ein Gitter ψ von Kontrollpunkten $\{\phi_{i,j,k}\}$ zu parametrisieren. Die Verrückung $\varphi : \mathbb{R}^3 \rightarrow \mathbb{R}^3$ eines Punktes $\boldsymbol{x} = (x, y, z)$ ergibt sich zu

$$\varphi(\boldsymbol{x}) = \sum_{l=0,m=0,n=0}^{3,3,3} \beta_l(u(\boldsymbol{x}))\beta_m(v(\boldsymbol{x}))\beta_n(w(\boldsymbol{x}))\phi_{i+l,j+m,k+n}. \tag{3}$$

Dabei sind die Indizes i, j und k der Gitterpunkte $\{\phi_{i,j,k}\}$ gegeben durch $i = \lfloor x/\delta_x^\psi \rfloor$, $j = \lfloor y/\delta_y^\psi \rfloor$, $k = \lfloor z/\delta_z^\psi \rfloor$ mit den relativen Koordinaten $u = x/\delta_x^\psi - i$, $v = y/\delta_y^\psi - j$, $w = z/\delta_z^\psi - k$. Die Kopplung von φ und c erfolgt durch die Minimierung der Zielfunktion

$$\mathcal{J}(\varphi; c) = c(\boldsymbol{x}, t) + \lambda \mathcal{S}(\varphi) \xrightarrow{\varphi} \min, \quad \lambda \in \mathbb{R}. \tag{4}$$

Analog zu Rueckert et al. [10] ist $\mathcal{S}$ ein, über den Lagrange-Multiplikator λ gewichteter, Strafterm. Dieser bestraft singuläre Verrückungen und ist über die Frobenius-Norm $\|\cdot\|_F$ der Hesse-Matrix $\mathrm{H}(\varphi)$ definiert durch

$$\mathcal{S}(\varphi) = \int_{\mathbb{R}^d} \| \mathrm{H}(\varphi) \|_F^2 d\boldsymbol{x}. \tag{5}$$

3.3 Bilddaten und Parameterwahl

Die Gewebeinformationen liefert der auf dem synthetischen MNI Datensatz [11] (Auflösung $\delta_x, \delta_y, \delta_z = 1$ mm) basierende Atlas. Die lokalen Diffusionstensoren werden einem DTI-Datensatz[1] entnommen und mit Hilfe der frei erhältlichen *MedINRIA* Software [12] räumlich normalisiert.

Zur Lösung von (1) verwenden wir ein Spacing von $0.5 \times [\delta_x, \delta_y, \delta_z]$. Weiter verwenden wir folgende Parameter: Startwert $c_0 = 1$, Diffusionskoeffizienten $\alpha = 0.2$ und $\beta = 0.01$ [4], Zellvermehrungsrate $\rho = 0.012$ [3]. $\boldsymbol{x}_S$ wird interaktiv bestimmt. Für den Lagrange-Multiplikator λ in (4) wählen wir einen Wert von 0.1 bei einem äquidistanten Gitterabstand von $\delta_x^\psi, \delta_y^\psi, \delta_z^\psi = 10$ mm. Für die Optimierung von (4) wird ein Gradienten-Abstiegsverfahren verwendet.

[1] http://gforge.inria.fr

4 Ergebnisse

In diesem Abschnitt werden erste qualitative Ergebnisse der vorgestellten Kopplung der Reaktionsdiffusionsgleichung an ein parametrisches Deformationsmodell dargestellt. Abb. 1(a)-(c) zeigt neben der Deformation die zugrunde liegende Zellkonzentration $c \in \Xi$ zu unterschiedlichen Iterationsschritten n. Entsprechend ist in Abb. 1(d)-(f) die Volumenänderung des Tumors anhand der Jacobi-Determinanten abgebildet (rot/blau: Volumenzunahme/-abnahme). Gut zu erkennen ist der diffuse Charakter des Tumors, sowie die damit verbundene, weitreichende Infiltration des Gewebes (blauer Bereich). Besonders auffällig manifestiert sich der Masseeffekt nahe des linken Ventrikels sowie im Bereich der Großhirnrinde.

5 Diskussion

In der vorliegenden Arbeit wurde ein deterministisches Diffusions-Proliferations-Modell vorgestellt, das die Kopplung der Reaktionsdiffusionsgleichung an die raumfordernde Wirkung des Tumors über die Beschreibung des Problems als Bildregistrieraufgabe ermöglicht. Es wurde gezeigt, dass der vorgestellte Ansatz es generell erlaubt, den Masseeffekt lokal plausibel zu approximieren. Desweiteren eignet sich das entwickelte Verfahren inbesondere zur Modellierung der raumfordernden Wirkung von nicht-konvexen, multifokalen Tumoren. Die Formulierung der Zielfunktion ermöglicht voraussichtlich eine direkte Integration

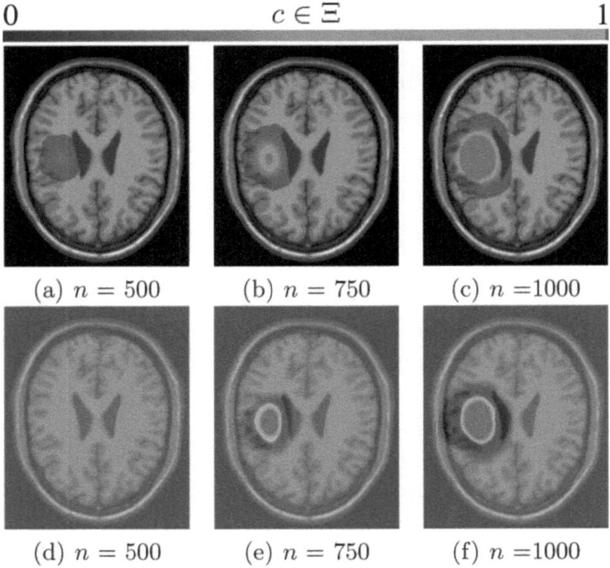

Abb. 1. Zeitverlauf der Modellierung. Darstellung (axialer Schnitt) der berechneten Deformation unter Einblendung der Konzentrationsverteilung $c \in \Xi$ (a)-(c) und der Volumenveränderung des Tumors (d)-(f). n markiert den jeweiligen Iterationsschritt.

der Methode in einen kombinierten Ansatz aus Tumorwachstumsmodellierung und Bildregistrierung [9].

Es besteht kein Zweifel, dass die vorgestellte Arbeit eine Machbarkeitsstudie darstellt. Die Validierung eines auf der Reaktionsdiffusionsgleichung basierenden Tumorwachstumsmodells gestaltet sich schwierig, ist immer noch aktueller Gegenstand der Forschung [1] und verbleibt auch in der vorgestellten Arbeit zunächst ungelöst.

Durch die Verwendung eines grobaufgelösten FFD-Gitters können sich leichte Deformationen am Schädel ergeben (vgl. Abb. 1(f)). Daher wollen wir uns zukünftig mit physikalisch motivierten Ansätzen zur Gewebedeformation befassen. Das hier vorgestellte Verfahren soll mit diesen Ansätzen, unter verschiedenen Gesichtspunkten, verglichen werden. Einen weiteren Forschungsschwerpunkt werden wir auf die Lösung des inversen Problems legen. Dieses erlaubt eine direkte Adaption des Modells an patientenspezifische Daten [1, 5].

Literaturverzeichnis

1. Angelini ED, Clatz O, Mandonnet E, et al. Glioma dynamics and computational models: A review of segmentation, registration, in silico growth algorithms and their clinical applications. Curr Med Imaging Rev. 2007;3(4):262–276.
2. Kansal AR, Torquato S, Harsh GR, et al. Simulated brain tumor growth dynamics using a three-dimensional cellular automaton. J Theor Biol. 2000;203(4):367–382.
3. Swanson KR, Bridge C, Murray JD, et al. Virtual and real brain tumors: Using mathematical modeling to quantify glioma growth and invasion. J Neurol Sci. 2003;216:1–10.
4. Clatz O, Sermesant M, Bondiau PY, et al. Realistic simulation of the 3-D growth of brain tumors in MR images coupling diffusion with biomechanical deformation. Trans Med Imaging. 2005;24(10):1334–1346.
5. Hogea C, Davatzikos C, Biros G. An image-driven parameter estimation problem for a reaction-diffusion glioma growth model with mass effects. J Math Biol. 2008;56(6):793–825.
6. Swanson KR, Alvord EC, Murray JD. A quantitative model for differential motility of gliomas in grey and white matter. Cell Profil. 2000;33(5):317–329.
7. Jbabdi S, Mandonnet E, Duffau H. Simulation of anisotropic growth of low-grade gliomas using diffusion tensor imaging. Magn Reson Med. 2005;54(3):616–624.
8. Zacharaki EI, Hogea CS, Biros G, et al. A comparative study of biomechanical simulators in deformable registration of brain tumor images. IEEE Trans Biomed Eng. 2008;55(3):1233–1236.
9. Zacharaki EI, Shen D, Lee SK, et al. ORBIT: A multiresolution framework for deformable registration of brain tumor images. IEEE Trans Med Imaging. 2008;27(8):1003–1017.
10. Rueckert D, Sonoda LI, Hayes C, et al. Nonrigid registration using free-form deformations: Application to breast MR images. IEEE Trans Med Imaging. 1999;18(8):712–721.
11. Collins DL, Zijdenbos AP, Kollokian V, et al. Design and construction of a realistic digital brain phantom. IEE Trans Med Imaging. 1998;17(3):463–468.
12. Yeo BTT, Vercauteren T, Fillard P, et al. DTI registration with exact finite-strain differential. In: Biomedical Imaging: From Nano to Macro; 2008. p. 700–703.

Long Bone X-ray Image Stitching Using C-arm Motion Estimation

Lejing Wang[1], Joerg Traub[1], Sandro Michael Heining[2], Selim Benhimane[1], Ekkehard Euler[2], Rainer Graumann[3], Nassir Navab[1]

[1]Chair for Computer Aided Medical Procedures (CAMP), TU Munich, Germany
[2]Trauma Surgery Department, Klinikum Innenstadt, LMU Munich, Germany
[3]Siemens SP, Siemens Medical Solutions, Erlangen, Germany
wangle@in.tum.de

Abstract. In this paper, we propose a novel method to generate panoramic X-ray images intra-operatively by using the previously introduced camera augmented mobile C-arm by Navab et al. [1]. This advanced mobile C-arm system acquires registered X-ray and optical images by construction, which facilitates the generation of panoramic X-ray images based on the motion estimation of the X-ray source. Visual marker tracking is employed to estimate the camera motion and this estimated motion is also applied to the X-ray source. Our proposed method is suitable and practical for intra-operative usage generating panoramic X-ray images without the requirement of a fronto-parallel setup and overlapping X-ray images. The results show that the panoramic X-ray images generated by our method are accurate enough (errors less than 1%) for metric measurements and promise suitability for intra-operative clinical applications in trauma surgery.

1 Introduction

Mobile C-arms are an everyday tool to acquire X-ray images in the operating room during surgery. Currently, long bone fracture fixation heavily relies on intraoperative X-ray images. The limited field of view is a drawback of mobile C-arm imaging. In long bone fracture fixation surgery, surgeons need to measure the length of the bone to be reconstructed and align the bone fragments. Single X-ray image can not visualize the entire long bone. Surgeons are required to acquire several individual X-ray images and correlate them.

Panoramic X-ray images can be obtained by stitching many X-ray images. For obtaining an X-ray panoramic image intra-operatively one method was proposed by Yaniv and Joskowicz [2] using a standard mobile C-arm. This method introduces an orthopaedic radiolucent X-ray ruler placed along and parallel to the bones. It uses the graduations of the ruler in the images to estimate the planar transformation by a feature-based alignment method and requires the user to manually select the reconstruction plane in order to compensate for parallax effects on that plane. However, this method requires overlapping areas between two consecutive X-ray images to estimate the planar transformation and thus requires additional radiation. Furthermore, it requires a frontal parallel C-arm setup, i.e. the ruler plane must be parallel to the detector plane of C-arms.

The CamC system that extends a regular mobile C-arm by a video camera [1] was proposed for X-ray and video image overlay. By construction and one time calibration of the device, the X-ray system and the camera have the same projection geometry. Using the video images for estimating the X-ray motion facilitates the creations of panoramic X-ray images. The major advantages over previous proposed solutions are the reduction of ionizing radiation since no overlapping regions of X-ray images are required, not requiring frontal parallel C-arm setup, and enabling metric measurements.

2 Methods

During the one time calibration of the CamC system, the X-ray source and the camera optical center are aligned, and then a planar homography is estimated for X-ray and video image overlay. This one time calibration results in that the X-ray source and the video camera have the same intrinsic and extrinsic parameters [1]. Therefore, all the poses and motions estimated using the video camera directly correspond to the X-ray.

The key step of image stitching is the estimation of the planar transformation to align images. The camera pose of acquiring the first image is defined as the world coordinate system, and the second image is obtained after a rotation $R \in \mathbb{R}^{3\times3}$ and a translation $t \in \mathbb{R}^3$ of the camera. In [2], the planar homography that aligns the first camera image to the second camera image is defined by

$$H = KRK^{-1} + \frac{1}{d}Ktn^TK^{-1} \tag{1}$$

where $K \in \mathbb{R}^{3\times3}$ is the intrinsic matrix of the camera. H is valid for all image points whose corresponding space points are on the same plane, called stitching plane, defined by the normal vector $n \in \mathbb{R}^3$ and distance d to the origin in the world coordinate system. However, any structure that is not within this stitching plane in 3D space will get ghosting or blurring effects also refered to as parallax.

Thanks to the CamC system, we can make use of the video images in combination of a visual square marker tracking system [3] for C-arm pose estimation. In our implementation, we designed a planar marker pattern, in which all the square markers can be uniquely detected. The corners of the square marker can be extracted with subpixel accuracy and used as feature points. Having the marker pattern with known geometries and uniquely detectable markers, we are able to establish point correspondences between the 2D image points and 3D space points in the marker plane. Based on these point correspondences, the pose of the video camera (the X-ray) with respect to the marker pattern is computed by using OpenCV libraries [4].

To generate panoramic images, the first acquired X-ray image is defined as the reference image, and all others will be registered into coordinate system of this first image. The homography that transforms the i-th images to the first image coordinate system will be calculated according to equation 1. The intrinsic parameter K was obtatined during the calibration of the CamC system. Let $R_i^p \in \mathbb{R}^{3\times 3}$ and $t_i^p \in \mathbb{R}^3$ be the X-ray source pose in the marker coordinate system for the i-th X-ray image. The X-ray source motion, R_i and t_i, from the pose of the i-th image to the pose of the first image can be computed by

$$\begin{bmatrix} R_i & t_i \\ 0 & 1 \end{bmatrix} = \begin{bmatrix} R_1^p & t_1^p \\ 0 & 1 \end{bmatrix} \begin{bmatrix} R_i^p & t_i^p \\ 0 & 1 \end{bmatrix}^{-1} \tag{2}$$

To obtain the homography, the plane parameters are still missing. The parameters of the marker plane in the marker coordinate system are known and represented by $\hat{n}$ and $\hat{d}$. Let n_i and d_i be the parameters of this marker plane in the camera coordinate system of acquiring the i-th image. In [5], we have

$$\begin{bmatrix} n_i \\ d_i \end{bmatrix} = \begin{bmatrix} R_i^p & t_i^p \\ 0 & 1 \end{bmatrix}^{-T} \begin{bmatrix} \hat{n} \\ \hat{d} \end{bmatrix} \tag{3}$$

So far, we are able to establish a homography, transforming the i-th image to the first image coordinate system, which is valid only for image points whose corresponding space points are on the exact marker plane. To obtain the homography valid for the bone plane (i.e. the tibial plane or the nail plane in the intramedullary tibial fracture reduction surgery), which is used for panoramic X-ray images and metric measurements, our method relies on two constraints: 1) the bone plane is placed roughly parallel to the marker plane; 2)The distance between the marker plane and the bone plane is known or estimated. The first constraint provides us the normal of the bone plane and the second constraint gives the distance of this bone plane to the origin in the world coordinate system. With these two constraints, we have the plane equation for the bone plane, and thus the homography valid for the bone plane is calculated and parallax effects on this plane is reduced.

For metric measurements, let $P = [x, y, z]^T$ be a 3D space point on the space plane defined by normal n and distance d in the camera coordinate system, and m be its image projection expressed in homogeneous coordinates. In the camera coordinate system, we have

$$P = (dK^{-1}m)/(n^T K^{-1} m) \tag{4}$$

With the known plane parameters in the camera coordinate system, we can derive the coordinates of space points within this plane from their projections. Therefore, metric measurements on the image are possible for this plane. In our stitching algorithm, all images are registered into the first image coordinate system. Therefore the bone plane parameters in the first camera coordinate system are needed for metric measurements.

3 Experiments and results

The phantom (Fig. 1) used throughout all our experiments is constructed to have two parallel planes. On the upper plane, the marker plane for motion

Table 1. Actual and measured distances/angles between the spherical X-ray markers on the panoramic images in mm/degrees.

Distances			Angles		
actual	measured	error	actual	measured	error
240	238.8533	1.1467 ± 0.5423	90	90.2657	0.2657 ± 0.0369
480	477.7680	2.2320 ± 0.1556	161.0754	161.3224	0.2470 ± 0.0577

estimation, the marker pattern is attached. On the lower plane, the bone plane, we placed X-ray markers with known distances for metric measurements or a bone phantom for feasibility tests.

The distance is defined by clicking two points on the image (three points for an angle). To determine the accuracy of metric measurements, we used spherical X-ray markers instead of a bone, since we can extract the center of a circle with sub-pixel accuracy. The ground truth of metric measurements is built by attaching X-ray markers on a pattern with known metric properties. The accuracy of the attachments was controlled by a ruler, thus the error in the ground truth was confirmed to be below 1mm. Our phantom with the X-ray marker was placed on the operating table (Fig. 1(b)) such that the stitching plane deviates several degrees from the image intensifier to simulate the general cases. While acquiring video and x-ray images, the operating table was moved through the C-arm and the panoramic image was created. Then we did the measurements on the generated panoramas. The same experiment was repeated ten times. Table 1 shows the distance and angle measurement results on the panoramic images. In order to investigate the clinical value, we performed preclinical experiments and generated panoramic X-ray images of a bone phantom. Figure 2 shows

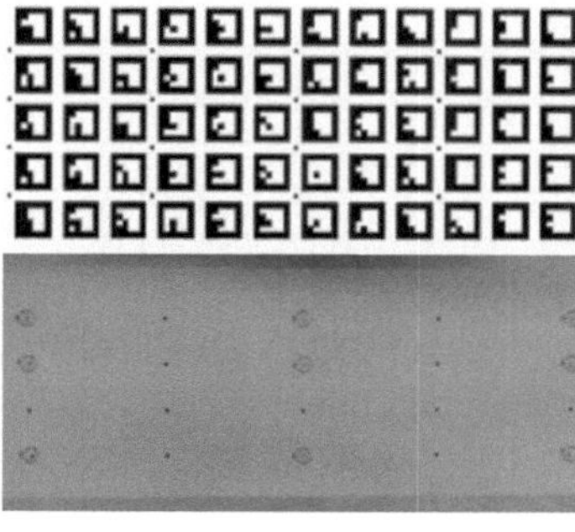

(a) The marker pattern (top) and X-ray markers (bottom).

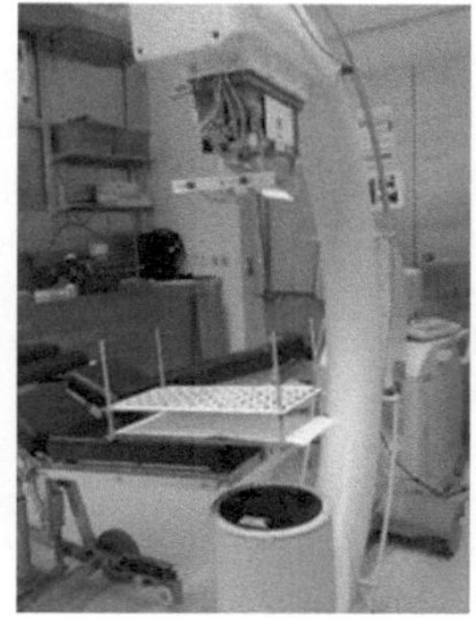

(b) The system setup for metric measurements.

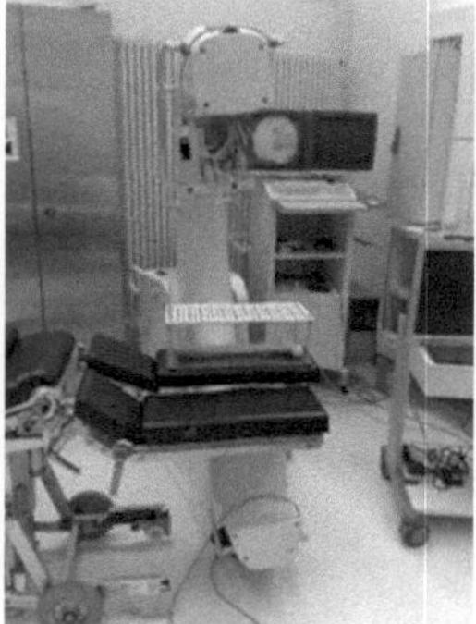

(c) The system setup for feasibility tests.

Fig. 1. Our designed phantom for experiments. The marker pattern is attached on the upper plane. The X-ray marker and the bone are placed on the lower plane.

Fig. 2. The panoramic X-ray image generated from four X-ray images by our method.

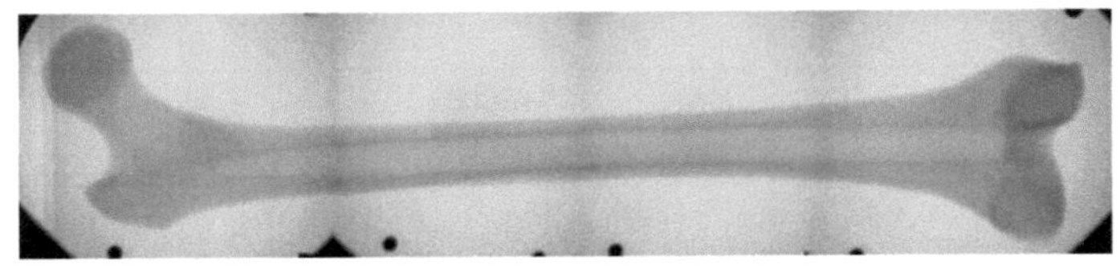

the panoramic X-ray image generated from four individual X-ray images by our method.

4 Discussion and conclusion

We presented a new method to generate panoramic radiographs intra-operatively by using the CamC system and a planar maker pattern. The proposed solution integrates smoothly into the surgical procedure as the square marker pattern is only needed during generation of panoramic X-ray images and removed from the complete surgical task. Our method is independent from overlapping X-ray regions and does not require a frontal parallel C-arm setup. However, the accuracy of estimating the transformation valid for the bone plane depends on the estimated distance between the marker plane and the bone reconstruction plane. In general, this distance is not trivial to recover. In our preclinical phantom setup we can directly measure this distance. Appropriate methods have to be incorporated to define the bone plane. Clinical tests in the near future will show the feasibility and the advantage of metric distance and angle measurements within the surgery room based on a standard C-arm. This will allow surgeons to ensure and validate during trauma reduction surgery the quality of their treatment.

References

1. Navab N, Mitschke M, Bani-Hashemi A. Merging visible and invisible: Two camera-augmented mobile C-arm (CAMC) applications. In: Proc. IEEE and ACM Int'l Workshop on Augmented Reality. San Francisco, CA, USA; 1999. p. 134–141.
2. Yaniv Z, Joskowicz L. Long bone panoramas from fluoroscopic x-ray images. IEEE Trans Med Imaging. 2004;23(1):26–35.
3. Zhang X, Fronz S, Navab N. Visual marker detection and decoding in AR systems: A comparative study. Proc IEEE ISMAR), October 2002. 2002.
4. OpenCV. http://opencvlibrary.sourceforge.net/wiki-static/.
5. Hartley R, Zisserman A. Multiple View Geometry in Computer Vision. New York, NY, USA: Cambridge University Press; 2003.

Evaluation of Approaches for Tracking Virus Particles in Fluorescence Microscopy Images

W. J. Godinez[1], M. Lampe[2], S. Wörz[1], B. Müller[2], R. Eils[1], K. Rohr[1]

[1]University of Heidelberg, BIOQUANT, IPMB, and DKFZ Heidelberg,
Dept. Bioinformatics and Functional Genomics, Biomedical Computer Vision Group,
Im Neuenheimer Feld 267, 69120 Heidelberg, Germany
[2]University of Heidelberg, Dept. of Virology,
Im Neuenheimer Feld 324, 69120 Heidelberg, Germany
wgodinez@ieee.org

Abstract. Tracking virus particles in fluorescence microscopy image sequences enables the characterization of the dynamical behavior of these objects. Several approaches have been developed for the task of virus tracking. However, few studies have quantitatively evaluated the performance of the different approaches. Such a comparison is essential to predict the performance of the approaches under realistic conditions. In this paper, we present a quantitative evaluation of eight approaches for tracking virus particles. We have investigated deterministic and probabilistic approaches. The evaluation is based on nine real microscopy image sequences of virus particles, for which ground truth was obtained by manual tracking.

1 Introduction

Tracking single virus particles in fluorescence time-lapse microscopy images yields quantitative information that describes their dynamical behavior. Such information can be employed to characterize the influence of antiviral drugs. To obtain statistically sound conclusions, a large number of particles must be tracked. Therefore, automatic tracking approaches are required to efficiently handle the large amount of image data.

Several approaches for virus tracking have been described. Typically, deterministic approaches have been employed (e.g., [1, 2]). More recently, probabilistic approaches (e.g., [3, 4]) have been introduced. However, few studies have quantitatively compared the performance of virus tracking approaches. Such a comparison is needed to predict the performance of the approaches for real images. The most detailed comparison of tracking approaches for fluorescent particles has been presented in [5]. There, the authors evaluate the performance of four deterministic tracking approaches using synthetic images with a focus on object localization. One main finding is that the performance of the tracking approaches declines as the signal-to-noise ratio (SNR) decreases. While the study is relatively detailed, it has three shortcomings. First, the performance measure is based on the localization error, and the influence of errors in correspondence finding is ignored. Second, no real images have been used. Third, only deterministic approaches are considered.

In this work, we present a quantitative performance evaluation of approaches for tracking multiple virus particles in microscopy image sequences. In total, we have evaluated eight tracking approaches. We have analyzed two deterministic approaches as well as six probabilistic approaches. The deterministic approaches are based on either the spot-enhancing filter [6] or 2D Gaussian fitting for particle localization, and a global nearest neighbor approach for motion correspondence. The probabilistic approaches are based on Kalman filters, mixture of particle filters (MPF), and independent particle filters (IPF). The approaches have been applied to synthetic image sequences displaying virus-like objects, as well as to 9 different real microscopy image sequences (each comprising between 150 and 400 frames) displaying HIV-1 particles. In comparison to [5], the employed performance measure reflects more comprehensively the performance of the evaluated tracking approaches.

2 Materials and methods

2.1 Deterministic tracking approaches

The deterministic approaches follow a two-step paradigm consisting of object localization and motion correspondence. For object localization, we employed two approaches: an approach based on the spot-enhancing filter (SEF), and an approach using 2D Gaussian fitting (GaussFit). For motion correspondence, we used a global nearest neighbor (GNN) approach [2]. By combining the localization schemes with the motion correspondence scheme we obtain two deterministic approaches: 1) spot-enhancing filter with global nearest neighbor (SEF&GNN), and 2) 2D Gaussian fitting with global nearest neighbor (GaussFit&GNN).

2.2 Probabilistic tracking approaches

The probabilistic approaches follow a Bayesian paradigm, where the aim is to estimate the state $\mathbf{x}_t$ of a virus particle at time step t given a sequence of measurements $\mathbf{y}_{1:t}$. A solution to this problem involves computing the posterior distribution $p(\mathbf{x}_t|\mathbf{y}_{1:t})$ using stochastic propagation and Bayes' theorem:

$$p(\mathbf{x}_t|\mathbf{y}_{1:t}) \propto p(\mathbf{y}_t|\mathbf{x}_t)\, p(\mathbf{x}_t|\mathbf{y}_{1:t-1}). \tag{1}$$

Given certain assumptions on the form of the distributions, the recursion can be solved analytically using a Kalman filter. More generally, the recursive relation can be solved via approximation using a particle filter. The idea behind this filter is to approximate the posterior distribution using a set of weighted random samples. When tracking multiple objects, multiple modes arise in the posterior distribution. The multimodality can be modeled via a non-parametric M-component mixture model, which can be computed using a mixture of particle filters [7]. Alternatively, one may track multiple objects by instantiating one independent particle filter per object (e.g., [8]). To prevent the problem of filter coalescence, the IPF includes a penalization scheme [4]. Similarly, one may use one Kalman filter per object to track multiple objects.

For all probabilistic approaches, we employed the two localization schemes described above to detect virus particles. Note that the approaches using a mixture of particle filters can only track a fixed number of objects. For the approaches using independent particle filters and Kalman filters, the motion correspondence problem, i.e., the problem of assigning the position measurements computed by the localization schemes to each spatial-temporal filter, is addressed using a global nearest neighbor approach. The combination of the two localization algorithms with the different filters yields the following tracking approaches: 3) spot-enhancing filter and Kalman filters (SEF&Kalman), 4) spot-enhancing filter and a mixture of particle filters (SEF&MPF), 5) spot-enhancing filter and independent particle filters (SEF&IPF), 6) 2D Gaussian fitting and Kalman filters (GaussFit&Kalman), 7) 2D Gaussian fitting and a mixture of particle filters (GaussFit&MPF), and 8) 2D Gaussian fitting and independent particle filters (GaussFit&IPF).

2.3 Performance assessment

To quantitatively assess the performance of each approach in each image sequence, we have employed the tracking accuracy $P_{\text{track}} = \frac{n_{\text{track,correct}}}{n_{\text{track,total}}}$, which reflects the ratio between the number of correctly computed trajectories $n_{\text{track,correct}}$ and the number of true trajectories $n_{\text{track,total}}$. The value $n_{\text{track,correct}}$ is computed as the weighted sum of the percentage of tracked time steps $r_{\text{tracked},i}$ for each i-th true trajectory: $n_{\text{track,correct}} = \sum_{i=1}^{n_{\text{track,total}}} w_i r_{\text{tracked},i}$, where the weight w_i is given by a Gaussian function $G(\cdot)$, which takes as its argument the number of correctly computed trajectories $n_{\text{track,i}}$ corresponding to each i-th true trajectory: $w_i = G(n_{\text{track},i}; \mu = 1, \sigma = 1)$. The weighting scheme is introduced to penalize computed trajectories that are broken. A computed trajectory is assumed to be correct if the Euclidean distance between the measured object position and the true object position is below 2 pixels.

3 Results

We have applied all eight approaches to synthetic as well as real microscopy images. Below, we present the results for nine real microscopy image sequences. In these sequences, fluorescently labeled HIV-1 particles were imaged using a fluorescence wide-field microscope; movies were recorded with a frequency of 10Hz. Ground truth for the virus positions was obtained by manual tracking using the commercial software MetaMorph. For all sequences, we have employed fixed parameter values for all approaches. Similarly, the noise parameters for the dynamical model of the Kalman filter were set analogously as the ones employed for the particle filter. Details for each sequence are given in Table 1. The quantitative experimental results for the nine sequences are presented in Table 2. As an example, results for the real image sequence "Seq. 7" are shown in Fig. 1.

Table 1. Description of real microscopy image sequences.

	Dimensions [pixels]	No. of time steps	No. of objects
Seq. 1	256×256	250	23
Seq. 2	256×256	250	10
Seq. 3	256×256	250	5
Seq. 4	256×256	150	21
Seq. 5	512×512	200	15
Seq. 6	512×512	400	29
Seq. 7	512×512	400	31
Seq. 8	512×512	400	43
Seq. 9	512×512	400	24

Table 2. Tracking accuracy P_{track} for real microscopy image sequences.

	SEF& GNN	SEF& Kalman	SEF& MPF	SEF& IPF	GaussFit& GNN	GaussFit& Kalman	GaussFit& MPF	GaussFit& IPF
Seq. 1	75.24	81.12	84.82	86.73	71.29	81.30	81.95	82.61
Seq. 2	60.78	68.70	71.93	83.52	30.79	44.64	63.49	84.67
Seq. 3	45.07	32.29	76.67	42.55	40.69	60.18	60.00	80.00
Seq. 4	61.71	68.89	28.52	71.10	70.53	74.59	23.81	83.39
Seq. 5	93.54	93.54	84.64	93.54	81.09	93.54	85.64	93.54
Seq. 6	57.79	74.59	39.64	63.98	55.18	67.97	41.73	62.10
Seq. 7	64.65	80.60	48.26	82.48	53.21	77.47	31.23	77.67
Seq. 8	74.61	74.09	50.62	74.64	75.10	74.11	49.04	67.76
Seq. 9	72.55	82.55	48.51	73.55	67.78	80.55	52.61	76.89
Mean	67.33	72.93	59.29	74.68	60.63	72.71	54.39	78.74
Std. Dev.	13.68	17.08	20.62	15.00	16.82	13.99	20.96	9.32

4 Discussion

Our experimental results in Table 2 indicate that the performance of the deterministic approaches is not very good (e.g., for the best deterministic approach, namely SEF&GNN, we obtain a mean tracking accuracy of $\bar{P}_{\text{track}} = 67.33\%$). The reason for this is that localization errors (e.g., detection failures) as well as errors in correspondence finding (e.g, incorrect assignments) reduce the number of correctly computed trajectories. The approaches based on the Kalman filter, in comparison to the deterministic approaches, yield an improved performance (e.g., $\bar{P}_{\text{track}} = 72.93\%$ for the best Kalman-based approach, namely SEF&Kalman). This suggests that the inclusion of a spatial-temporal filtering step enhances the performance. For the approaches using particle filters, it turned out that those using independent particle filters (IPF) outperform those using a mixture of particle filters (MPF). The reason for this result is twofold:

Fig. 1. Tracking results for four approaches for the real image sequence "Seq. 7" (time step $t = 110$).

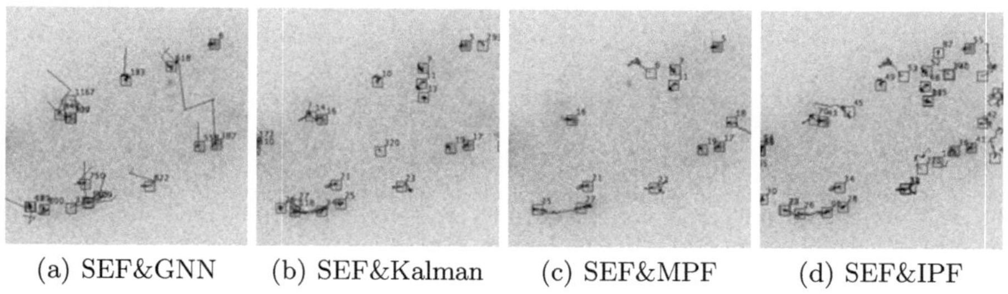

(a) SEF&GNN (b) SEF&Kalman (c) SEF&MPF (d) SEF&IPF

first, MPF cannot track a variable number of objects (whereas in the real images, the number of objects varies over time); second, the MPF uses a variable number of samples to estimate each mixture component. As such, the estimation accuracy decreases for those components for which few samples have been assigned. Among all approaches, the best tracking accuracy is obtained by GaussFit&IPF ($\bar{P}_{\text{track}} = 78.74\%$). The superior performance is mainly due to the comprehensive tracking machinery of the particle filter, which includes the steps of particle localization, motion correspondence, and position estimation. In summary, the quantitative results suggest that the probabilistic approaches are more accurate than the deterministic schemes.

Acknowledgement. Support of the BMBF (FORSYS) project VIROQUANT is gratefully acknowledged.

References

1. Schutz GJ, Schindler H, Schmidt T. Single-molecule microscopy on model membranes reveals anomalous diffusion. Biophys J. 1997;73(2):1073–1080.
2. Sbalzarini IF, Koumoutsakos P. Feature point tracking and trajectory analysis for video imaging in cell biology. J Struct Biol. 2005;151(2):182–195.
3. Arhel N, Genovesio A, Kim K, et al. Quantitative four-dimensional tracking of cytoplasmic and nuclear HIV-1 complexes. Nat Methods. 2006;3(10):817–824.
4. Godinez WJ, Lampe M, Wörz S, et al. Probabilistic tracking of virus particles in fluorescence microscopy images. Proc ISBI. 2008; p. 272–275.
5. Cheezum MK, Walker WF, Guilford WH. Quantitative comparison of algorithms for tracking single fluorescent particles. Biophys J. 2001;81:2378–2388.
6. Sage D, Neumann FR, Hediger F, et al. Automatic tracking of individual fluorescence particles: Application to the study of chromosome dynamics. IEEE Trans Image Process. 2005;14(9):1372–1382.
7. Vermaak J, Doucet A, Pérez P; IEEE. Maintaining multi-modality through mixture tracking. Proc ICCV. 2003; p. 1110–1116.
8. Qu W, Schonfeld D, Mohamed M; IEEE. Real-time interactively distributed multi-object tracking using a magnetic-inertia potential model. Proc IEEE ICCV. 2005;1:535–540.

1D-Messungen physiologischer Bewegungen am Hals mit optischer Kohärenztomographie

M. Dämgen, B. Schwab, Th. Lenarz, M. Leinung

Medizinische Hochschule Hannover
Klinik und Poliklinik für Hals-Nasen-Ohrenheilkunde
(Direktor: Prof Dr. med. Th. Lenarz)
Carl-Neuberg-Str. 1 30625 Hannover
daemgen.michael@mh-hannover.de

Kurzfassung. In der Chirurgie insbesondere bei onkologischen Fragestellungen kommt es zu Grenzsituationen, in denen es gilt, Gewebeverbände mit hoher Genauigkeit aufzutrennen, z.B. bei Infiltration von Gefäßwänden oder Nervenstrukturen durch Tumorausläufer. Oft könnte eine physiologisch funktionell wichtige Struktur erhalten werden, wenn ein chirurgisches Instrument existierte, das mit einer überaus hohen Präszision arbeitet. Hierfür ist ein (ultra-)kurzgepulster Laser geeignet, der bei kleinem Focus und minimalen thermischen Wechselwirkungen lediglich vernachlässigbare Kollateralschäden im umgebenden Gewebe erzeugt. Allerdings ist ein solches System nicht mehr allein durch den Operateur kontrollierbar. Daher wurde die Idee entwickelt, ein automatisiertes Assistenzsystem zu designen, das mit einem in entsprechender Genauigkeit arbeitenden Sensor (optische Kohärenztumographie, OCT) und einem Femtosekunden(fs)-Laser als Aktor teilautonom kritische Schritte des operativen Eingriffs unter der Kontrolle des Operateurs vornimmt. Die Vorbedingung eines solchen Systemes jedoch ist die Anpassung an physiologische Bewegungen im OP-Gebiet. Zur Messpooletablierung müssen diese physiologischen Bewegungen aufgezeichnet werden mit der den Dimensionen erforderlichen Präzision.

1 Einleitung

Bei der Weichgewebschirurgie treten unvermeidliche physiologische, zumeist periodische Bewegungen des Operationssitus auf. Durch Effekte wie Pulsation oder Atmung verlagert sich der Zielpunkt des Lasereingriffs kontinuierlich. Somit ist es erforderlich, dass zur suffizienten Regelung des oben beschriebenen Operationssystems diese physiologischen Bewegungen erfasst und quantifiziert werden. Dies leistet die Optische Kohärenz Tomography und darüber hinaus die Bereitstellung zusätzlicher intraoperativer Informationen [1] und [2]. Hierfür wurden punktuelle 1D-OCT-Messungen sowohl an Probanden als auch intraoperativ vorgenommen.

2 Methoden

Bei dem verwendeten OCT-Gerät, handelt es sich um ein System der Fa. *Light-Lab Imaging.* Als Lichtquelle dient eine Superlumineszenzleuchtdiode der Fa. *Opto Speed*, deren Zentralwellenlänge bei $\lambda_c = 1278\ nm$ liegt mit einer spektralen Breite von $\Delta\lambda = 39,45\ nm$. Die Leistung der Lichtquelle liegt bei $6\ mW$, die nach Passieren eines optischen Zirkulators zu je 50% in Referenz- und Probenlicht aufgeteilt wird. Das von Probe und Referenzspiegel zurückgeworfene Licht überlagert sich bei Durchgang durch einen Faserkoppler und erzeugt ein um $\frac{\pi}{2}$ phasenverschobenes Interferenzsignal. Die beiden Signale werden elektronisch subtrahiert, ein Verfahren das als dual balanciertes Detektionsverfahren bekannt ist [3].

Eine schematische Darstellung der Einzelkomponenten eines OCT Systems ist in Abbildung 1 gegeben.

Diese OCT-Einheit wurde mit einem Operationsmikroskop der *Fa. Zeiss*, Typ S21 gekoppelt. Hierbei sind in einem separaten Gehäuse OCT-Scanner, Linsen und Tubus, in den die lichtführende Faser mündet, direkt unter dem Operationsmikroskop untergebracht. Ein Zielstrahl definiert das Arbeitsfeld des OCT-Scanners, das mit dem Sichtfeld des Operationsmikroskops korreliert werden muss. Ferner müssen die Foci von OCT-Strahl und OPMI in Übereinstimmung gebracht werden, da ansonsten keine genügende simultane Kontrolle zwischen Mikroskopbild und OCT realisiert werden kann.

Mit diesem funktionellen Aufbau wurden nun nicht nur die Lebensfunktionen Respiration und Puls aufgenommen sondern auch Störvorgänge, wie etwa Husten. Eine Schwierigkeit liegt in dem geringen Tiefensichtfeld der OCT-Einheit, dass rd. 3,5 mm beträgt. Die Bewegung des Messobjektes, die bei einer in vivo

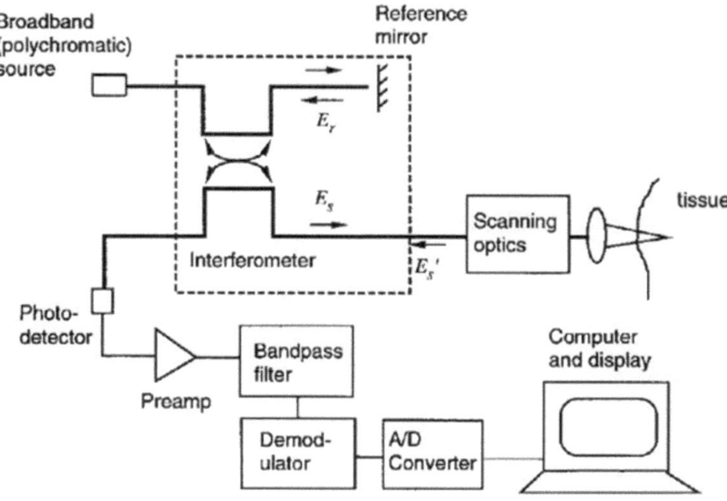

Abb. 1. Funktionelle Komponenten eines OCT-Systems

Messung grundsätzlich der Fall ist, lässt das Messobjekt leicht aus dem darstellenden Messfenster herauswandern, zumal ein konstanter Abstand von rd. 170 mm zwischen Messobjekt und Scannerspiegel eingehalten werden muss.

Wir haben bei 5 Probanden 1D-OCT-Messungen im Halsbereich über die Zeit aufgezeichnet, um Verlagerungen des Operationssitus in in Richtung der Messachse zu dokumentieren. Hierbei wurde sowohl bei Atmung als auch bei Respirationpausen gemessen sowie Messpunkte direkt auf den arteriellen und venösen Blutleitern, bzw. in verschiedenen Entfernungen zu diesen erfasst. Mithilfe eines auf der Programmierplattform *LabVIEW* editierten Algorithmus' erfolgte anschließend die Extrapolation der Gewebeoberfläche aus den Schnittbildern, Artefakteliminierung sowie die Auswertung der generierten Kurven hinsichtlich Amplitude und Geschwindigkeit der physiologischen Bewegungsmuster.

Zum vereinfachten Auffinden des korrekten Arbeitsabstandes der OCT/Mikroskop Einheit zum Messpunkt wurden zwei Laserpointer an beiden Seiten des Gehäuses befestigt Abbildung 2. Die Fokusebene ist dann durch die Überlagerung der beiden Laserspots gegeben. Im Folgenden wird der OCT Scanner deaktiviert, sodass der OCT Strahl lediglich stationär genutzt wird und weshalb diese Methode eindimensional (1D in Sichtachse) genannt wird.

3 Ergebnisse

Die gewonnenen Daten zeigten selbst im Ruhezustand (keine Atmung, Messpunkt in größtmöglichem Abstand von Blutgefäßen) eine mittlere Amplitude

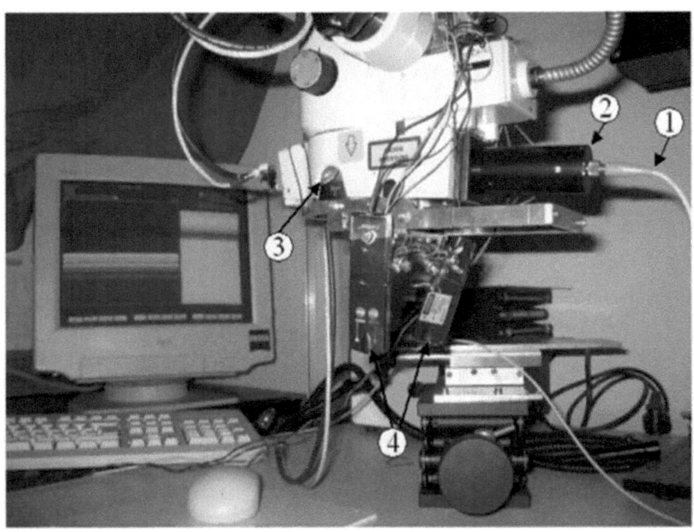

Abb. 2. Experimenteller Aufbau: Microskopkopf mit OCT und Laserzieleinrichtung. Die lichtführende Faser (1) führt in den Tubus (2). Der Strahl wird weitergeführt zum Scannerkopf mit Spiegel (3). Am Metallrahmen sind seitlich zwei Laserpointer befestigt (4), die sich im Fokus des OCT Strahles überlagern.

von 0,22 mm mit einer maximalen Geschwindigkeit (= Anstiegssteilheit der Kurve) von 2,13 mm/s. Hier zeigte sich eine doppelgipflige Pulskurve, wie sie aus intraarterieller Druckmessung bekannt ist. Wurde nun ein Punkt direkt über der Bifurkation der Arteria carotis (Halsschlagader) als Messpunkt gewählt, so blieb die Amplitude mit 0,21 mm annähernd konstant bei einer signifikant höheren mittleren Geschwindigkeit von 5,54 mm/s. Dies muss somit durch ein geeignetes Nachfahren des Laserfokus in alle drei Raumrichtungen kompensiert werden.

Eine deutlich größere Amplitude ergab die Messung respiratorischer Bewegungen mit einer Amplitude von 1,71 mm bei einer Geschwindigkeit von 3,45 mm. Bei der Messung des Hustenimpulses wurde der Darstellungsbereich des Visualisierungsfensters überschritten, sodass die sehr große Amplitude auf etwa 7 mm geschätzt werden musste.

Schematisch dargestellt in Abbildung 3 an einem gesunden Probanden.

Große Atembewegungen finden sich demnach entsprechend brustkorbnah und im kaudalen Halsbereich, einzelne Pulsspitzen über der den Aa. carotis communis, externa und interna, wie in Abbildung 4 dargestellt.

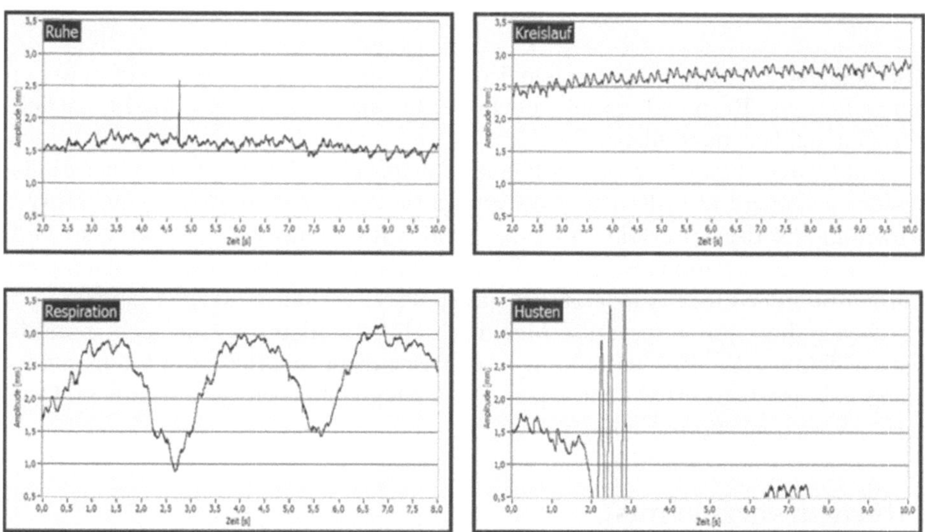

Abb. 3. Messkurven der physiologischen Bewegungen der Halsweichteile in 3 cm Entfernung (li. oben) und über der Bifurkation (re. oben). An der Aa. Carotis konnte der charakteristische Doppelpuls registriert werden. Der Doppelpuls konnte ebenfalls trotz Überlagerung durch die Atemkurve (li. unten) festgestellt werden. Ein Hustenereignis (re. unten) überschreitet den Erfassungsbereich des genutzten OCT.

Abb. 4. a) Position der 36 Messpunkte am Hals auf der Hautoberfläche b) Kartierung der Halsweichteile unter Benutzung des beschriebenen Messaufbaues: das farbcodierte Diagramm zeigt eine größere Amplitude während des Atemvorganges bei vergleichsweise zur Pulsation niedrigerer Geschwindigkeit.

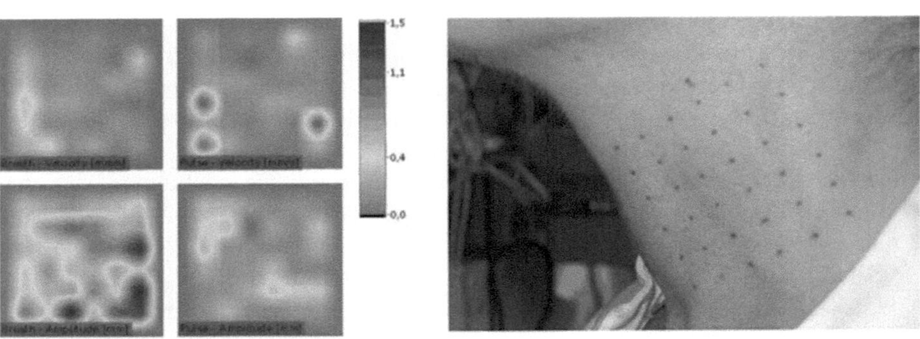

4 Fazit und Ausblick

Mit dem OCT lassen sich physiologische Bewegungsmuster von Weichgeweben auf Grund von Respiration und Puls in der für die Aufgabenstellung hinreichenden Genauigkeit darstellen.

Auf Grund dieser Datenbasis können für das oben beschriebene Operationssystem zwingend erforderliche Leistungsparameter (Arbeitsraum, Nachführgeschwindigkeit des Laserfokus in x-, y- und z-Richtung) definiert werden. Ggf. wird über die Periodizität dieser Bewegungen diese mathematisch modelliert werden und der Laser entsprechend (prospektiv) verfahren werden können.

Ferner dient die vorgestellte Messmethodik zur Identifikation nicht periodischer Effekte (z.B. Hustenstoß), die – sofern sie nicht in Echtzeit mit genügender Sicherheit kompensiert werden können – zu einem Abbruch des autonomen Operationsvorganges führen müssen.

Literaturverzeichnis

1. Huang D, Swanson E, Lin C, et al. Optical coherence tomography. Science. 1985;254:1178–1181.
2. Swanson E, Huang D, Hee M, et al. High speed optical coherence domain reflectometry. Opt Lett. 1992;17:151–153.
3. Drexler W, Morgner U, Kärtner F, et al. In vivo ultrahigh-resolution optical coherence tomography. Opt Lett. 1999;24:1221–1223.

Vorhersage des Krankheitsverlaufes von leichten kognitiven Beeinträchtigungen durch automatisierte MRT Morphometrie

Klaus H. Fritzsche[1], Sarah Schlindwein[1], Bram Stieltjes[2], Marco Essig[2], Hans-Peter Meinzer[1]

[1]Abteilung für Medizinische und Biologische Informatik, DKFZ Heidelberg
[2]Abteilung Radiologie, DKFZ Heidelberg
k.fritzsche@dkfz-heidelberg.de

Kurzfassung. Die leichte kognitive Beeinträchtigung (LKB) gilt als Anzeichen für ein erhöhtes Risiko der Entwicklung einer Alzheimerdemenz. Eine fundierte klinische Prognose für den Krankheitsverlauf kann aber bis dato nicht gegeben werden. Das Ziel dieser Arbeit besteht darin, eine möglichst präzise Vorhersage mittels automatisierter Morphometrie des Hippokampus im MRT-Bild zu treffen. In einer Studie mit 18 Probanden mit LKB wurde eine Prädiktionsgenauigkeit für die Entwicklung einer späteren Demenz von 83.3% erzielt. Eine manuelle Vergleichsmethode erreichte mit 55.6% Trefferquote keine signifikante Vorhersagegenauigkeit. Das automatische Verfahren erfüllt viele wichtige Voraussetzungen für den routinemäßigen klinischen Einsatz mit dem Potential, die klinische Vorhersage des Krankheitsverlaufes bei der LKB zu verbessern.

1 Einleitung

Die leichte kognitive Beeinträchtigung (LKB) und im speziellen die amnestische LKB (aLKB) gelten als erhöhtes Risikostadium der Alzheimer Demenz (AD) [1]. Die Konversionsrate zur AD bei der LKB liegt in einem Zeitraum von drei Jahren bei 50%. In der Untergruppe der aLKB findet sich sogar eine Konversionsrate von 80%. Die Konversion kann im Frühstadium bis heute klinisch nicht vorhergesagt werden. Eine frühzeitige Diagnose noch vor einer manifestierten Demenz wird jedoch gerade aufgrund neuartiger therapeutischer Möglichkeiten bei der AD immer wichtiger.

Die strukturelle MR-Bildgebung ist weit verfügbar und gehört mittlerweile zum Standardrepertoire der klinischen Untersuchung von entsprechenden Patienten. Insbesondere ist sie auch wichtig, um andere Krankheitsursachen auszuschließen. Ihr Potential für die Demenzdiagnose selbst ist jedoch noch nicht ausgeschöpft. Frühere Studien zeigen, dass sich AD Patienten anhand von morphometrischen Analysen gut von gesunden Probanden unterscheiden lassen [2]. Bei Patientengruppen mit LKB hat sich die Unterscheidung von AD Patienten oder gesunden Probanden als schwieriger herausgestellt [3]. Klinisch am relevantesten ist es, innerhalb der LKB Gruppe zwischen später konvertierenden

(LKBc) und nicht konvertierenden Patienten (LKBn) unterscheiden zu können. Dies ist jedoch zusätzlich auch die schwierigste Herausforderung. Aktuell relevante Arbeiten zu diesem Thema finden sich im Literaturverzeichnis [4, 5, 6, 7].

Mögliche Messmethoden müssen auf der einen Seite die feinen morphologischen Unterschiede robust detektieren und bewerten. Um im klinischen Alltag anwendbar zu sein, müssen sie aber auch schnell durchführbar und gut reproduzierbar sein. Ziel dieser Arbeit ist es, eine möglichst präzise Vorhersage mittels automatisierter Morphometrie des Hippokampus im MRT-Bild zu treffen.

2 Material und Methoden

Um bei Patienten mit LKB möglichst präzise vorhersagen zu können, ob diese in Zukunft eine Alzheimerdemenz entwickeln werden, wurden ein manuelles (Abschn. 2.2) und ein automatisches Verfahren (Abschn. 2.3) zur Klassifikation getestet. Als Goldstandard standen hierfür Bilder von Probanden zur Verfügung, deren spätere klinische Entwicklung bekannt war. Außerdem stand eine gesunde Kontrollgruppe sowie eine Gruppe von Probanden zur Verfügung, bei denen zum Einschlusszeitpunkt schon eine Alzheimerdemenz diagnostiziert war (Abschn. 2.1).

2.1 Datenakquisition

Die Rekrutierung der Probanden erfolgte von der Abteilung für geriatrische Psychiatrie in der Universitätsklinik Heidelberg. Die klinische Evaluation folgte einem ausführlichen Testprotokoll. Insgesamt wurden 48 Personen in die Studie eingeschlossen, 15 gesunde Kontrollprobanden (66 ± 7 Jahre), 18 LKB (70 ± 5 Jahre) und 15 AD Patienten (72 ± 7 Jahre). *Levy's criteria of Aging-associated cognitive decline* bildeten die Grundlage für die LKB Diagnose. Die milde bis moderate Alzheimerdemenz wurde nach den Kriterien der NINCDS-ADRDA definiert. 10 der Probanden mit LKB entwickelten im späteren Verlauf eine Alzheimerdemenz (LKBc), die restlichen 8 Probanden blieben im Status der LKB (LKBn). Die MR Aufnahmen stammen von einem klinischen 1,5 Tesla Scanner (Magnetom Vision, Siemens Medical Solutions, 128 T1-gewichtete koronare Schichtbilder, TR=4ms, Flip=13°, FOV=250mm, Matrix=256×256, Schichtabstand 1.0 mm).

2.2 Manuelles Klassifikationsverfahren

Mittels manueller Morphometrie wurde die Weite der unteren Hirnventrikelhörner bestimmt. Wie in Gao et al. beschrieben [8], wurde hierbei zunächst eine transversale Schicht kaudal zu der interkommissuralen Linie eingestellt. Die Weite des Temporalhornes wurde als Distanz zweier paralleler Tangenten definiert, die die Spitze des Temporalhorns begrenzen (Zhang et al., Fig. 1 [9]).

Zur Klassifikation wurden die Weiten des linken und rechten Temporalhorns addiert und ein einfacher Schwellwertklassifikator angewendet. Es wurde hierbei für die beiden Klassifikationsaufgaben „AD/Gesund“ und „LKBn/LKBc“ jeweils ein Schwellwert bestimmt, der die Gruppen optimal trennt. Die Validierung erfolgte mittels Leave-One-Out Cross Validation Protokoll.

2.3 Vollautomatisiertes Klassifikationsverfahren

Mittels einer vollautomatischen Serie von Bildanalyseschritten wurde, wie in Fritzsche et al. [10] beschrieben, eine Extrahierung von Atrophieindizes in der Hippokampusregion durchgeführt. Zur Vorverarbeitung wurden die Bildvolumina mittels nichtlinearer Registrierung in ein gemeinsames Koordinatensystem gebracht. Hierbei kam in zwei Schritten zuerst eine affine Transformation und dann eine auf diskreten Kosinusbasisfunktionen basierende, nichtlineare Deformation zum Einsatz. Es folgten eine MR Inhomogenitätskorrektur und eine landmarkenbasierte Histogrammnormalisierung. Das gemeinsame Koordinatensystem und die vergleichbaren Voxelintensitäten erlauben den Vergleich verschiedener Hirnregionen direkt auf den Bildinformationen. Verschiedene Krankheitsmuster können so charakterisiert und quantifiziert werden. Für jedes Bildvolumen wurde zu diesem Zweck ein z-Score Volumen berechnet, welches in jedem Bildpunkt die patientenindividuelle Abweichung der Bildinformation von einer gesunden Vergleichspopulation enthält. Eine Integration der Werte in bestimmten Zielregionen erlaubt eine lokale Bestimmung von Atrophieindizes [10]. Zur Klassifikation wurde analog zu Abschnitt 2.2 die Summe der linken und rechten Indizes im Bereich des Hippokampus berechnet und mittels optimalem Schwellwert klassifiziert.

3 Ergebnisse

Tabelle 1 stellt die Klassifikationsergebnisse der beiden Ansätze gegenüber. Die Korrelation der beiden Verfahren ergab einen Pearson Korrelationskoeffizienten von $r = 0.62$. Eine genauere Betrachtung der einzelnen Probandengruppen ergab, dass die Verfahren in der Gruppe der AD Patienten mit $r = 0.68$ besser korrelieren. In den restlichen Gruppen, jeweils für sich betrachtet, korrelierten die Verfahren hingegen nicht mehr signifikant. Der Zeitaufwand für die manuelle Morphometrie betrug zirka 3-5 Minuten pro Proband. Der automatische Ansatz benötigt keine Interaktion und eine Rechenzeit von zirka einer Minute.

4 Diskussion

Die Ergebnisse zeigen, dass ein erhöhter Wert des vollautomatisch bestimmten Indizes für Atrophie im Hippokampusbereich ein valider Indikator für eine spätere Konversion des Patienten zur Alzheimerdemenz ist. In früheren Studien wurde bereits nachgewiesen, dass das Verfahren eine gute Trennschärfe zwischen den Gruppen *Alzheimer* und *Gesund* liefert. Eine robuste Klassifikation zwischen gesunden Probanden und Patienten mit LKB gelang jedoch nicht. Auch die interaktiven Referenzverfahren verzeichneten hier keine guten Ergebnisse [11]. Die

Tabelle 1. Korrektklassifikationsraten für die Unterscheidung von AD Patienten von gesunden Probanden sowie die Unterscheidung von später zur Alzheimerdemenz konvertierenden Patienten mit LKB (LKBc) von nicht konvertierenden Patienten (LKBn).

	AD/Gesund	LKBn/LKBc
Manuelle Morphometrie:		
Temporalhornweite	80.0%	55.6%
Automatische Morphometrie:		
Atrophieindex Hippokampus	90.0%	83.3%

hier vorliegende Studie demonstriert, dass sich die Gruppe der Patienten mit LKB signifikant in zwei Untergruppten aufteilen lässt, die der konvertierenden und die der nicht konvertierenden Patienten.

Mittels der zeitlich aufwändigeren, interaktiven Bestimmung der Temporalhornweite, die auf den gleichen Datensätzen durchgeführt wurde, konnten keine signifikanten Prognosen getroffen werden. Die Korrelation der beiden Verfahren ist nur bei der Gruppe der Alzheimerpatienten signifikant. Dies könnte darauf zurückführbar sein, dass die Atrophie im hippokampalen Bereich zwar messbar, aber noch nicht ausgeprägt genug ist, um eine Weitung der Ventrikelhörner zu verursachen. Außerdem ist die manuelle Vermessung bei ausgeprägten Ventrikelhörnern leichter und eindeutiger durchführbar.

Die Vorhersagegenauigkeit der automatischen Auswertung ist im Vergleich zu aktuellen Publikationen zu dieser Fragestellung sehr hoch. Nestor et al. geben keine Trefferwahrscheinlichkeiten an, erreichen aber über die semiautomatische Vermessung der Ventrikelvolumina ein Signifikanzniveau von $p = 0.027$ (n=18 konvertierende Patienten mit LKB) [7]. Mittels manueller Volumetrie erreichten Eckerström et al. nur in weniger als der Hälfte der Probanden mit LKB eine aussagekräftige Vorhersage des Krankheitsverlaufes [5]. Fan et al. beschränkten sich bei der Evaluation ihres Verfahrens auf die reinen Mini-Mental-Status-Testergebnisse (MMST) der Probanden im Verlauf eines Jahres. Die klinische Konversion zur Demenz wurde nicht in Betracht gezogen. Mit Hilfe hochdimensionaler Patternanalyse konnten so mit 87 prozentiger Treffsicherheit Personen identifiziert werden, deren MMST sich über die Grenzen eines bestimmten Schwellwertes hinaus verschlechterte [4]. Die besten Ergebnisse unter vergleichbaren Bedingungen erreichten Teipel et al. mit Trefferwahrscheinlichkeiten von bis zu 80% anhand von automatisierten Deformationsfeldanalysen segmentierter und registrierter CSF-Karten (n=9 konvertierende Patienten mit LKB) [6].

Die in dieser Arbeit erreichte Vorhersagegenauigkeit von 83.3% stellt im Vergleich zum aktuellen Stand der Forschung ein sehr gutes Ergebnis dar. Im Vergleich zu [7, 5] zeichnet es sich durch seine volle Automatisierung aus. Die einzelnen Verarbeitungsschritte sind anschaulich nachvollziehbar und visualisierbar. Sie stellen also nicht, wie es bei hochdimensionalen Klassifikationsverfahren oft der Fall ist, eine Blackbox dar, welche ein nicht nachvollziehbares Ergebnis berechnet (vergleiche [4, 6]). Die räumliche Integration der zugrundeliegenden z-

Score Karte und die einfache Schwellwertklassifikation haben den Vorteil, dass eventuell unstimmige Ergebnisse immer auf das zugrundeliegende Bildmaterial zurückgeführt werden können.

Der Zeitaufwand für die hier präsentierte Auswertung ist mit zirka einer Minute pro Bildvolumen äußerst gering. Die grundsätzlichen Voraussetzungen für den routinemäßigen Einsatz im Bereich der computergestützten Diagnose sind somit gegeben. Der nächste Schritt ist die Validierung der Methode anhand einer größeren, multizentrischen Datenbasis wie sie beispielsweise von der Alzheimer's Disease Neuroimaging Initiative (ADNI, www.loni.ucla.edu/ADNI) zur Verfügung gestellt wird.

Literaturverzeichnis

1. Petersen R, Stevens J, et al. Practice parameter: Early detection of dementia: Mild cognitive impairment (an evidence-based review). Report of the quality standards subcommittee of the american academy of neurology. Neurology. 2001;56(9):1133–1142.
2. Lehéricy S, Marjanska M, et al. Magnetic resonance imaging of Alzheimer's disease. Eur Radiol. 2007;17(2):347–362.
3. Albert M, DeCarli C, et al. The Use of MRI and PET for Clinical Diagnosis of Dementia and Investigation of Cognitive Impairment: A Consensus Report; 2004. Available at: http://www.alz.org/Research/Papers/Imaging.
4. Fan Y, Batmanghelich N, et al. Spatial patterns of brain atrophy in MCI patients, identified via high-dimensional pattern classification, predict subsequent cognitive decline. Neuroimage. 2007.
5. Eckerström C, Olsson E, et al. Small baseline volume of left hippocampus is associated with subsequent conversion of MCI into dementia: The Göteborg MCI study. J Neurol Sci. 2008;272(1-2):48–59.
6. Teipel S, Born C, et al. Multivariate deformation-based analysis of brain atrophy to predict Alzheimer's disease in mild cognitive impairment. Neuroimage. 2007;38(1):13–24.
7. Nestor S, Rupsingh R, et al. Ventricular enlargement as a possible measure of Alzheimer's disease progression validated using the Alzheimer's disease neuroimaging initiative database. Brain. 2008;131(Pt 9):2443–2454.
8. Gao F, Black S, et al. A reliable MR measurement of medial temporal lobe width from the Sunnybrook dementia study. Neurobiol Aging. 2003;24(1):49–56.
9. Zhang Y, Londos E, et al. Usefulness of computed tomography linear measurements in diagnosing Alzheimer's disease. Acta Radiol. 2008;49(1):91–97.
10. Fritzsche K, von Wangenheim A, et al. A computational method for the estimation of atrophic changes in Alzheimer's disease and mild cognitive impairment. Comput Med Imaging Graph. 2008;32(4):294–303.
11. Fritzsche K, Giesel F, et al. Quantifizierung neurodegenerativer Veränderungen bei der Alzheimer Krankheit - Evaluierung eines automatischen Verfahrens. Proc BVM. 2008; p. 363–67.

Klassifikation von Standardebenen in der 2D-Echokardiographie mittels 2D-3D-Bildregistrierung

Christoph Bergmeir[1], Navneeth Subramanian[1]

[1]GE Global Research, Bangalore, India
navneeth.s@ge.com

Kurzfassung. Zum Zweck der Entwicklung eines Systems, das einen unerfahrenen Anwender von Ultraschall (US) zur Aufnahme relevanter anatomischer Strukturen leitet, untersuchen wir die Machbarkeit von 2D-US zu 3D-CT Registrierung. Wir verwenden US-Aufnahmen von Standardebenen des Herzens, welche zu einem 3D-CT-Modell registriert werden. Unser Algorithmus unterzieht sowohl die US-Bilder als auch den CT-Datensatz Vorverarbeitungsschritten, welche die Daten durch Segmentierung auf wesentliche Informationen in Form von Labeln für Muskel und Blut reduzieren. Anschließend werden diese Label zur Registrierung mittels der Match-Cardinality-Metrik genutzt. Durch mehrmaliges Registrieren mit verschiedenen Initialisierungen ermitteln wir die im US-Bild sichtbare Standardebene. Wir evaluierten die Methode auf sieben US-Bildern von Standardebenen. Fünf davon wurden korrekt zugeordnet.

1 Einleitung

Ultraschall (US) ist eine wichtige Bildgebungsmodalität in der medizinischen Diagnostik und Therapie. Nicht zuletzt durch neueste Trends in Herstellung und Miniaturisierung finden 2D-Ultraschall-Scanner immer größere Verbreitung. Ihr allgegenwärtiger Gebrauch wird damit vor allem noch durch eingeschränkte Bildqualität und die dadurch schwierige Interpretation der Aufnahmen verhindert. Bisher wird dieses Problem durch ausgedehntes Training und Erfahrung im Rahmen der Ausbildung von Spezialisten gelöst, so dass der Arzt mit kritischen Parametern umzugehen lernt, z. B. welches Schallfenster zu wählen ist oder wie eine Standardebene aufgenommen werden kann.

Wir untersuchen die Machbarkeit eines bildbasierten Ansatzes, um diese Informationen zu erhalten. Schlussendlich soll der unerfahrene Anwender interaktiv durch die Anzeige eines 3D-Modells zur Aufnahme der relevanten anatomischen Strukturen geleitet werden. Wir verwenden rigide 2D-3D-Registrierung, um in der 2D-Echokardiographie Aufnahmen von Standardebenen zu lokalisieren. Es wurde jedoch darauf geachtet, dass der Ansatz auf Nicht-Standardebenen und andere Organe (durch die Verwendung eines geeigneten 3D-Modells) übertragbar ist.

In der Literatur finden sich einige Arbeiten zu Klassifikation von Standardebenen und Registrierung von US zu anderen Modalitäten. Penney et al. [1]

entwickelten eine Methode, um 3D-Freehand-US zu MR-Bildern der Leber zu registrieren. Sie nutzen dabei Gefäße als Landmarken. Wein et al. [2] entwickelten effektive Ähnlichkeitsmaße für 3D-US zu CT Registrierung. Lu et al. [3] extrahierten Standardebenen aus 3D-US-Datensätzen mit Hilfe von Lernalgorithmen. All diese Ansätze arbeiten mit 3D-US- oder 3D-Freehand-US-Daten.

Neben den Studien von Wachowiak et al. [4], welche sich auf Teilprobleme beschränkten, wurden unseres Wissens nach bislang keine Versuche unternommen, reine 2D-US-Daten zu 3D-Daten anderer Modalitäten zu registrieren. Denn die spärlich vorhandene Information in den 2D-US-Datensätzen macht eine genaue Registrierung schwierig bis unmöglich. Wir untersuchen die Registrierung jedoch nicht im Hinblick auf hohe Genauigkeit, sondern hinsichtlich brauchbarer Orientierungsinformationen.

2 Material und Methoden

Die vorgestellte Methode arbeitet in zwei Stufen. Zuerst wird die US-Aufnahme mit Hilfe von Vorwissen über mögliche Aufnahmepositionen grob ins lokale Koordinatensystem des Modells positioniert. Dann wird aufbauend auf dieser Initialisierung eine verfeinernde Registrierung durchgeführt.

2.1 Generierung des 3D-Modells

Eine kontrastverstärkte CT-Aufnahme des Herzens wird als 3D-Modell verwendet. Dass die CT-Aufnahme und das US-Bild weder vom selben Patienten, noch vom gleichen Zeitpunkt des Herzzyklus stammen, scheint mit Blick auf den Zweck der Registrierung vertretbar. Ein Radiologe segmentiert in diesem CT-Datensatz die vier Ventrikel und die Aorta manuell. Ein weiterer Radiologe definiert drei Ebenen mit jeweils zwei unterschiedlichen Ursprungspunkten, welche den sechs Standardansichten des Herzens entsprechen: parasternaler Langachsenblick (plx), parasternaler Kurzachsenblick (psx), apikaler Langachsenblick (alx), apikaler Vierkammerblick (afc), subkostaler Kurzachsenblick (ssx) und subkostaler Vierkammerblick (sfc), siehe Abb. 1. Die Bereiche zwischen den einzelnen Segmentierungen werden mit Hilfe einer Erosionsoperation vergrößert. Das Modell wird für alle durchgeführten Registrierungen verwendet.

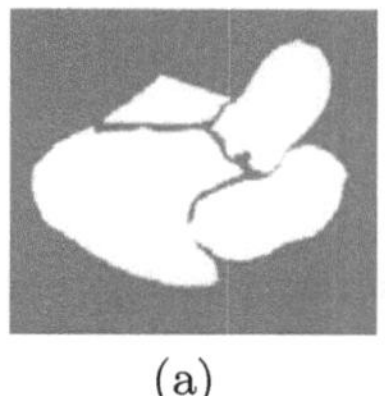
(a)

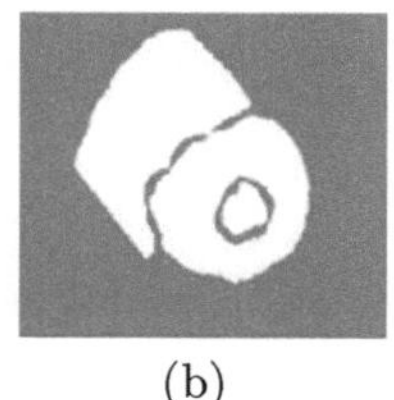
(b)

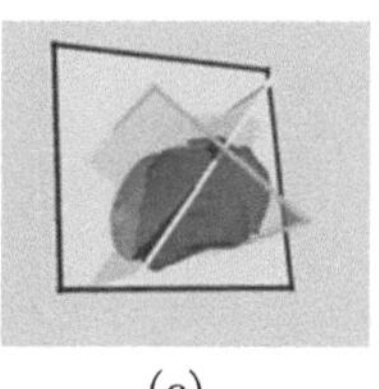
(c)

Abb. 1. Generierung des 3D-Modells und Extraktion der Standardebenen. (a) plx. (b) psx. (c) 3D-Modell der Segmentierungen mit den definierten Standardebenen.

2.2 Vorverarbeitung des Ultraschallbildes

Die gesamte Vorverarbeitung wird auf Rohbildern vollzogen, d. h. vor der Scan-Konvertierung, wodurch Methoden verwendet werden können, welche die Bilder entlang des Ultraschallstrahls bearbeiten. Die Vorverarbeitung verfolgt erstens das Ziel, markante Strukturen (Muskeln, Blut) zu identifizieren, zweitens soll sie Artefakte im Nah- und Fernfeld eliminieren (siehe Abb. 2). Zuerst wird eine Bildmaske erzeugt, welche die Bildbereiche identifiziert in denen wir die relevanten Strukturen erwarten. Dazu nutzen wir die von Penney et al. [1] vorgeschlagene Methode, welche die Maske durch zwei Parameter definiert. Der erste Parameter gibt eine Distanz d von der Sonde aus an und definiert damit eine Region im Nahfeld, welche von der Maske entfernt wird. Diese Region enthält mit hoher Wahrscheinlichkeit nur Aufnahmen der Haut. Wir verwenden $d = 2,5\ cm$. Der zweite Parameter definiert einen Schwellwert th. Beginnend am Ende eines jeden Ultraschallstrahls werden Pixel so lange aus der Maske entfernt, bis der Grauwert eines Pixels einmalig th überschreitet. Dieses Vorgehen ist dadurch motiviert, dass Reflexionen (im Bild sehr hell zu sehen) den Ultraschallstrahl

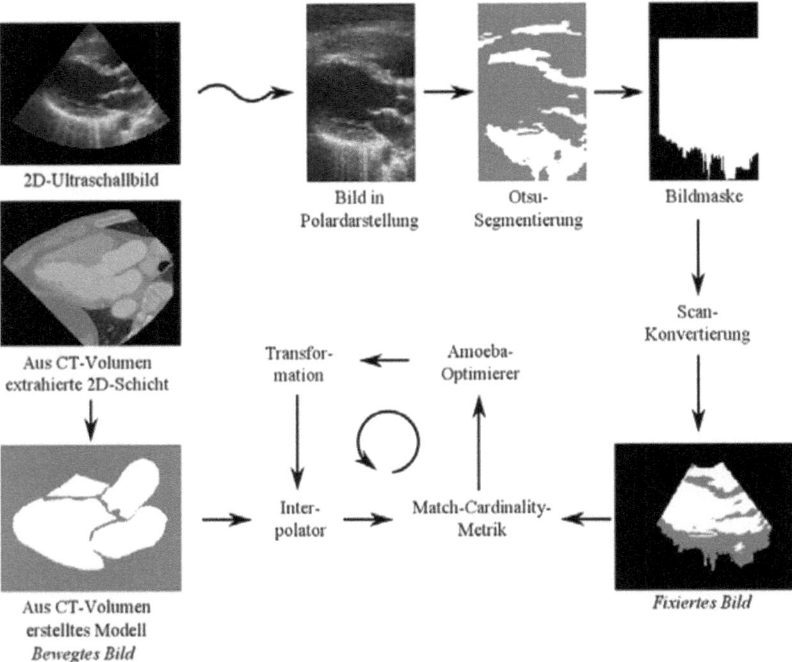

Abb. 2. Flussdiagramm des Algorithmus. Sowohl das US- als auch das CT-Bild werden in einer Weise vorverarbeitet, dass nur die prominentesten Strukturen erhalten bleiben. Dann wird die Registrierung mit der Position einer Standardebene initialisiert und anschließend durchgeführt.

Tabelle 1. Ergebnisse der Registrierung. Wenn das Ergebnis der Methode mit der Ground Truth übereinstimmt, dann ist der Algorithmus in der Lage, die 2D-US-Aufnahme korrekt im 3D-Modell zu lokalisieren.

Datensatz	1	2	3	4	5	6	7
Ground Truth	plx	plx	plx	plx	psx	psx	psx
Unsere Methode	plx	plx	plx	alx	plx	psx	psx

so stark schwächen, dass er dahinterliegende Strukturen nicht mehr hinreichend abbildet. Wir wählen $th = 150$ für unsere Experimente.

Schließlich glätten wir das Bild mit einem anisotropischen Diffusionsfilter und segmentieren es durch einen Otsu-Schwellwertfilter. Damit wird das Bild in zwei Klassen eingeteilt, die wir als Muskel und Blut interpretieren (siehe Abb. 2).

2.3 Registrierung

Durch die extrahierten Standardebenen des Modells sind sechs Initialisierungen für die Registrierung möglich. Wir starten die Registrierung nacheinander von allen diesen Positionen. Die Endposition derjenigen Registrierung, welche den besten Endwert der Metrik liefert, wird anschließend als die korrekte Position angenommen. Die Registrierungsparameter sind so eingestellt, dass die Registrierung das US-Bild lokal gut mit dem Modell zur Deckung bringt; sie soll (und kann) jedoch keine so starke Fehlpositionierung ausgleichen, dass die Endposition im Bereich einer anderen Standardebene liegt.

Da durch die Vorverarbeitungsschritte sowohl aus dem CT- als auch aus den US-Datensätzen Binärbilder entstehen, wird das Registrierungsproblem auf ein Zuordnen von Muskel zu Muskel und Blut zu Blut reduziert. Hierfür nutzen wir die Match-Cardinality-Metrik als Ähnlichkeitsmaß. Sie bringt Regionen mit gleichem Label zur Deckung, indem sie die Anzahl der übereinstimmenden Pixel zählt und anschließend mit Hilfe der Anzahl betrachteter Pixel (der Pixel in der Maske) normalisiert. Zur Optimierung verwenden wir den Amoeba-Optimierer.

3 Ergebnisse

Wir evaluierten unsere Methode mit Hilfe von vier plx- und drei psx-Aufnahmen, alle von verschiedenen Patienten. Ergebnisse, die korrekte Aufnahmeansicht zu finden, d.h. den besten Wert der Metrik in der korrekten Ansicht zu erhalten, zeigt Tab. 1. Repräsentative Einzelfälle (mit korrekter Zuordnung) zeigt Abb. 3.

4 Diskussion

Unser System kann zwischen verschiedenen Standardansichten des Herzens unterscheiden und findet die korrekte Ansicht in fünf von sieben Fällen. Werden nur

Abb. 3. Registrierungsergebnisse. Linke Spalte: 2D-Eingabebilder. Mittlere Spalte: 2D-Schicht des CT-Datensatzes nach der Registrierung. Rechte Spalte: Visualisierung der Schichtposition im 3D-Modell. (a-c) psx. (d-f) plx.

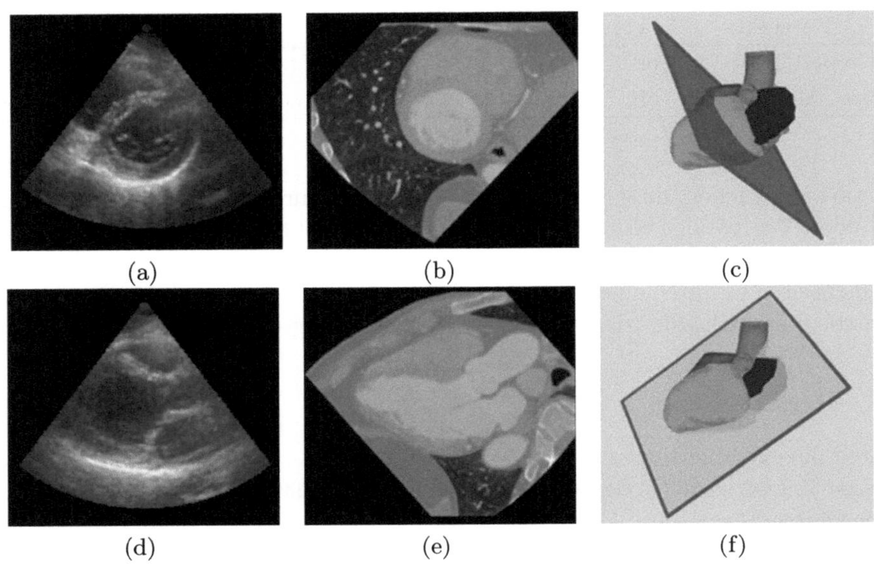

Standardansichten betrachtet, so könnten Klassifikationsalgorithmen oder 2D-2D-Registrierung u. U. bessere Ergebnisse liefern. Das eigentliche Ziel unserer Arbeit ist es jedoch, das vorgestellte Verfahren auch für Nicht-Standardebenen zu nutzen, um den Anwender dann zu einer Standardebene zu führen. Hierfür ist 2D-3D-Registrierung sinnvoll. Da wir Interpatientenvariabilität, unterschiedliche Modalitäten und mit dem Herz ein sehr dynamisches Organ zu Grunde legen, scheint eine Registrierung mit guter Genauigkeit schwierig bis unmöglich. Dass eine Registrierung dennoch sinnvolle Informationen zur Navigation und Orientierung liefern kann, zeigt unser Ansatz. Weitere geplante Arbeiten bestehen im Testen des Systems auf mehr Datensätzen und anderen Standard- und Nicht-Standardansichten, wofür auch ein Ultraschallphantom zur Verfügung steht.

Literaturverzeichnis

1. Penney G, Blackall J, Hamady M, et al. Registration of freehand 3D ultrasound and magnetic resonance liver images. Med Image Anal. 2004;8:81–91.
2. Wein W, Roper B, Navab N. Integrating diagnostic B-mode ultrasonography into CT-based radiation treatment planning. IEEE Trans Med Imgaging. 2007;26:866–879.
3. Lu X, Georgescu B, Zheng Y, et al. AutoMPR: Automatic detection of standard planes in 3D echocardiography. Proc ISBI. 2008; p. 1279–1282.
4. Wachowiak MP, Smolikova R, Elmaghraby AS. Hybrid optimization for ultrasound and multimodal image registration. Eng Med Biol Soc. 2001;3:2418–2421.

Generierung korrespondierender Schichtbilder zur verbesserten lokalen Analyse des linken Ventrikels in 4D-MRT-Bildsequenzen

D. Säring[1], K. Müllerleile[2], M. Groth[3], H. Handels[1]

[1]Institut für Medizinische Informatik, Universitätsklinikum Hamburg-Eppendorff
[2]Klinik und Poliklinik für Kardiologie/Angiologie, UKE
[3]Klinik und Poliklinik für Diagnostische und Interventionelle Radiologie, UKE
d.saering@uke.uni-hamburg.de

Kurzfassung. Die genaue Erfassung lokaler Veränderungen des linken Ventrikels insbesondere bei der Verlaufskontrolle nach einem Infarkt erfordert die Extraktion lokaler Form- und Funktionsparameter. Die für den Inter- und Intrapatientenvergleich notwendige räumliche Korrespondenz der MRT-Schichtbilder ist durch die manuelle Planung der Schichtpositionen beim Aufnahmeverfahren i.A. nicht gewährleistet. In dieser Arbeit wird daher ein Verfahren vorgestellt, das unter Berücksichtigung der anatomischen Grenzen des linken Ventrikels räumlich korrespondierende Positionen bestimmt, zu denen anschließend unter Verwendung der originären Daten und der strukturerhaltenden Interpolation neue Schichtbilder generiert werden. Dadurch wird eine bessere Übereinstimmung der räumlichen Position der zu vergleichenden Schichten erzielt. Das Verfahren wurde an zu Evaluationszwecken generierten Probandendatensätzen getestet. Dabei konnte gezeigt werden, dass die Generierung korrespondierender Kurzachsen-MRT-Schichtbilder zu einer verbesserten Extraktion lokaler Parameter führt.

1 Einleitung

Der Herzinfarkt ist eine der häufigsten Erkrankungen und eine der Hauptursachen vorzeitiger Sterblichkeit bei Menschen in industrialisierten Ländern [1]. Von besonderer Bedeutung für die Beurteilung eines Patienten mit akutem Infarkt ist die quantitative Beschreibung der linksventrikulären Form- und Funktionsveränderungen. Dabei kommt es im Krankheitsverlauf häufig zu Veränderungen im infarzierten und im gesunden linksventrikulären Herzmuskel. So versucht beispielsweise der gesunde Herzmuskelbereich den entstandenen Leistungsverlust zu kompensieren, was zu einer lokalen kompensatorischen Hypertrophie führen kann. Um dies quantitativ zu beschreiben, müssen globale und lokale Parameter extrahiert und analysiert werden. Hierzu werden in der Klinik räumlich-zeitliche 4D-Cine-MRT-Bildsequenzen in kurzer und langer Achse sowie kontrastmittelgestützte 3D-DE-MRT-Bildsequenzen aufgenommen. Die Extraktion globaler Parameter, wie das end-diastolische Volumen (EDV) oder die linksventrikuläre

Ejektionsfraktion (LVEF), ist Gegenstand vieler veröffentlichter Forschungsarbeiten [2, 3]. Spezielle Bildgebungstechniken, wie Tagged-MRT [4], ermöglichen die nicht-invasive Schätzung lokaler Bewegungen aus der zeitlichen Veränderung eines mittels Magnetisierung künstlich erzeugten Gittermusters. Sind diese Markierungen nicht vorhanden, so werden häufig Verfahren eingesetzt, die auf Basis von Segmentierungen den linken Ventrikel in den MRT-Schichtbildern (Kurzachse) in kleinere Segmente unterteilen und für jedes Segment mittels Punktkorrespondenzen lokale Parameter extrahieren [5]. Eine Zuordnung korrespondierender Segmente zur Beurteilung der Veränderung der Parameter z.B. bei der Verlaufskontrolle, erfordert die Aufnahme der MRT-Schichtbilder an korrespondierenden Positionen, welche durch die interaktive Positionierung während der MRT-Aufnahmeprozedur häufig nicht gegeben ist [6]. Dadurch können bei der Verlaufskontrolle im Baseline- zum Follow-up-Datensatz die Anzahl der Schichten und deren Positionen im Raum unterschiedlich sein (Abb. 1).

In dieser Arbeit wird daher ein Verfahren vorgestellt, welches unter Berücksichtigung der Lage der Mitralklappe und der Herzspitze anatomisch korrespondierende Positionen bestimmt und unter Verwendung einer strukturerhaltenden Interpolation [7] auf Basis der originären MRT-Schichtbilder zu diesen Positionen neue Schichtbilder generiert. Abschließend werden die zuvor erstellten Segmentierungsergebnisse auf die neuen Schichten übertragen und lokale Parameter extrahiert [5].

2 Methoden und Evaluation

Ziel dieser Arbeit ist eine Verbesserung der lokalen Analyse des linken Ventrikels in 4D-Bildsequenzen für den Inter- und Intrapatientenvergleich. Hierzu wird ein 3D-Volumen zu einem bestimmten Zeitpunkt im 4D-Datensatz selektiert. In diesem werden dann im Gegensatz zu den bestehenden Verfahren neue Schichtbilder zu korrespondierenden räumlichen Positionen relativ zur Länge des linken Ventrikels geneiert. Dadurch soll erreicht werden, dass für jedes 3D-Volumen die Anzahl und die relative räumliche Position der für die lokale Analyse verwendeten Schichten identisch ist. Diesem Ansatz liegt die Annahme zu Grunde, dass

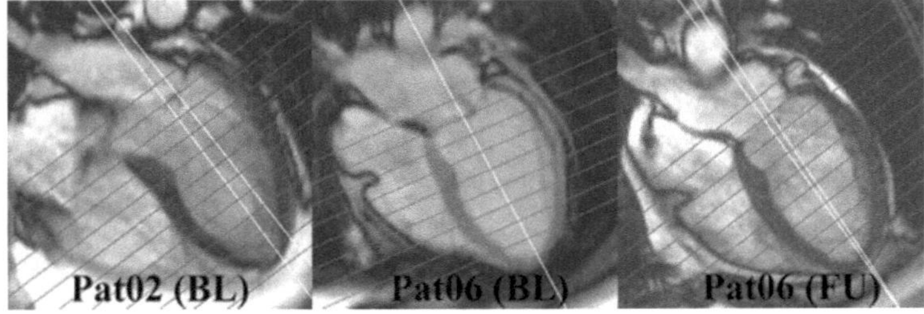

Abb. 1. Anzahl, Position und Orientierung der Kurzachsen-MRT-Schichtbilder von drei Datensätzen in Baseline (BL) und Follow-up (FU) überlagert auf der jeweiligen Langachsen-MRT (4-Kammer-Blick).

MRT-Schichtbilder aus unterschiedlichen Datensätzen an der gleichen relativen Position zwischen der Herzspitze und der Mitralklappe zueinander korrespondieren.

2.1 Methoden

In einem Vorverarbeitungsschritt werden Lang- und Kurzachsen-MRT-Schichtbilder auf Basis ihrer DICOM Informationen in ein gemeinsames 3D Koordinatensystem transformiert. Zusätzlich wird die Position der Mitralklappe und der Herzspitze manuell sowie die Segmentierung der inneren und äußeren Begrenzung des Myokards, dem so genannten Endo- bzw. Epikard, semi-automatisch bestimmt [8].

Auf Basis dieser Daten wird im Rahmen dieser Arbeit zunächst der Abstand zwischen Mitralklappe und Apex berechnet. Entlang einer virtuelle Linie von Mitralklappenmittelpunkt zur Herzspitze werden sowohl die Schnittpunkte mit den originären Kurzachsen-MRT-Schichtbildern bestimmt als auch eine Menge von n äquidistanten Punkten $P_i(x)$ mit $i = (1, \ldots, n)$ und $x \in \mathbb{R}^2$ konstruiert. Die Punkte P_i definieren die relativen Positionen, an denen die neuen Schichtbilder interpoliert werden (Abb. 2). Für die Interpolation wird das Verfahren der strukturerhaltenden Interpolation verwendet [7]. Dabei wird zwischen den beiden räumlich benachbarten MRT-Schichtbildern ein Bewegungsfeld geschätzt welches anschließend für die Generierung des neuen Schichtbildes verwendet wird. Dadurch werden in den neu generierten Bilddaten bestehende Strukturen wie die Objektgrenzen des Myokards erhalten. Anschließend werden die Konturen des Endo- und Epikards aus den originären MRT-Schichtbildern unter Verwendung des Bewegungsfeldes auf die neu generierte Schicht adaptiert.

Für die Extraktion der lokalen Parameter wird das Myokard, repräsentiert durch die adaptierten myokardialen Konturen, in den interpolierten Schichten in 100 Segmente unterteilt. Dann wird für jedes Segment in der Phase der maximalen Kontraktion (Endsystole) und der maximalen Relaxion (Enddiastole) die lokale Dicke des Herzmuskels und die Position des Endokards extrahiert. Auf Basis dieser Werte kann dann die myokardiale Kontraktion und die endokardiale Bewegung für jedes Segment berechnet werden.

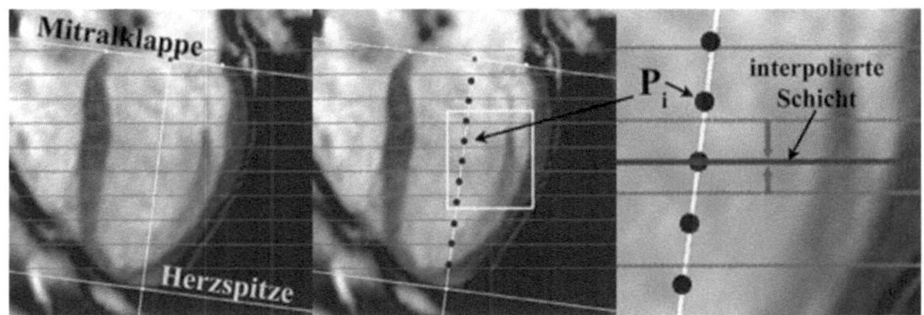

Abb. 2. Definition äquidistanter Punkte auf einer virtuellen Linie zwischen Mitralklappe und Herzspitze sowie die Generierung von n korrespondierender Schichten auf Basis der räumlich benachbarten originären Schichten.

2.2 Evaluation

Für die Evaluation des vorgestellten Verfahrens wurde ein Datensatz D_{Proband} mit 6mm Schichtabstand in zwei neue Datensätze D_1, D_2 aufgeteilt, wobei jeweils alle ungeraden und alle geraden Schichten verwendet wurden (Abb. 3). Die resultierenden Datensätze D_1 und D_2 haben somit einen Schichtabstand von 12mm, was in etwa dem klinischen Standard von 10mm entspricht. In D_1 und D_2 wurde von erfahrenen Radiologen das Myokard segmentiert und visuell korrespondierende Schichten in D_1 und D_2 bestimmt. Anschließend wurden die oben beschriebenen lokalen Parameter aus den originären (D_1, D_2) und den interpolierten Schichten (D_1^{ip}, D_2^{ip}) extrahiert, jeweils der erste Datensatz (D_1 bzw. D_1^{ip}) als BL und der zweite (D_2 bzw. D_2^{ip}) als FU definiert und schichtweise die mittlere Differenz über alle Segmente berechnet.

3 Ergebnisse

In Absprache mit den klinischen Kooperationspartner wurde die Anzahl der interpolierten Schichten auf $n = 10$ festgelegt, wobei die Nummerierung der Schichten vom apikalen zum basalen Bereich aufsteigend gewählt wurde. In Abbildung 4 sind schichtweise die über alle lokalen Segmente gemittelten Differenzen für die myokardiale Kontraktion (MK) dargestellt. Es wurde gemittelt über alle Schichten eine Reduktion der mittleren Differenzen von $1,3$cm auf $0,3$cm (MK) bzw. $1,0$cm auf $0,4$cm (endokardiale Bewegung) erzielt. Wobei für die Schichten 1 und 10 keine Differenzen berechnet wurden, da in den originären Bilddaten im basalen und im apikalen Bereich keine korrespondierenden Schichten definiert werden konnten.

4 Diskussion

Durch die Verwendung der Datensätzen eines Probanden sollten im optimalen Fall die mittleren Differenzen 0 sein. Somit zeigen die präsentierten Ergebnisse, dass mit dem vorgestellten Verfahren zur Generierung korrespondierender

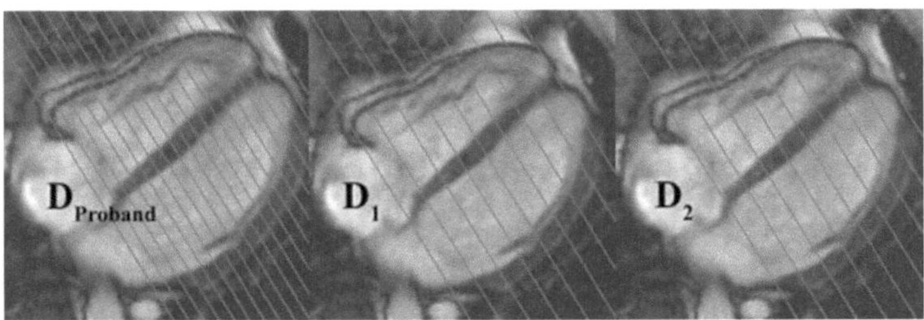

Abb. 3. Position und Orientierung der Kurzachsen-MRT-Schichtbilder eines Probanden mit einem geringem Schichtabstand von 6mm (links) und die daraus generierten Datensätze D_1 und D_2 mit einem von Schichtabstand 12mm.

Abb. 4. Schichtweise Gegenüberstellung der mittleren Differenzen auf Basis der originären (dunkel) und der interpolierten (hell) Daten. Vergleich der originären und der interpolierten MRT-Schichtbilder (BL, FU) im basalen Bereich des linken Ventrikels.

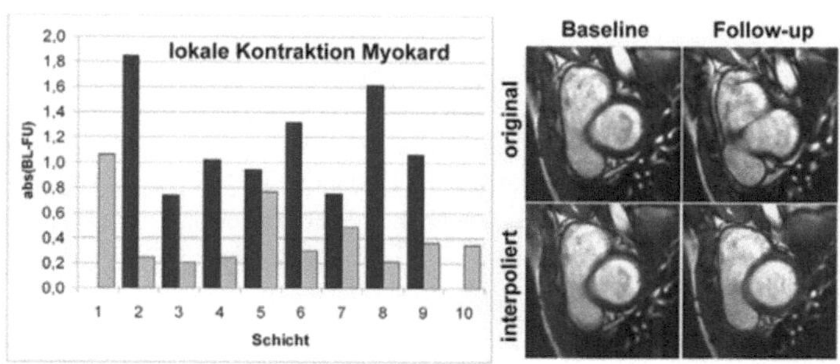

MRT-Schichtbilder die quantitative Auswertung der lokalen Parameter verbessert werden kann. Eine visuelle Beurteilung der Korrespondenz bestätigt die quantitativen Ergebnisse. Insbesondere im basalen Bereich des linken Ventrikels konnte die Ähnlichkeit der Daten erhöht werden. Abbildung 4 zeigt die als korrespondierend definierten Schichten (BL zu FU) aus den originären und die zu korrespondierenden Positionen generierten Bilddaten.

In näherer Zukunft sollen weitere MRT-Datensätze von Probanden analysiert werden, um die erzielten Ergebnisse zu verifizieren. Darüber hinaus ist geplant, die Interpolation der Schichten zu erweitern, so dass korrespondierende Schichten nicht nur parallel zu den originären MRT-Schichtbildern sondern auch parallel zur Mitralklappenebene generiert werden können. Es wird erwartet, dass dadurch die Extraktion lokaler Parameter weiter verbessert werden kann.

Literaturverzeichnis

1. Schelhase T, Weber S. Mortality statistics in Germany. Bundesgesundheitsblatt. 2007;50(7):969–976.
2. Alfakih K, et al. Normal human left and right ventricular dimensions for MRI as assessed by turbo gradient echo and steady-state free precession imaging sequences. J Magn Reson Imaging. 2003;17(3):323–329.
3. Montagnat J, et al. 4D deformable models with temporal constraints: application to 4D cardiac image segmentation. Med Image Anal. 2005;9(1):87–100.
4. Axel L, Montillo A, Kim D. Tagged magnetic resonance imaging of the heart: A survey. Med Image Anal. 2005;9(4):376–393.
5. Säring D, et al. Computer-assisted analysis of 4D cardiac MR image sequences after myocardial infarction. Methods Inf Med. 2006;45(4):377–383.
6. Lelieveldt BP, et al. Automated observer-independent acquisition of cardiac short-axis MR images: a pilot study. Radiology. 2001;221(2):537–542.
7. Ehrhardt J, Säring D, Handels H. Structure-preserving interpolation of temporal and spatial image sequences using an optical flow based method. Methods Inf Med. 2007;46(3):300–307.
8. Säring D, et al. Combination of short- and longaxis MR image sequences for 3D segmentation of the left ventricle. Procs MIE. 2008.

Ermittlung einer kranial-kaudalen Korrespondenz in MR-Aufnahmen

Andrea Fränzle[1], Armin Stoll[1], Rolf Bendl[1,2]

[1]Abteilung für Medizinische Physik in der Strahlentherapie, DKFZ Heidelberg
[2]Fakultät für Informatik, Hochschule Heilbronn
a.fraenzle@dkfz-heidelberg.de

Kurzfassung. Grundlage einer Bestrahlungsplanung ist ein dreidimensionales Modell der individuellen Patientenanatomie, das auf Basis von Schichtbildaufnahmen durch Segmentierung erstellt wird. Manuelle Segmentierungsverfahren sind zeitaufwendig, aus diesem Grund besteht der dringende Bedarf an möglichst vollautomatischen Verfahren. Bekannte Segmentierungsverfahren brauchen geeignete Initialisierungen, um bestimmte Strukturen zu extrahieren. Dazu ist es notwendig zu wissen, welche Strukturen ein Bild enthält. Mit Hilfe des hier präsentierten Verfahrens ist eine automatische Zuordnung eines Bildes zu einer Körperregion möglich. Dazu wird zunächst der Körper des Patienten vom Hintergrund getrennt und anhand von Eigenschaften aus der Grauwertverteilung und eines Formmerkmals mit Hilfe eines Random-Forest-Klassifikators für jede Schicht die zugehörige Körperregion ermittelt. Dieses Wissen kann zu einer anschließenden automatischen Segmentierung von Risikoorganen in MR-Aufnahmen weiterverwendet werden.

1 Einleitung

Bei der Strahlentherapieplanung sind Risikoorgane zu berücksichtigen, die im Umfeld des zu bestrahlenden Tumors liegen und vor Strahlung zu schützen sind. Für die Planung zur Verfügung stehende semiautomatische Segmentierungsverfahren benötigen häufig Saatpunkte, Startpunkte oder Bounding Boxen und setzen zumindest rudimentäre Bildverarbeitungskenntnisse voraus. Daher werden diese Verfahren in der Praxis oft nicht eingesetzt und die Segmentierung von Hand bevorzugt.

Mit Hilfe von wissensbasierten Methoden können semiautomatische Segmentierungsverfahren automatisiert werden, indem Wissen, das man zur Ausführung dieser Verfahren benötigt, automatisch aus den Aufnahmen extrahiert wird. Dazu gehört zunächst die Zuordnung einer Transversalschicht zu einer Körperregion, die Analyse der sogenannten kranial-kaudalen Korrespondenz. Mit dem Wissen über die Lage einer Transversalschicht im Körper ist auch bekannt, welche Organe in dieser Bildschicht zu erwarten sind.

In der Arbeit von Stoll [1] wird die Ermittlung der kranial-kaudalen Korrespondenz in CT-Aufnahmen vorgestellt. Hierfür wird zunächst der Körper des Patienten vom Hintergrund extrahiert und anhand des Verhältnisses von Höhe zur Breite der Anatomie sowie von verschiedenen Gewebeanteilen, charakterisiert durch ihre Hounsfield-Units, mit Mustererkennungsverfahren einer Körperregion zugeordnet.

Im MR kann solch eine Zuordnung von absoluten Grauwerten zu Geweben nicht als Merkmal dienen, da hier ein Äquivalent zur Hounsfield-Skala im CT fehlt. In diesem Beitrag wird ein alternativer Ansatz zur Ermittlung der kranial-kaudalen Korrespondenz im MR vorgestellt.

2 Material und Methoden

Für die Zuordnung von Bildschichten zu einer Körperregion wird zunächst der Körper des Patienten vom Bildhintergrund getrennt. Auf Grundlage dieser anatomischen Maske werden Merkmale bestimmt, die die Transversalschichten charakterisieren. Anschließend erfolgt eine Klassifikation der Bildschichten mit Random Forests. Im Folgenden wird das Vorgehen zur Erstellung der anatomischen Maske und der Klassifikation mit Random Forests erläutert.

2.1 Erstellung der anatomischen Maske

Aufgrund vielfältiger Artefakte ist die Information in MR Bildern häufig verfälscht und die Trennung des Patienten vom Hintergrund deutlich komplexer als im CT. Eine grobe Segmentierung der Anatomie wird im MR durch eine Binarisierung mit einem dynamischen Schwellwert erreicht. Das in der Arbeit von Stoll [1] eingesetzte Verfahren nach Otsu [2] hat sich bei MR-Bildern als ungeeignet erwiesen, da es z.B. im Bereich des Beckens durch Setzen einer zu hohen Schwelle zu viel von der Anatomie entfernt. Als Schwellwert im MR ist die erste Minimal-Stelle nach dem ersten Maximum im Median-gefilterten Histogramm als erster Schritt geeignet [3], aber nicht ausreichend. Nach der Binarisierung müssen kleinere Objekte, verursacht durch Bildrauschen, entfernt und Löcher innerhalb der Anatomie geschlossen werden.

2.2 Klassifikation der Bildschichten

Um die Bildschichten den Körperregionen Kopf, Hals, Thorax, Abdomen und Becken zuordnen zu können, müssen möglichst aussagekräftige Merkmale der Anatomie bestimmt werden. Ebenso wie bei Stoll [1] wird hier das Verhältnis der Höhe zur Breite der Anatomie als Merkmal verwendet, da dieses charakteristisch für die genannten Körperregionen und unabhängig von der Aufnahmemodalität ist. Da im MR keine eindeutige Zuordnung von Grauwertbereichen zu Geweben existiert, können die von Stoll [1] verwendeten Merkmale, die sich aus den Anteilen der Gewebe anhand ihrer Hounsfield-Units-Bereiche ergeben, nicht exakt übernommen werden. Es hat sich jedoch gezeigt, dass sich die Anteile von Grauwertbereichen, die sich durch die Aufteilung des Histogramms in 10 Säulen ergeben, als Merkmale für die Klassifikation im MR eignen. Zusätzlich verbessert das Hinzufügen des Grauwert-Medians das Klassifikationsergebnis. Abbildung 1 bietet eine Übersicht der hier zur Charakterisierung von Transversalschichten verschiedener Körperregionen verwendeten Merkmale.

Zur Klassifikation der Bildschichten wird ein robuster Klassifikator benötigt, dessen Leistung nicht zu sehr von der Qualität jedes einzelnen Merkmals abhängt. Ebenso sollte eine schnelle Klassifizierung erfolgen können, um die Dauer der Klassifizierung auch bei größeren Datenmengen gering zu halten. Für die genannte Aufgabenstellung hat sich der Random-Forest-Klassifikator [4] als geeignet erwiesen. Er zeichnet sich dadurch aus, dass ein zu klassifizierendes Element durch eine Menge von Entscheidungsbäumen klassifiziert wird und als endgültiges Klassifikationsergebnis die am häufigsten gewählte Klasse betrachtet wird. Daraus resultiert eine robuste Klassifizierung, da sich das Klassifikationsergebnis nicht auf das Resultat eines einzelnen Klassifikators stützt. Jeder der n Entscheidungsbäume wird hier nach dem CART-Algorithmus [5] mit einer Bootstrap-Stichprobe aus der Trainingsmenge erstellt. Für jeden zu spaltenden Baumknoten wird aus k Merkmalen, die zufällig ohne Zurücklegen aus der Menge der Merkmale gezogen werden, das am besten trennende Merkmal ermittelt. Da hier bereits eine Merkmalsauswahl getroffen wird, ist eine Untersuchung, welche Merkmale tatsächlich entscheidend für eine gute Klassifikation sind, praktisch unnnötig. Ein Element kann schnell klassifiziert werden, da hier lediglich Entscheidungsbäume durchlaufen werden müssen und nicht wie z.B. beim k-Nächste-Nachbarn-Verfahren für die Klassifikation jedes einzelnen Elements sämtliche Muster der Trainingsstichprobe zu berücksichtigen sind.

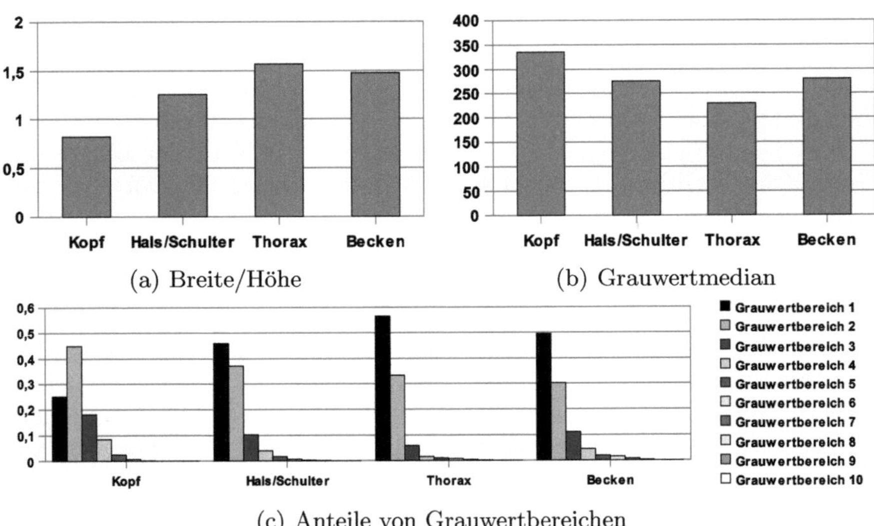

(a) Breite/Höhe

(b) Grauwertmedian

(c) Anteile von Grauwertbereichen

Abb. 1. Durchschnittliche Werte für das Verhältnis von Breite zur Höhe der Anatomie, den Grauwertmedian und für Anteile von Grauwertbereichen eines in 10 Bereiche aufgeteilten Histogramms von Transversalschichten der Körperregionen Kopf, Hals/Schulter, Thorax und Becken.

Tabelle 1. Fehlerraten bei Klassifikation von Testdaten mit Random Forests bei unterschiedlicher Baumanzahl n und Merkmalsanzahl k.

$n\backslash k$	1	2	3	4	5	6	7	8	9	10	11	12
10	0,20	0,22	0,20	0,16	0,15	0,13	0,13	0,17	0,13	0,16	0,15	0,16
25	0,39	0,21	0,21	0,20	0,16	0,16	0,13	0,13	0,14	0,13	0,17	0,17
50	0,42	0,22	0,18	0,15	0,16	0,12	0,13	0,13	0,13	0,15	0,15	0,18
100	0,42	0,21	0,18	0,16	0,17	0,16	0,15	0,15	0,15	0,15	0,16	0,17
250	0,37	0,21	0,21	0,17	0,15	0,15	0,15	0,15	0,14	0,16	0,16	0,18

3 Ergebnisse

Für die Erstellung der Random Forests wurde für $n = [10, 25, 50, 100, 250]$ und k von 1-12 gewählt. Mit jeder Kombination von n und k wurden 10 Random Forests erstellt und daraus durchschnittliche Fehlerraten ermittelt. Die zugrunde liegenden Trainingsdaten umfassen 2529 T1-gewichtete, manuell klassifizierte Bildschichten (SE-Sequenz), davon sind 1386 Schichten von 9 Kopf-Hals-Bildserien und 1143 Schichten von 9 Prostata-Bildserien. Für einen ersten Test wurden 3 von der Trainingsmenge unabhängige Bildserien verwendet, darin enthalten sind 110 Schichten aus 2 Kopf-Hals-Bildserien und 69 Schichten einer Prostata-Bildserie. Diese Schichten wurden manuell und mit den Random Forests klassifiziert. Anschließend wurden die Fehlerraten, die in Tabelle 1 aufgelistet sind, ermittelt. Die geringste Fehlerrate (0,12) und damit das beste Klassifikationsergebnis liefert hier ein Random-Forest-Klassifikator mit $n = 50$ und $k = 6$.

4 Diskussion

Das von Stoll [1] entwickelte Verfahren zur Bestimmung der kranial-kaudalen Korrespondenz in CT-Aufnahmen kann nicht direkt für MR-Bildserien übernommen werden, da hier Merkmale zur Klassifikation verwendet werden, die auf Gewebeanteilen, die durch ihre Hounsfield-Units-Bereiche charakterisiert sind, basieren. In diesem Beitrag wurde ein alternatives Verfahren vorgestellt, mit dem eine Zuordnung von Bildschichten zu Körperregionen in MR-Bildserien erfolgen kann. Dieses Wissen kann zu einer anschließenden automatischen Segmentierung von Risikoorganen verwendet werden, da mit der Kenntnis der Bildschicht auch die darin zu erwartenden Organe bekannt sind.

Mit einer Binarisierung anhand eines dynamischen Schwellwerts und daran anschließenden, automatisch durchgeführten Bildverarbeitungsschritten erhält man eine Maske, die die Anatomie des Patienten bei ausreichend ausgeleuchteten Aufnahmen zuverlässig wiedergibt. Ausgehend von dieser anatomischen Maske können Merkmale, die die Transversalschichten charakterisieren, bestimmt werden.

Die Zuordnung von Transversalschichten zu einer Körperregion erfolgt hier durch eine Klassifikation mit Random Forests. Anhand der ermittelten Fehlerraten scheinen hier Random Forests mit $n \geq 50$ und k zwischen 3 und 10 für die Klassifikation von Bildschichten geeignet zu sein. Die geringste Fehlerrate und damit das beste Klassifikationsergebnis wird hier mit $n = 50$ und $k = 6$ erzielt. Einzelne Fehlzuordnungen treten bei den Kopfhals-Serien hauptsächlich im Übergangsbereich von Hals/Schulter zum Kopf auf. Schichten im Kopfbereich werden nahezu vollständig richtig klassifiziert. Im Beckenbereich erfolgt die Klassifikation ebenfalls recht zuverlässig. Fehlzuordnungen treten hier hauptsächlich aufgrund von schlechter Ausleuchtung im unteren Bereich der Bildserie auf. Ebenso wie bei [1] beschrieben, lassen sich auch im MR einzelne falsch zugeordnete Bildschichten mit einer Medianfilterung korrigieren. Dabei werden jeweils fünf aufeindanderfolgende Bildschichten betrachtet und der mittleren Bildschicht die Körperregion zugeordnet, die dem Median der Körperregionen der betrachteten Bildschichten entspricht.

Die Klassifikation der Bildschichten mit Random Forests erfolgt sehr schnell. Eine Bildserie wird hier in weniger als 1s vollständig klassifiziert.

Die gewählten Merkmale und die Klassifikation mit Random Forests sind grundsätzlich zur Ermittlung der kranial-kaudalen Korrespondenz im MR geeignet. Um jedoch eine fundiertere Aussage über die Güte des Klassifikationsverfahrens treffen zu können, ist das Verfahren auf Basis einer größeren Menge von Test- und eventuell auch von Trainingsdaten zu validieren.

Literaturverzeichnis

1. Stoll A, Wetter T, Bendl R. Wissensakquisition mit Methoden der Mustererkennung zur wissensbasierten Segmentierung von Risikoorganen in CT-Bilddaten. Proc BVM. 2008; p. 39–45.
2. Otsu N. A Threshold Selection Method from Gray-Level Histograms. IEEE Trans Syst Man Cybern. 1979;SMC-9(1):62–66.
3. Spiliotis IM, van Ormondt D, Mertzios BG. Prior Knowledge for Improved Image Estimation from Raw MRI Data. In: Procs 2nd Int Workshop Image Signal Process; 1995. p. 8–10.
4. Breiman L. Random Forests. Machine Learning. 2001;45(1):5–32.
5. Hastie T, Tibshirani R, Friedman J. The elements of statistical learning. New York: Springer; 2007.

Automatische Qualitätsmessung von Retina-Fundusbildern

Jan Paulus[1], Jörg Meier[1], Rüdiger Bock[1], Joachim Hornegger[1], Georg Michelson[2]

[1]Lehrstuhl für Informatik 5 (Mustererkennung), Universität Erlangen-Nürnberg
[2]Augenklinik Erlangen, Universität Erlangen-Nürnberg
joerg.meier@informatik.uni-erlangen.de

Kurzfassung. Zur frühzeitigen Diagnose von Erkrankungen am Augenhintergrund existieren automatische Bildverarbeitungsmethoden. Für die Effektivität solcher Verfahren und für die ärztliche Bewertung ist die Bildqualität der Eingabedaten entscheidend. Wir stellen einen neuen segmentierungsfreien Algorithmus zur automatischen Qualitätsmessung einzelner Fundusbilder vor, der Clustering-Merkmale, Schärfemaße und globale Bildstatistiken kombiniert. Die Güte der Methode wird mit einem etablierten Verfahren zur Qualitätsmessung von Retina-Fundusbildern verglichen, das nur Clustering-Merkmale auf gefilterten Bildern verwendet. Der neue Algorithmus zeigt dabei auf 302 Fundusfotos mit einer Klassifikationsgenauigkeit von 90,3% eine deutlich höhere Zuverlässigkeit als das Vergleichsverfahren mit 69,5%.

1 Einleitung

Retina-Fundusbilder stellen die Grundlage für die Diagnose von Erkankungen am Augenhintergrund, wie Glaukom oder diabetische Retinopathie, dar. Zur frühzeitigen Erkennung existieren automatische Bildverarbeitungsmethoden, die den Arzt unterstützen sollen. Entscheidend für die Zuverlässigkeit solcher Methoden ist die Bildqualität. Um diese automatisch und sicher zu bestimmen, wird hier ein neues Verfahren vorgeschlagen. Im Gegensatz zu anderen Methoden (wie z. B. [1]) kommt die Methode ohne fehleranfällige Segmentierung von Bildstrukturen aus und bestimmt die Bildqualität eines Eingabebildes ohne ein Referenzbild zu benötigen.

Nach Wissen der Autoren gibt es drei relevante Arbeiten im Bereich von Retinabildqualitätsbewertung. Fleming et al. [1] verwenden einen segmentierungsbasierten Ansatz, bei dem zunächst die Erkennbarkeit der Gefäße im Bereich der Makula (Punkt des schärfsten Sehens) zur Messung der Qualität dient. Außerdem wird der anatomische Ausschnitt bestimmt, den das Bild zeigt. Bilder guter Qualität zeigen die Papille (Sehnervkopf) sowie den Augenhintergrund in einem Bereich der Größe des doppelten Papillendurchmessers um die Makula.

Lalonde et al. [2] berechnen die Qualität eines Eingabebildes segmentierungsfrei über das Histogramm des Gradientenmagnitudenbildes und über lokale Histogramminformationen der Grauwerte. Die Klassifikation erfolgt über Vergleiche mit einem Referenzhistogramm entwickelt aus Bildern guter Qualität.

Niemeijer et al. [3] schlagen "Image Structure Clustering" (ISC) als ebenfalls segmentierungsfreie Methode vor. Die Qualität einer Retinaaufnahme wird dabei durch die Verteilung von Clustern charakterisiert, die das Aussehen bestimmter Strukturen auf den Bildern modellieren. Hierzu wird das Eingabebild in das Gauge-Koordinatensystem transformiert, das in jedem Punkt durch die Richtung seiner Gradienten definiert ist. Nach einem k-Means-Clustering werden die Clustergrößen sowie jeweils ein 5-Bin-Histogramm jedes Farbkanals als Merkmale verwendet. Durch die Verwendung der unterschiedlich gefilterten Gauge-Koordinaten, gehen bei diesem Verfahren hauptsächlich lokale Kanteninformationen in die Merkmalsberechung ein. Globale Bildstatistiken fehlen.

Unser Verfahren verwendet ebenfalls ein unüberwachtes Clustering, das jedoch direkt auf den Grauwerten arbeitet und so versucht, strukturelle Komponenten zu finden. Als Merkmale dienen zusätzlich zu den Clustergrößen die Inter-Cluster-Differenzen, um die Trennbarkeit der Strukturen zu messen. Außerdem führen wir ein Schärfemaß ein und berechnen drei Haralick-Merkmale [4]. Damit verbindet es lokale mit globalen Bildmerkmalen.

2 Methoden

Der Beurteilung der Bildqualität liegen vier Qualitätskriterien zu Grunde: (i) Homogene Ausleuchtung, (ii) Erkennbarkeit der Papillenstruktur, (iii) Erkennbarkeit der Gefäßstrukturen und (iv) heller bzw. kontrastreicher Hintergrund.

Der Algorithmus berechnet drei Merkmalsgruppen. Im ersten Teil wird ein unüberwachtes Clustering durchgeführt, das die Bildkomponenten in Clustern zusammenfasst. Es werden die Clustergrößen und Inter-Cluster-Differenzen bestimmt. So wird Erkennbarkeit und Differenzierung der einzelnen Strukturen bewertet. Im zweiten Teil wird ein Schärfemaß berechnet, das mit einem Schwellwertverfahren die Kantengüte schätzt. Es bewertet, wie deutlich die Strukturen abgegrenzt sind. Im dritte Teil werden durch Haralick-Merkmale die Homogenität, der Kontrast und die allgemeine Bildschärfe gemessen. Schließlich werden die drei Merkmalsgruppen zu einem Vektor kombiniert.

2.1 Clustering

Es erfolgt ein k-Means-Clustering des Eingabebildes B der Größe $n \times m$ mit k Clustern C_i, wobei $i \in \{1, \ldots, k\}$. Es wird nur der Grünkanal der Bilder betrachtet, da dieser den besten Kontrast aufweist. Die Grauwerte b_{xy}, mit $x \in \{1, \ldots, n\}$ und $y \in \{1, \ldots, m\}$, werden zu Clustern zusammengefasst. Damit stützt sich das Verfahren nicht auf lokale Kanteninformationen. Das Clustering soll verschiedene Strukturen des Augenhintergrundes detektieren. Dazu werden die Clusterzentren durch gemittelte Werte für die k zu findenden Strukturen aus *guten* Bildern (nach Goldstandard durch Arzt festgelegt) initialisiert. Das Verhältnis c_i der Pixel b_{xy} jedes Clusters C_i zur Gesamtanzahl der Pixel wird als Kennzahl für die Größe der jeweiligen Struktur verwendet und im folgenden *Clustergröße* genannt. Als entscheidende Merkmale kommen nun die Inter-Cluster-Differenzen hinzu. Je deutlicher Strukturen erkennbar und separierbar sind, desto höher ist der Kontrast zwischen ihnen, der durch die Inter-Cluster-Differenzen gemessen wird. Dafür wird für die Differenz aus dem Mittelwert m_i des jeweiligen Clusters C_i mit den Mittelwerten der anderen Cluster d_{ij} gebildet.

$$c_i = \frac{\#\{b_{xy} | b_{xy} \in C_i\}}{n \cdot m} \tag{1}$$

$$d_{ij} = m_i - m_j, i \in \{1, \ldots, k\}, j \in \{1, \ldots, k\}, i > j \tag{2}$$

Die Clustergrößen c_i und die Inter-Cluster-Differenzen d_{ij} beurteilen somit die strukturelle Erkennbarkeit der einzelnen Bildkomponenten, wie z. B. der Papille.

2.2 Schärfemessung

Zur Messung der Bildschärfe wird eine Blind-SNR-Schätzung vorgenommen. Zunächst wird die Gradientenmagnitude G des Eingabebildes B berechnet.

$$G = \sqrt{B_x^2 + B_y^2} \; mit \; B_x = \frac{\partial B}{\partial x}, \; B_y = \frac{\partial B}{\partial y} \tag{3}$$

Die Grauwerte g_{xy} des Gradientenbildes G werden auf den Bereich $[0 \ldots 1]$ skaliert. Zusätzlich zur Anzahl s_1 wird die Summe s_2 der Grauwerte g_{xy} berechnet, die über einem Schwellwert $\alpha \in [0 \ldots 1]$ liegen. Die beiden Kennzahlen werden zur Normalisierung durch die Gesamtanzahl der Bildpunkte dividiert.

$$s_1 = \frac{\#\{g_{xy} | g_{xy} \geq \alpha\}}{n \cdot m} \quad und \quad s_2 = \frac{\sum_{i=1}^{n \cdot m} v_{xy}}{n \cdot m}, \; v_{xy} = \begin{cases} 0 & g_{xy} < \alpha \\ g_{xy} & g_{xy} \geq \alpha \end{cases} \tag{4}$$

Der Schwellwert α wurde auf 0.5 festgelegt. s_1 beschreibt nun die Anzahl der Kantenpunkte und s_2 die durchschnittliche Kantenstärke. Beide Merkmale messen damit die Abgrenzung der einzelnen Strukturen.

2.3 Haralick-Merkmale

Es werden die drei Haralick-Merkmale [4] Entropie h_1, Energie h_2 und Kontrast h_3 verwendet.

2.4 Kombination der Merkmale

Die Clustergrößen c_i der k Clustern, die Cluster-Abstände d_{ij}, die beiden Schärfekennzahlen s_1, s_2 und die drei Haralick-Maße h_1, h_2 und h_3 werden zu einem Merkmalsvektor zusammengefasst. Durch Evaluierung der Klassifikationsleistung wählten wir $k = 5$. Strukturell wird somit eine Aufteilung des Bildes in Gefäße, zwei Papillen- und zwei Hintergrundbereiche ermöglicht. Die Cluster korrelieren also gut mit den genannten Qualitätskriterien. Der resultierende 20-dimensionale Merkmalsvektor kann ohne weitere Dimensionsreduktion klassifiziert werden.

Tabelle 1. Klassifikation von *guten* Bildern: neues Verfahren und ISC

Verfahren	Klassifikationsgenauigkeit	Sensitivität	Spezifität
neues Verfahren	90,3%	95,1%	70,9%
ISC	69,5%	69,0%	70,0%

3 Ergebnisse

Zur Evaluierung diente eine Menge von 302 Retinaaufnahmen (Kowa non-myd, 22,5° FOV, linke und rechte Augen), die von drei unabhängigen Bewertern, darunter ein Augenarzt, anhand der in Abschnitt 3 genannten vier Kriterien bewertet wurden. Es erfolgte eine Einteilung in zwei Klassen *gut* und *schlecht*. Ein Bild gilt als *gut*, wenn mindestens 2 Kriterien positiv bewertet wurden. Der vorgestellte Algorithmus wurde mit dem selbst nachimplementierten ISC-Verfahren verglichen. Bei allen Tests wurde eine Support Vector Machine mit radialer Basisfunktion $k(\boldsymbol{u}, \boldsymbol{v}) = \exp(-\gamma \cdot |\boldsymbol{u} - \boldsymbol{v}|^2)$ als Klassifikator verwendet. Die Parameter γ und der Bestrafungsfaktor C wurden auf einer Teilung der Bilder in Trainings- und Testmenge optimiert. Zur Evaluierung der Klassifikation wurden je zwei Teilmengen der Bildmenge in 10 Iterationen kreuzvalidiert und daraus der Mittelwert ermittelt.

Das neue Verfahren erreicht eine Klassifikationsgenauigkeit von 90,3%. ISC erzielt 69,5% (Tab. 1). Die Sensivität des neuen Algorithmus liegt bei 95,1% und die des ISC bei 69,0%. Die Spezifität beider Verfahren unterscheidet sich mit 70,9% beim neuen Verfahren und 70,0% bei ISC nur wenig.

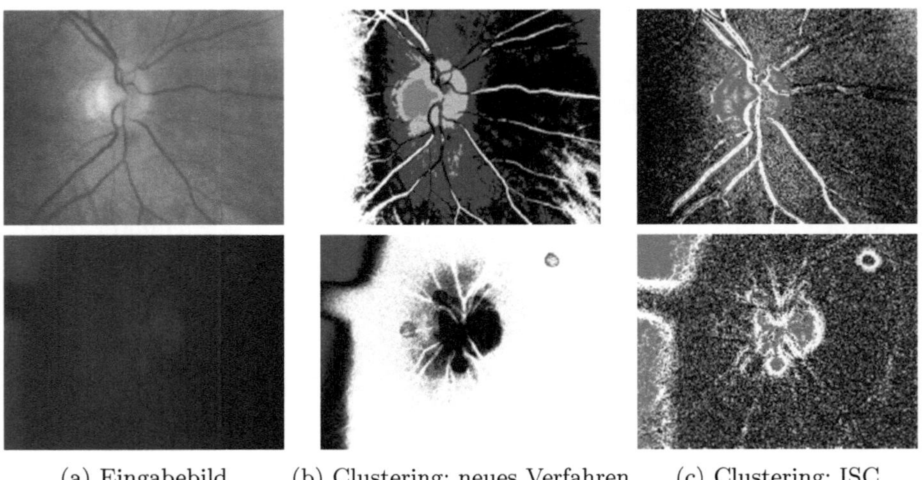

(a) Eingabebild (b) Clustering: neues Verfahren (c) Clustering: ISC

Abb. 1. Bildbeispiele: *Gute*, *schlechte* Retinabilder (erste, zweite Zeile) und Cluster-Ergebnis kodiert durch Grauwerte.

4 Diskussion

Trennt man die etablierten Haralick-Merkmale von den neuen Cluster- und Schärfemerkmalen, errreichen die Haralick-Maße eine Sensivität von 92,7% (Spezifität von 67,0%). Die beiden neuen Cluster- und Schärfemerkmale kombiniert erzielen eine Sensivität von 74,7% (Spezifität 85,7%). Die Haralick-Merkmale alleine neigen also dazu, Bilder eher als *gut* einzustufen. Die neuen Clustering- und Schärfemerkmale dagegen identifizieren die *schlechten* Bilder besser. Kombiniert ergibt sich dadurch die Klassifikationsgenauigkeit von 90,3%. Das neue Verfahren zeigt damit eine deutlich bessere Klassifikationsgenauigkeit als das ISC. Es gibt mehrere Gründe, weshalb die publizierten Ergebnisse von ISC auf dem hier benutzten Datensatz nicht verifiziert werden konnten. In [3] wurde ISC auf Bildern mit größerem FOV als in unserem Datensatz getestet. Auch das Goldstandard Qualitätskriterium war dort anders. Trotz der niedrigeren Klassifikationsgenauigkeit, sind die Gefäße in den ISC-Clustern deutlich besser separiert (visuelle Einschätzung, siehe Abb. 1). ISC eignet sich also z. B. als Initialisierung für ein Segmentierungsverfahren besser.

Wir erreichen die hohe Klassifikationsgenauigkeit mittels Modellierung der hier geforderten Qualitätskriterien durch das neue Verfahren in den fünf Clustern und durch die Ergänzung mit globalen Bildstatistiken. Wir konnten also zeigen, dass diese Kombination von globalen und lokalen Merkmalen für die automatische Qualitätsmessung den verwendeten Goldstandard gut abbildet.

Literaturverzeichnis

1. Fleming AD, Philip S, Goatman KA, et al. Automated assessment of diabetic retinal image quality based on clarity and field definition. Invest Ophthal Vis Sci. 2006;47(3):1120–1125.
2. Lalonde M, Gagnony L, Boucher MC. Automatic visual quality assessment in optical fundus images. Proc Vis Interface. 2001; p. 259–264.
3. Niemeijer M, Abràmoff MD, van Ginneken B. Image structure clustering for image quality verification of color retina images in diabetic retinopathy screening. Med Image Anal. 2006;10(6):888–898.
4. Haralick RM, Shanmugam K, Dinstein I. Textural features for image classification. IEEE Trans Syst Man Cybern. 1973;3(6):610–621.

Fuzzy Multiscale Region Growing for Segmentation of MR Images of the Human Brain

Karin Engel[1], Frederik Maucksch[1], Anja Perlich[1], Matthias Wolff[1], Klaus Toennies[1], André Brechmann[2]

[1]Otto von Guericke University, Magdeburg, Germany
[2]Leibniz Institute for Neurobiology, Magdeburg, Germany
engel@isg.cs.uni-magdeburg.de

Abstract. We propose an automatic region growing technique for the segmentation of the cerebral cortex and white matter in MRI data. Our method exploits general anatomical knowledge and uses an iterative multi resolution scheme for the estimation of intensity distributions to compensate for artifacts within the data. We present a comparison to segmentation results created by the neuroimaging software Brainvoyager QX and show advantages of our approach based on a qualitative and quantitative evaluation.

1 Introduction

A precise segmentation of the cortical grey and white matter in anatomical MR images is necessary for a large number of medical applications, including morphometry, visualisation and the analysis of the functional organisation of the human brain as assessed by anatomical and functional MRI. An automatic segmentation of the cortex is difficult because the inter–subject variability of the human brain anatomy restricts the use of anatomical knowledge. Furthermore, image artifacts, such as noise, partial volume effects and inhomogeneities of the scans, complicate the separation between grey and white matter regions and also the identification of the boundaries of the cortex.

Several methods have been applied in recent years to estimate grey and white matter regions on MRI. The most popular methods separate intensity histograms which are assumed to be composed of distributions for the different tissue types. The data is then classified directly[1], or the parameters of the distributions determine the intensity range for region growing approaches [2]. Other methods include computationally expensive active contours and surfaces [3, 4, 5]. Here, the segmentation of thin gyral folds poses a problem due to partial volume effects and numerical issues (e.g., related with the curvature–based energy terms). In the presence of magnetic field inhomogeneities traditional region growing as well as active contours may underestimate, e.g. the upper part of the frontal lobe[6].

Our algorithm resolves the complex task utilising general anatomical knowledge. It combines an iterative region growing with fuzzy labels and estimation of the intensity distributions of the grey and white matter using a Gaussian pyramid of the data. This multi resolution strategy allows to compensate for artifacts within the data and provides automatic, accurate and fast segmentations of the grey and white matter regions.

2 Fuzzy multiscale region growing

Our algorithm for separation of the cortical grey and white matter is based on a region growing, which uses histogram analysis for estimating the probability density functions (PDF) for the intensity of these different brain tissue types. The estimates are represented by Gaussian distributions P_ρ and P_ω, with $\mu_\omega > \mu_\rho$, and dynamically updated during a fuzzy region growing. The algorithm uses multiple scales of resolution of the data until the estimates for the inner and outer cortical surface (i.e. the grey–white matter boundary and pial surface) converge. The result of our algorithm is a segmentation in 3D where each voxel x of the 3D MRI data set is assigned one of three labels. These labels are l_ω for white matter, l_ρ for grey matter and l_b for background.

For segmentation we assume that the data sets are AC/PC–rotated such that pons and corpus callosum can be located in a set of sagittal slices. We further assume that the white matter is a single connected component, and is surrounded by the cortical grey matter which has an average thickness of $2.5 \pm 0.7mm$ [7]. For estimating the cortical grey matter based on the white matter, the cerebellum which is connected to the cerebrum via the brainstem, has to be removed.

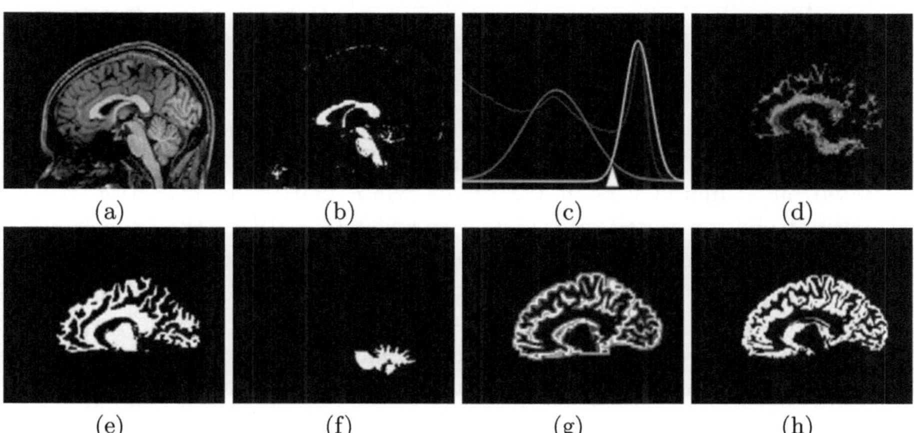

Fig. 1. Overview of the Fuzzy Multiscale Region Growing algorithm. (a) sagittal MR slice containing the interhemispheric fissure, (b) binarised version of (a), (c) histogram with estimated PDF P_ρ and P_ω, and threshold θ (arrow), (d) probability mask $\mathbf{P}_\omega$, (e) white matter segment W, (f) stripped cerebellum and brain stem, (g) probability mask $\mathbf{P}_\rho$ in terms of a normalised distance transform of W, (h) grey matter segment G.

2.1 Segmentation of the white matter

We obtain the desired seed points for the region growing within the white matter by selecting pixels that belong to the corpus callosum and pons (fig. 1(a)). Therefore, the sagittal slice that is most likely to contain the interhemispheric fissure is binarised using a threshold θ for separating grey and white matter (fig. 1(b)). Here, we use the grey value which represents the intersection of the estimated PDF, P_ρ and P_ω (fig. 1(c)). Seed points are obtained randomly by selecting points that survive a morphological erosion of the binarised volume.

Next, we compute a Gaussian pyramid $\{L(t), t = 0, ..., N\}$ of the data. A region growing is performed starting at lowest scale of resolution, $t = N$. The resulting segmentation is then propagated to the next scale in terms of a probability mask $\mathbf{P}_\omega(t)$, which determines for each voxel the probability of being included into the white matter region (fig. 1(d)). (Note that $\mathbf{P}_\omega(N) = 0$.) Therefore, the parameters μ and σ of the PDF, P_ω, are estimated by a histogram analysis at the current scale of resolution. We let

$$\hat{\mu} = \frac{1}{k} \sum_{i=1}^{k \leq K} h_i g_i(x), \hat{\sigma} = \frac{1}{K-1} \sum_{i=1}^{k \leq K} h_i (g_i(x) - \bar{g})^2, \tag{1}$$

given that grey value g_i occurs with frequency h_i. The $K = |\{x \in L(t) = l_\omega\}|$ samples are obtained by estimating an interval around the white matter PDF peak in the histogram. Here, we introduce a scaling factor $s \in \mathbb{R}$, such that $\hat{P_\omega} = sP_\omega$, and high values for s lead to less fuzzy segmentations of the white matter region. The result of this step is a binary mask, $W(x) = 1 \leftrightarrow x = l_\omega$ (fig. 1(e)).

2.2 Segmentation of the cortical grey matter

First, we use the AC/PC points to introduce a plug for separating the brainstem (truncus cerebri) and cerebellum from cerebrum using region growing (fig. 1(f)).

Based on a dilated version W_d of the white matter segmentation W, we calculate an approximated grey matter segment $G = W_d - W$, from which a random set of seed points is obtained for segmentation of the cortical grey matter. Here, we include a simplified model of the cortex thickness reported in [7] into the algorithm and use a normalised distance transform w.r.t. the grey–white matter boundary to initialise the probability mask $\mathbf{P}_\rho$ (fig. 1(g)). (Initially, the outer cortical surface is allowed to deviate by $4mm$ from the grey–white matter boundary.) Again, the parameters μ and σ of the PDF P_ρ are estimated by a histogram analysis based on samples from G, i.e. $K = |\{x \in L(t) = l_\rho\}|$ in equation 1. A fuzzy region growing based on these parameters results in the final grey matter segment, $G(x) = 1 \leftrightarrow x = l_\rho$ (fig. 1(h)).

3 Results

We evaluated the above algorithm using 20 MR data sets with (256^3) $1mm$ iso–voxels acquired on a 3 Tesla scanner. The quality of the data varied w.r.t.

signal–to–noise ratio and intensity inhomogeneities. For of a subset of 10 data sets, results of our algorithm have been compared with segmentations created by Brainvoyager QX (BVQX), a commercial software for the analysis of MRI (`http://brainvoyager.com`). These segmentations have been created with interaction by an experienced user and are more exact than an automated segmentation using BVQX. Segmentation includes rotation of the data into the AC/PC–plane, inhomogeneity correction, isolation of the cerebrum by applying standard masks, spatial smoothing, region growing (using a user–specified threshold θ) and morphological operations[2]. Note that our algorithm was also applied to the AC/PC–rotated data to allow for a comparison of both methods.

Examples of segmentation results using both algorithms are given in figure 2. A visual inspection by neurobiologists suggests that the grey–white matter boundary found by our algorithm is usually more exact, especially in regions of low contrast, e.g. the lower temporal lobe (figs. 2(g), 2(h)) and occipital lobe. Overall, the BVQX segmentations underestimate the white matter and miss white matter of gyri which can be easily identified (figs. 2(e)-2(h)). Since the outer cortical surface given by the commercial software is simply an estimate based on a the grey–white matter boundary and average cortex thickness of $3mm$, the results are usually inexact. Again, a visual inspection proved the correctness of our results.

For a quantitative analysis we used a set of manually labelled landmarks in visual and auditory regions as ground truth. These anatomical landmarks

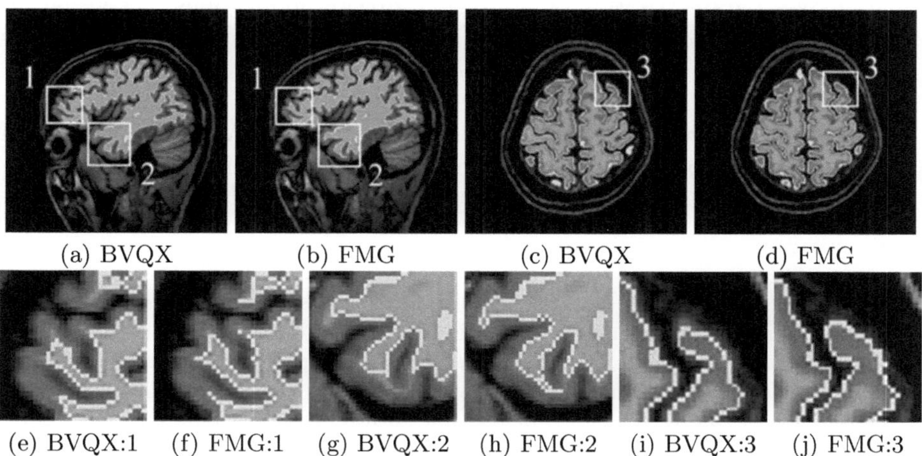

(a) BVQX (b) FMG (c) BVQX (d) FMG

(e) BVQX:1 (f) FMG:1 (g) BVQX:2 (h) FMG:2 (i) BVQX:3 (j) FMG:3

Fig. 2. Comparison of segmentation results using BVQX and our proposed algorithm (FMG). Note the underestimation of the white matter in the BVQX results. Differences in the resulting inner cortical surface (a-b) are visible in the enlarged areas within the frontal (1) and lower temporal lobe (2) in (e-h). While our algorithm actually segments the cortical grey matter, BVQX computes an estimate by constant dilation of the white matter segmentation. The resulting outer cortical surfaces (c-d) are usually less exact for the BVQX segmentations, as visible in the frontal lobe (3) in (i).

contribute to the inner cortical surface, λ_i (voxels within the grey matter that border white matter) and outer cortical surface, λ_o (background voxels that border grey matter). Our segmentations identified at average an absolute distance of $\delta = 0.37 \pm 0.74mm$ and a maximum distance of $d = 5.91mm$ to the ground truth λ_i (BVQX: $\delta = 1.3 \pm 1.18mm, d = 8.37mm$), and $\delta = 1.15 \pm 1mm$, $d = 5.83mm$ for the ground truth λ_o (BVQX: $\delta = 1.43 \pm 1.3mm, d = 7.07mm$).

Our algorithm requires no user interaction, and due to the multi resolution strategy the same set of parameters ($s = 1.0, N = 5$) could be used for all data sets without the need for further pre–processing, e.g. inhomogeneity correction. A visual inspection of segmentation results in 10 uncorrected MR data sets suggests that even in the presence of strong magnetic field inhomogeneities our algorithms gives satisfactory results. In contrast, using the BVQX software, small variations in the parameter values led to significant alterations in the segmentations, while segmentation failed in the uncorrected data sets. The computational time of our algorithm on a data set is about 68 seconds (3GHz Core2Duo, 4Gb RAM), which clearly outperforms the semi–automatic segmentation process with BVQX.

4 Discussion

We presented a region growing approach for the accurate and fast segmentation of cortical grey and white matter in MRI data. The proposed algorithm does not require any user interaction, and utilises an iterative multi resolution scheme which makes parametrisation of the region growing more robust. A visual inspection by neurobiologists and quantitative evaluation confirmed the accuracy in the estimated cortical surfaces.

Acknowledgement. The authors would like to thank Andreas Fügner and Jochem Rieger for providing the segmentation results used in this study.

References

1. Mangin J, et al. Robust brain segmentation using histogram scale-space analysis and mathematical morphology. Proc MICCAI. 1998; p. 1230–1241.
2. Kriegeskorte N, Goebel R. An efficient algorithm for topologically correct segmentation of the cortical sheet in anatomical MR volumes. Neuroimage. 2000;14:329–346.
3. Davatzikos C, Bryan N. Using a deformable surface model to obtain a shape representation of the cortex. IEEE Trans Med Imaging. 1996;15(6):785–795.
4. Dale A, et al. Cortical surface–based analysis 1. segmentation and surface reconstruction. Neuroimage. 1999;9:179–194.
5. Goldenberg R, et al. Cortex segmentation: A fast variational geometric approach. IEEE Trans Med Imaging. 2002;21(12):1544–1551.
6. Sokoll S, et al. Dynamic segmentation of the cerebral cortex in MR data using implicit active contours. Proc MIUA. 2008; p. 184–188.
7. Fischl B, Dale A. Measuring the thickness of the human cerebral cortex from magnetic resonance images. Proc Nat Acad Sci. 2000;97:11044–11049.

Modellbasierte Segmentierung von differenzierten Lymphknoten in CT-Daten

Lars Dornheim[1,2], Jana Dornheim[2]

[1] Dornheim Medical Images, Magdeburg
[2] Institut für Simulation und Graphik, Otto-von-Guericke-Universität Magdeburg
lars@dornheim-medical-images.de

Kurzfassung. Für die computerbasierte Diagnoseunterstützung bei Tumorerkrankungen ist Wissen über Lage, Ausdehnung und Art der Lymphknoten für die TNM-Klassifikation nötig. Für die computergestütze Planung nachfolgender Eingriffe wie der Hals-Lymphknoten-Ausräumung, ist dieses Wissen ebenfalls von Bedeutung. Deshalb ist ein effizientes und exaktes Segmentierungsverfahren für Lymphknoten in CT-Datensätzen erforderlich, das besonders auch mit pathologisch veränderten Lymphknoten zurechtkommt. Basierend auf früheren Arbeiten präsentieren wir in dieser Arbeit ein deutlich weiterentwickeltes, modellbasiertes Segmentierungsverfahren für Lymphknoten in CT-Datensätzen, mit dem nun besonders auch vergrößerte sowie nekrotische Lymphknoten adressiert werden. Unser Verfahren wurde an 21 Lymphknoten aus 5 CT-Datensätzen getestet, darunter mehrere vergrößerte und nekrotische. Die Ergebnisse liegen im Bereich der Inter-Personen-Varianz und verbessern die Ergebnisse früherer Arbeiten noch einmal spürbar.

1 Einleitung

Die Einschätzung einer Tumorerkrankung (TNM-Klassifikation) und nachfolgende Operationen (z. B. Neck Dissections) hängen zu einem bedeutenden Teil von der Situation der Lymphknoten (Größe, Befall, Infiltrationen von Nachbargewebe) ab. Daher ist es im Rahmen der Computerunterstützung von Tumordiagnose und -operationsplanung wichtig, diese Informationen zu erheben. Sollen im Computer exakte Analysen, Visualisierungen oder Vermessungen möglich sein, so müssen die Lymphknoten segmentiert werden (z. B. in CT-Daten), was einer der zeitaufwendigsten Schritte ist.

In [1] wird festgestellt, daß die Lymphknotensegmentierung nur mit erheblichem Modellwissen zuverlässig möglich ist. Eine Fast-Marching-Variante aus [2] benötigt deutliche Nutzereingriffe (Barrieren, etc.) für ein stabiles Verhalten und die Aktive Oberfläche aus [3] nutzt zwar deutlich komplexeres Modellwissen, jedoch neben Kanten- keine Grauwertinformationen. Zudem wird sie nicht auf realen Daten evaluiert (nur auf idealisierten Phantomen). Das erste relativ robuste Verfahren [4] nutzt ein zweischaliges Stabiles Feder-Masse-Modell (SMSM), das Form- und Grauwertwissen integriert und lediglich einen Startpunkt benötigt. Vergrößerte, nekrotische Lymphknoten oder solche mit unklaren Grenzen werden nicht addressiert, obwohl gerade sie für die Tumordiagnostik von besonderer Bedeutung sind. Relativ neu ist ein ähnliches Verfahren [5], das ein statistisches Formmodell einsetzt, das jedoch nur sehr wenig Form-Modi nutzt, um die Form auf Ellipsoide einzuschränken. Die Ergebnisse sind im Vergleich zu [4] nur knapp schlechter, jedoch ist deutlich mehr Benutzerinteraktion (ungefähres Nachzeichnen der Lymphknotenkontur) erforderlich und z. T. wird eine manuelle Nachkorrektur eingesetzt.

2 Material und Methoden

Wir stellen ein Segmentierungsverfahren für Lymphknoten in CT-Daten vor, das das Verfahren aus [4] hinsichtlich Genauigkeit und der Unterstützung für vergrößerte, nekrotische und stark deformierte Lymphknoten erweitert, da diese von besonderer anwendungsspezifischer Relevanz sind. Wir setzen dazu ein SMSM ([6]) ein, das zu Beginn aus zwei kugelförmigen Schalen (Abb. 1 (a)) besteht. Die äußere Schale ist mit Kantensensoren an den Knotenpunkten besetzt, die in den CT-Daten zu Kanten mit modelloberflächen-paralleler Ausrichtung streben. Die Knotenpunkte der inneren Schale tragen Intensitätssensoren, die den typischen Grauwertbereich von Lymphknotengewebe anstreben.

2.1 Plateau-Filterung

Im Gegensatz zu [4] filtern wir die CT-Datensätze (ihre Intensitäten) mittels Plateau-Transformationen, bevor die Sensoren des Modells darauf zugreifen. Für die Intensitätssensoren wird eine Transformationsvariante genutzt, die den Lymphknoten-Hounsfield-Bereich (bei unseren Daten 1050 bis 1100) auf 1050 nivelliert, den Wertebereich darunter nicht ändert und den Wertebereich darüber an der Intervallmitte nach unten spiegelt (Abb. 1 (b)). Auf diese Weise ist garantiert, das alle Gradienten in Richtung des Lymphknotengrauwertbereichs zeigen und innerhalb dieses Bereiches keine Gradienten existieren. Dadurch streben die gradientenbasierten Intensitätssensoren immer in die Lymphknoten, erzeugen aber innerhalb der Lymphknoten keine störenden, eventuell deformierenden Kräfte. Gerade bei nekrotischen Lymphknoten (zu sehen in Abb. 2 und 3) ist

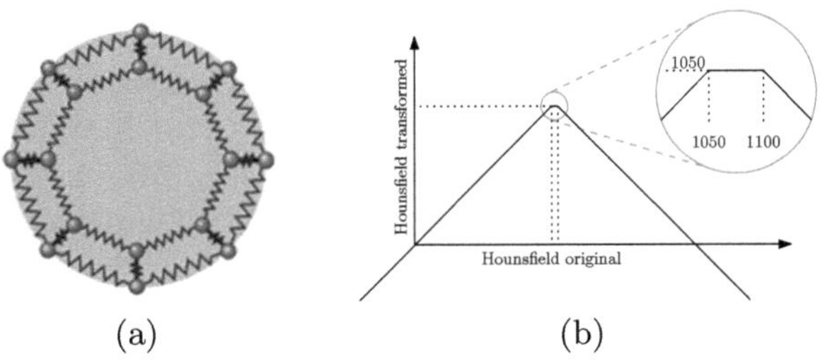

Abb. 1. (a): Schema des doppelschaligen Lymphknoten-Modells (SMSM). (b): schematischer Funktionsverlauf einer Plateau-Filterfunktion.

Abb. 2. (a): plateau-transformierter Datensatz. (b): Modellanpassung bei binär gefiltertem Grauwertbereich für die Intensitätssensoren. (c), (d): Modellanpassung in (c) ohne und in (d) mit Plateau-Filterung für die Kantensensoren.

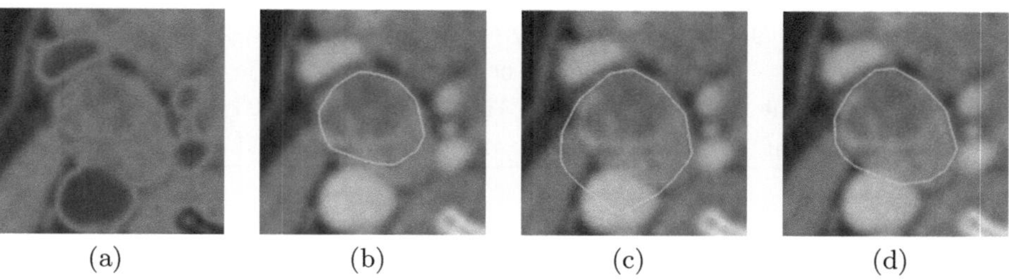

dieses Verhalten wichtig, da ihr Inneres starke Grauwertschankungen aufweist, die das Modell nicht ablenken dürfen.

Die Kantensensoren setzen statt auf dem Originaldatensatz auch auf einem speziellen plateau-gefilterten Datensatz auf, dessen Plateau zu einer Spitze am oberen Ende des Lymphknotengrauwertbereichs (bei uns 1100) zusammengeschoben ist. Dadurch wird erreicht, daß alle Bildkanten im Grauwertbereich oberhalb 1100 ihre Richtung umkehren, aber ihre Stärke und Kontinuität nicht verändert wird. Nach dieser Plateau-Filterung ist der Lymphknotengrauwertbereich der hellste Bereich im Bild, so daß man davon ausgehen kann, daß alle Lymphknotenrandgradienten nach innen zeigen, auch wenn sie im orginalen Datensatz an ein helleres, kontrastiertes Gefäß angrenzen (Abb. 2 (a) im Vergleich zu (b)). Auf diese Weise können die Kantensensoren auf immer die gleiche oberflächenrelative Kantenrichtung eingestellt werden.

2.2 Multi-Modell-Segmentierung

Tumorrelevante Lymphknoten sind oft vergrößert, deformiert oder nekrotisch und bilden damit im Sinne der Bildanalyse verschiedene Klassen von Objekten unter den Gesichtspunkten Skalierung, Formvarianz und Textur. SMSMs sind prototypische Modelle und nachweislich gut dazu geeignet, eine Klasse von Objekten zu segmentieren. Statistische Modelle (ASMs, etc.) können theoretisch

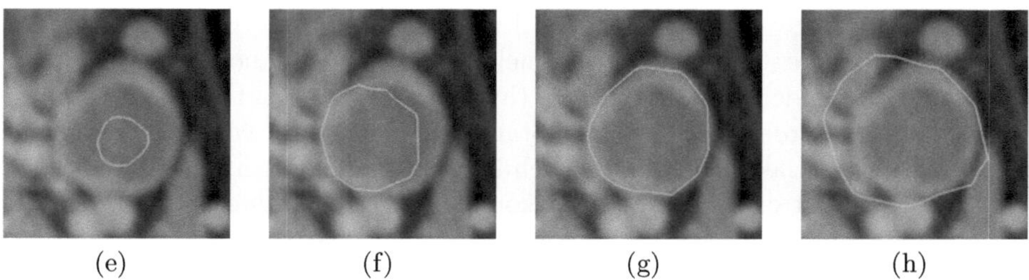

Abb. 3. Multi-Modell-Segmentierungsergebnisse mit Modellen verschiedener Skalierungsstufe: (a): Faktor 3, (b): Faktor 5, (c): Faktor 7, (d): Faktor 9.

Tabelle 1. Ergebnisse der Multi-Modell-Segmentierung mit Modellen verschiedener Skalierungsstufe auf einem großen, nekrotischen Lymphknoten.

Skalierungsfaktor	1	2	3	4	5	6	7	8	9	10
Anpassungsqualität	0.572	0.570	0.572	0.757	0.769	0.834	0.835	0.841	0.791	0.763
visuell akzeptabel	nein	nein	nein	nein	nein	ja	ja	ja	nein	nein
mittl. Ob.-dist. [mm]	8.85	8.80	8.35	3.65	3.53	1.19	1.23	1.03	1.98	1.97
Tanimoto-Koeffizient	0.012	0.012	0.046	0.428	0.445	0.733	0.731	0.760	0.620	0.591

verschiedene Objektklassen abbilden, praktisch gibt es jedoch Probleme wenn diese Klassen zu stark von einander abweichen. Für einzelne Klassen liefern speziell zugeschnittene Modelle bessere Ergebnisse als ein solch allgemeine Modelle.

Daher nutzen wir eine Reihe auf spezielle Lymphknotentypen zugeschnittene SMSMs in einer konkurrierenden Segmentierungsstrategie. Dabei werden diese Modelle, die in unserem Fall verschiedene Größen (Abb. 3) bzw. Grauwertbereiche von Lymphknoten modellieren, parallel an gleicher Position gestartet und das am besten angepaßte Modell wird im Nachhinein als Segmentierungsergebnis ausgewählt. Die Güte der Anpassung wird über eine Funktion ermittelt, die sowohl die Übereinstimmung des angepaßten Modells mit den Daten (über die Sensorwerte des Modells) als auch seine Verformung (über die vorhandenen innere Formkräfte des Modells) berücksichtigt und zu einem Wert zwischen 0 (nicht angepaßt) und 1 (sehr gut angepaßt) vereint [7].

3 Ergebnisse

Die Versuche wurden an 21 Lymphknoten in 5 CT-Datensätzen von Geräten drei verschiedener Hersteller mit Schichtabständen von 1 bis 3 mm und einer Auflösung von 0,28 bis 0,47 mm durchgeführt. Für das korrekte Funktionieren gradientenbasierter Modelle war ein isotropisches Resampling (auf die Schichtauflösung) nötig, so daß kleine, kubische Voxel vorlagen. Als Goldstandard diente eine von einem Radiologen bestätigte Expertensegmentierung.

Der Effekt der Multi-Modell-Segmentierung wurde mit Modellen verschiedener Größe (Grundmodell mit 3 mm Durchmesser und Skalierungsstufen dieses Modells) auf den vier vorhandenen vergrößerten Lymphknoten (Durchmesser > 10 mm) quantitativ evaluiert. Tabelle 1 zeigt exemplarisch die repräsentativen Ergebnisse für einen besonders großen nekrotischen Lymphknoten (Durchmesser > 20 mm). Besonders gute Ergebnisse (hier korrespondierend mit hoher Anpassungsqualität) werden hier für einem Startskalierungsfaktor von 6 bis 8 erreicht, bei denen das Initialmodell gerade noch in den Lymphknoten hineinpaßte.

Tabelle 2 zeigt die Ergebnisse der kompletten Evaluierung. Hier werden die Ergebnisse zweier menschlicher Experten mit dem Basisverfahren nach [4] und dem aktuell vorgestellten Verfahren verglichen. Im Gegensatz zu dem alten Verfahren ist das neue um ca. 23 % besser (bzgl. der mittleren Oberflächendistanz) und liegt komplett innerhalb des Varianzbereichs der menschlichen Anwender.

Tabelle 2. Segmentierungsergebnisse über alle 21 Lymphknoten im Vergleich von zwei menschlichen Experten, dem Verfahren nach [4] und dem vorgestellten Verfahren.

Verfahren	Anwender 1	Anwender 2	Basisverf. nach [4]	neues Verf.
mittl. Oberfl.-dist. [mm]	0.418	0.442	0.535	0.412
Hausdorff-Dist. [mm]	3.258	3.243	3.514	3.153

4 Diskussion

Das hier vorgestellte Verfahren ist erstmals in der Lage, tumorrelevante Lymphknoten verschiedener Klassen (vergrößert, nekrotisch) mit minimalen Interaktionsaufwand (ein Klick in die Lymphknotenmitte) in CT-Datensätzen zu segmentieren. Die Ergebnisse verbessern selbst gute, bisherige Verfahren und liegen im Bereich menschlicher Experten. Da die Laufzeiten des Verfahrens im Sekundenbereich liegen, ist es für reale Aufgaben im klinischen Umfeld geeignet. Komplizierte Deformationen oder starke Nekrosen werden u. U. aber nicht in jedem Fall befriedigend segmentiert werden können, da in diesen Fällen keine Modellinformation vorliegt, um fehlende Datensatzinformation auszugleichen.

Die eingeführten Plateau-Filterungen können auch für andere Segmentierungsaufgaben von Interesse sein, da hier allgemeine Probleme adressiert werden (objektinnere Grauwertbereiche und unnütze, ablenkende Kanteninformation). Gleiches gilt für das Prinzip der Multi-Modell-Segmentierung, dessen Effekt theoretisch motiviert und im Test klar bestätigt werden konnte.

Literaturverzeichnis

1. Rogowska J, et al. Evaluation of selected two-dimensional segmentation techniques for computed tomography quantification of lymph nodes. Invest Radiol. 1996;13:138–145.
2. Yan J, et al. Lymph node segmentation from CT images using fast marching method. Comput Med Imaging Graph. 2004;28:33–38.
3. Honea D, Snyder WE. Three-dimensional active surface approach to lymph node segmentation. Proc SPIE. 1999;3361:1003–1011.
4. Seim H, Dornheim J, Preim U. Ein 2-Fronten-Feder-Masse-Modell zur Segmentierung von Lymphknoten in CT-Daten des Halses. Porc BVM. 2006.
5. Maleike D, et al. Lymph node segmentation on CT images by a shape model guided deformable surface method. proc SPIE. 2008.
6. Dornheim L, et al. Stable dynamic 3D shape models. Proc IEEE ICIP. 2005.
7. Dornheim L. Quality of fit of stable mass-spring models. Pattern Recogn Image Anal. 2008;18(2):359–364.

Polyp Segmentation in NBI Colonoscopy

Sebastian Gross[1,2], Manuel Kennel[1], Thomas Stehle[1], Jonas Wulff[1], Jens Tischendorf[2], Christian Trautwein[2], Til Aach[1]

[1]Institute of Imaging & Computer Vision, RWTH Aachen University, Germany
[2] Medical Department III, RWTH Aachen University Hospital, Germany
sebastian.gross@lfb.rwth-aachen.de

Abstract. Endoscopic screening of the colon (colonoscopy) is performed to prevent cancer and to support therapy. During intervention colon polyps are located, inspected and, if need be, removed by the investigator. We propose a segmentation algorithm as a part of an automatic polyp classification system for colonoscopic Narrow-Band images. Our approach includes multi-scale filtering for noise reduction, suppression of small blood vessels, and enhancement of major edges. Results of the subsequent edge detection are compared to a set of elliptic templates and evaluated. We validated our algorithm on our polyp database with images acquired during routine colonoscopic examinations. The presented results show the reliable segmentation performance of our method and its robustness to image variations.

1 Introduction

Colorectal cancer is the second most common form of cancer in Germany for both women with 36,000 new incidents and men with 37,000 new incidents each year [1]. Endoscopic screening of the colon (colonoscopy) is aimed at locating and classifying polyps.

Colorectal polyps can be divided up into three classes: benign hyperplasias, malignant carcinomas, and adenomas which are benign polyps developing into cancer over a period of about 10 years. While hyperplasias should remain in the colon as polyp removal (polypectomy) may cause side-effects like severe bleeding or colon wall perforation, adenomas are removed by the medical practitioner during colonoscopy to prevent the development of cancer. Carcinomas have to be excised together with their neighbouring colon section during additional surgical interventions because of the high risk of spreading cancer. Tischendorf et al. applied Narrow-Band imaging (NBI) to highlight blood vessels structures which are an indicator for adenomatous tissue in a recent study [2].

A crucial step in an automatic colon polyp classification system is segmentation which will be discussed in this paper. To our best knowledge there are no publications on polyp segmentation in NBI colonoscopy available. However some approaches have been made to analyze white light endoscopic video images of the colon.

Bourbakis et al. detected abnormal regions including gastrointestinal bleeding [3]. Kang et al. used the Hough Transform on Canny Edge Detector results to locate colorectal polyps [4]. Hwang et al. used elliptical shape features on binary edge maps acquired by watershedding [5]. These two methods do not meet our requirements for the segmentation area in terms of ruling out colon wall segmentation.

The remainder of the paper is organized as follows. In Section 2 the proposed method for the segmentation of polyp surfaces in colonoscopic NBI image material is described. The validation setup is highlighted in Section 3 and results are summarized in Section 4. A closing discussion and future research are presented in Section 5.

2 Method

We developed a computer-aided system for the classification of polyps in images acquired by Narrow-Band Imaging [6]. During screening the investigator observes a polyp and activates NBI illumination. A screenshot picturing the polyp is taken and the proposed algorithm segments the polyp area. If the result is approved by the examiner the area is used as a region of interest for a classification algorithm based on NBI blood vessel features. The system provides an objective classification decision and reduces intra-investigator and inter-investigator variability. Segmenting polyps in colonoscopic NBI images is complicated because of variability and an individual angle of view. Figure 1 illustrates variations of polyp appearance. After examining various other options we decided to locate polyp surface via its outer boundary edges. We chose the Canny Edge Detector as it preserves long, connected edges. However NBI illumination causes an increased amount of edges in the edge maps because of the blood vessel enhancement. Thus to decrease noise and to eliminate minor edges in preparation for the segmentation all images were reduced in size to 147x126 pixels by subsampling. Resizing lowers processing time and memory requirements as well. We use Non-Linear Diffusion Filtering (NLDF) [7, 8] which is based on Fick's law of diffusion to reduce noise, to subdue smaller blood vessels, and to emphasize major edges. The NLDF is applied iteratively which increases its effect. In figure 2 the edge detection results with and without prior filtering are illustrated.

We store the results after 10, 15, and 20 NLDF iterations. Edges detected after 25 iterations are dilated and eroded N times to close gaps. In our experi-

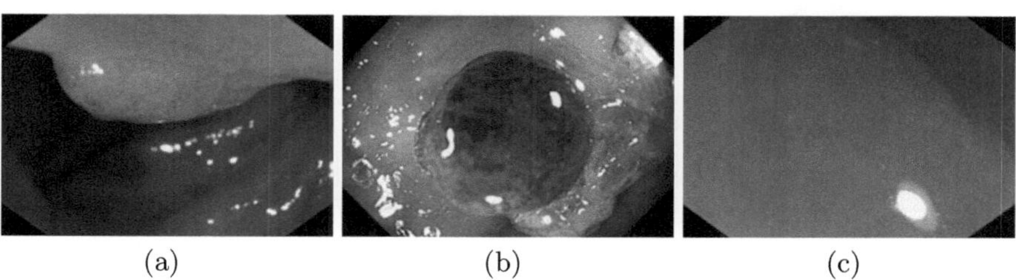

(a) (b) (c)

Fig. 1. Lateral view of a polyp (a), top view of a polyp with characteristic texture for potentially malignant polyp (b), no distinct texture (c).

Fig. 2. Original image (a), Canny edge detector without prior filtering (b), results with prior filtering (c).

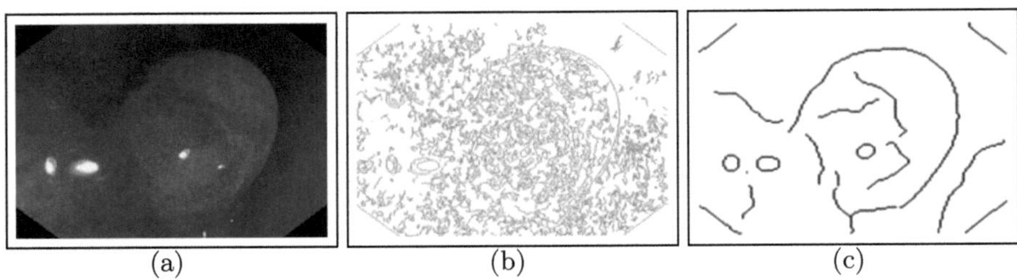

(a) (b) (c)

ments $N = 4$ was used. Subsequently the results are elongated by adjacent edge pixels from the 10 iterations edge map. If there are no edges found after 25 iterations, the results recorded after 20, 15, and 10 iterations are used successively instead.

We use a template matching approach to analyze the two longest resulting edges which we found to have a very high probability of being part of the polyp contour. The varying forms of the templates are generated by rotating a 3D ellipsoid while observing its projection onto a 2D plane. The projection result is subsequently scaled, rotated, shifted, and dilated to yield our template set.

The templates are evaluated by the rating function $r = \frac{n_{\text{over}}^3}{n_{\text{templ}}}$ where n_{over} is the number of overlapping pixels of template and edge image. n_{templ} is the number of pixels forming the template. r is the rating value by which the template is compared to other templates. The template with the highest score is combined with the potentially disjoint edge detection result. However the outcome is still a closed contour. The results are upsampled to match the original image size and the enclosed area as illustrated in figure 3 is used for classification. Our polyp classification algorithm requires a representative minimum area of 64×64 pixels to operate. However classification accuracy is obviously improved by using more input data. Thus it is desirable but not necessary to segment the entire polyp. On the other hand segmentation of colon wall (benign tissue) could cause misclassification of malignant polyps and needs to be ruled out.

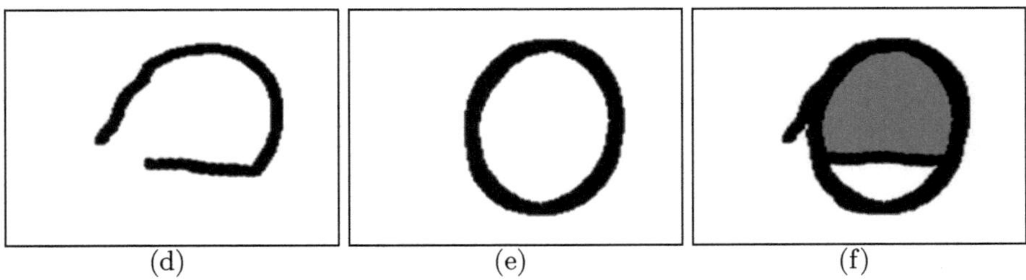

(d) (e) (f)

Fig. 3. Artificial results of the filtering and edge detection process (a), template with highest rating (b), combined outcome and the segmented polyp area (c).

Table 1. Localization results for a preselected test set with 56 genuine polyp images

Detected area	$\geq 90\%$	$50\% - 90\%$	$\leq 50\%$	Wall inclusioon	False detection
Number of polyps	18	25	7	6	-
Category rate	32.14 %	44.64 %	12.5 %	10.72 %	-
Cumulative rate			89.28 %		10.72 %

3 Validation

We formed two test sets for the polyp classification software [6] with images taken from our polyp database which is maintained and extended in cooperation with our medical partners. The database consists of more than 1500 images of varying sizes from 320 polyps observed during routine colonoscopies. The first test set consists of 56 images which were selected because the polyps were completely pictured, the image quality was high and we had reliable histological results as goldstandard. The second test set includes images from all polyps that had reliable corresponding histological data available. Some show only small, distant polyps or parts thereof. Some images are unsharp and noisy. This test set represents a variety of 209 images taken during routine examinations.

4 Results

The polyp classification results are arranged into five categories. Category 1 includes segmentations with more than 90 % of the polyp area segmented. Category 2 consists of polyps with more than 50 % but less than 90 % segmented polyp area. Less than 50 % of the polyp area (but still enough for classification) was segmented for polyps in category 3. The fourth category 4 includes results where minor parts of the segmented area belonged to the colon wall. Results with large area of segmented colon wall are in category 5. The results of the first experiment with 56 preselected polyps presented in table 1 indicate a reliable polyp area detection. In less than 11 % of the cases we would expect the medical practitioner to reject the results. Possible reactions are to repeat the process or to manually select a region of interest for classification. More than 89 % of the segmentation results can be used as input for our polyp classification algorithm.

Table 2 illustrates complementary results for the extended test set with all 209 polyps which still yield more than 80 % positive detection rate proving the robustness of the approach.

5 Discussion

We presented a novel template matching approach for the segmentation of polyps in NBI colonoscopy. The performed tests suggest robust segmentation results for subsequent classification. In the future we will establish a quantitative analysis

Table 2. Localization results for an extended test set with 209 genuine polyp images

Detected area	$\geq 90\%$	$50\% - 90\%$	$\leq 50\%$	Wall inclusion	False detection
Number of polyps	25	70	75	22	17
Category rate	11.96 %	33.49 %	35.89 %	10.53 %	8.13 %
Cumulative rate			81.34 %		18.66 %

method for our algorithm to complement our qualitative evaluation. In addition we will continue to improve our algorithm. Possible ideas for enhancement include the creation of better edge maps by considering results from different colour channels and the replacement of the template matching steps by particle filter based methods or ellipse fitting. Furthermore we intend to implement our algorithm in C++ code as it is currently written for Matlab. This will enable us to run it on the real time demonstrator platform "RealTimeFrame" [9].

References

1. Gesundheitsberichterstattung des Bundes. Krebs in Deutschland 2003-2004: Häufigkeiten und Trends. 8th ed. Robert Koch Institut, Gesellschaft der epidemiologischen Krebsregister in Deutschland e.V.; 2008.
2. Tischendorf JJW, Wasmuth HE, Koch A, et al. Value of magnifying chromoendoscopy and narrow band imaging (NBI) in classifying colorectal polyps: A prospective controlled study. Endoscopy. 2007;39(12):1092–6.
3. Bourbakis N. Detecting abnormal patterns in WCE images. Procs IEEE BIBE. 2005; p. 232–238.
4. Kang J, Doraiswami R. Real-time image processing system for endoscopic applications. In: Canadian Conference on Electrical and Computer Engineering (IEEE CCECE). vol. 3; 2003. p. 1469–1472.
5. Hwang S, Oh J, Tavanapong W, et al. Polyp detection in colonoscopy video using elliptical shape feature. Procs ICIP. 2007;2:II–465–II–468.
6. Stehle T, Gross S, Behrens A, et al. Classification of colon polyps in NBI endoscopy using vascularization features. Procs SPIE. 2009;To appear.
7. Perona P, Malik J. Scale-space and edge detection using anisotropic diffusion. IEEE Trans Pattern Anal Mach Intell. 1990;12(7):629–639.
8. Weickert J. Anisotropic Diffusion in Image Processing. Universität Kaiserslautern; 1996. Available from: http://www.mia.uni-saarland.de/weickert/Papers/diss.ps.gz.
9. Gross S, Stehle T, Behrens A, et al. RealTimeFrame: A real time image processing solution for medical environments. In: 41. DGBMT-Jahrestagung Biomedizinische Technik (BMT). Aachen; 2007.

Surface-Based Respiratory Motion Classification and Verification

Kerstin Müller[1], Christian Schaller[1], Jochen Penne[1], Joachim Hornegger[1]

[1]Chair of Pattern Recognition, Department of Computer Science, Friedrich-Alexander University Erlangen-Nuremberg, Martensstr. 3, 91058 Erlangen, Germany
christian.schaller@informatik.uni-erlangen.de

Abstract. To ensure precise tumor irradiation in radiotherapy a stable breathing pattern is mandatory as tumors are moving due to respiratory motion. Consequentially, irregularities of respiratory patterns have to be detected immediately. The causal motion of tissue also differs due to different physiological types of respiration, e.g., chest- or abdominal breathing. Currently used devices to measure respiratory motion do not incorporate complete surface deformations. Instead only small regions of interest are considered. Thereby, valuable information to detect different breathing patterns and types are lost. In this paper we present a system that uses a novel camera sensor called Time-of-Flight (ToF) for automatic classification and verification of breathing patterns. The proposed algorithm calculates multiple volume signals of different anatomical regions of the upper part of the patient's body. Therefore disjoint regions of interest are defined for both, the patient's abdomen and thorax. Using the calculated volume signals the type of respiration is determined in real-time by computing an energy coefficient. Changing breathing patterns can be visualized using a 2-D histogram, which is also used to classify and detect abnormal breathing phases. We evaluated the proposed method on five persons and obtained a reliable differentation of chest- and abdominal breathing in all test cases. Furthermore, we could show that the introduced 2-D histogram enables an accurate determination of changing breathing patterns.

1 Introduction

Improving cancer treatment in radiotherapy is an important topic. To minimize damnification of healthy tissue during treatment sessions techniques like gating or tumor tracking [1, 2] are applied. For so called external gating an adaptive surrogate respiratory signal is used to represent the patient's breathing over time as there is a correlation between the actual tumor movement and the patient's respiration [3].

Independent of the type of an external surrogate signal, there are always uncertainties in the correlation between external surrogates and internal target positions during respiratory cycles. This is mainly caused by the variation of this correlation due to changing breathing patterns and different types of respiration, e.g., chest- or abdominal breathing.

Khamene et al [4] present a method to establish the correlation between a surrogate signal and an internal target prior to the treatment session. Using this method it is possible to compute a mapping between a known reference breathing cycle and the current breathing of a patient. Once the patient changes his type of respiration in any way a new mapping has to be established. Breathing can change in various ways, e.g. chest vs. abdominal breathing or in speed or depth. Detecting all these changes in a respiratory signal requires a fast real-time surface-based method to measure respiratory motion.

Nowadays a common way to acquire a breathing signal is to use a pressure sensor integrated into a belt to generate a 1-D respiratory signal [5]. Another approach is to observe the patient's surface either with or without markers to obtain information about respiration [5, 6]. Unfortunatly most of these systems do not provide the required properties to perform analysis including the just mentioned issues. Recently, a system using an emerging technology called ToF was proposed to measure respiratory motion [7]. Such a system enables markerless real-time surface monitoring for respiratory motion gating. Furthermore, there are already several other applications within medical imaging where ToF sensors are suggested to improve medical procedures, like 3-D endoscopy or patient positioning [8, 9].

Using a ToF camera it is possible to acquire a 3-D point cloud containing more than 25k points in real-time with 50 Hz and above. ToF cameras emit light in the near infra-red range which is reflected by the surface of an object, e.g., a patient's body. The emitted signal is modulated by a cosine-shaped signal of frequency f. By calculating the phase shift ϕ of both the outgoing and incoming signal, the distance to the camera can be calculated in the following way, where f denotes the modulation frequency of the camera and c is the speed of light:

$$d = \frac{c}{2f} \cdot \frac{\phi}{2\pi} \quad (1)$$

Current available ToF cameras operate at a modulation frequency of about 20 MHz. Thus, the unambiguousness for observable distances of the camera systems is approx. 7.5 m, which is sufficient for respiratory motion tracking.

2 Materials and methods

In the following we will give a brief overview how a ToF sensor enables surface-based respiratory motion classification and verification of multidimensional respiratory signals. Please note, that in the following indices can be considered to be integer values. We denote $\mathbf{P}$ as the $K \times L$ 3-D points of interest acquired by a ToF camera.

$$\mathbf{P} = [\mathbf{p}_{i,j}], i \in \{0, 1, .., K-1\}, j \in \{0, 1, ..L-1\} \quad (2)$$

Furthermore we assume, the ToF camera is rigidly mounted above the patient table. To reduce the amount of data we segment the upper part of the patient's body using the method described in Schaller et al [9]. As a result for further computations only relevant 3-D points $\hat{\mathbf{P}} \subseteq \mathbf{P}$ ($\subseteq$ denotes a subset of points) have to be considered after the segmentation.

We want to compute a certain region of interest $\mathbf{I} \subseteq \hat{\mathbf{P}}$ and partition this region into n sub-regions $\mathbf{I} = \{\mathbf{S_1} \dot{\cup} \mathbf{S_2} \dot{\cup} .. \dot{\cup} \mathbf{S_n}\}$ and $\mathbf{S_q} \cap \mathbf{S_w} = \emptyset$, where $q \in \{0, 1, .., n-1\}, w \in \{0, 1, .., n-1\}$. Using these n regions of interest we can compute anatomical adaptive respiratory signals of the patient's chest and abdomen. We assume that the coarse orientation of the patient is known and apply a Karhunen-Loève-Transformation to all remaining 3-D points $\hat{\mathbf{P}}$. Resulting, the origin of the coordinate system is placed in the center of gravity of the point cloud $\hat{\mathbf{P}}$ and the axis are aligned with the axial, sagittal and coronal plane of the patient. By applying this transformation an accurate and stable computation of the volume signal can be assured.

To calculate accurate volume signals for each sub-region $\mathbf{S_k}$ ($k \in \{0, 1, .., n-1\}$) each point $\mathbf{p}_{i,j} \in \mathbf{S_k}$ has to be clipped against the 2-D border lines of $\mathbf{S_k}$. This algorithm is necessary to compute the exact volume of each sub-region as the borders of each region intersect the 3-D points arbitrary. We are using the Cohen-Sutherland clipping algorithm to perform this task [10]. By using this approach the partition is always consistent and independent from the patient's position. To calculate the volume of $\mathbf{S_k}$ we take a triangle of three neighboring points $\mathbf{p}_{i,j}$, $\mathbf{p}_{i,j+1}$, $\mathbf{p}_{i+1,j} \in \mathbf{S_k}$ and the distance between the segmentation plane [8] and the mean z-coordinate of these three points to calculate the partial volume. If one or more triangle points are not present in $\mathbf{S_k}$ points computed by the clipping algorithm are used. All particular triangle volumes are summed up to obtain the whole volume value for a specific subregion $\mathbf{S_k}$. By plotting the volume values for each subregion $\mathbf{S_k}$ over time n respiratory graphs can be generated.

We now can use the computed volume signals to distinguish between chest and abdominal breathing. Therefore the signal energy $\mathbf{E_k}$ of each subregion $\mathbf{S_k}$ is calculated over a certain timespan T, where $A_k(t)$ denotes the volume values of subregion $\mathbf{S_k}$.

$$E_k = \sum_{t=-T}^{0} |A_k(t)|^2 \tag{3}$$

After computing the energy for every subregion an energy coefficient α is calculated. Therefore the signal values of the subregions assigned to the chest area E_{chest} and the signal energy of the subregions assigned to the abdominal area $E_{abdominal}$ are summed up. The relation α of the energies is achieved by dividing the abdominal energy by the overall computed energy E_{all}. For the classification an appropriate border λ has to be set:

$$\text{Abdominal Respiration} : \alpha > \lambda \mid \text{Chest Respiration} : \alpha \leq \lambda \tag{4}$$

Furthermore, we analyse the minima and maxima of each volume signal. A 2-D histogram where the time between two minima, which equals the duration of one breathing cycle is plotted on one axis and the maximum amplitude of the

Table 1. α values (in percent) of classification with volume signals for chest and abdominal respiration of five test persons using data acquired by a SR-3000 ToF camera from MESA Imaging.

	1	2	3	4	5
α (chest)	65, 74	37, 62	39, 14	42, 59	64, 77
α (abdominal)	92, 85	91, 40	87, 11	89, 10	81, 30

same breathing cylce on the other axis is computed. Using this visualization, one can immediately detect a variation in the type of breathing of the patient, which is illustrated in more detail in the following.

3 Results

To evaluate the algorithm each part starting with the volume computation was gradually evaluated. Therefore a box with known geometry was placed in front of the camera and was observed from different positions with a distance of 80 cm. We could show, that the difference between the original size of the volume and the computed volume only differs marginal, preconditioned the segmentation prior to the calculation was performed accurately. The real volume of the box was 16368 cm^3, where the computed mean volume was 16501 cm^3 with a standard deviation of 35 cm^3.

Second, the reliability of the classification of chest or abdominal breathing was tested. We computed the signal energy over a time span of 8 sec. Five people were introduced to breath firstly with the thorax and thereafter with the abdomen (Tab. 1). By choosing $\lambda = 0.7$ a distinction between both breathing types in all cases can be achieved.

Finally, a test candidate was advised to perform four different types of breathing, including deep-slow, deep-fast, shallow-slow and shallow-fast breath-

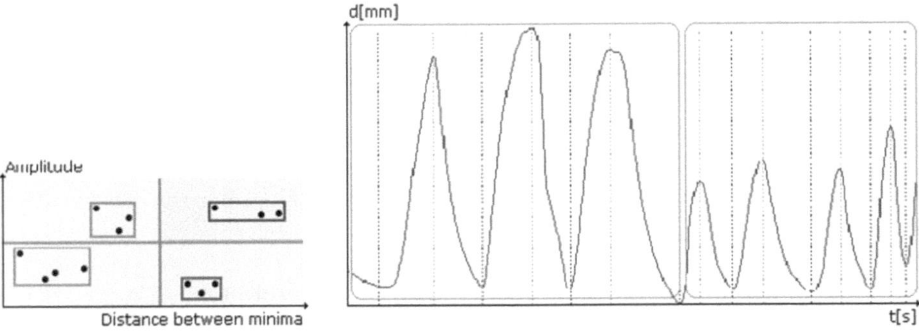

Fig. 1. Left: 2-D histogram showing the cluster formation. right: corresponding breathing cycles for the two left clusters.

ing. While observing the respiration of the test candidate, the above introduced 2-D histogram was successively computed. Figure 1 shows that it is possible to differentiate certain types of breathing. It can be observed, that for regular breathing a clustering in the histogram occurs.

4 Discussion

We introduced a new method to acquire and analyze a respiratory curve using a ToF Camera. The algorithm uses multiple volume signals in order to distinguish between chest and abdominal breathing. Furthermore, using the introduced 2-D histogram, a simple and intuitive way to classify changes in the respiration is introduced. Prospective, further algorithms will be developed to extract more information out of the introduced tools.

Acknowledgement. This work was supported by the International Max Planck Research School for Optics and Imaging (IMPRS-OI), Erlangen, Germany and the SAOT Erlangen, Germany.

References

1. Ue H, Haneishi H, Iwanaga H, et al. Nonlinear motion correction of respiratory-gated lung SPECT images. IEEE Trans Med Imaging. 2006;25(4):486–495.
2. Seppenwoolde Y, Berbeco RI, Nishioka S, et al. Accuracy of tumor motion compensation algorithm from a robotic respiratory tracking system: A simulation study. Med Phys. 2007;34(7):2774–2784.
3. Plathow C, Ley S, Fink C, et al. Analysis of intrathoracic tumor mobility during whole breathing cycle by dynamic MRI. Int J Radiat Oncol Biol Phys. 2004;59(4):952–959.
4. Khamene A, Schaller C, Hornegger J, et al. A novel image based verification method for respiratory motion management in radiation therapy. Proc IEEE ICCV. 2007; p. DVD Proceedings.
5. XA L, Stepaniak C, Gore E. Technical and dosimetric aspects of respiratory gating using a pressure-sensor motion monitoring system. Med Phys. 2006;33(1):145–54.
6. Tarte S, McCelland J, Hughes S, et al. A non-contact method for the acquisition of breathing signals that enable distinction between abdominal and thoracic breathing. Radiother Oncol. 2006;81(1):S209.
7. Schaller C, Penne J, Hornegger J. Time-of-flight sensor for respiratory motion gating. Med Phys. 2008;35(7):1861–6410.
8. Penne J, Höller K, Krüger S, et al. NOTES 3D: Endoscopes learn to see 3-D: Basic algorithms for a novel endoscope. Proc VISAPP. 2007; p. 134–139.
9. Schaller C, Adelt A, Penne J, et al. Time-of-flight sensor for patient positioning. Proc SPIE. 2009; p. online.
10. Foley J, van Dam A, Feiner S, et al. Computer Graphics Principles and Practice. Addison-Wesley Longman Publishing Co; 1996.

Computer-Assisted Navigation on the Arrested Heart During CABG Surgery

C. Gnahm[1], C. Hartung[1], R. Friedl[2], M. Hoffmann[3], K. Dietmayer[1]

[1]Institute of Measurement, Control and Microtechnology, University of Ulm
[2]Department of Cardiac Surgery, University Hospitals of Ulm and Lübeck
[3]Department of Diagnostic Radiology, University Hospital of Ulm
claudia.gnahm@uni-ulm.de

Abstract. Coronary artery bypass grafting (CABG) is the standard treatment for advanced coronary artery diseases (CAD). Optimal placement of the bypass graft on the diseased vessel is very important. To assist the surgeon in this matter, a computer assistance system has been developed facilitating navigation on the heart surface. After retrospective validation on patient data sets yielded good results, the system was successfully applied for in-vivo navigation on the front side of the heart during several CABG procedures. Postoperative evaluation confirmed that intraoperative navigation has been performed with adequate accuracy.

1 Introduction

The underlying pathology of CAD is intraluminal narrowing of the coronary arteries by wall plaque formations, severely limiting the blood flow to the myocardium. During CABG surgery, the blood flow is rerouted around a stenosis by a blood vessel graft. The position of the distal anastomosis on the diseased vessel is of great importance. Optimal placement of the anastomosis is a difficult task, especially as the target region may be covered with epicardial fat. To assist the heart surgeon in optimally placing the bypass graft, a computer assistance system facilitating navigation on the arrested heart during open heart CABG has been developed and tested.

2 Materials and methods

Nowadays, navigation systems are widely used in surgical disciplines such as neurosurgery and orthopaedic surgery [1, 2]. Concerning cardiac interventions, valuable research has been done in minimally invasive surgery [3]. In open heart surgery, the development of navigation systems is still at the beginning. The Cardio-Pointer project is the first approach to develop a surgical assistance system for open heart CABG with navigation at the beating [4] and the arrested heart. The system concept comprises preoperative planning of the optimal position for the anastomosis as well as intraoperative navigation to that position. Navigation is facilitated by registration of pre- and intraoperative data of the patient's heart. This is illustrated in fig.1 which also shows the intraoperative setup and the surgeon using the Cardio-Pointer (trackable pointing device).

2.1 Preoperative data set and preoperative planning

A cardiac MSCT (multi slice computed tomography) showing stenoses of the coronaries is recorded prior to surgery. For each diseased target vessel, the optimal distal anastomosis site is planned jointly by heart surgeon and diagnostic radiologist and marked in the MSCT data. Apart from forming the basis of the preoperative planning, the MSCT data are used as a basis for the registration and intraoperative visualisation. For the registration, 3D positions of coronary vessels and anatomical point landmarks potentially visible during surgery are extracted. For the visualisation, a volume rendered map of the coronaries is generated.

2.2 Intraoperative data set and registration

During surgery, the arrested heart is repositioned prior to grafting each bypass. As it is intended to represent the operating situs, intraoperative data have to be recorded after positioning the heart for subsequent bypass grafting. During the short period of data recording, registration and navigation, movement of heart or patient must be avoided. Intraoperative data are recorded with an infrared optical tracking system. Using the trackable Cardio-Pointer, the surgeon retraces visible parts of the vessels and points at anatomical point landmarks. In most patients, only a few point landmarks and vessel paths are actually visible on the heart surface due to epicardial fat. If the number of corresponding point landmarks is smaller than 3, additional landmarks can be generated in most cases. Then, all point landmarks are employed to coarsely match the data sets. The matching is then refined using the recorded vessel paths. Further improvement of the matching is achieved by a subsequent deformation correction. A more detailed description of the registration mechanism and the possibility of generating additional landmarks based on the vessel length was previously described in [5].

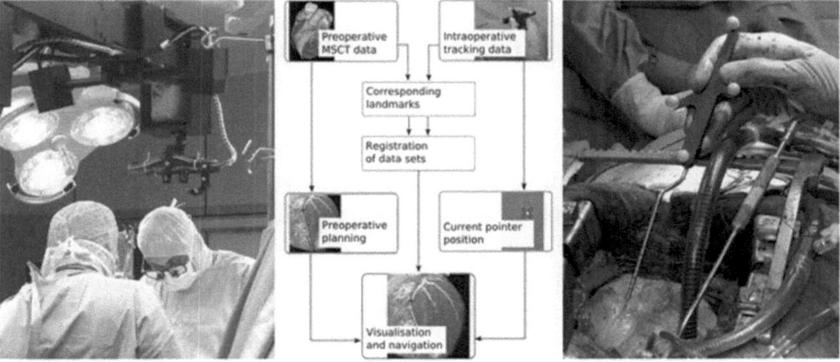

Fig. 1. From left: Intraoperative setup; Schematic view of the usage of pre- and intraoperative data for navigation; Cardio-Pointer on the heart surface.

Table 1. Overall errors and standard deviation for 16 vessels and 48 LMs

Point landmarks	
Mean RMS of point LMs (in mm)	2.4
RMS standard deviation of point LMs (in mm)	1.0
Vessel paths	
Mean RMS of vessel paths (in mm)	1.6
RMS standard deviation of vessel paths (in mm)	1.0

2.3 Image-guided navigation

Registration establishes a direct connection between the preoperative data including the planned anastomosis site and the intraoperative data representing the operating field. This allows for visualisation of the planned anastomosis site together with the current position of the pointer in the patient's coronary map. A video screen is used for visualisation. The displayed pointer position is continuously updated while the surgeon moves the pointer along the target vessel. Consequently, navigation to the preoperatively planned position is enabled.

3 Results

The registration mechanism developed for the arrested heart was validated in two phases: At first, intraoperative tracking data sets recorded during bypass grafting procedures have been registered retrospectively with preoperative CT data. The registration results obtained this way were very promising and justified subsequent in-vivo testing of the registration mechanism. Thus, the intraoperative modus operandi was altered to enable not only data recording but also immediate registration and subsequent navigation on the arrested heart.

3.1 Evaluation of retrospective registration

Retrospective registration was performed on 16 data sets from patients undergoing CABG surgery. Intraoperative data were recorded directly prior to bypass grafting after the heart was manually brought into a position exposing the target vessel in the centre of the operating field. Although considerable deformations of the heart were observed in each case, the registration mechanism for the arrested heart was able to match all data sets with sufficient accuracy, i.e. a similar accuracy is found for multiple measurements of the same anatomical landmark. 10 of the 16 data sets provided at least the minimally required number of 3 corresponding point landmarks, while 6 data sets didn't provide enough landmarks due to epicardial fat. For these data sets, 1 to 3 additional landmarks were generated on the basis of the unaltered vessel length. To evaluate the performance of the registration mechanism, both the RMS (root mean square) fiducial registration error of all corresponding landmark (LM) points and the average distance of corresponding vessel paths were calculated after registration (Tab. 1). Good results led to intraoperative live application of the system.

3.2 Intraoperative registration and navigation

Intraoperative navigation on target vessels on the front side of the heart has been performed during 7 bypass grafting procedures. Both, the complete registration mechanism and an alternative registration based on the vessel length [5] were used for live application. The resulting accuracies indicated no preference for either method. After successful registration, the surgeon performed navigation with the pointer on the arrested heart guided by the surgical assistance system. Target vessels on the front side of the heart were the LAD and its diagonal branches. In the patient's coronary map, the optimal position of the anastomosis as preoperatively planned by the heart surgeon and radiologist was displayed. After registration, the current position of the pointer was also displayed and continuously updated while the heart surgeon moved the pointer until its current position coincided with the planned anastomosis site (Fig. 2 (a)). This position was marked with a clip right beside the vessel and then, the bypass was grafted. Navigation on a target vessel including intraoperative data recording and registration takes about 3-4 minutes. During this short period of time, neither the heart nor the operating table must be moved. In two cases, successful registration was performed, but valid navigation was not possible due to unintendedly induced movement. This is attributed to the learning curve.To evaluate the navigation results, a postoperative MSCT of the patient was compared with the preoperative MSCT data. In both data sets, the same distinctive point on the target vessel path was used as reference point (Fig. 2b). The length of the vessel centreline from this reference point to the position of planned and grafted anastomosis respectively was determined. Comparison of both lengths shows how accurately the bypass was grafted to the preoperatively planned position. In case the position of the grafted anastomosis was not right beside the clip marking the navigation result, the clip position in the postoperative MSCT was evaluated. As a grafted anastomosis is several mm long, the centre of the anastomosis was

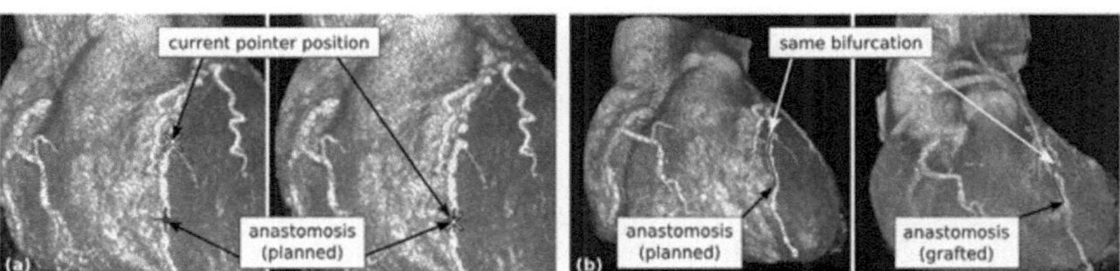

Fig. 2. (a) Intraoperative navigation: planned anastomosis site (dark +) and current pointer position (bright x) are displayed in the coronary map for one arbitrary moment during navigation and the end of navigation. (b) Evaluation of navigation result: preoperative and postoperative MSCTs with the distances from a bifurcation to the planned (left) and grafted (right) anastomosis respectively along the vessel centreline.

Table 2. Navigation results

Data No.	Target vessel	Distance from planned to grafted site (in mm)
1	LAD	0.0
2	LAD	3.1
3	LAD	4.6
4	LAD	2.2
5	LAD	2.6
6	LAD	3.4
7	D2	0.3

Table 3. Target vessels and errors

Target vessels	
Number of LAD bypass grafts	6
Number of bypass grafts on diagonal branches of the LAD	1
Navigation results	
Mean distance of planned and grafted anastomosis (in mm)	2.3
Standard deviation of the distances (in mm)	1.6

used for calculations. Measurement inaccuracies of up to ± 2 mm may occur. For the 7 target vessels, the distance between planned and grafted anastomosis was 2.3 ± 1.6 mm, confirming good accordance of planned positions and navigation results (Tab. 2 and 3). This navigation accuracy actually reaches the limiting measurement accuracy at the arrested heart which amounts to ± 2.2 mm.

3.3 Discussion

A surgical navigation system for computer assisted CABG on the arrested heart has been developed on patient data sets and its performance has been evaluated during several intraoperative live applications. The system successfully enabled intraoperative navigation on the surface of the heart during CABG surgery. The heart surgeon efficiently performed navigation with the Cardio-Pointer on the target vessels for bypass grafting. Postoperative evaluation shows that the intraoperative navigation correctly identified the planned anastomosis site in each case with sufficient accuracy. Navigation on all other target vessels for bypass grafting has been performed as well, the results currently being evaluated. The system developed within the Cardio-Pointer project is capable of matching pre- and intraoperative data sets from the patient's heart and provides precise intraoperative navigation assistance to a preoperatively planned position.

References

1. Peters TM. Image-guided surgery: From x-rays to virtual reality. Comput Meth Biomech Biomed Eng. 2000;4(1):27–57.
2. DiGioia AM, et al. Computer assisted navigation systems for hip and knee reconstructive surgery. In: DETEC. ASME 2001; 2001.
3. Coste-Manière E, et al. Optimal planning of robotically assisted heart surgery: First results on the transfer precision in the operating room. Int J Robot Res. 2004;23:539–548.
4. Hartung C, et al. Image guidance for coronary artery bypass grafting. Int J CARS. 2008;3(6):505–510.
5. Gnahm C, et al. A registration approach for cardiac MSCT and optical tracking data recorded at the ischaemic heart. Proc MIUA; 2008. p. 251–255.

Interpolation of Histological Slices by Means of Non-rigid Registration

Simone Gaffling[1,2], Florian Jäger[1,2], Volker Daum[1], Miyuki Tauchi[3], Elke Lütjen-Drecoll[3]

[1]Lehrstuhl für Mustererkennung
[2]SAOT Graduate School in Advanced Optical Technologies
[3]Institut für Anatomie, Lehrstuhl II
Friedrich-Alexander-Universität Erlangen-Nürnberg
simone.gaffling@informatik.uni-erlangen.de

Abstract. It is a common approach to create and inspect histological slices to investigate functional and morphological structures on a cellular level. For the easier analysis of the resulting data sets, the underlying 3-D structure has to be reconstructed and visualized. Due to mechanical stress imposed on the tissue during the slicing, some slices are damaged, leading to an unsatisfying reconstruction result. In this article we present a means to interpolate missing images. For this, a deformation field, calculated by a variational non-rigid registration method using adjacent slices as reference and template images, is partially applied to the template image. The approach is tested on a histological data set, and evaluated using visual inspection by experts. The resulting reconstruction is shown to be a significant improvement.

1 Introduction

3-D visualization of images is advantageously applied in a broad range of areas, especially for medical imaging modalities such as CT, MRI and Ultrasound. In functional morphology, however, the majority of images that is dealt with are still 2-D histological images. A problem is that in some cases it would be benefitial to be able to relate the displayed cellular features to the underlying 3-D structure of the tissue. As a consequence, several attempts are recently made to perform 3-D visualization of histological slices. For instance, the Neuroscanning Project of the Institute for Anatomy, University of Lübeck, aims to reconstruct human and animal brains based on series of high-resolution histological images. Their goal is to be able to remodel the neural distribution in the brain [1]. Furthermore, Weinhold et al. [2] reconstruct a series of histological slices of a rat liver, to be able to understand the capability of the liver to regenerate.

However, the data sets that have to be dealt with are afflicted with artifacts, stemming from the mechanical stress that was imposed on the tissue during the cutting of the slices and the following staining process, which includes exposure to heat, liquids and chemicals. As a result, the final digital images show artifacts like holes, blurred regions, and different inter-slice intensities. In particular, some slices are completely disrupted and cannot be used for reconstruction (Fig.1).

To our knowledge, no approach to deal with the problem of defect slices was proposed before. For a good 3-D reconstruction, though, complete data sets are a must, and depending on the specific case, a total loss of 5-30% of the images is possible. This is the reason why missing slices have to be interpolated. This work adresses this issue, by presenting a method to interpolate those images, and the performance of the proposed method is demonstrated on a histological data set.

2 Methods

The interpolation of images is performed by means of non-rigid registration. A deformation field between two neighboring slices is calculated, and the missing step(s) are created by partial application of the deformation field on one of the images. The non-rigid registration technique of choice is a variational approach, as proposed in [3].

2.1 Preprocessing

The digital images acquired from the histological slices show many artifacts that have to be taken into account, including intensity differences between slices, which makes an intensity normalization obligatory. Here, histogram matching provided by the Insight Toolkit (ITK) [4] is incorporated. After a gray-level conversion, a reference slice for the normalization is determined, and the associated image histogram is then used as reference to linearly match the histograms of the other slices, resulting in same intensities for same features. Afterwards, a rigid registration of all images is performed using an ITK multilevel rigid registration approach [4] to align the displayed tissue for the whole data set.

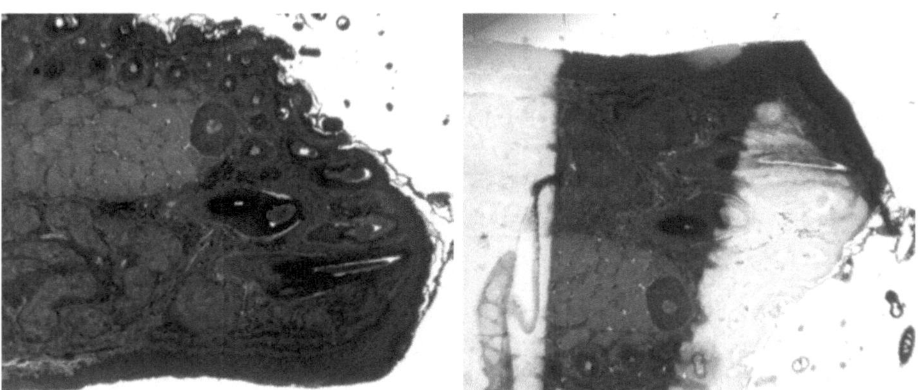

Fig. 1. Left: Intact histological slice. Right: Disrupted slice unsuitable for reconstruction.

2.2 Variational approach

After the preprocessing steps, the images adjacent to a missing slice are used as reference R and template image T, and a deformation field u transforming T to R is calculated, i.e. $R = T_u = T(x - u(x))$. The parameters of the previously performed rigid registration are used as initialization, and the following registration is performed on an overlapping region of both images, to prevent unrealistic deformations of the edges. The non-rigid registration method of choice is the variational formulation of the problem, introduced in [3]. The objective function to be minimized is given by

$$\mathcal{J}[u] := \mathcal{D}[R, T;\, u] + \alpha \mathcal{S}[u] \rightarrow min,$$

where $\mathcal{D}[R, T;\, u]$ is a distance metric used to evaluate the similarity between the reference image and the transformed template image. We choose mutual information (MI), measuring the amount of information one image contains about the other image. The second term $\mathcal{S}[u]$, called regularizer, is weighted by an adjustable parameter α, and keeps the deformation field smooth.

In general, an optimization problem of this kind is solved by calculating the Gâteaux-derivatives of the individual terms, and finding a root of the resulting equation. Hermosillo et al. [5] developed an expression for the gradient of the mutual information, with respect to a deformation field. For the estimation of the joint intensity probability that is used for the computation of the MI, Parzen windowing is applied, using a Gaussian kernel with $\sigma = 2.0$. As regularizer, the curvature regularizer as proposed in [3] is used. Also, in contrast to [3], an inexact Newton method is employed in the nonlinear optimization.

2.3 Interpolation

After performing the beforementioned steps, the missing slices are eventually interpolated. This avoids holes in the final reconstruction, cmp. Fig. 3. The deformation field u resulting from the non-rigid registration is divided into several parts, depending on the number of missing slices k in the respective gap. The final deformation field that has to be applied to the template image T to approximate the i-th intermediate slice S_i is then given by

$$u_i = \frac{i}{k+1} \cdot u,$$

and the interpolated slice itself is given by application on the template image, $S_i = T_{u_i}$.

2.4 Evaluation strategies

The approach was tested using a histological data set consisting of 42 images, with a size of 1300×1030 pixels. The images represent a tissue sample cut into 60 slices, where 18 were lost in the cutting process and unsuitable for further processing. An expert working prevalently with histological images was asked to inspect the results. The first task was to find out whether interpolated images can be identified if they are randomly mixed with original histological images. At the same time the quality of the images should be rated on a scale from 1 (very good) to 5 (very bad), deciding whether the images show the features of interest in a realistic way. Last, the smoothness of transition from reference to template image should be rated, where the image series consisted of the reference image, the template image, and the interpolated slices in between.

3 Results

Showing the results to an expert, 36.67% of the unaltered histological images and 50% of the interpolated images were correctly identified as original resp. interpolated images, and their overall quality was denoted to be good (2.1 resp. 2.0). For the smoothness of transition in an image series of five images (R, three interpolated, T), the interpolated series was graded with 2.0, where the original series was found to be very good (1.0). For two smaller image series consisting of three images, the interpolated series were found to be better (2.0 resp. 1.0) than the original series (3.0 resp. 2.0).

Fig. 2 compares our approach to a linear interpolation between two slices. On the left detail image showing the linear interpolation, the displayed structures are visible twice, leading to a blurred appearance. In contrast to that, the slice on the right hand side, interpolated by non-rigid registration, shows the structures only once, and in a more natural way.

Fig. 3 shows the reconstruction of a hair follicle contained in the histological data set. On the left hand, the original data set with missing images is shown. The parts where images are missing are clearly visible. On the right hand side, the same structure, reconstructed using interpolated images, is shown.

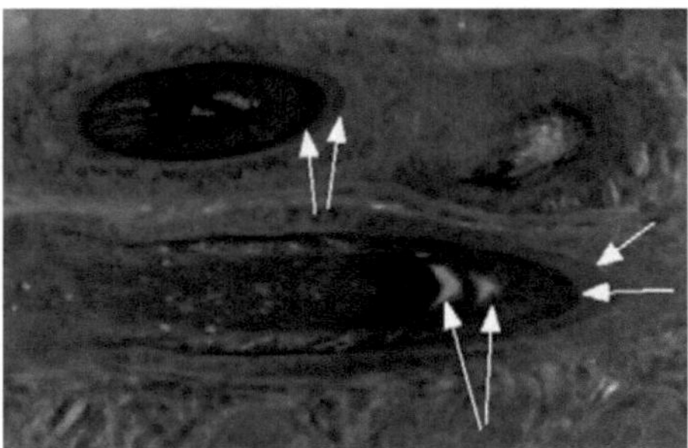
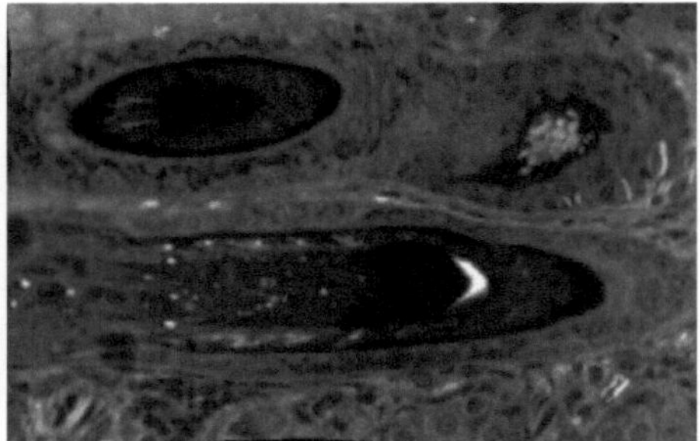

Fig. 2. Details of an interpolation. Left: Linear interpolation between R and T. Right: Our approach.

Fig. 3. Reconstructed hair follicle: original (left), interpolated (right

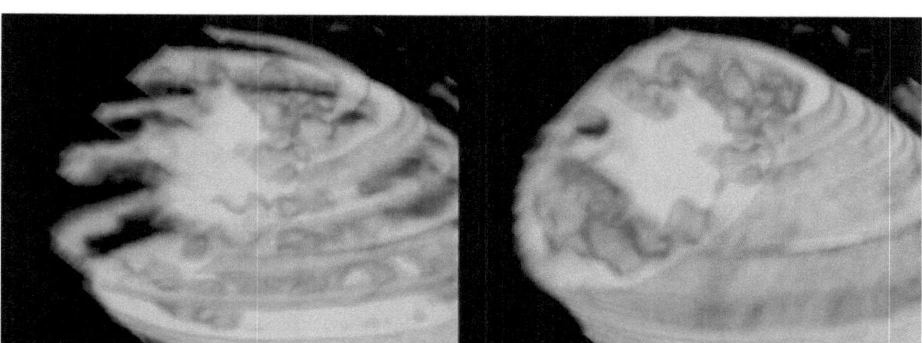

4 Discussion

It turned out that the interpolation of missing slices works well if the parameters of the non-rigid registration are chosen carefully. The overall quality of the interpolated images was found satisfying by experts, similar to the quality of the original images, and the reconstruction is significantly improved if missing slices were interpolated.

One drawback is the relatively large "gap" between the reference and first interpolated slice in the case of images with large differences, which requires further refinement of the approach. Still, the result prooves to be a more thorough and superior 3-D reconstruction than without the interpolated images.

For the future, an important task is to further evaluate the approach on other data sets. In addition, non-rigid registration of all slices of the data sets should be incorporated, to correct deformations of the tissue introduced during the cutting of the histological slices.

References

1. Schmitt O, Modersitzki J, Heldmann S, et al. Image registration of sectioned brains. Int J Computer Vis. 2007;73:5–39.
2. Weinhold A, Wirtz S, Schenk A, et al. Vollautomatische Vorverarbeitung und rigide Registrierung zur Rekonstruktion von Bildern histologischer Stufenschnitte der Rattenleber. Procs BVM. 2007; p. 419–423.
3. Modersitzki J. Numerical Methods for Image Registration. Oxford University Press; 2003.
4. Ibanez L, Schroeder W, Ng L, et al. The ITK Software Guide. 2nd ed. Kitware, Inc; 2005.
5. Hermosillo G. Variational Methods for Multimodal Image Matching. University of Nice Sophia Antipolis; 2002.

GPU-basierte Smart Visibility Techniken für die Planung von Tumor-Operationen

Christian Tietjen, Christoph Kubisch, Stefan Hiller, Bernhard Preim

Institut für Simulation und Graphik, Otto-von-Guericke-Universität Magdeburg
tietjen@isg.cs.uni-magdeburg.de

Kurzfassung. Bei der Planung von Tumoroperationen ist die Einschätzung von Abständen und Infiltrationen zu vitalen Strukturen wichtig. Im Bereich der medizinischen Visualisierung wurden hierfür bereits zahlreiche Techniken entwickelt, die unter dem Begriff Smart Visibility zusammengefasst werden. Zu diesen zählen Ghost Views und Section Views. In diesem Beitrag wird eine GPU-basierte Realisierung dieser Techniken für polygonale Daten vorgestellt. Die Parametrisierung der Techniken erfolgt automatisch, um einen klinischen Einsatz ermöglichen zu können.

1 Einleitung

Um die Lage von Tumoren in ihrer Umgebung beurteilen zu können, müssen vor allem Abstände und Infiltrationen in gesundes Gewebe korrekt eingeschätzt werden. Die Darstellung der direkten Umgebung des Tumors ist dabei entscheidend. Optimalerweise müssten alle Strukturen völlig opak gezeichnet werden, um Form und räumliche Lagebeziehungen einschätzen zu können. Problematisch sind dabei die Verdeckungen, die in 3D-Visualisierungen zwangsweise auftreten. Die transparente Darstellung umgebender Strukturen ist oft nicht hilfreich, da je nach Transparenzgrad der Tumor oder die umliegende Struktur nicht ausreichend sichtbar ist. Daher wurden Visualisierungstechniken entwickelt, die die Sichtbarkeit garantieren, ohne auf Transparenz angewiesen zu sein. Diese Techniken werden unter dem Begriff Smart Visibility zusammengefasst [1]. Im folgenden Beitrag wird eine GPU-basierte Realisierung zweier Techniken aus diesem Bereich für polygonale Daten vorgestellt, mithilfe derer die Sichtbarkeit von verdeckten Strukturen sichergestellt werden kann. Außerdem wird eine automatische Parametrisierung dieser Verfahren vorgestellt, sodass diese Techniken ohne Mehraufwand für den Nutzer verwendet werden können.

Von Zhou et al. wurde vorgeschlagen, einen kugelförmigen Bereich frei in einem direkten Volumen-Rendering (DVR) zu bewegen, um einen beliebigen Bereich hervorzuheben [2]. Die Sichtbarkeit wird hierbei nicht sichergestellt. Bei dem so genannten Ghost View wird die Sichtbarkeit eines ausgewählten Tumors garantiert, in dem Strukturen ausgeblendet werden, die direkt vor dem Tumor liegen. Alternativ kann die Sichtbarkeit einer segmentierten Struktur in einem DVR auch mithilfe einer Maximum Importance Projection gewährleistet werden [3]. Dabei werden verdeckende Strukturen kegelförmig (konisch) weggeschnitten, um die Tiefe des Schnittes und die umliegenden Strukturen sichtbar zu machen. Dies wird im weiteren Verlauf der Arbeit als Section View bezeichnet.

Für polygonale Oberflächennetze wurden ebenfalls Smart Visibility-Techniken entwickelt [4, 5]. Das Problem bei der Generierung von Section Views in polygonalen Szenen ist die Tatsache, dass die Dreiecksnetze nur die Oberfläche einer Struktur repräsentieren. Wenn diese Strukturen nicht parallel zur Sichtrichtung aufgeschnitten werden, ist keine Geometrie im Inneren zu sehen – die Strukturen sind „leer". Die bisher untersuchten Systeme haben dieses Problem unter Verwendung von Constructive Solid Geometry (CSG) behoben [6]. Im vorliegenden Beitrag wird ein Verfahren vorgestellt, das für diesen speziellen Anwendungsfall optimiert wurde und so wesentlich bessere Laufzeiten aufweist und leichter zu implementieren ist.

2 Material und Methoden

Zunächst wird der Ghost View vorgestellt. Die Umsetzung der Technik auf der GPU ist dabei trivial, der Fokus in diesem Abschnitt liegt auf der automatischen Parametrisierung des Schnittvolumens. Die Berechnung des Schnittvolumens ist auch für den im zweiten Teil vorgestellten Section View von Bedeutung. Voraussetzung für die Verfahren ist eine Segmentierung aller relevanten Strukturen zur Extraktion der polygonalen Oberflächen.

2.1 Ghost View

Beim Ghost View wird die Sichtbarkeit eines Tumors gewährleistet, indem Strukturen ausgeblendet werden, die zwischen dem Tumor und dem Betrachter liegen. Dabei wird ein Zylinder als Schnittvolumen verwendet, dessen Achse immer zum Betrachter ausgerichtet ist. Um die Schnittkante hervorzuheben, wird sie mit einer farblichen Umrandung versehen. Zusätzlich hebt sich der Schnitt durch seine gleichmäßige Form hervor, da die dargestellten anatomischen Modelle in der Regel eine unregelmäßige und unebene Form besitzen. Die Silhouette der ausgeblendeten Strukturen kann weiterhin angezeigt werden, um die Begrenzung von geschnittenen Strukturen zu betonen.

Zunächst werden der Mittelpunkt und der Radius des Tumors berechnet, der freigestellt – also sichtbar gemacht – werden soll. Geometrie innerhalb des so entstandenen Kreises wird ausgeblendet. Die vertikale Position des Zylinders richtet sich nach der Tiefe des hervorzuhebenden Tumors, so dass dahinter liegende Strukturen sichtbar bleiben.

Durch die Verwendung eines Fragment-Shaders können die betroffenen Fragmente einfach modifiziert werden. Bei einem Zylinder mit dem Mittelpunkt (x_M, y_M), Radius r_M und maximaler Tiefe z_M sowie einem Fragment mit der Position (x_F, y_F, z_F) gilt:

$$\sqrt{(x_M - x_F)^2 + (y_M - y_F)^2} - r_M \begin{cases} < 0 - \epsilon, \Rightarrow \text{Fragment ausblenden} \\ = 0 \pm \epsilon, \Rightarrow \text{farbliche Umrandung} \\ > 0 + \epsilon, \Rightarrow \text{Fragment normal behandeln} \end{cases}$$

Durch ϵ wird dabei die Breite der farblichen Umrandung angegeben. Zur Bestimmung des Zylinders müssen die Eckpunkte des Tumors zunächst auf den Bildschirm projiziert werden, um anschließend den Mittelpunkt der 2D-Punktmenge bestimmen zu können. Die Größe des kleinsten umschließenden Kreises wird auf der CPU bestimmt [7]. Der am weitesten hinten liegende projizierte Punkt wird dabei als z_M für die vertikale Platzierung des Zylinders verwendet.

Zur Beschleunigung der Berechnung wird die dreidimensionale konvexe Hülle des Tumors ermittelt, da nur diese Punkte zur weiteren Verarbeitung interessant sind [8]. Durch diese einmalige Berechnung kann die Zahl der zu projizierenden Punkte stark reduziert werden.

2.2 Section View

Beim Section View wird ein vorn abgerundeter Kegel als Schnittgeometrie verwendet, um zu entscheiden, welches Fragment ausgeblendet werden soll und welches nicht. Dadurch werden die Schnittflächen zwischen dem Kegel und den Strukturen sichtbar. Durch die gleichmäßige Form des Kegels hebt sich der Schnitt gut hervor, sodass die Manipulation der Szene deutlich wird. Die Abrundung verhindert, dass die Spitze des Kegels als Feature in den Daten missverstanden wird. Der Kegel wird dabei genauso positioniert wie der Zylinder des Ghost Views. Die abgerundete Spitze wird an z_M ausgerichtet. An der Stelle, an der er von der Halbkugel zum normalen Kegel übergeht, beträgt der Radius des Kegels r_M.

Der grobe Ablauf des Algorithmus ist wie folgt: Zunächst muss bestimmt werden, welche Strukturen von dem Kegel geschnitten werden. Bei dem Schnitt mit dem Kegel können drei Fälle auftreten:

1. die Struktur liegt komplett außerhalb des Kegels,
2. die Struktur liegt komplett innerhalb des Kegels oder
3. die Struktur wird vom Kegel geschnitten.

Genau genommen muss von allen geschnittenen Strukturen diejenige bestimmt werden, dessen Vorderseite am nächsten zur Schnittfläche liegt. Dieser Test wird pro Fragment durchgeführt. Die Fragmente, die den Test bestanden haben, werden anschließend so manipuliert, dass der Farbwert mit der Normalen des Schnittkegels berechnet wird. Die vorhandene Geometrie wird also genutzt, um einen Eindruck einer CSG-Berechnung zu simulieren.

Zunächst wird einmalig die Schnittgeometrie in eine Textur mit Größe des Ausgabebildes gerendert. Die RGB-Werte speichern hierbei die Richtung der Normalen der Schnittgeometrie, in unserem Fall des Kegels. Der α-Kanal speichert die Tiefe der Schnittgeometrie.

Die benötigten Fragmente werden über eine Kombination aus Stencil- und Depthtest ermittelt. Getestet werden ausschließlich die Fragmente, die innerhalb der Schnittgeometrie liegen. Der Stencilbuffer wird so parametrisiert, dass er beim Rendern einer Vorderseite inkrementiert, bzw. beim Rendern einer Rückseite dekrementiert wird. Wenn der Stencilbuffer einen positiven Wert aufweist, wird der Depthbuffer an dieser Stelle auf die Tiefe der Vorderseite gesetzt. An dieser Position wird die Struktur vom Kegel angeschnitten, da sie hier nicht durch eine Rückseite geschlossen wird. Dieser Test wird pro Struktur durchgeführt, da sonst nicht differenziert werden kann, ob eine Struktur komplett innerhalb des Kegels liegt, bzw. welche Struktur vom Kegel geschnitten wird.

Der Stencilbuffer wird nach dem Rendern jeder Struktur wieder gelöscht. Der Depthbuffer wird jedoch erhalten, da nur so bestimmt werden kann, welche Vorderseite am nächsten an der Schnittgeometrie liegt. Der Depthtest wird dazu im Gegensatz zum normalen Rendering invertiert (Lower Equal), d.h. es wird immer der z-Wert der weiter entfernten Struktur gespeichert.

Durch den Aufbau der Stencil- und Depthtest-Kombination wird der Depthbuffer nur an den Positionen verändert, an denen die Strukturen vom Kegel geschnitten werden. Die Beleuchtung der Fragmente an diesen Positionen muss manipuliert werden, um den Schnitt mit dem Kegel zu simulieren. An allen anderen Positionen wird die Szene in einem zweiten Rendering-Schritt normal gerendert. Das Rendering wird dabei auf Fragmente eingeschränkt, die außerhalb des Kegels liegen. Dadurch werden alle Strukturen verworfen, die komplett innerhalb des Schnittvolumens liegen.

3 Ergebnisse

Beide Verfahren wurden auf einer NVIDIA GeForce 9600 GT Grafikkarte getestet. Bei der Laufzeituntersuchung des Ghost Views konnten keine nennenswerten Unterschiede in der Frame-Rate im Gegensatz zum Rendering ohne Ghost View festgestellt werden, der Section View konnte mit $500 fps$ gerendert werden.

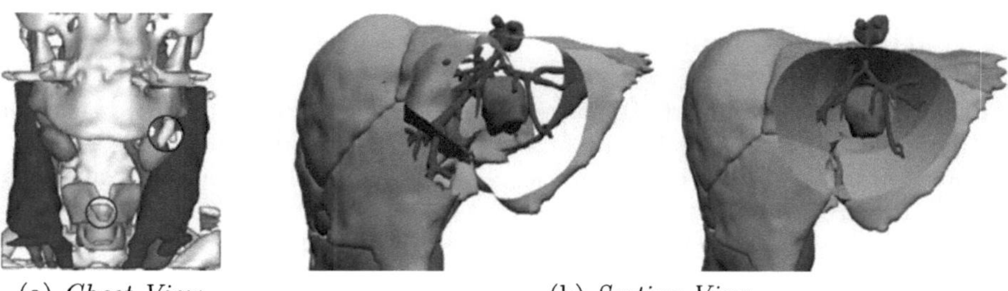

(a) *Ghost View* (b) *Section View*

Abb. 1. (a) Mithilfe des Ghost Views werden ein Tumor und ein vergrößerter Lymphknoten hervorgehoben, welche sonst verdeckt wären. (b) Darstellung einer Leber mit den portalvenösen Versorgungsgebieten sowie der Portalvene. Links sind die „leeren“ Strukturen nach dem Schnitt mit dem Kegel zu sehen. Rechts wird die CSG-Simulation angewendet. Die Szene beinhaltet ca. 70000 Dreiecke und wird inkl. Section View mit ca. $500 fps$ gerendert.

4 Diskussion

Die Einsatzmöglichkeiten dieser Techniken liegen vor allem in der Therapieplanung. Für ausgewählte Fragestellungen, z.B. operative Entfernung von Halstumoren, ist eine Evaluierung geplant, um zu untersuchen, ob die Zielgruppe die räumlichen Verhältnisse schneller und genauer einschätzen kann.

Der Ghost View eignet sich sehr gut zur Hervorhebung eines oder mehrerer Tumoren, da nur eine kleine Region um den Tumor verändert wird. Bei dem Ghost View ist leider nicht zu erkennen, wie weit hinten der Tumor liegt, da alle davor liegenden Strukturen entfernt werden. Der Abstand zu direkt angrenzenden Strukturen kann ebenfalls nicht eingeschätzt werden, da diese ebenfalls entfernt werden.

Um diesen Nachteil zu beheben, wurde die Technik zu einem Section View erweitert. Durch den Section View kann die Umgebung eines Tumors sehr gut exploriert werden. Voraussetzung für den beschriebenen Ansatz ist, dass die Oberfläche geschlossen ist, da sonst nicht bestimmt werden kann, ob sich die jeweilige Struktur mit dem Kegel schneidet. Zurzeit ist es nicht möglich, den Section View mit transparenten Oberflächen zu nutzen, da sonst für jede einzelne Struktur die Schnittinformation gespeichert werden muss. Eine Kombination mit einem Depth Peeling-Ansatz ist daher geplant [9]. Da der Stenciltest für jede Struktur einzeln durchgeführt werden muss, wären auch einzelne Schnittgeometrien pro Struktur möglich, um die verdeckende Geometrie zwiebelartig entfernen zu können.

Mit Ausnahme der Ermittelung der Zylinder- bzw. Kegelparameter werden alle auszuführenden Berechnungen direkt auf der Grafikkarte ausgeführt. Die Techniken sind relativ einfach zu implementieren und haben ein sehr gutes Laufzeitverhalten.

Literaturverzeichnis

1. Viola I, Gröller ME. Smart visibility in visualization. In: Proc. of EG Workshop on Computational Aesthetics in Graphics, Visualization and Imaging; 2005.
2. Zhou J, Hinz M, Tönnies KD. Hybrid focal region-based volume rendering of medical data. Proc BVM. 2002; p. 113–116.
3. Viola I, Kanitsar A, Gröller ME. Importance-driven volume rendering. Proc IEEE Vis. 2004; p. 139–145.
4. Diepstraten J, Weiskopf D, Ertl T. Interactive cutaway illustrations. Computer Graphics Forum. 2003;22(3):523–532.
5. Li W, Ritter L, Agrawala M, et al. Interactive cutaway illustrations of complex 3D models. Procs SIGGRAPH. 2007; p. 31.
6. Kirsch F, Döllner J. OpenCSG: A library for image-based CSG rendering. In: Proc. of the USENIX Annual Technical Conference. USENIX; 2005. p. 129–140.
7. Welzl E. Smallest enclosing disks (balls and ellipsoids). LNCS. 1991;555:359–370.
8. Preparata FP, Shamos MI. Computational Geometry: An Introduction. Springer; 1985.
9. Everitt C. Interactive Order-Independent Transparency. NVIDIA; 2001.

Feature Processing for Automatic Anatomical Landmark Detection Using Reservoir Networks

Benjamin Roeschies, Susanne Winter

Institut für Neuroinformatik, Ruhr-Universität Bochum, 44780 Bochum, Germany
Benjamin.Roeschies@neuroinformatik.rub.de

Abstract. We present an approach to the combination of an arbitrary number of image features to produce more sophisticated features for anatomical landmark detection. The combination was done using reservoir networks. The results were compared to Gabor wavelet features on single point detection in 2D slices of MR image data to show behavior and potential quality of the combined features.

1 Introduction

The automatic detection of anatomical landmarks in medical data is a challenging task [1, 2]. Many computer assisted procedures in modern medicine use landmarks e. g. for intraoperative registration in navigated surgery. They can also serve as starting points in image segmentation for automatic diagnosis. Recently, a landmark detection techniqe for CT data has been proposed [3], that is based on a bunch graph matching [4] with Gabor wavelet features [5], which are used frequently for recognition tasks in computer vision. This method, however, failed in our experiments on MR image data, which is probably because the Gabor features are not adequate in this case.

The graph matching algorithm performs a global search for several landmarks at once by combining them in a pre-defined topology. This initial global search leads to a starting position for each landmark, which should be already close to the correct position. Thus, features are needed that produce local similarity maxima at the correct target positions within a limited area. A global similarity maximum for the correct point is not a requirement, because a global search for possible regions in which certain points are located is solved by the consideration of topology during the bunch graph matching.

In our approach we started with the extraction of features from an input image. Afterwards, these features served as input for a two-dimensional recurrent neural network as a processing unit. This network was composed of 4 identical neuron layers. Each layer processed the input in a different direction. One point was processed at a time by feeding its scalar feature values – i.e. the elements of the feature tensors at that given point – into the network. This way of image processing using recurrent neural networks has been introduced recently [6]. In contrast to that approach, however, we use a different network type, introduced as echo state networks [7] or liquid state machines [8]. The basic idea of this network concept is to use a comparably large recurrent network and randomly initialize the interconnection weights, which remain untrained. This principle is referred to as reservoir computing.

For comparison of two points or landmarks, a similarity measure was then applied to the network's outputs corresponding to these points.

2 Materials and methods

2.1 Image data

For our experiments we used T2 weighted MRT sequences of 4 different patient vertebrae. For faster calculation slices were rescaled to a resolution of 128×128 pixels, where 1 pixel corresponds to 1 mm.

2.2 Feature extraction

We considered a two-dimensional image $\mathbf{I} \in \mathbb{R}^{N \times M}$, where N is the height and M the width of the image. In the first step, we extracted F feature tensors $\mathcal{F}_1 \ldots \mathcal{F}_F$ with $\mathcal{F}_f \in \mathbb{R}^{N \times M \times L_f}$, where L_f is the length of the f-th feature response. Before features were fed into the neural network, they were normalized to accomodate for different scales. In our experiments we extracted Gabor wavelet features on 5 scales with 8 orientations, and used the local gray level as a second type of feature.

2.3 Feature integration by a reservoir network

Each of the 4 network layers is a time-discrete network model with a state vector $\mathbf{x} \in \mathbb{R}^X$, where X is the number of neurons, which was set to 100 in our experiments. The state update equation at time step t is given by

$$\mathbf{x}(t+1) = \mathbf{W} \cdot g(\mathrm{diag}(\mathbf{a})\mathbf{x}(t) + \mathbf{b}) + \mathbf{W}_u \mathbf{u}(t)\,. \tag{1}$$

The matrix $\mathbf{W} \in \mathbb{R}^{X \times X}$ gathers the weights of the connections. The vector $\mathbf{u}(t)$ resembles the external input at time step t and $\mathbf{W}_u$ is the input weight matrix. The activation function g is applied component-wise to the vector $\mathbf{x}(t)$ to calculate the firing rates of the neurons and is given by

$$g(x) = \frac{1}{1 + \exp(-x)}\,. \tag{2}$$

The vectors $\mathbf{a}, \mathbf{b} \in \mathbb{R}^X$ allow for adjustment of a neuron's firing rate. Before the network was used for image interpretation, weights were initialized by drawing uniformly from [-0.02, 0.02] and $\mathbf{a}$ and $\mathbf{b}$ were optimized by intrinsic plasticity [9], which drives the firing rate distribution of the network towards an exponential distribution with fixed mean μ and maximizes the neurons' output entropy under the constraint of the fixed mean. Plasticity was performed by presenting a typical input image once and update **a** and **b** in every time step t according to

$$\Delta b_i(t) = \zeta \cdot \left(1 - \left(2 + \frac{1}{\mu}\right) g(x_i(t)) + \frac{1}{\mu} g(x_i(t))^2\right) , \tag{3}$$

$$\Delta a_i(t) = \zeta \cdot \left(\frac{1}{a} + x_i(t) - \left(2 + \frac{1}{\mu}\right) x_i(t) g(x_i(t)) + \frac{1}{\mu} x_i(t) g(x_i(t))^2\right) , \tag{4}$$

where μ is the target mean and ζ the learning rate. We use $\mu = 0.2$ and $\zeta = 0.001$ in our experiments.

Using update equation (1) we then collected X neuron states for each layer at each point of the image. Every time step t resembles one point of the image if they are sequentially fed into the network. These neuron states defined a combined feature tensor $\mathcal{X} \in \mathbb{R}^{N \times M \times 4X}$.

2.4 Similarity measure and experimental setup

To compare two points $P_1 = (x_1, y_1)$ and $P_2 = (x_2, y_2)$ we calculated their similarity S as the reciprocal of the squared error of the respective features:

$$S([\mathcal{X}]_{x_1 y_1}, [\mathcal{X}]_{x_2 y_2}) = \frac{1}{\sum_k \left([\mathcal{X}]_{x_1 y_1 k} - [\mathcal{X}]_{x_2 y_2 k}\right)^2} \tag{5}$$

The task in our experiments was to calculate similarities for 6 distinct landmarks of a labelled vertebra in a target image, by calculating the respective similarities for every point in the target image using either Gabor wavelet features only, or Gabor wavelet features and the local gray level combined by the neural network. Fig. 1 shows the points that were to be detected and the test image.

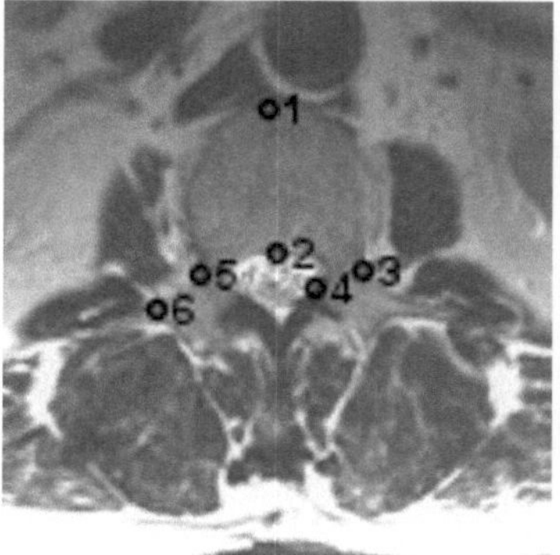

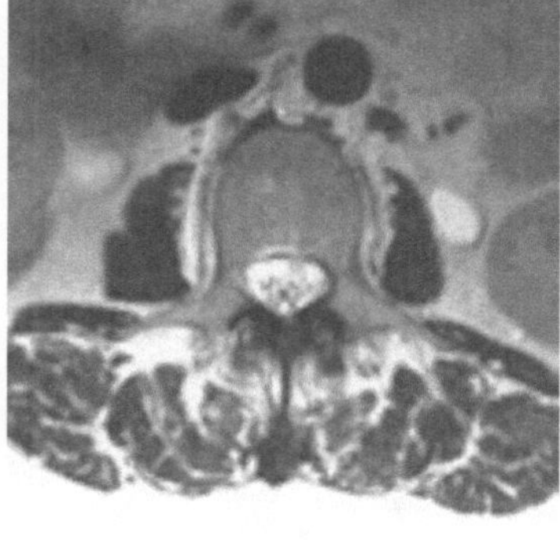

Fig. 1. The labelled image on the left hand side shows the points that were to be detected in the image on the right hand side.

3 Results

We display the results by overlaying similarity images and input images to show where high similarities are present (see Fig. 2). For better viewability we applied a threshold to the similarity images to only show the location of local similarity maxima. The threshold was selected in a way that 99% of the gray values in the similarity image were below the threshold. For both experiments local similarity maxima were at least close to the correct location for points 1, 2, 4, and 5. The Gabor wavelets did not produce a maximum near the correct locations for points 3 and 6, while the network processed features were able to detect those points.

4 Discussion

The results show that Gabor wavelet similarity pictures usually produce broad maxima, which correspond to the Gaussian nature of the Gabor wavelets, while the inclusion of gray level as a second feature and the processing by the recurrent

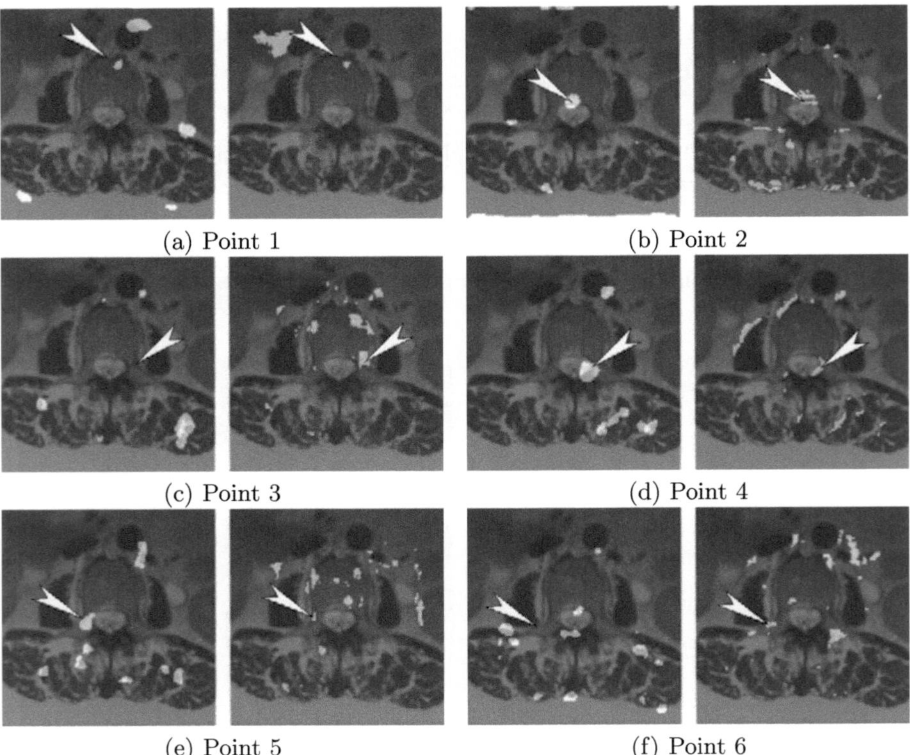

(a) Point 1 (b) Point 2 (c) Point 3 (d) Point 4 (e) Point 5 (f) Point 6

Fig. 2. Similarity images for the six points (marked by arrows) of the labelled image. Results for Gabor wavelets are on the left hand side, results for the neural network integration are on the right hand side.

network results in locally bounded maxima. Our experiments indicate that combination of several feature types using a neural network might enable a bunch graph matching algorithm to work on MR data as well as it does on CT data. The improvement over Gabor wavelets alone is based on the combination process by the reservoir, which basically does two things: First, it transforms the original features into random higher-dimensional, and potentially higher-order features, and second, it integrates context into the feature vector of a single point, i.e. features of neighboring points are considered as well. The size and influence of the considered context is implicit within the random weights of the network.

A problem with this approach, however, is the large amount of calculation time required by the neural network as complexity grows quadratically with network size X. This is bothersome, because much larger reservoirs, which are commonly used in reservoir computing, usually produce even better results.

Even though feature quality is hard to judge based on our limited experiments, the results are promising and motivate further research in this direction. In the next step we will expand our evaluation to more data sets as well as to different MR sequences. Performance might further be improved by using even more than two feature types. Additionally, supervised training of the reservoir might overcome the problems with the small network size.

References

1. Liu J, Gao W, Huang S, et al. A model-based semi-global segmentation approach for automatic 3-D point landmark localization in neuroimages. IEEE Trans MI. 2008;27(8):1034–1044.
2. Wörz S, Rohr K. Localitaion of anatomical point landmarks in 3D medical images by fitting 3D parametric intensity models. Med Image Anal. 2004;10(1):41–58.
3. Roeschies B, Winter S. Detection of vertebrae in CT slices by bunch graph matching. Proc Eur Congress Med Biomed Eng. 2008;22:2575–2578.
4. Wiskott L, Fellous JM, Kruger N, et al. Face recognition by elastic bunch graph matching. IEEE Trans PAMI. 1997;19(7):775–779.
5. Gabor D. Theory of communication. J IEE. 1946;93(26):429–457.
6. Graves A, Fernández S, Schmidhuber J. Multi-dimensional recurrent neural networks. CoRR. 2007;abs/0705.2011.
7. Jaeger H. The "echo state" approach to analysing and training recurrent neural networks. German National Research Center for Information Technology; 2001. 148.
8. Natschläger T, Maass W, Markram H. The liquid computer - A novel strategy for real-time computing on time series. Special Issue on Foundations of Information Processing of TELEMATIK. 2002;8(1):39–43.
9. Triesch J. Synergies between intrinsic and synaptic plasticity in individual model neurons. In: Saul LK, Weiss Y, Bottou L, editors. Advances in Neural Information Processing Systems 17. MIT Press; 2005. p. 1417–1424.

4D MRT Lungen-Volumetrie und funktionale Analyse mittels deformierbarer Formmodelle

Tobias Schwarz[1], Ralf Tetzlaff[2], Tobias Heimann[1], Monika Eichinger[2], Ivo Wolf[3], Hans-Peter Meinzer[1]

[1]Medizinische und Biologische Informatik, Deutsches Krebsforschungszentrum
[2]Abteilung Radiologie, Deutsches Krebsforschungszentrum
[3]Institut für Medizinische Informatik, Hochschule Mannheim
tobias.schwarz@dkfz-heidelberg.de

Kurzfassung. Segmentierung mit Hilfe von deformierbaren modellbasierten Ansätzen hat sich zu einer gängigen Praxis in der medizinischen Bildanalyse entwickelt, da sie eine schnelle und robust Methode zur semi- oder vollautomatischen Detektion von Strukturen darstellt, also z.B. Organen. In diesem Paper wird die Anwendung eines deformierbaren Formmodells zur funktionalen Analyse der Atmung aus MR-Bildern vorgestellt. Die Segmentierungsergebnisse stimmen sehr gut mit gleichzeitig aufgenommenen Spirometriedaten überein, bei einem mittleren Fehler des Gesamtvolumens von etwa 70ml. Zusätzlich erlaubt der Formmodell-Ansatz jedoch eine unabhängige Analyse beider Lungenflügel und ermöglicht damit eine Detektion von lokalen Bewegungseinschränkungen. Weiterhin zeigen wir, dass die Kalibrierung der Segmentierungsergebnisse auf das Respirationsvolumen weitestgehend durch Subtraktion eines konstanten Faktors möglich ist.

1 Einleitung

Eingeschränkte Atemmechanik ist eine wichtige Charakteristik der meisten Erkrankungen der Lunge. Viele Erkrankungen jedoch, sowohl solche, die vorwiegend das Parenchym als intestinale Fibrose betreffen, als auch chronische obstruktive Pulmonal-Erkrankungen (COPD), entwickeln sich inhomogen und sind ungleichmäßig verteilt. Die Spirometrie als Goldstandard für Lungenfunktionsanalyse ist jedoch ein von Natur eine globale Messmethode und misst den kombinierten Atemfluss beider Lungen. Für viele Untersuchungen, insbesondere in der Strahlentherapie und zum Tumor-Monitoring, wird deshalb 4D CT unterstützend hinzugenommen [1, 2]. Um Strahlenbelastung des Patienten zu vermeiden, wird für Standarduntersuchungen verstärkt dynamische Magnetresonanztomographie (dMRT) des Thorax verwendet. Auch hier können spirometrische Indizes und Volumenänderungen der Gesamtlunge sowie Lungenflügelspezifisch mit guter Korrelation extrahiert werden [3, 4, 5, 6]. Diese Ansätze erfordern allerdings alle ein hohes Maß an Benutzerinteraktion und Erfahrung. Wir stellen deshalb hier ein weitgehend automatisiertes Verfahren vor, das auf der semiautomatischen Segmentierung der MRT Daten beruht.

2 Material und Methoden

2.1 Deformierbare Formmodelle

Deformierbare Formmodelle, wie zuerst von Cootes et al. 1995 vorgeschlagen [7], bieten die Möglichkeit, medizinische Bilder nahezu vollautomatisch zu segmentieren. Das hier verwendete Formmodells [8] ist eine Anwendung basierend auf dem Medical Imaging Interaction Toolkit (MITK) [9]. Die einzig nötige Nutzerinteraktion ist eine grobe Platzierung des initialen Modells an einer geeigneten Startposition für die Segmentierung; der Zeitaufwand hierfür liegt unter 10 Sekunden. Modelle wurden unabhängig für beide Lungenflügel erstellt. Eine zeitaufgelöste Segmentierung wurde erreicht, indem das Ergebnis eines Zeitschritts als Startlösung für den nächsten weiterpropagiert wurde. Dadurch konnte eine den ganzen Atemzyklus umfassende Serie in weniger als 5 Minuten Rechenzeit segmentiert werden.

2.2 Lungen-MRT-Volumen

Die Trainingsdaten für das Lungenformmodell bestehen aus Datensätzen von 10 Patienten, die jeweils 20 Zeitschritte des kompletten Atemzyklus enthielten. Die Bilder wurden in einer FLASH3D Sequenz aufgenommen und haben eine räumliche Auflösung von 3.75 x 3.75 x 3.8 mm, eine zeitliche Auflösung von 1 Sekunde. Da Bilder aus allen Stadien des Respirationszyklus in das Modell eingeflossen sind, repräsentiert die erste Variationsmode größtenteils die Atembewegung.

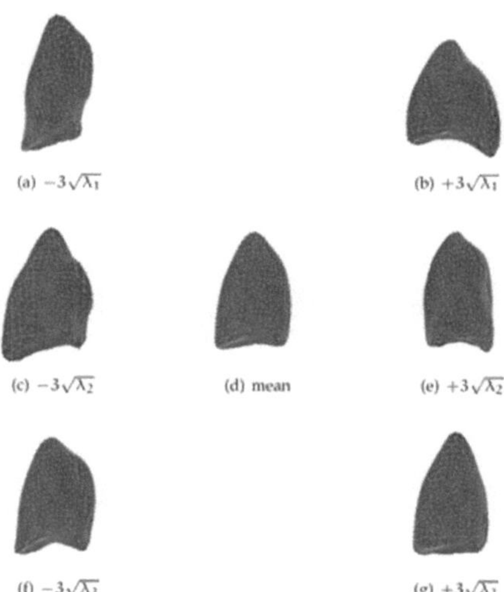

Abb. 1. Die drei stärksten Variationsmoden des Lungenformmodells. Für jede Mode ist die Form in einem Abstand von drei Standardabweichungen dargestellt [8].

Die Daten für die Evaluation bestanden aus TWIST4D Sequenzen von vier Probanden, die jeweils 101 Zeitschritte beinhalteten. Auflösung war hier 3.52 x 3.52 x 8mm räumlich, 0.5 Sekunden zeitlich.

2.3 Spirometrie

Die Spirometriedaten wurden zeitgleich während der Aufnahme der MRT Daten akquiriert. Hierfür wurde ein spezielles MRT kompatibles Spirometer verwendet [10].

2.4 Volumetrie

Das physikalische Lungenvolumen wurde für alle Zeitschritte aus den Segmentierungsergebnissen berechnet. Die Segmentierungsqualität und volumetrische Genauigkeit wurde gegen die gleichzeitig aufgenommene Spirometrie als Goldstandard evaluiert. Die Segmentierung allerdings umfasst jeweils einen kompletten Lungenflügel, also auch Blut und Gewebe und nicht nur das Luftvolumen. Wie erwarten deshalb, dass das berechnete Volumen auf das tatsächlichen Atemvolumen geeicht werden muss, im Idealfall jedoch nur ein konstanter Faktor zur Kalibrierung nötig ist, da das mit eingeschlossene Gewebe und Blut in erster Näherung konstant Volumina über den Atemzyklus behält.
Das totale segmentierte Volumen, also die Summe der Einzelvolumen der Lungenflügel, wurde gegen die Spirometriedaten normiert wie folgt:

$$x' = \frac{(x - \min)}{(\max - \min)} (\max_{\mathrm{norm}} - \min_{\mathrm{norm}}) + \min_{\mathrm{norm}} \tag{1}$$

Hierbei beziehen sich die Indizes norm auf das Zielintervall, min und max sind die jeweils kleinsten und größten Volumina in der Zeitserie. Man sieht hier, dass sich die Korrektheit der Annahme eines konstanten Volumenbias aus der Abweichung des linearen Normierungsterms von 1.0 ergibt.

3 Ergebnisse

Die Volumen-Zeit-Kurven der drei Probanden sind in den Abbildungen 2 und 3 dargestellt. Die Zeitschritte 56 und 57 mussten wegen eines Datenfehlers in den Originaldaten bei allen drei Auswertungen weggelassen werden, da eine Segmentierung hier unmöglich war. Die Mittelwerte der volumetrischen Differenzen zwischen den geeichten Segmentierungsergebnissen und der Spirometrie sind in Tabelle 1 dargestellt, ebenso der lineare Korrekturfaktor $\frac{\max_{\mathrm{norm}} - \min_{\mathrm{norm}}}{\max - \min}$.

4 Diskussion

Die aus der Segmentierung mit deformierbaren Formmodellen extrahierten Volumendaten zeigen sehr gute Übereinstimmung mit den gemessenen Spirometriedaten. Der Mittelwert der volumetrischen Abweichung aller drei Probanden

Tabelle 1. Mittelwerte und Standardabweichungen der volumetrischen Abweichung zwischen Segmentierung und Spirometrie bei den drei Probanden, sowie der lineare Korrekturfaktor, der die Abweichung von einer konstanten Korrektur darstellt (1).

Proband	Absoluter Volumenfehler [ml]	Relativer Volumenfehler [%]	Korrekturfaktor
1	46.09 ± 34.04	1.20 ± 0.98	1.029
2	77.31 ± 41.84	1.91 ± 1.32	1.115
3	85.48 ± 90.35	3.90 ± 4.24	1,036

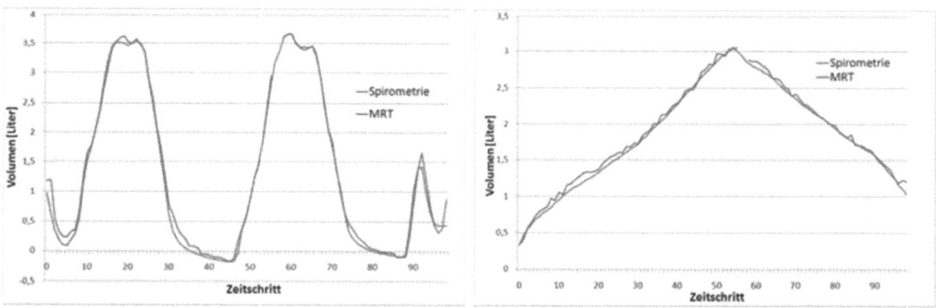

Abb. 2. Volumenverlaufskurven der ersten beiden Probanden

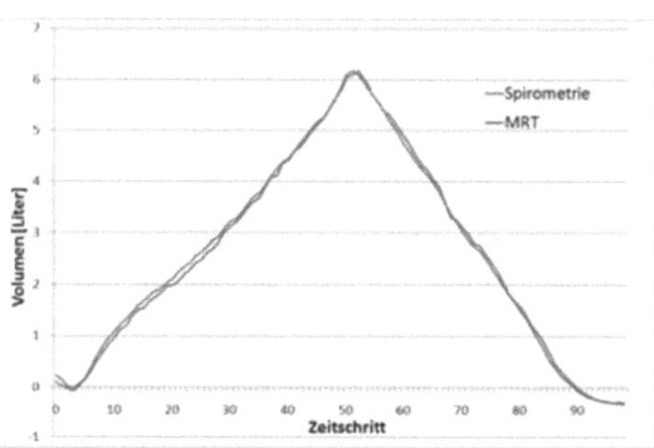

Abb. 3. Volumenverlaufskurve des dritten Probanden

liegt bei ca. 70 ml. Auch hat sich gezeigt, dass eine lineare Eichung der Daten nicht nötig erscheint, da der lineare Korrekturfaktor bei allen Probanden nahe bei eins lag und somit nur eine Korrektur um einen konstanten Betrag erforderlich macht. Ein konstanter Normierungsfaktor lässt sich sehr schnell und einfach durch eine Messung der Vitalkapazität bestimmen. Weiterhin erlaubt die bereits vorhandene Segmentierung eine unabhängige Analyse der beiden Lungenflügel, sowie durch eine zeitaufgelöste Analyse auch eine direkte Berechnung und Visualisierung der Lungen-Oberflächenbewegung und damit eine lokale Detektion von Bewegungseinschränkungen. Wir hoffen, durch unsere Ergebnisse die klinische Akzeptanz von MRT zur volumetrischen und funktionalen Analyse der Lunge weiter zu erhöhen und den Einsatz zu erleichtern.

Literaturverzeichnis

1. Ehrhardt J, Schmidt-Richberg A, Handels H. Generation of a Mean Motion Model of the Lung using 4D CT Data. In: Botha CP, Kindlmann G, Niessen J, et al., editors. Eurographics Workshop on Visual Computing for Biomedicine. Delft: Eurographics Association; 2008. p. 69–76.
2. Xu S, Taylor R, Fichtinger G, et al. Lung deformation estimation and four-dimensional CT lung reconstruction. Acad Radiol. 2006;13(9):1082–1092.
3. Plathow C, Ley S, Fink C, et al. Evaluation of chest motion and volumetry during the breathing cycle by dynamic MRI in healthy subjects: Comparison with pulmonary function tests. Invest Radiol. 2004;42:202–209.
4. Swift AJ, Woodhouse N, Fichele S, et al. Rapid lung volumetry using ultrafast dynamic magnetic resonance imaging during forced vital capacity maneuver - correlation with spirometry. Invest Radiol. 2007;42:37–41.
5. Tetzlaff R, Eichinger M, Schoebinger M, et al. Semiautomatic assessment of respiratory motion in dynamic MRI–comparison with simulta-neously acquired spirometry. Rofo. 2008;180(11):961.
6. Suga K, Tsukuda T, Awaya H, et al. Impaired respiratory mechanics in pulmonary emphysema: Evaluation with dynamic breathing MRI. J Magn Reson Imaging. 1999;10:510–520.
7. Cootes TF, Taylor CJ, Cooper DH, et al. Active shape models - Their training and application. Comput Vis Image Underst. 1995;61(1):38–59.
8. Heimann T. Statistical shape models for 3D medical image segmentation. University of Heidelberg; 2008.
9. Wolf I, Vetter M, Wegner I, et al. The medical imaging interaction toolkit. Med Image Anal. 2005 Dec;9(6):594–604.
10. Eichinger M, Puderbach M, Smith HJ, et al. MR-compatible spirometry: Principle, technical evaluation and application. Eur Respir J. 2007;30(5):972–981.

Model-Based Characterization of Mammographic Masses

Sven-René von der Heidt[1], Matthias Elter[2], Thomas Wittenberg[2], Dietrich Paulus[1]

[1]Institut für Computervisualistik, Universität Koblenz-Landau
[2]Abteilung Bildverarbeitung und Medizintechnik, Fraunhofer-Institut für Integrierte Schaltungen
agas@uni-koblenz.de

Abstract. The discrimination of benign and malignant types of mammographic masses is a major challenge for radiologists. The classic eigenfaces method was recently adapted for the detection of masses in mammograms. In the work at hand we investigate if this method is also suited for the problem of distinguishing benign and malignant types of this mammographic lesion. We furthermore evaluate two extended versions of the eigenfaces approach (fisherface and eigenfeature regularization extraction) and compare the performance of all three methods on a public mammography database. Our results indicate that all three methods can be applied to discriminate benign and malignant types of mammographic masses. However, our ROC analysis shows that the methods still require combination with other features to allow for reliable classification.

1 Introduction

Mammography is the most effective technique for the early detection and diagnosis of breast cancer available today. One of the most difficult tasks in the context of mammogram interpretation is the discrimination of benign and malignant mass lesions, which are defined as space-occupying lesions that can be seen in at least two different projections [1]. Recently, Oliver et al. [2] have proposed to apply the classic eigenface method to a related task, the detection of mammographic masses. Their results indicate that the eigenface method is a promising approach to the detection of masses, or more precisely, the discrimination of normal tissue and mammographic masses. In the work at hand, we investigate if the eigenface method is also suited to discriminate between benign and malignant types of mammographic masses. Furthermore, we have implemented two extended versions of the eigenface method: the fisherface and the eigenfeature-regularization-extraction methods. We compare the receiver operating characteristic curve performance of all three approaches on a public mammography database. There has been considerable interest in the classification of mammographic masses in the last decade. Due to the broad variety of approaches that have been published in the last years, we can mention only some representative examples of state of the art methods here. In contrast to the three approaches that we propose in this work, most of the work that can be found in literature follows the classic pattern recognition chain: segmentation of a mass from the background tissue, feature extraction and classification. Good examples are the work of Shi et al. [3] who apply level-sets for the segmentation of masses and propose several features specifically designed for the task of mass characterization. Varela et al. [4] have developed features that measure the degree of sharpness and microlobulation of the mass margin to improve their previously proposed CAD approach. Drukker et al. [5] extract mass features from both mammograms and ultrasound images and thus have proposed a promising multi-modal approach for the discrimination of masses. Timp and Karssemeijer [6] have developed a segmentation method based on dynamic programming to improve the classification performance of their previously proposed system for mass characterization.

The rest of this work is organized as follows: in Sec. 2 the eigenface, fischerface and eigenfeature regularization extraction methods (ERE method) are briefly described. Furthermore, details on the database of mammograms that we use to develop and evaluate the proposed approach are provided. In Sec. 3 the experiments and their results that we have performed to evaluate the classification performance of the proposed approaches are described. Finally, we close this work with a discussion of our results and provide possible directions for future research (Sec. 4).

2 Materials and methods

We use the digital database for screening mammography (DDSM) [7] for our experiments. It is a widely used public reference database for computer-aided detection and diagnosis of mammographic lesions. For this study we have randomly selected 206 regions of interest (ROIs) containing mammographic masses from the DDSM. 114 ROIs contained malignant and 92 ROIs benign masses. In the following we will apply eigenface techniques to the input images. This requires that each image has the same size. We crop ROIs from the mammograms and normalize them to a standard size. Another major problem are the different intensity ranges for the ROIs. Hence, we rescale each region to a normalized distribution of gray-levels. The principal component analysis (PCA) provides the basis for the following mathematical approaches. It is also called the Karhunen-Loeve transform (KLT) [8].

- The eigenface method was introduced by Turk and Pentland [9] for face recognition. It requires a set of images that have each the same size. For faces the method works best if the images are aligned (e.g. the nose is in the center of each image). Eigenfaces (or eigenvectors) are obtained from the covariance matrix of the probability distribution of the vector space of possible faces (in our case mammographic masses) using the PCA.
- Another approach used in face recognition is due to Fisher [10]. It extends the eigenface method by a LDA (linear discriminant analysis). The input

images are divided into subsets for each class. Two covariance matrices are computed for intra-class features and inter-class distances. A linear transform is computed that simultaneously de-correlates the feature vectors and class separation. The fisherface method is known to be less sensitive to variation in lighting and pose of the object than the eigenface method.

– The ERE method [11] further extends the eigenface method and particularly inspects those eigenvectors who's eigenvalues are zero.

3 Results

For the experiments we normalize and pre-process the input images as outlined in Sect. 2. We have evaluated and compared the classification performance of the three proposed approaches using 10-fold cross validation and receiver operating characteristic (ROC) curve analysis. We use the area under the ROC curve A_z as a performance metric. The classification is done using the k-nearest neighbors (kNN) classifier with Euclidean distance metric in eigenfeature space. We use the program ROCKIT by Charles E. Metz, PhD, to determine A_z based on the output of the ckNN classifier [12]. Fig. 1 shows ROC-curves for eigen- and fisherfaces and the ERE method. Fig. 1 shows results for the DDSM-database with uniform size for input images of 80×80 pixels. The training set for all tests consisted of 206 ROIs. The A_z values are 0.5256 for the Fisherfaces, 0.5617 for

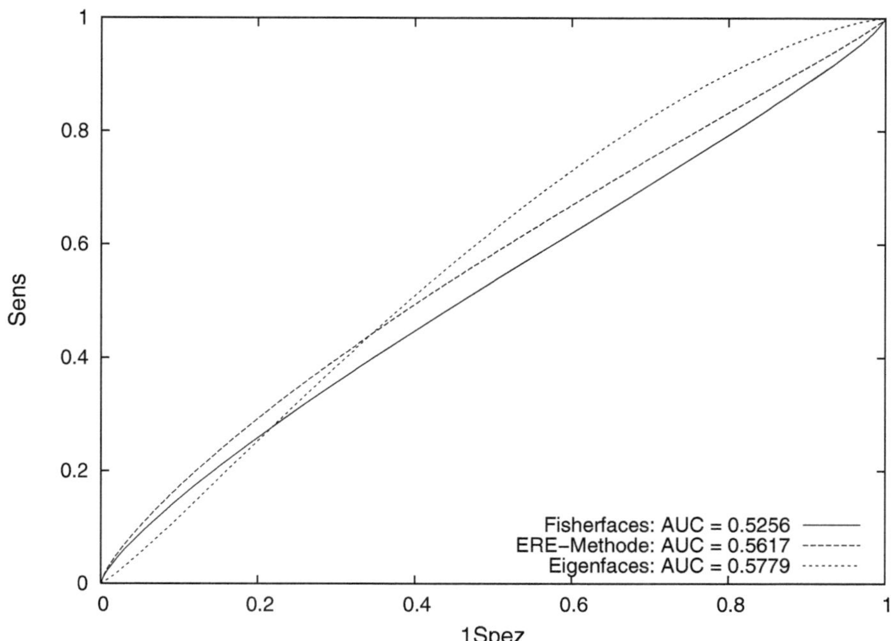

Fig. 1. Tests with uniform scaling to 80×80 pixel using 206 ROIs

Table 1. Results with uniform scaling to 80 × 80 pixel and 206 ROIs for different numbers of eigenfeatures.

	AUC values		
Number of eigenfeatures	Eigenfaces	Fisherfaces	ERE method
10	0.6017	0.5623	0.5496
40	0.6017	0.5161	0.5559
all	0.5941	0.5155	0.5406

Table 2. Results with grouping by ROI size instead of scaling and 206 ROIs for different numbers of eigenfeatures.

	AUC values		
Number of eigenfeatures	Eigenfaces	Fisherfaces	ERE method
10	0.5916	0.5152	0.5713
40	0.6000	0.5016	0.5735
all	0.5988	0.5527	0.5422

the ERE-Method, and 0.5779 for eigenfaces. Table 1 and Table 2 summarize AUC results for different experiments. For Table 2 we grouped the ROIs of similar sizes and avoided resizing.

4 Discussion

We have proposed to apply the eigenface method to the discrimination of benign and malignant mass. We showed that the eigenface method and two extended approaches can be used for discriminating benign and malignant mammographic masses. However, the AUC values show that the methods are not reliable enough, yet, for diagnosis. Interestingly, the classic eigenface method seems to be better suited for mass classification than the two extended approaches, which are known to be superior in other applications [10, 11]. We tested different preprocessing approaches and came to the result that scaling as required for eigenfaces actually reduces the classification performance. We are confident that manual selection of the examples used for the estimation of the covariance matrices will yield better values.

Acknowledgement. The authors are also grateful to Charles E. Metz, PhD, for providing the ROCKIT program for ROC analysis. This work was supported in part by the Bayerische Forschungsstiftung within the scope of the project Mammo-iCAD.

References

1. American College of Radiology. Breast Imaging Reporting and Data System BI-RADS Atlas; 2006.

2. Oliver A, Marti J, Bosch A, et al. A new approach to the classification of mammographic masses and normal breast tissue. In: The 18th International Conference on Pattern Recognition (ICPR'06); 2006. p. 707–710.
3. Shi J, Sahiner B, Chan HP, et al. Characterization of mammographic masses based on level set segmentation with new image features and patient information. Med Phys. 2008;35(1):280–290.
4. Varela C, Timp S, Karssemeijer N. Use of border information in the classification of mammographic masses. Phys Med Biol. 2006;51(2):425–441. Available from: http://dx.doi.org/10.1088/0031-9155/51/2/016.
5. Drukker K, Horsch K, Giger ML. Multimodality computerized diagnosis of breast lesions using mammography and sonography. Acad Radiol. 2005;12(8):970–979. Available from: http://dx.doi.org/10.1016/j.acra.2005.04.014.
6. Timp S, Karssemeijer N. A new 2D segmentation method based on dynamic programming applied to computer aided detection in mammography. Med Phys. 2004;31(5):958–971.
7. Heath M, Bowyer K, Kopans D, et al. The digital database for screening mammography. Procs Int Workshop on Digital Mammography. 2001; p. 212–218.
8. Kessler W. Multivariante Datenanalyse: Für die Pharma-, Bio- und Prozessanalyse. WILEY-VCH Verlag GmbH & Co. KGaA, Weinheim; 2007.
9. Turk M, Pentland A. Eigenfaces for Recognition. J Cognitive Neuroscience. 1991;3(1):71–86.
10. Belhumeur PN, Hespanha JP, Kriegman DJ. Eigenfaces vs. fisherfaces: Recognition using class specific linear projection. IEEE Trans PAMI. 1997;19(7):711–720.
11. Jiang X, Mandal B, Kot A. Eigenfeature regularization and extraction in face recognition. IEEE Trans PAMI. 2008;30(3):383–394.
12. Metz CE, Herman BA, Shen JH. Maximum-likelihood estimation of ROC curves from continuously-distributed data. Stat Med. 1998;17:1033–1053.

Spatio-temporal Analysis of Unstained Cells In-vitro

Nico Scherf[1,2], Jens-Peer Kuska[3], Ulf-Dietrich Braumann[2], Katja Franke[4], Tilo Pompe[4], Ingo Röder[1]

[1]Inst. f. Medizinische Informatik, Statistik u. Epidemiologie, Universität Leipzig
[2]Translationszentrum für Regenerative Medizin, Universität Leipzig
[3]Interdisziplinäres Zentrum für Bioinformatik, Universität Leipzig
[4]Leibniz-Inst. f. Polymerforschung, Max-Bergmann-Zentr. f. Biomaterialien, Dresden
nscherf@imise.uni-leipzig.de

Abstract. The tracking of individual cells in time-lapse microscopy facilitates the assessment of certain characteristics of different cell types. Since manual tracking of an adequate number of cells over a considerable number of frames is tedious and sometimes not feasible, there is a vital interest in automated methods. We present a rather minimalistic approach for the tracking of unstained cells in cell culture assays. The proposed approach comprises background subtraction, an object detection method based on discrete geometrical feature analysis together with a validation of the resulting graph-structures. The main advantage of this approach lies in its computational efficiency.

1 Introduction

A proper way of understanding biological systems necessarily incorporates not only spatial organisation but also their dynamic development. Therefore, experiments assessing the spatio-temporal aspects of a biological system provide a promising way to unravel the underlying organisational principles. It is natural to extend the established methods of microscopy by taking a series of images in order to assess the temporal development. This so called *time-lapse imaging* will become a valuable tool in biological and medical research. The potential benefits are discussed in the review found in [1] and an overview of the technical aspects of time-lapse imaging and object tracking in a biomedical context can be found in [2].

A variety of different approaches to the analysis of time-lapse image data exists, where three main classes of approaches to object tracking can be distinguished according to [3]: (i) correspondence-based, (ii) transformation-based and (iii) contour-based methods. The latter two classes could also be subsumed into one. Correspondence-based methods base upon the detection of objects in a frame-by-frame manner. The correspondences between the detected objects are subsequently established. Transformation- or contour-based techniques focus on tracking the changes of initial objects over time. Here the contour-based aproaches became very popular over the last years [4, 3, 5, 6], especially in biomedical applications. Similar to [7], we decided to take the first approach of correspondence-based tracking since such methods are usually computationally more efficient. This is in particular true for cases when a great number of objects needs to be tracked.

We are interested in analysing the migration and proliferation of unstained cells in a cell-culture assay. The cells are not stained to rule out the effects of the staining agents on the behaviour of the cells. Usually phase-contrast microscopy is the common method of choice with the known drawbacks e.g. the typical halos and differences in the visual appearance of normal and mitotic cells [4]. Thus, we decided to use transmitted light microscopy and enhance the visibility of the cells by exploiting the effect, that slightly defocussed cells appear as rather bright objects (Fig. 1(a)).

The experiments are desgined to assess the behaviour of hematopoietic stem-cells (HSCs) *in vitro*. The cells are cultured on a 3D silicone-substrate consisting of microcavities of different diameter, coated with certain molecules like fibronectin, heparin, collagen etc. to model the interactions between cells and extracellular matrix. The aim is to analyse the effects of these parameters (different proteins, spatial structure) on the behaviour of the cells. We are in particular interested in analysing the frequency and location of cell-divisions, different aspects of cell motility and also the structure of the obtained cellular genealogies (e.g. [1, 7]).

2 Materials and Methods

The main problem of tracking unstained cells is the low signal-to-noise ratio. As can be seen from the image histograms, there is no clear distinction between the gray-level distribution of the cells and the background. This problem is further complicated by the visible structures of the substrate. As an example the gray-level profile along two different line is shown for a sample image in Fig 1(b). To alleviate this problem we subtract the background from every frame. The mean background image can be either obtained by taking a series of images

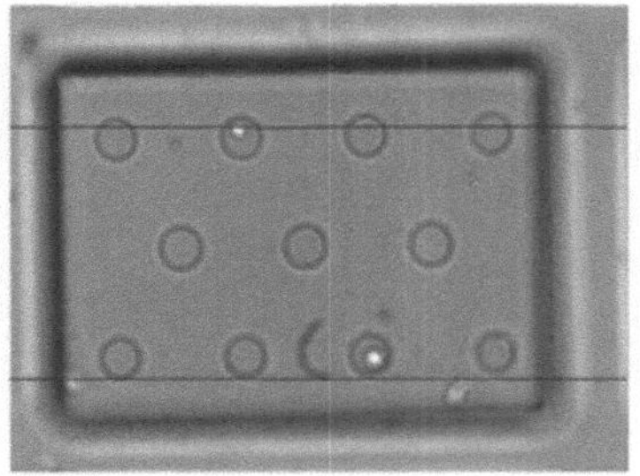

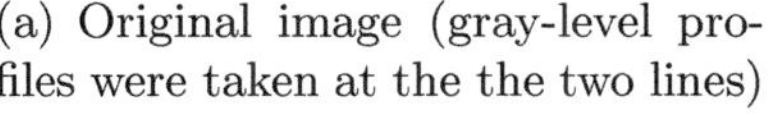

(a) Original image (gray-level profiles were taken at the the two lines)

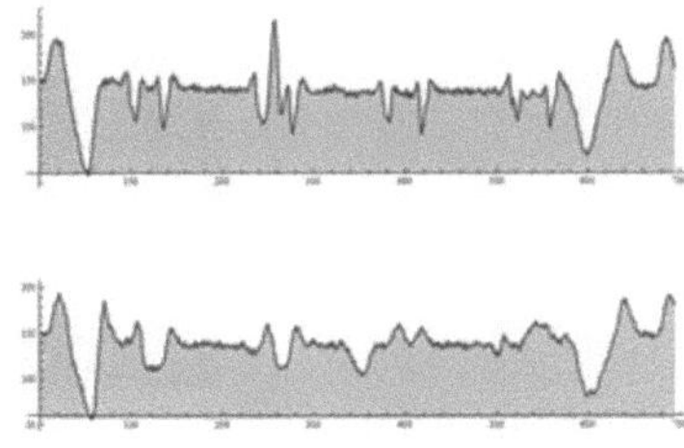

(b) Corresponding gray-level profiles

Fig. 1. Example of an image and its characteristic gray-level profiles

before the cells are applied on the substrate or, if this is not possible, the mean intensity for every pixel must be estimated from the data. This simple approach to background estimation is computationally more efficient compared to more sophisticated methods (e.g. Gaussian mixture modelling, eigenbackgrounds etc.) and is sufficiently robust under the given image characteristics.

The pre-processed images are then segmented by thresholding and detection of connected foreground-components. Different geometrical features are calculated for the obtained objects to further remove falsely detected background structures. The most important features used here are the area, the largest and smallest object diameter as well as the discrete compactness and solidity of the objects. Deviations from typical values of compactness and solidity are used to detect objects that are likely to correspond to partially occluding or touching cells. Such objects are subsequently splitted into smaller structures. By taking the endpoints of a graph-based description of the objects [8] we obtain the center points to find a suitable splitting.

The results are depicted in Fig 2. The described method scales linearly with the number of foreground pixels. Thus, it is not as sensitive to the number of cells in the image as an approach based on active contours (e.g. [5]).

After object detection, the correspondence between consecutive frames needs to be established. To achieve this, we calculate the overlap of the objects in the previous and in the current frame. Ambiguities arise when an object overlaps with more than one object in the next frame. These cases are solved by detecting one-to-one mappings, removing the corresponding objects and then re-analysing the remaining objects. Such an approach critically depends on whether or not the sampling-theorem is met by image acquisition (for a detailed discussion see [2]). However, in some cases this requirement is not met and hence, errors in the cell correspondences can occur. In these cases we relax the requirements and allow correspondences between two objects that are a distance of not more than twice of the object diameter away. Furthermore, cells can be lost, in particular at the corners of the substrate structures. Thus, we need to keep track of such

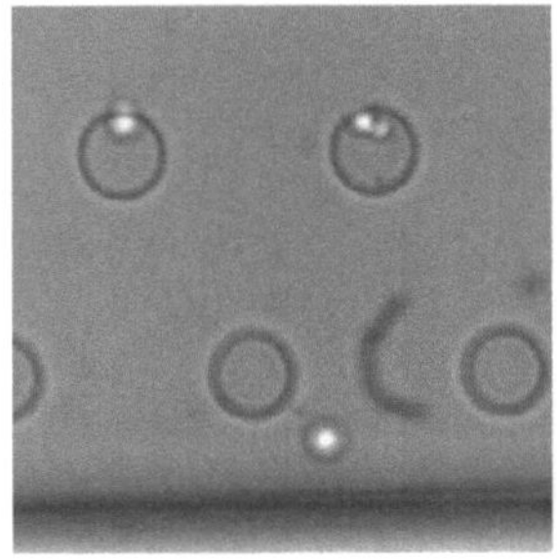
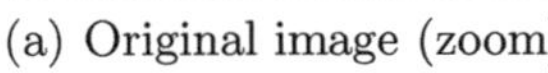
(a) Original image (zoom)

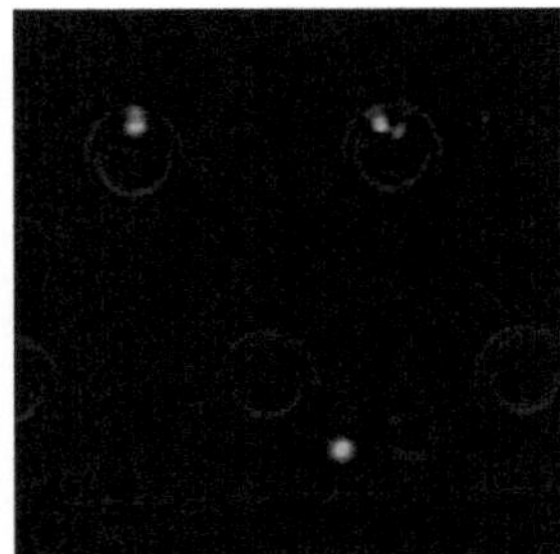
(b) Image with mean background removed

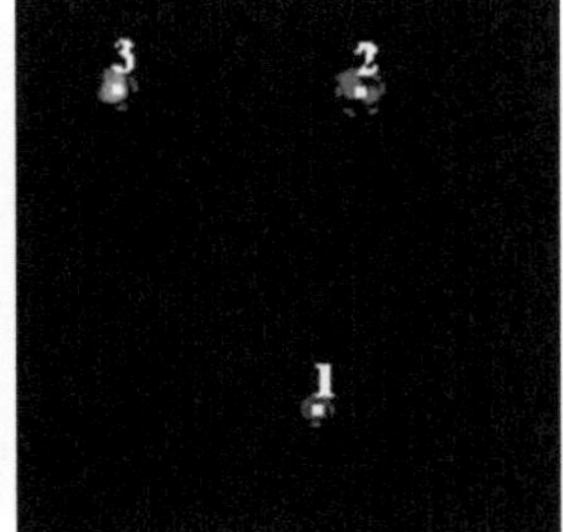

(c) Segmented objects

Fig. 2. Image preprocessing and segmentation

lost cells. If a cell cannot be detected in the current frame, its position is stored and it is re-considered in the next frames for a certain period of time.

Sometimes cells overlap and consequently are falsely detected as a single object. If the fused object cannot be splitted as described above, the object is marked. When the cells eventually diverge, the correspondence is calculated between these newly seperated objects and the objects before the fusion.

3 Results

This work is still in progress, so presently only some preliminary, qualitative results are available to illustrate our propsed method. As an example an image sequence consisting of 4000 frames (examples shown here) taken every 60 sec is analysed. Here we were in particular interested in the detection of cell divisions. Fig 3(b) shows the places, where cell divisions were detected. All of the mitotic events that occured during the observation time were successfully found. There was only one *false positive* detected cell division. It can be seen, that most of the cell divisions took place in the cavities or near the border structures of the substrate. The migrating behaviour of the cells was also analysed. In Fig 3(a) two examples of reconstructed cell tracks (over a period of 4000 frames) can be seen, showing different characteristics of migration patterns. In Fig 3(b) all places are marked, where a cell has been detected in the analysis. Here a tendency of the cells to move towards the upper left corner is apparent, which is most likely due to an incline of the petri-dish. And in Fig 3(c) a visualisation of reconstructed spatio-temporal cell-tracks is shown, where the track of one cell is marked in white showing both the migration pattern over time and the division events in a tree-like structure.

4 Discussion

We presented an approach to the problem of the spatio-temporal tracking of unstained cells *in vitro*. The results on the testing sequences are very promising

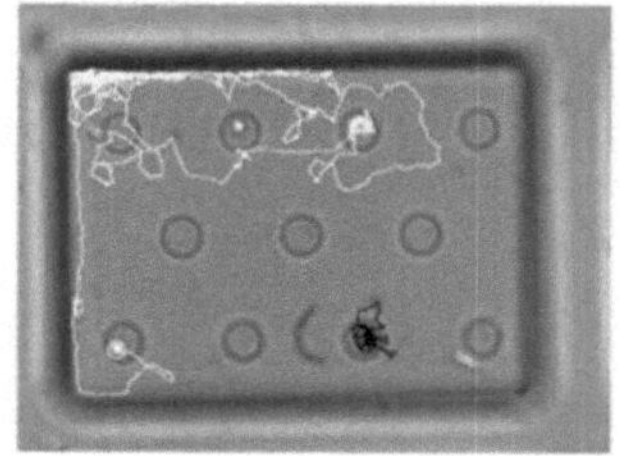

(a) Example tracks of two cells

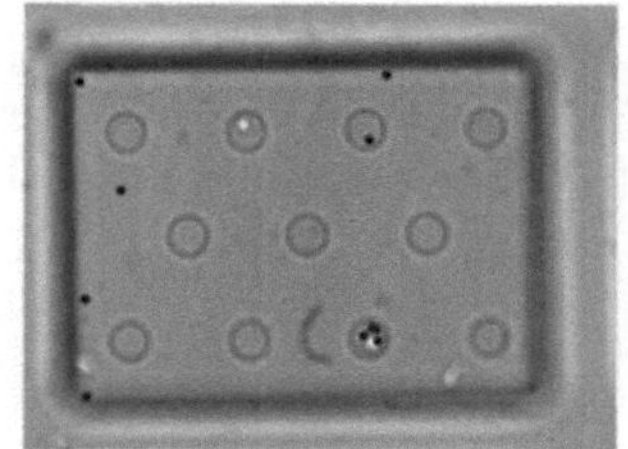

(b) All places of detected mitotic events (black spots)

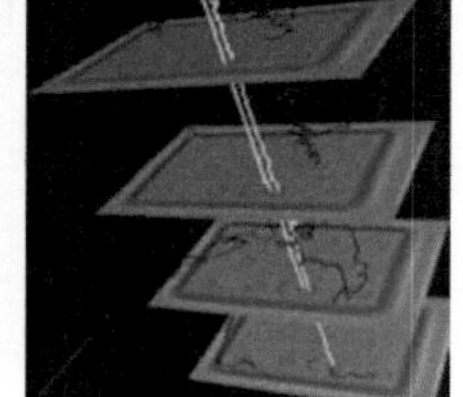

(c) Example of a reconstructed spatio-temporal trajectory (shown in white)

Fig. 3. Examples of information to be extracted from the time-lapse data

and allow for an automated (or at least semi-automated) analysis of a variety of features of the spatio-temporal behaviour of the hematopoietic stem-cells in the presented culture-assays, which otherwise would not be feasible. The main advantage is that the presented approach is computationally attractive, thus allowing for an analysis in real-time. One important drawback is its sensitivity to segmentation errors and the resulting complications for object-linking. Some of the problems might be alleviated by a contour-based approach, which on the other hand would considerably increase the computational costs. As a next step, an objective validation of the method is needed as e.g. in [9] to evaluate the robustness of the method with respect to several parameters (e.g. cell density). It is to be expected that human interaction will be needed to correct for inevitably occuring errors during tracking, so a crucial point will be the optimisation of these interactions in order to obtain reliable results from the large amounts of data. Last but not least further measures for analysing the spatio-temporal trajectories need to be assessed.

References

1. Schroeder T. Imaging stem cell driven mammalian regeneration. Nature. 2008;453:345–351.
2. Meijering E, Smal I, Dzyubachyk O, et al. Microscopic Image Processing; 2008.
3. Yilmaz A, Li X, Shah M. Object contour tracking using level sets. Procs ACCV. 2004.
4. Li K, Miller E, Weiss L, et al. Online tracking of migrating and proliferating cells imaged with phase-contrast microscopy. Procs CVPRW. 2006; p. 65 – 72.
5. Nath SK, Bunyak F, Palaniappan K. Robust tracking of migrating cells using four-color level set segmentation. Lect Notes Comput Sci. 2006;4179:920–932.
6. Padfield DR, Rittscher J, Sebastian T, et al. Spatio-temporal cell cycle analysis using 3D level set segmentation of unstained nuclei in line scan confocal fluorescence images. Procs ISBI. 2006; p. 1036–1039.
7. Al-Kofahi O, Radke RJ, Goderie SK, et al. Automated cell lineage construction: A rapid method to analyze clonal development established with murine neural progenitor cells. Cell Cycle. 2006;5(3):327–335.
8. Braumann U, Franke H, Hengstler J, et al. Graph-based quantification of astrocytes. Procs BVM. 2006; p. 379–383.
9. Godinez W, Lampe M, Wörz S, et al. Probabilistic tracking of virus particles in fluorescence microscopy image sequences. Procs BVM. 2008; p. 448–452.

Computergestützte Patchplanung für Aortenerweiterungsplastiken

Urte Rietdorf[1], Eugénie Riesenkampff[2], Ivo Wolf[1], Mathias Seitel[1], Nicole Engel[1], Titus Kühne[2], Michael Hübler[2], Tobias Schwarz[1], Hans-Peter Meinzer[1]

[1]Abteilung für Medizinische und Biologische Informatik, DKFZ Heidelberg
[2]Abteilung Kinderkardiologie und Angeborene Herzfehler , DHZB Berlin
u.rietdorf@dkfz-heidelberg.de

Kurzfassung. Stenosen der Aorta betreffen 5-8% aller Neugeborenen mit Herzfehlern und führen unbehandelt meist zum Tod. Liegt die Indikation für einen chirurgischen Eingriff vor, hängt die Wahl der Operationsmethode maßgeblich von der Anatomie der Aorta sowie dem Erfahrungsschatz des Operationsteams ab. Ein Verfahren hierbei ist die Patcherweiterungsplastik, bei der ein Patch in das Gefäß eingefügt wird, um das Lumen zu erweitern. Bisher erfolgt die Patchplanung intraoperativ auf Grundlage der Erfahrung des Operateurs. Wir haben eine Applikation entwickelt, mit der bereits präoperativ ein individueller Patchvorschlag angefertigt werden kann. Dadurch wird die Operationszeit verkürzt und postoperative Komplikationen wie Re- bzw. Reststenosen und Aneurysmen reduziert. Um die Applikation zu evaluieren wurde die Stenosenquantifizierung unseres Ansatzes mit der eines Kinderkardiologen verglichen und zeigt eine Abweichung im Durchmesser von lediglich $(2,33 \pm 1,43)$ mm.

1 Einleitung

Stenosen der Aorta (Coarctation of Aorta, CoA) betreffen 5-8% aller Neugeborenen mit angeborenen Herzfehlern (AHF). Unbehandelt verursachen sie, je nach Schweregrad, starke Organschäden und führen meist zum Tod innerhalb des ersten Lebensjahres. Ist als Therapie ein chirurgischer Eingriff indiziert, so hängen die Operationstechnik und der Operationserfolg maßgeblich von der Anatomie der Aorta und dem Erfahrungsschatz des Operateurs ab. Eine Operationsmethode stellt hierbei die plastische Erweiterung der Aorta durch einen Patch, die sogenannte Patchaortoplastie, dar. Hierbei wird ein Patch in die Engstelle der Gefäßwand eingefügt, um das Lumen durch Vergrößerung des Gefäßdurchmessers zu erweitern.

Das Patchmaterial, das zum Erweitern des Lumens eingesetzt wird, muss dabei in Form und Größe so gestaltet sein, dass es das Gefäß auf den gewünschten Durchmesser abändert [1]. Bei einer komplizierten, irregulären CoA ist dies oft schwer zu planen. Derzeit wird der dafür notwendige Patch vom Operateur auf

Grundlage seiner Erfahrung in Form und Größe intraoperativ frei angefertigt und eingesetzt, wofür zusätzliche Operationszeit eingeplant werden muss.

Ein weiteres großes Problem der Patchaortoplastie stellen die häufig auftretenden, und ebenfalls von der Erfahrung des Operateurs abhängigen, postoperativen Komplikationen der Re- bzw. Reststenose (20-30 %) und Aneurysmen (24%) dar [2].

Daher wurde eine Applikation entwickelt, mit der, basierend auf MRT-Daten, die Aorta inklusive Stenose quantifiziert, und ein individueller Patchvorschlag erstellt wird. Durch diese präoperative Planungsmöglichkeit wird nicht nur die Operationszeit verkürzt, sondern auch postoperative Komplikationen sollen durch die hohe Präzision minimiert werden.

2 Methoden

Das Softwarewerkzeug, mittels dessen ein möglichst optimaler Patch zur Gefäßerweiterung bei Stenosen der Aorta ermittelt werden kann, arbeitet in mehreren Schritten. Zuerst muss die Aorta aus dem Datensatz extrahiert werden, um sie anschließend in zur Quantifizierung geeignete Modelle umwandeln zu können. Die Quantifizierung erfolgt durch Ermittlung der Radien entlang der Aorta, aus deren Differenz zum größten ermittelten Radius der Patchvorschlag erfolgt. Die Applikation, welche die interaktive Korrektur sämtlicher Zwischenschritte ermöglicht, wurde auf Grundlage des Medical Imaging Interaction Toolkits (MITK), einem C++-basierten Framework, erstellt [3].

2.1 Gefäßsegmentierung mittels Graph-Cut

Um die Aorta möglichst schnell und genau aus dem Datensatz zu extrahieren, wurde eine Segmentierung mit dem Graph-Cut-Algorithmus [4] angewendet. Wie in Abb. 1 dargestellt, werden innerhalb einer zuvor definierten Region of Interest (ROI) bestimmte Bereiche dem Gefäß zugeordnet, andere dem Hintergrund. Als Resultat entsteht eine binäre Segmentierung der Aorta. Falls das Segmentierungsergebnis nicht den Anforderungen entspricht, kann es durch die Definition weiterer Objekt- oder Hintergrundbereiche interaktiv verändert werden.

2.2 Quantifizierung der Aorta

Zur Quantifizierung der Aorta werden aus der Segmentierung zwei Modelle erstellt: Ein Polygonnetz (Surface) mittels des Marching-Cube-Algorithmus [5], und ein Gefäßbaum mittels einer Skelettierung [6]. Die Surface liefert die Oberflächenkoordinaten der Aorta, während durch die Skelettierung die Mittellinie des Gefäßes, die Centerline, definiert wird.

Die Durchmesser entlang der Aorta werden errechnet, indem zu jedem Punkt auf der Centerline die gemittelte Entfernung zu n Punkten auf der Oberfläche in

360° um den Centerlinepunkt herum gemessen werden. Dazu wird das Oberflächenmodell diffusionsbasiert parametrisiert [7], indem die Punkte des Polygonnetzes, wie in Abb. 2 dargestellt, in n Längengrade eingeteilt werden. Anschließend lässt sich jeder Punkt auf der Oberfläche einem Längensegment zuordnen.

Der mittlere Radius um einen Centerlinepunkt herum wird ermittelt, indem zu jedem Punkt auf der Centerline jeweils der nächstliegende Punkt innerhalb eines der n Segmente zugeordnet wird.

Wie in Abb. 3 links abgebildet, entsteht dadurch für jeden Punkt auf der Centerline die Zuordnung von n Punkten der Surface, was einem Ring mit kleinstem gemitteltem Gefäßradius um die Aorta entspricht.

Als optimaler Gefäßradius wird hier der größte Radius innerhalb des quantifizierten Gefäßabschnitts definiert. Das Verhältnis zwischen den einzelnen mittleren Radien um die Centerlinepunkte und dem größten ermittelten Radius definiert die Stärke des Stenosegrades an den Centerlinepunkten. Umgewandelt in Umfänge ergibt sich hieraus die Fläche, die als Patch in die Aorta eingesetzt werden muss, um die Stenose auszugleichen. Abb. 3 zeigt in der Mitte die Abbildung der mittleren Radien entlang einer Aorta als Graphen und rechts den daraus resultierenden Patchvorschlag.

2.3 Studiendesign

Um die Quantifizierung der Aorta zu evaluieren wurden bei neun Testpatienten die rechnergestützt ermittelten minimalen Aortendurchmesser mit den ermittelten Werten eines Kinderkardiologen verglichen. Dazu wurden die neun MRT-Daten der Patienten analysiert. Der Radius der applikationsgestützen Quantifizierung wurde in n = 18 Sektoren ermittelt. Die Auflösung der Datensätze betrug 1x1x1.2 mm^3.

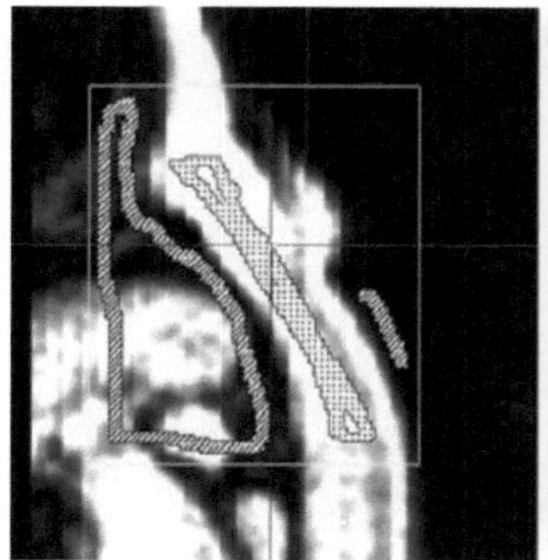

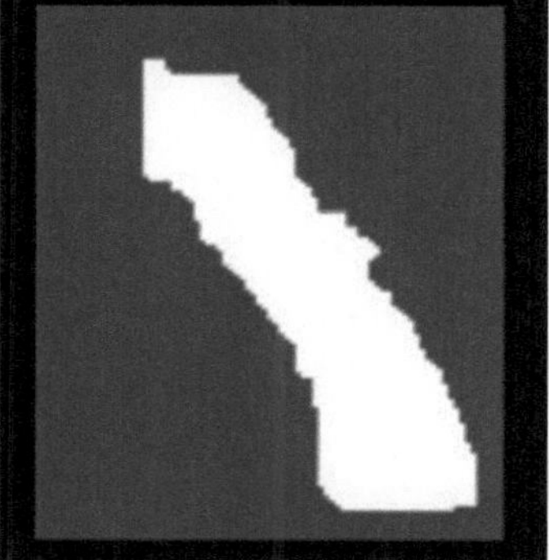

Abb. 1. Aortensegmentierung mittels Graph-Cut. Links: Innerhalb einer zuvor definierten ROI (helles Quadrat) werden Bereiche der Aorta (gepunktet) und des Hintergrundes (schraffiert) markiert. Ergebnis ist eine binäre Segmentierung (rechts).

3 Ergebnisse

Der mittlere Aortendurchmesser der neun Testpatienten, gemessen durch den Kinderkardiologen, betrug $(11,86 \pm 2,4)$ mm $(\mu \pm \sigma)$. Unsere Applikation ermittelte $(9,54 \pm 2,2)$ mm. Die durchschnittliche absolute Differenz zwischen der manuellen Messung und unserer Annäherung betrug $(2,33 \pm 1,43)$ mm.

Die Zeit des Anwenders, die für die manuelle Durchmesserermittlung benötigt wurde, lag bei $(3,6 \pm 1,5)$ min (gemessen bei 7 Patienten), sowie $(4,1 \pm 2,2)$ min bei Quantifizierung mittels der Applikation.

In allen neun Fällen konnte ein Patchvorschlag ermittelt werden. Abb. 3 rechts zeigt den Patchvorschlag für einen Patienten als Beispiel. Der Patch gleicht die fehlenden Umfänge entlang der Aorta im Vergleich zum größten Umfang aus.

4 Diskussion und Ausblick

Die genaue Form und Größe eines Patches ist bei einer komplizierten, irregulären CoA vom Chirurgen oft schwer zu planen. Wir stellen eine neue Methode zur präoperativen Aortenquantifizierung vor, mit der die Stenose der Aorta ermittelt und ein Patchvorschlag erstellt werden kann. Mit Hilfe des individuellen Patchvorschlages kann bereits präoperativ ein Patch erstellt werden, der in Form und Größe den stenotischen Abschnitt auf den gewünschten Durchmesser erweitert. Dadurch kann zum einen die Operationszeit reduziert, und somit das Operationsrisiko für den Patienten minimiert werden, zum anderen können optimale Patches die postoperativen Komplikationen der bei dieser chirurgischen Therapieform häufig auftretenden Re- bzw. Reststenosen und Aneurysmen reduzieren. Bei neun Testpatienten betrug die Differenz zwischen den manuell durch einen Kinderkardiologen ermittelten Radien an der engsten Stelle der Aorta und den applikationsermittelten Werten durchschnittlich $(2,33 \pm 1,43)$ mm, was ungefähr der Größe von zwei Pixeln der MRT-Datensätze entspricht.

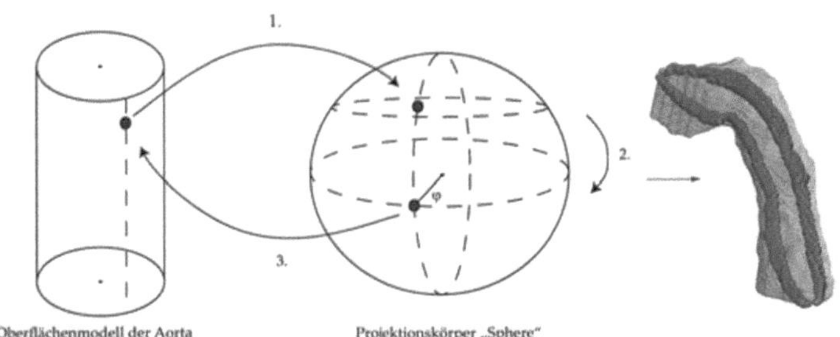

Abb. 2. Surfaceparametrisierung. Die Surface wird in n Längengrade eingeteilt, indem die Punkte des Polygonnetzes auf eine Kugel projiziert (1.) und in Grade eingeteilt werden (2.). Nach der Rückprojektion (3.) lässt sich jeder Punkt auf der Oberfläche genau einem Längengrad zuordnen. Rechts abgebildet: Eine Surface mit den Punkten zweier Längengradbereiche.

Abb. 3. Ermittlung des mittleren Radius für einen Centerlinepunkt (CP) und daraus resultierender Patchvorschlag. Jedem CP werden die Surfacepunkte (SP) zugeordnet, die innerhalb eines Sektors am nächsten liegen. Aus den Entfernungen der n Punkte zum CP errechnet sich der mittlere Radius. An der Stelle des geringsten mittleren Radius ist die Stenose lokalisiert. In der Mitte ist die Abbildung aller ermittelten Radien entlang der Aorta. Aus der Differenz des mittleren Radius zum größten innerhalb der Aorta ermittelten Radius errechnet sich anschließend der Patchvorschlag (rechts).

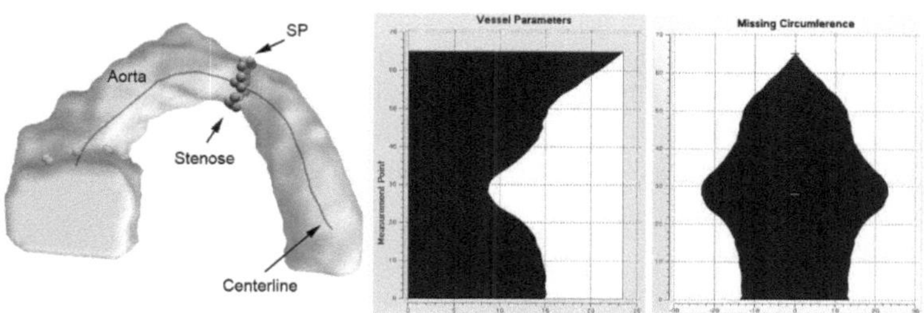

Derzeit wird der optimale Gefäßradius automatisch als der größte ermittelte Radius definiert, was bei Aneurysmen oder hypoplastischen Aorten problematisch ist. Daher ist eine Erweiterung geplant, in der der Kardiologe auf die Definition des optimalen Gefäßdurchmessers Einfluss nehmen kann. Zudem soll bei der Patchform die Krümmung der Aorta, insbesondere im Aortenbogen, mit berücksichtigt werden. Dies ist als Erweiterung der Applikation zusammen mit Studien zur Evaluierung der Patchform und -größe geplant. Außer für Patchplanungen an Stenosen der Aorta soll die Applikation auch für Stenosen anderer Gefäße, wie beispielsweise an Pulmonalbifurkationen eingesetzt werden.

Literaturverzeichnis

1. Smaill BH, McGiffin DC, LeGrice IJ, et al. The effect of synthetic patch repair of coarctation on regional deformation of the aortic wall. J Thoracic Cardiovasc Surg. 2000;120(6):1053–1063.
2. Schumacher G, Hess J, Bühlmeyer K. Klinische Kinderkardiologie: Diagnostik und Therapie der angeborenen Herzfehler. Springer Verlag, 4. Auflage; 2007.
3. Wolf I, Vetter M, Wegner I, et al. The medical imaging interaction toolkit (MITK). Med Image Anal. 2005;9:594–604.
4. Boykov J, Jolly MP. Interactive graph cuts for optimal boundary and region segmentation of objects in n-d images. Procs ICCV. 2001;1:105–112.
5. Lorensen WE, Cline HE. Marching cubes: A high resolution 3D surface construction algorithm. Computer Graph. 1987;21(4):163–169.
6. Zhou Y, Kaufmanand A, Toga AW. Efficient Skeletonization of Volumetric Objects. IEEE Trans Vis Computer Graph. 1999;5(3):196–209.
7. Brechbühler C, Gerig G, Kübler O. Parametrization of closed surfaces for 3-D shape description. Computer Vis Image Underst. 1995;61:154–170.

Interfractional Displacement Analysis of the Spinal Cord for 21 Head & Neck Cases in Radiation Therapy Planning

Armin Stoll[1], Kristina Giske[1], Eva Stoiber[2], Rolf Bendl[1,3]

[1]Medical Physics in Radiation Oncology, DKFZ Heidelberg
[2]Clinical Cooperation Unit Radiation Oncology, DKFZ Heidelberg
[3]Medical Informatics, Heilbronn University
a.stoll@dkfz-heidelberg.de

Abstract. A monomodal slice-based displacement analysis of the spinal cord for three-dimensional computer tomography imaging in radiation therapy planning is presented. In total, 21 head and neck cases with tumor indications close to the spinal cord are studied and evaluated. Two-dimensional cross-correlation is applied to propagate manually segmented contours of the spinal cord from a high-resolution planning CT to subsequently acquired control CTs. The method and the fully automatic implementation turned out to be reliable and robust. A very few manual corrections on the resulting contours remained necessary in single transversal slices.

1 Introduction

A main effort to fractional radiation therapy is to achieve high tumor control probability with minimal risk of side effects during several weeks of cancer treatment with ionizing radiation [1]. Adaptive radiation therapy is therefore in the focus of research to conform precise radiation dose distributions to a cancerous target volume [2, 3]. To overcome inter- and intrafractional motion uncertainties, margins of the gross tumor volume are increased and adapted according to physicians' expertise. A monomodal displacement analysis of the spinal cord in computer tomography imaging along the longitudinal axis is presented in this contribution. As a result, a multiplicity of non-rigid interfractional organ motions are seen, even though individually adjusted immobilization techniques are applied. The displacement of the spinal cord is automatically determined by propagating manually segmented contours of the spinal cord from the treatment planning computer tomogram (TPCT) to several control computer tomograms (CCTs) by applying two-dimensional cross-correlation per transversal slice [4].

2 Material and methods

Twenty-one head and neck cases are studied in this retrospective investigation and the displacement of the spinal cord in lateral (L) and anterior-posterior

(AP) direction during several weeks of radiation therapy treatment is evaluated. Variances along L and AP directions are additionally derived.

Each case comprises one TPCT and several CCTs (4-11; mean $\mu = 6.6$). All TPCTs (acquired by a Toshiba Aquilion© CT scanner) and CCTs (mainly acquired by a Siemens Somatom Emotion© CT scanner – within the treatment room) have spatial resolutions of 512×512 voxels (voxel size: $1 \times 1 \times 3$ mm). A TPCT covers the whole volume of interest from the human anatomy (> 100 slices) while all CCTs only focus on a specific volume of interest (~ 50 slices) – primarily on the target volume (see Fig. 1). The maximum value of the normalized cross-correlation coefficient $\Theta_{CC} \in [-1, 1]$ is evaluated as a measure for similarity between a template patch A from the TPCT and a search region B within the CCTs after transformation T:

$$\Theta_C = \sum_{\boldsymbol{x} \in \Omega^T_{A,B}} (A(\boldsymbol{x}) - \overline{A})(B^T(\boldsymbol{x}) - \overline{B}) \tag{1}$$

Apart from the substraction of the image mean values $\overline{A}$ and $\overline{B}$, the cross-correlation coefficient Θ_C in equation (1) describes a convolution of two images. A convolution can be calculated in an efficient way in its Fourier domain. Both image-patches (the zero-padded template from the TPCT and the search region from a given CCT) are therefore transformed into the Fourier domain. The calculation then turns into a multiplication of both images. The inverse Fourier transformation leads to all correlation coefficients and enables an fast estimation of the displacement of the spinal cord within the CCT:

$$\Theta_C = \mathbf{FFT}^{-1}(\mathbf{FFT}(\Omega_A) \cdot \mathbf{FFT}(\Omega_B)^*) \tag{2}$$

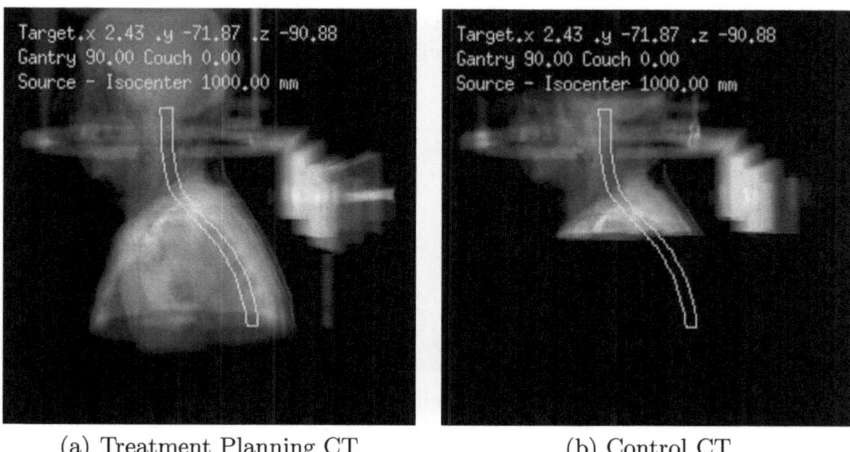

(a) Treatment Planning CT (b) Control CT

Fig. 1. Visualization: digitally reconstructed radiographs (DRR) in lateral direction

Finally, the correlation coefficients Θ_C are divided by the square root of the auto-correlation product of both images, to obtain normalized correlation coefficients:

$$\Theta_{CC} = \frac{\Theta_C(A, B^T)}{\sqrt{\Theta_C(A, A) \cdot \Theta_C(B^T, B^T)}} \tag{3}$$

All rectangular templates, with image contents according to the manually segmented contours of the spinal cord in the TPCT, are derived from minimum and maximum vertices along L and AP direction. The template size is constantly increased in both direction by 20 voxels (~20mm), with intention to enhance robustness of the cross-correlation calculation (see Fig. 2(a)).

Since all CCTs per case are stereotactically registered according to the TPCT, a global coordinate system is given for every CCT and therefore the relative template position in the TPCT serves as initial search region within the CCTs, too. The initial search region in each CCT is additionally enlarged by 15 voxels (~15mm) in L and AP direction (see Fig. 2(b)). This area seemed to be suitable to cover large displacements without overestimating the search volume. The maximum cross-correlation coefficient finally indicates similar image content in the TPCT and CCT and therefore implicitly enables to estimate the displacement of the spinal cord within a slice (see Fig. 2(c)).

3 Results

Using this approach, 7573 contours of the spinal cord from 21 head and neck cases were adapted to 138 CCTs in every single transversal slice (see Table 1). Seventeen false propagation results within single transversal slices were immediately identified during the calculations and instantly reported for subsequent manual corrections. As error criterion, a displacement > 13 mm in one directions was assumed. After three-dimensional visualization of all resulting contours, 14

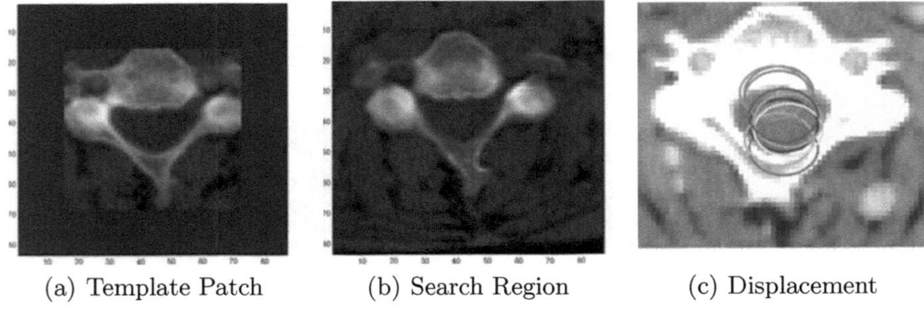

(a) Template Patch (b) Search Region (c) Displacement

Fig. 2. Examples: Fig. 2(a) shows a zero-padded template patch. It is identified in every transversal slice of the TPCT around the spinal cord. Fig. 2(b) demonstrates that a similar pattern is expected to occur in the CCTs within an extended search region. Fig. 2(c) gives an example of the displacement of the spinal cord within one slice.

Table 1. Detailed evaluation of all 21 head and neck cases without error correction

Case	#CCTs	Err. Det.	Man. Cor.	$\overline{x}$ [mm]	$\overline{y}$ [mm]	σ_x^2 [mm]	σ_y^2 [mm]	#Contours
1	5	0	0	-0,12	-0,61	0,22	0,87	292
2	7	0	0	0,39	2,67	0,95	10,32	388
3	8	0	0	-3,12	0,12	4,07	2,24	432
4	9	0	1	-2,20	-2,06	2,93	10,8	451
5	4	1	3	-0,55	-0,01	1,66	2,73	262
6	7	0	0	-0,36	-0,42	0,83	1,97	426
7	8	2	2	3,70	-0,22	5,44	1,67	446
8	4	0	0	-0,96	-0,85	1,16	0,62	182
9	7	0	0	-1,84	-0,83	1,46	1,40	411
10	6	0	0	-1,43	2,15	0,99	1,94	301
11	6	0	3	0,71	-1,79	1,02	5,64	343
12	8	0	2	-0,34	-0,99	1,55	1,28	440
13	5	0	0	0,71	-0,17	4,87	0,95	255
14	11	0	0	-1,72	0,37	1,84	1,04	599
15	7	0	0	0,08	-0,47	0,81	2,21	327
16	5	0	3	-0,07	-0,62	0,15	0,98	265
17	5	0	0	-1,23	-1,13	6,57	5,80	323
18	9	12	14	0,72	0,02	5,65	10,65	459
19	6	2	3	0,05	-0,20	2,21	3,56	296
20	5	0	0	2,20	-0,56	2,41	1,90	314
21	6	0	0	-0,89	-0,27	1,71	2,37	361
Sum	138	17	31					7573

additional false propagation results were identified in a few slices and necessary to manually correct. In summary, 31 outliers are corrected manually after the fully automatic propagation. These outliers occurred due to image artifacts, CCT range limitations or crucial superior-interior displacements of a vertebral body.

4 Conclusion

A multiplicity of non-rigid L and AP displacements along the spinal cord are observed (see Fig. 3). For this reason, patient positioning after rigid image registration can remain insufficient for head and neck cases in radiation therapy treatment. Single non-rigid displacements could eventually cause serious adverse effects when the spinal cord extends high radiation dose volumes. In particular, when target volumes and spinal cord are located in close proximity to each other. It is therefore considered to apply elastic image registration algorithms in this body region [5, 6, 7] instead of rigid ones. Elastic image registration

Fig. 3. One head and neck case with severe non-rigid displacements of the spinal cord in AP direction – along the longitudinal axis.

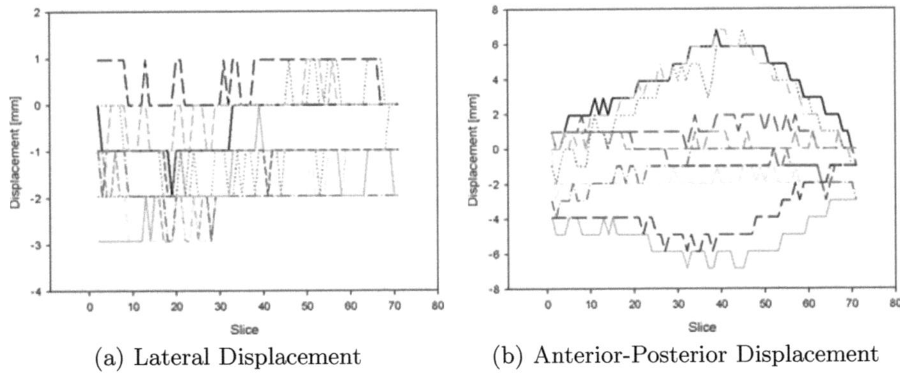

(a) Lateral Displacement (b) Anterior-Posterior Displacement

eventually can reveal non-rigid displacements of the spinal cord and help to correct them. An other strategy could be to apply spine segmentation [8] to detect displacements at an early stage and correct them if necessary, too.

References

1. Schlegel W, Mahr A. 3D conformal radiation therapy. Berlin Heidelberg New York: Springer Verlag; 2001. A multimedia introduction to methods and techniques.
2. Hysing LB, Skorpen TN, Alber M, et al. Influence of organ motion on conformal vs. intensity-modulated pelvic radiotherapy for prostate cancer. Int J Radiat Oncol Biol Phys. 2009;71(5):1496–503.
3. Moser T, Biederer J, Nill S, et al. Detection of respiratory motion in fluoroscopic images for adaptive radiotherapy. Phys Med Biol. 2008;53(12):3129–45.
4. Maintz JB, Viergever MA. A survey of medical image registration. Med Image Anal. 1998;2(1):1–36.
5. Li P, Malsch U, Bendl R. Combination of intensity-based image registration with 3D simulation in radiation therapy. Phys Med Biol. 2008;53(17):4621–4637.
6. Malsch U, Thieke C, Bendl R. Fast elastic registration for adaptive radiotherapy. Comput Assist Interv. 2006;9(2):612–9.
7. Floca RO, Metzner R, Wirtz CR, et al. Entwicklung und Optimierung eines elastischen Registrierungsverfahrens für CTA und RA Daten. Procs BVM. 2008; p. 133–137.
8. Klinder T, Wolz R, Lorenz C, et al. Spine segmentation using articulated shape models. Proc MICCAI. 2008; p. 227–234.

Semi-automatic Epileptic Hot Spot Detection in ECD Brain SPECT Images

Laszlo Papp, Maaz Zuhayra, Eberhard Henze

Department of Radiology and Nuclear Medicine, UK-SH Campus Kiel, Kiel, Germany
lpapp@nuc-med.uni-kiel.de

Abstract. A method is proposed to process ECD brain SPECT images representing epileptic hot spots inside the brain. For validation 35 ictal - interictal patient image data were processed. The images were registered by a normalized mutual information method, then the separation of the suspicious and normal brain areas were performed by two threshold-based segmentations. Normalization between the images was performed by local normal brain mean values. Based on the validation made by two medical physicians, minimal human intervention in the segmentation parameters was necessary to detect all epileptic spots and minimize the number of false spots inside the brain.

1 Introduction

Epileptic foci detection is a major field in neuroimaging which is mostly performed by obtaining and comparing an ictal and an interictal ECD brain SPECT image about the patient representing an epileptic event and a normal stage of the brain respectively [1]. Since these images are never acquired at the same time, registration between them is necessary, as well as the normalization of them, due to the different dose and biological uptake represented by these images. While registering the image pairs is generally performed with a high confidence [2], normalization methods can strongly affect the result of the ictal-interictal subtraction [3], since they can erase existing hot spots or generate false positive ones. By the other hand even if the chosen normalization method is desired, the subtraction image might represent positive false spots where a non-epileptic normal brain region was brighter in the ictal image than in the interictal one (Fig. 1). Our goal was to develop a program representing our method for detecting true hot spots and minimizing positive false spots by performing local normalization inside the brain only at epileptic suspicious areas.

2 Materials and methods

2.1 Patient data

35 epileptic ictal-interictal ECD brain SPECT patient were identified in the Picture Archiving and Communication System (PACS) of our clinic and their raw

image pairs were collected. The raw data were reconstructed by Geometric Mean (GMA) iterative reconstruction. Conversion of the reconstructed images to Analyze format was performed for being compatible with our program implemented in IDL 7.0

2.2 Image registration

Both ictal and interictal images were duplicated, and the grey values of the copied images were down sampled between 0 and 255. For similarity measurement the normalized mutual information (NMI) cost function was calculated [4] in the auto registration algorithm (equation 1). For function minimization Downhill-Simplex method was applied with functional tolerance 0.0001 [5]. The byte scaled ictal A image was the reference of the registration and the byte scaled interictal image B was transformed to find the desired transformation parameters. A rigid transformation (shifting and rotation) determined by the auto registration was performed between the original images to superimpose them.

$$\frac{(H(A) + H(B))}{H(A,B)} \tag{1}$$

Where $H(A)$ is the Shannon entropy [4] of the image A, and $H(A,B)$ is the Shannon entropy of the joint probabilities of images A and B.

2.3 Normalization and hot spot detection

Two default threshold values were determined for both A and B images (lowThresh$_A$, highThresh$_A$ and lowThresh$_B$, highThresh$_B$). The low and high thresh values were 40% [3] and 75% of the maximum value of the corresponding image. All voxels in image A higher than highThresh$_A$ were marked as epileptic-suspicious areas (ESA_A). All voxels between the corresponding lowThresh and

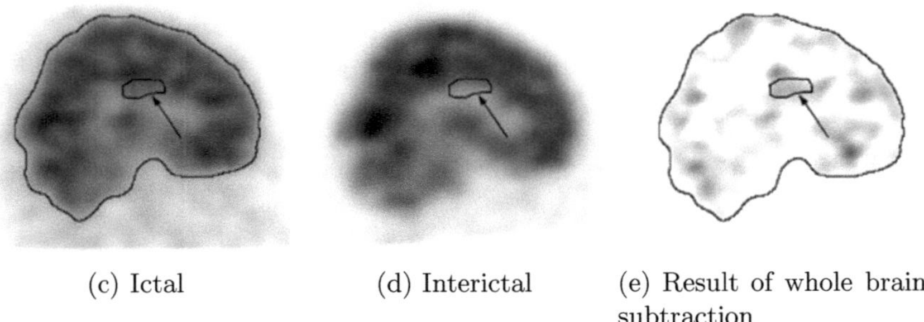

(c) Ictal (d) Interictal (e) Result of whole brain subtraction

Fig. 1. Sagittal slices of a whole brain subtraction example. The region signed by arrows represents a normal brain area in the ictal image (a). Relatively it has a lower uptake in the interictal image (b) which produces a positive false spot on the subtraction (c).

highThresh values were marked as normal brain activity areas in both images (NBA_A, NBA_B). The mean values (M_A and M_B) of NBA_A and NBA_B were computed for both images respectively. For all v_A ictal voxel values inside ESA_A a weighting for the given v_A voxel value was determined based on equation 2:

$$\left(\frac{v_A - \text{highThresh}_A}{M_A} - \frac{v_B - \text{highThresh}_B}{M_B}\right) * v_A \tag{2}$$

where v_A and v_B were ictal and interictal voxel values respectively at positions defined by ESA_A region in both brain images. In the result image all negative values were modified to 0.

2.4 Visualization

A binary image from the ictal image based on lowThresh_A was generated, where all values higher than lowThresh_A were modified to 1, other values were modified to 0. A morphological gradient was performed on the binary image to generate a one voxel thick boundary [6]. The result of the hot spot detection was merged with the boundary image for better visualization and hot spot localization.

2.5 Validation

Validation was done by two medical physicians independently. The transformation parameters given by the NMI auto registration was validated in the first step by visual assessment. Modification of the auto-determined transformation parameters was provided to allow necessary corrections. Every manual correction in the NMI transformation parameters was recorded for further registration error analysis. To validate the correctness of the default threshold values the manual threshold modification was provided in the program. For better foci localization the ictal-interictal image pairs, the classic subtraction of them and the result of our method was represented in parallel (Fig. 2).

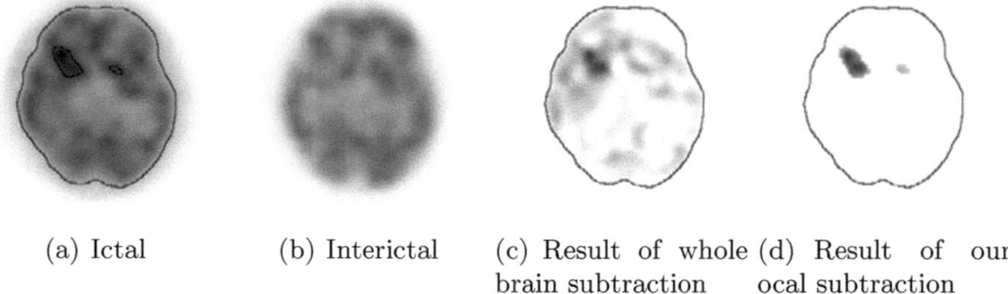

(a) Ictal (b) Interictal (c) Result of whole brain subtraction (d) Result of our ocal subtraction

Fig. 2. Comparison of the whole brain subtraction (c) with our method (d) on axial slices. Our local filtered result (d) represents hop spots only inside area defined by highThresh_A.

3 Results

The average registration error was 1.2 mm of shifting and 0.37 degrees of rotation. Modification of the auto registration-given transformation parameters was necessary in 2 cases, where the misregistrations were between 2-4 mm for translation and 1-3 degrees for rotation. Modification of the threshold values was necessary in 7 cases of the input images, hence the default threshold values were correct in 80% of the patient image pairs. Due to the possibility of the threshold value modifications it was possible to detect all epileptic foci of all patients.

4 Conclusion

The most trivial way of detecting hop spots inside the brain is subtracting the interictal image from the ictal one, although this step generates many false positive spots in the subtraction hence the multiple examination of the subtraction and ictal image is necessary. Since our method excludes the normal brain area from the visualization by building on the fact that hotspots always have a high activity, the number of false positive hot spots occurrences in the result is minimized. Due to the possibility of modifying the threshold values our tool is flexible enough to generate a specific result for all the patients. Our normalization step operates with local brain values instead of global ratios between the images. Due to the local normalization the global grey value stretching of the images is avoided which would not lead to a sophisticated normalization [2]. The clinical evaluation of our method is still under investigation, since higher number of inputs is needed, although based on our present 35 patient data the first results show that our program may become a useful tool for epileptic patient investigations.

References

1. Koo CW, Devinsky O, Hari K, et al. Stratifying differences on ictal/interictal subtraction SPECT images. Epilepsia. 2003;44(3):379–386.
2. Radau PE, Slomka PJ, Julin P, et al. Evaluation of linear registration algorithms for brain SPECT and the errors due to hypoperfusion lesions. Med Phys. 2001;28:1660–1668.
3. Boussion N, Houzard C, Ostrowsky K, et al. Automated detection of local normalization areas for ictal-interictal brain SPECT. J Nucl Med. 2002;43(11):1419–1425.
4. Pluim JPW, Maintz JBA, Viergever MA. Mutual-information-based registration of medical images: A survey. IEEE Trans Med Imaging. 2003;22(8):986–1004.
5. Bernon JL, Mariano-Goulart D, Zanca A. A comparative study of Powell's and Downhill simplex algorithms for a fast multimodal surface matching in brain imaging. Comput Med Imaging Graph. 2001;25(4):287–297.
6. Peng J, Rusch PH, Herrmann T, et al. Morphological filters and edge detection application to medical imaging. Procs IEEE EMBS. 1991;13:251–252.

Vollautomatische Einzelzellerkennung auf fluoreszenten Gewebeschnitten humaner Epidermis

Thora Pommerencke[1], Hartmut Dickhaus[1], Niels Grabe[1]

[1]Institut für Medizinische Biometrie und Informatik, Universitätsklinikum Heidelberg
thora.pommerencke@med.uni-heidelberg.de

Kurzfassung. Wir stellen hier ein vollautomatisches Verfahren zur Einzelzellerkennung auf fluoreszenten Gewebeschnitten humaner Epidermis vor. Das Ziel dieser Arbeit war es, Expressionsverschiebungen von beispielsweise Zellmembran zu Nucleus detektieren zu können. Diese können bei pathologischen Veränderungen des Gewebes auftreten. Im Vergleich zu anderen existierenden Segmentierungen werden hier die Zellgrenzen in einem kombinierten Ansatz sowohl auf Basis einer Membranfärbung als auch anhand detektierter Zellkerne mittels Watershed ermittelt. Wir konnten zeigen, dass wir mit unserem Verfahren eine Membranfärbung deutlich von einer Zellkernfärbung unterscheiden können. Somit ermöglicht die von uns entwickelte Einzelzellerkennung eine Detektion von Translokationen in der Expression.

1 Einleitung

Die Unterscheidung von pathologisch verändertem und gesundem Gewebe geschieht meist anhand geeigneter Biomarker, mit denen ein Gewebe angefärbt wird. In [1] wurde bereits gezeigt, wie die Proteinexpression in einem fluoreszent gefärbten Gewebeschnitt räumlich, vollautomatisch und quantitativ vermessen werden kann. Hierbei wurde jedoch bisher die subzelluläre Lokalisation der Expression vernachlässigt. Pathologische Veränderungen im Gewebe können sich jedoch auch in einer Verschiebung des Expressionsmusters innerhalb der Zelle widerspiegeln [2]. Ohne diese subzelluläre Auflösung könnten daher wichtige Informationen verloren gehen.

Die uns bekannten Einzelzellerkennungen auf epithelialen Geweben sind entweder nur semiautomatisch [3] oder approximieren die Zellgrenzen anhand der Lokalisation der Zellkerne über Voronoi oder Watershed [4]. Letztere Verfahren bieten nicht die von uns gewünschte Genauigkeit für eine subzelluläre Expressionsanalyse. Vor diesem Hintergrund haben wir eine vollautomatische Zellerkennung mit Detektion der Zellkerne auf fluoreszent gefärbten Gewebeschnitten entwickelt, welche die Zellgrenzen auf Basis einer Membranfärbung detektiert.

2 Material und Methoden

2.1 Färbung

Experimentell wurden Schnitte cryokonservierter in vitro Hautkulturen (EFT, Mattek) über eine fluoreszente Dreifachfärbung angefärbt. Dabei wurden die Zellmembranen mittels eines Antikörpers gegen E-Cadherin über indirekte Immunfluoreszenz mit Alexa 488 (grün) und die Zellkerne direkt chemisch mit DAPI (Diamidinophenylindol) blau gefärbt. Der später zu untersuchende Biomarker wurde über indirekte Immunfluoreszenz mittels Alexa 594 (rot) gekennzeichnet.

2.2 Bildakquise

Die Bildakquise erfolgte mithilfe des Hamamatsu NanoZoomer Digital Pathology (NDP) System in einer Auflösung von 0,23 μm/Pixel (40x Vergrößerung) und in drei Ebenen, d.h. Z-Höhen, in einem Abstand von jeweils 2 μm. Abbildung 1 zeigt exemplarisch einen Bildausschnitt aufgenommen mit 40x Vergrößerung.

2.3 Bildanalyse

Die zu untersuchenden Gewebebereiche wurden entweder automatisch oder manuell aus einem Übersichtsbild selektiert. Für die nachfolgenden Analysen wurde für jeden Farbkanal jeweils diejenige Bildebene aus dem Z-Stapel ausgewählt, bei der die gefärbten Strukturen die größte Schärfe aufwiesen. Diese kann je nach Bildregion unterschiedlich sein. Auf jedem der extrahierten Teilbilder erfolgte dann die Einzelzellerkennung, welche sich in drei größere Analyseblöcke unterteilen lässt: die Erkennung des Epithels, die Detektion der Zellkerne und schließlich die Segmentierung der einzelnen Zellen. Alle drei Blöcke werden im Folgenden nun kurz beschrieben.

Für die Segmentierung des Epithels wurde zunächst der Kontrast im Bild der Membranfärbung mit einer Intensitätsanpassung und adaptiver Histogrammangleichung erhöht. Anschließend erfolgte die automatische Segmentierung anhand der Membranfärbung über ein Schwellwertverfahren und morphologische Operationen wie „Schließen“ und „Öffnen“. Zur Performanzsteigerung erfolgte dieser Schritt bei einer Vergrößerung von 10x.

Die Detektion der Zellkerne erfolgte nach Kontrasterhöhung über ein iteratives und adaptives Schwellwertverfahren und anschließender Watershedtransformation bei einer Vergrößerung von 20x. Über einen Größenfilter wurden Cluster von Zellen identifiziert, auf denen zur Trennung der Zellen eine Watershedtransformation auf Basis lokaler Maxima durchgeführt wurde. Potentielle Artefakte wurden mittels Diskriminanzanalyse anhand zuvor ermittelter Erwartungswerte für Merkmale wie Fläche, Rundheit, Rauheit, Kontrast und Kompaktheit ausgeschlossen.

Die Zellgrenzen wurden bei einer Vergrößerung von 40x auf dem Bild der Membranfärbung ermittelt. Hierbei kam eine weitere Watershedtransformation zum Einsatz. Die Schwierigkeit bei der Ermittlung der Zellgrenzen besteht insbesondere darin, dass bei den uns vorliegenden Schnittbildern starke Überlagerungen der Zellstrukturen auftraten und einige Zellen im Präparat nicht in ihrer Mitte durchgeschnitten, sondern entlang ihrer Oberfläche geschnitten wurden. In diesem Fall ist anstelle einer gefärbten Zellkontur eine gefärbte Fläche zu sehen, welche für die Anwendung der Watershedtransformation ungeeignet ist. Daher wurden Minima nicht nur in der Ebene gesucht, die im Mittel das schärfste Bild zeigt, sondern auch in der darüber und darunter liegenden, da eine flächig gefärbte Zelle in einer anderen Ebene evtl. als Kontur zu sehen ist. Anschließend wurden die Minima aus allen Ebenen sowie die detektierten Zellkerne zu einer Maske vereint und mit dieser das Bild der Membranfärbung so durch morphologische Rekonstruktion modifiziert, dass regionale Minima nur in den Maskenbereichen vorlagen bzw. dort erzwungen wurden. Auf diesem veränderten Bild der Membranfärbung wurden schließlich die Zellgrenzen mittels einer letzten Watershedtransformation ermittelt. Zellflächen außerhalb des zu erwartenden Größenbereichs wurden verworfen.

Alle Algorithmen zur Bildanalyse der digitalisierten Schnitte wurden mithilfe von Matlab R2008a unter Verwendung der Image Processing Toolbox entwickelt.

3 Ergebnisse

Für die Validierung der Zellsegmentierung wurde die Anzahl manuell segmentierter Zellen mit der detektierten Anzahl von Zellen verglichen. Bei der auto-

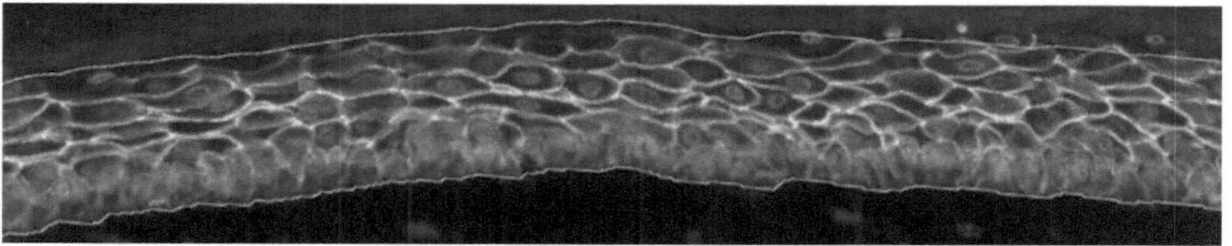

(a) Segmentierung des Epithels

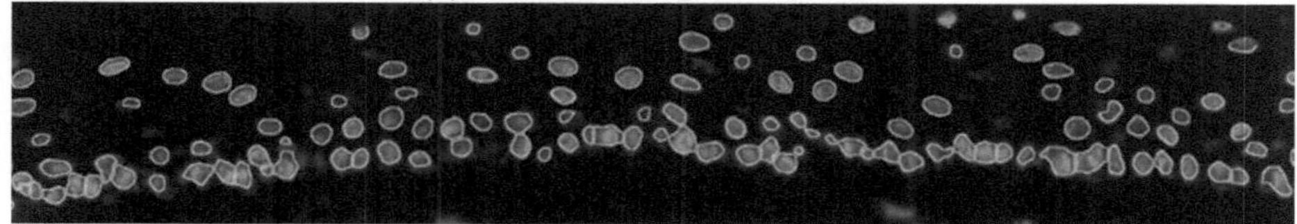

(b) Detektion der Zellkerne

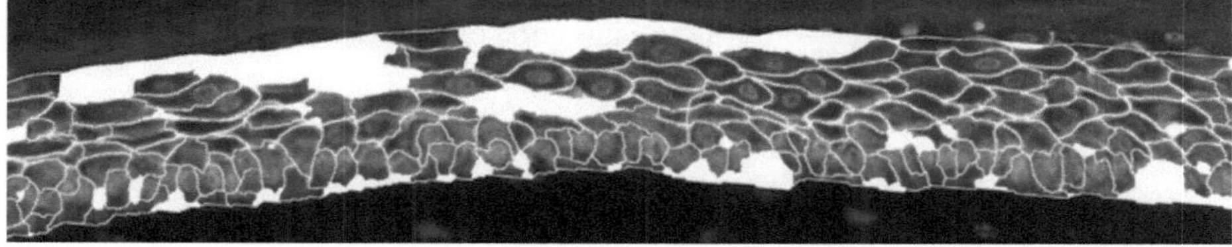

(c) Segmentierung der Zellen

Abb. 1. Ablauf der Segmentierung

matischen Zellsegmentierung wurden statt 277 Zellen 297 Zellen (d.h. eine Übersegmentierung von ca. 7%) ermittelt. Weiterhin wurde getestet, ob es mit dieser Segmentierung möglich ist, eine membranständige Färbung von einer Zellkernfärbung zu unterscheiden. Für diesen Test wurde für 1150 Zellen das Verhältnis der mittleren Färbungsintensität im betrachteten Kompartiment (Nucleus bzw. Membran) zur Färbungsintensität der Gesamtzelle berechnet. Für die Zellkernfärbung wurde ein Verhältnis von 3,3 für Nucleus zu Zelle und 0,7 für Membran zu Zelle berechnet. Und für die Membranfärbung ein Verhältnis von 0,9 für Nucleus zu Zelle und 1,4 für Membran zu Zelle ermittelt. Ein exemplarisches Segmentierungsergebnis ist in Abbildung 2 zu sehen.

4 Diskussion

Das Ziel dieser Arbeit war die Entwicklung einer Einzelzellerkennung auf fluoreszent gefärbten Gewebeschnitten, um subzelluläre Kompartimente voneinander unterscheiden zu können. Als eine wichtige Anwendung sei hier die Translokation der Expression von ß-Catenin von der Membran in den Zellkern im Frühstadium des Colon-Karzinoms genannt, welche nur über eine subzelluläre Expressionsanalyse sichtbar wird.

Der Vergleich des von uns entwickelten Verfahrens mit der manuellen Segmentierung zeigt nur eine Übersegmentierung von knapp 7%, welche hauptsächlich darauf zurückzuführen ist, dass bei der manuellen Segmentierung in unklaren Fällen keine Kontur gezeichnet wurde, während die automatische Segmentierung immer nach einer Lösung sucht.

Die von uns durchgeführte Expressionsanalyse zeigt, dass mit der automatischen Zellsegmentierung eine membranständige Expression deutlich von einer Expression im Zellkern unterschieden werden kann. Es scheint daher hinreichend für eine vollautomatische Analyse subzellulärer Expressionsverschiebungen zwischen den Kompartimenten Zellkern, Membran und Cytoplasma geeignet. Im Vergleich zu den uns bekannten Segmentierungsverfahren, welche die Zellgrenzen anhand der Lokalisation der Zellkerne z.B. durch Voronoi-Graphen setzen, ist bei uns eine weitaus höhere Genauigkeit zu erwarten, da wir uns direkt an den Membranen orientieren. Weiterhin können wir auch bei einer lückenhaften Zellkernverteilung robuste Ergebnisse liefern. Die ersten hier beschriebenen Ergebnisse der Segmentierung wurden auf Gefrierschnitten durchgeführt. Insbesondere durch Verwendung dünner präparierbarer histologischer Schnitte aus Paraffineingebettetem Gewebe erwarten wir noch erheblich klarere Membranstrukturen. Das vorgestellte Verfahren sollte dann eine noch erheblich verbesserte Detektion der Zellgrenzen zeigen.

Literaturverzeichnis

1. Grabe N, Pommerencke T, Steinberg T, et al. Reconstructing protein networks of epithelial differentiation from histological sections. Bioinformatics. 2007;23:3200–3208.
2. Kobayashi M, Honma T, Matsuda Y, et al. Nuclear translocation of beta-catenin in colorectal cancer. Br J Cancer. 2000;82:1689–1693.
3. Baggett D, Nakaya M, McAuliffe M, et al. Whole cell segmentation in solid tissue sections. Cytometry. 2005;67:137–43.
4. Landini G, Othman I. Estimation of tissue layer level by sequential morphological reconstruction. J Microscopy. 2002;209:118–125.

Robuste Verzweigungserkennung von Gefäßen in CTA-Datensätzen zur modellbasierten Extraktion der Centerline

Thomas Beck[1,2], Dominik Fritz[2], Christina Biermann[2,3], Rüdiger Dillmann[1]

[1]Institut für Technische Informatik ITEC, Universität Karlsruhe (TH)
[2]Siemens Healthcare, Forchheim
[3]Abteilung für Diagnostische und Interventionelle Radiologie, Eberhard-Karls-Universität Tübingen
thomas.beck.ext@siemens.com

Kurzfassung. Bei der Befundung und Visualisierung von Blutgefäßen ist deren Centerline von zentraler Bedeutung. Die Unterscheidung zwischen unverzweigten Abschnitten des Gefäßes und Verzweigungsbereichen ermöglicht den Einsatz spezialisierter und sehr effizienter Algorithmen zur modellbasierten Extraktion der Centerline. In diesem Artikel wird ein robustes Verfahren zur Verzweigungserkennung vorgestellt. Das Verfahren beruht auf einem Front-Propagation-Ansatz mit dynamisch angepassten Schwellwerten und einer anschließenden Clusteranalyse. Die vorgestellte Methode zur Verzweigungserkennung wurde als Komponente einer Architektur zur Extraktion der Centerline auf handannotierten Datensätzen getestet. Erste Ergebnisse sind sehr vielversprechend und ermöglichen auch bei pathologischen Gefäßen eine robuste Detektion von Gefäßverzweigungen.

1 Einleitung

Erkrankungen des Blutkreislaufs gehören zu den am weitesten verbreiteten Krankheiten in den Industrienationen. So starben alleine in Deutschland im Jahr 2001 insgesamt 290.000 Personen an Erkrankungen des Herz-Kreislauf-Systems und davon knapp 14.000 Personen an Atherosklerose [1]. Daher sind zuverlässige Diagnose-Systeme und eine Verbesserung bestehender Verfahren von großer Bedeutung.

Moderne Mehrschicht-CT-Scanner sind in der Lage, hochauflösende Abbildungen des menschlichen Körpers zu erstellen. Zur verbesserten Darstellung des Gefäßapparates wird dem Patienten Kontrastmittel appliziert. Durch die kontrastierte Abbildung wird eine automatische Segmentierung der Gefäße ermöglicht.

Die robuste Extraktion der Centerline von Gefäßen bildet die Grundlage zahlreicher Visualisierungen und ermöglicht eine präzise Vermessung zur quantitativen Gefäßuntersuchung. Durch den Einsatz modellbasierter Verfahren und die hierdurch ermöglichte Verwendung von Hintergrundwissen zur Bestimmung der

Centerline, lässt sich die Robustheit der Berechnung verbessern [2]. Eine differenzierte Modellierung von Verzweigungen erfordert eine zuverlässige Detektion verzweigter, beziehungsweise unverzweigter Abschnitte. In der Literatur finden sich hierfür verschiedene Verfahren, so untersuchen Flasque et al. die Durchstoßbereiche des Gefäßes durch eine lokale Bounding-Box [3]. Ein auf Region-Growing basierendes Verfahren auf MRT-Daten, das als Motivation des hier vorgestellten Verfahrens dient, beschreiben Eiho et al. [4]. Allerdings wird die Methode mit dem Ziel eingesetzt, den gesamten Gefäßbaum in einer Schädel-MRT zu segmentieren. Die benötigte Laufzeit von 5 Minuten verhindert jedoch den praktischen Einsatz der vorgeschlagenen Implementierung. In diesem Beitrag werden neben einer deutlichen Reduktion erforderlicher Zusammenhangsanalysen weitere Verbesserungen zur Erhöhung der Robustheit des Verfahrens von Eiho vorgestellt.

Eine effiziente Architektur zur modellbasierten Bestimmung der Centerline, in der das vogestellte Verfahren integriert ist, beschreiben Beck et al. [5]. Iterative Segmentierungsverfahren dieser Art stellen das beabsichtigte Einsatzgebiet des hier vorgestellten Verfahrens zur Verzweigungserkennung dar.

2 Material und Methoden

Vor der Untersuchung eines Gefäßabschnitts auf eine vorliegende Verzweigung werden lokale Schwellwerte bestimmt. Hierdurch fließen lokale Informationen über die Homogenität des Hintergrunds bzw. des Vordergrunds ein, wodurch die Robustheit des Verfahrens verbessert wird. So wird beispielsweise erzielt, dass das anschließend durchgeführte Front-Propagation-Verfahren deutlich seltener in Umgebungsstrukturen ausläuft. Das vorgeschlagene Verfahren besteht aus zwei Schritten, der dynamischen Schwellwertanpassung und der anschließenden Untersuchung eines Gefäßabschnitts durch das Front-Propagation-Verfahren.

2.1 Dynamische Schwellwertanpassungen

Die Schwellwertanpassung verwendet ein lokales Histogramm, berechnet aus der aktuell zu untersuchenden Umgebung. Mit Hilfe eines Maximum-Likelihood-

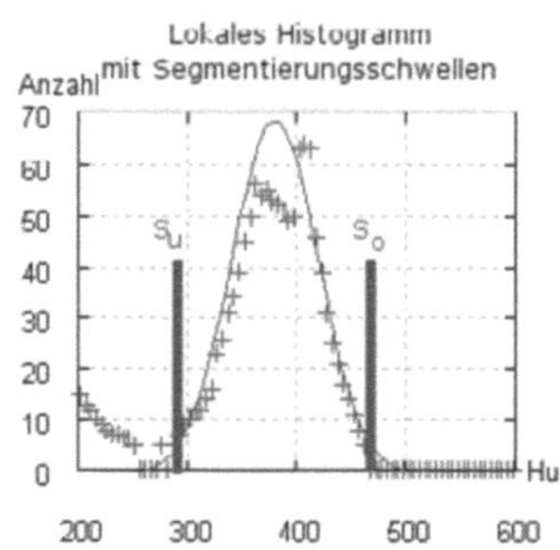

Abb. 1. Lokales Histogramm mit berechneter Normalverteilung und daraus extrahierten Schwellwerten s_u und s_o für die Segmentierung

Schätzers wird, wie in Abb. 1 dargestellt, eine Gaußkurve in das Histogramm eingepasst. Hierzu wird die Likelihood-Funktion aus Gl. 1 aufgestellt und, wie in Gl. 2 angegeben, deren Maximum bestimmt. Eine Beschränkung auf typische Histogrammbereiche von kontrastiertem Blut ermöglicht die vereinfachte Histogrammuntersuchung durch eine Normalverteilung (Abb. 1). Von der hierdurch bestimmten Normalverteilung wird angenommen, dass sie auftretende Hounsfield-Werte von kontrastiertem Blut der aktuellen Umgebung wiederspiegelt. Für die Durchführung der Verzweigungserkennung werden daraus Schwellwerte s_u und s_o für die Segmentierung extrahiert (Gl. 3).

$$\begin{aligned} L(\mu, \sigma^2|y) &= \prod_{i=1}^{N} \left[\frac{1}{\sigma\sqrt{2\pi}} e^{-\frac{(y_i-\mu)^2}{2\sigma^2}} \right] \\ &= \left(\frac{1}{\sigma\sqrt{2\pi}} \right)^N e^{-\frac{\sum_{i=1}^{N}(y_i-\mu)^2}{2\sigma^2}} \end{aligned} \tag{1}$$

$$\Rightarrow \quad \hat{\mu} = \frac{\sum_{i=1}^{N} y_i}{N} \qquad \hat{\sigma}^2 = \frac{\sum_{i=1}^{N}(y_i - \hat{\mu})^2}{N} \tag{2}$$

$$\Rightarrow \quad s_u = \hat{\mu} - 2\hat{\sigma} \qquad s_o = \hat{\mu} + 2\hat{\sigma} \tag{3}$$

2.2 Verzweigungsdetektion innerhalb eines Gefäßabschnitts

Die zuvor extrahierten Schwellwerte bilden die Grundlage der nun folgenden Verzweigungsdetektion. In Abb. 3(a) mit Nummer “1“ markierte Voxel stellen das Ende des bereits modellierten Gefäßabschnitts dar. Ausgehend von dieser Menge an Voxeln wird das Front-Propagation-Verfahren schichtweise fortgesetzt. Nach Erreichen einer gewünschten Wachstumstiefe (Voxel mit Nummer “12“) wird eine Historie von mehreren Schichten auf Zusammenhang analysiert. Sind die äußeren Schichten zusammenhängend, so wird angenommen, dass sich im untersuchten Abschnitt keine Verzweigung befindet. Für eine robustere Verzweigungsdetektion werden extrahierte Zusammenhangskomponenten im Folgenden noch weiter untersucht.

Neben der Untersuchung einer Historie von Schichten wurde das Verfahren zur Erhöhung der Robustheit um zwei weitere Bedingungen erweitert. Zum Einen wird eine Mindestanzahl an Voxeln gefordert, damit eine extrahierte Zusammenhangskomponente als abzweigendes Gefäß erkannt wird. Zum Anderen ist ein Mindestabstand zwischen benachbarten Zusammenhangskomponenten (single linkage distance) erforderlich.

Zur Durchführung von Tests wurden 18 manuell annotierte CTA-Datensätzen verschiedener Körperregionen verwendet. Es handelte sich um Aufnahmen von Patienten, bei denen Stenosen, Aneurysmen oder auch Kalzifizierungen diagnostiziert wurden. Darüber hinaus waren in zwei Datensätzen deutliche sichtbare, strahlenförmige Bildartefakte durch Zahnimplantate enthalten. Das Verfahren dieses Beitrags wurde innerhalb der MeVisLab-Plattform [6] entwickelt und auch getestet.

Abb. 2. Untersuchung eines Gefäßabschnitts mit dem Front-Propagation-Verfahren. Die Zusammenhangsanalyse der äußeren Wachstumsschicht detektiert eine Verzweigung (a). Durch Verwendung einer Historie von Schichten können fehlerhaft detektierte Gefäßverzweigungen vermieden werden (b).

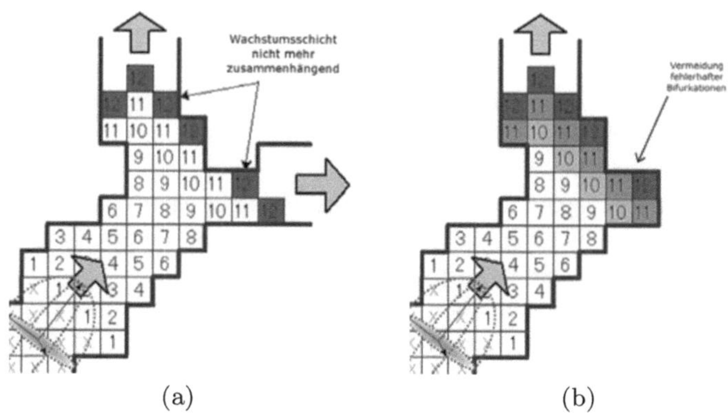

3 Ergebnisse

In Abb. 3 werden exemplarische Ergebnisse der Verzweigungserkennung dargestellt. Wird für die Zusammenhangsanalyse ausschließlich die äußere Schicht der Front-Propagation betrachtet, so ist das Verfahren sehr sensibel gegenüber Störungen. Diese können durch Unebenheiten der Gefäßwand, beziehungsweise Kalzifikationen oder Bildartefakte hervorgerufen werden.
Die Anzahl falsch positiv klassifizierter Verzweigungen lässt sich durch die Betrachtung mehrerer Schichten besonders im Bereich von Kalzifikationen sehr stark verringern. Die dynamische Anpassung der Schwellwerte wirkt sich bei

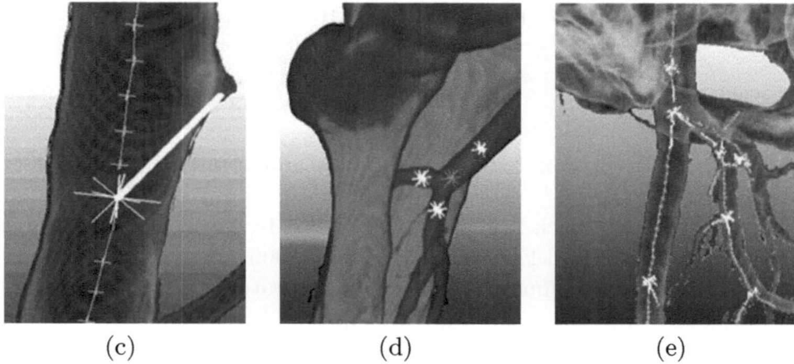

Abb. 3. Durch ausschließliche Betrachtung der äußeren Wachstumsschicht ist das Verfahren sehr sensibel (c). Für einen untersuchten Gefäßabschnitt liefert das Verfahren den Verzweigungsschwerpunkt und Centerlinepunkte angrenzender Gefäße (d). Der Einsatz des Verfahrens in einer modellbasierten Architektur zur Centerline-Extraktion ermöglicht eine Untersuchung des gesamten Gefäßbaums (e).

ungleichmäßiger Kontrastierung der Gefäße und in direkter Nähe zu Knochen positiv auf die Robustheit aus.

4 Diskussion

In diesem Beitrag wurde ein robustes Verfahren zur Detektion von Gefäßverzweigungen vorgestellt. Durch die Erweiterung eines Front-Propagation-Ansatzes mit einer dynamischen Schwellwertanpassung kann der Ansatz erfolgreich auf verschiedenen Bildern eingesetzt werden. Insbesondere bei der Untersuchung langer Gefäßabschnitte wie beispielsweise in RunOffs, aber auch wenn sich das Gefäß in direkter Nähe von schwer zu differenzierenden Bildbereichen befindet, lassen sich dadurch deutlich robustere Ergebnisse erzielen.

Bei der Detektion von Verzweigungen erweist sich eine ausschließliche Betrachtung der äußeren Wachstumsschicht als zu fehleranfällig (Abb. 3(c)). Die Robustheit des Verfahrens lässt sich durch vorgeschlagene Erweiterungen verbessern. Lediglich bei der Untersuchung dünner Gefäße werden hierdurch teilweise schlechtere Ergebnisse erzielt.

Bei der Bewertung der Testfälle erwiesen sich die Schwerpunkte der Zusammenhangskomponenten als zuverlässige Centerlinepunkte der angrenzenden Gefäße (Abb. 3d). Diese Beobachtung ist kein direkter Bestandteil der Verzweigungserkennung, jedoch lassen sich diese zusätzlichen Informationen für die Initialisierung der weiteren Gefäßsegmentierung verwenden.

Die durchgeführten ersten Tests haben gezeigt, dass durch das Verfahren eine robuste Detektion von Gefäßverzweigungen bei geringer Laufzeit erreicht werden kann. Darüber hinaus lassen sich aus der Lage von Gefäßverzweigungen und angrenzenden Gefäßen Informationen extrahieren, die eine weitergehende Untersuchung des Gefäßbaums ermöglichen. Für die nähere Zukunft ist es geplant, diese Komponente als Teil einer größeren Architektur zur Segmentierung und Interpretation des gesamten Gefäßbaums einzusetzen. Hierzu werden zunächst weitere quantitative und qualitative Tests durchgeführt.

Literaturverzeichnis

1. World Health Organization. Health Statistics and Health Information Systems; 2008. http://www.who.int/.
2. Lesage D, Angelini E, Bloch I, et al. A Review of 3D Vessel Segmentation Techniques: Models, Features and Extraction Schemes; 2006.
3. Flasque N, Desvignes M, Constans JM, et al. Accurate detection of 3D tubular tree structures. IEEE Proc Image Process. 2000;3.
4. Eiho S, Sekiguchi H, Sugimoto N, et al. Branch-based region growing method for blood vessel segmentation. Proc ISPRS. 2004.
5. Beck T, Biermann C, Fritz D, et al. Robust model-based centerline extraction of vessels in CTA data. Proc SPIE. 2009;7259:in press.
6. MeVis Research GmbH. MeVisLab: Medical Image Processing and Visualization; 2008. http://www.mevislab.de.

Segmentierung des Femurs aus MRT-Daten mit Shape-Based Level-Sets

Claudia Dekomien[1], Martin Busch[2], Wolfram Teske[3], Susanne Winter[1]

[1]Institut für Neuroinformatik, Ruhr-Universität Bochum, 44780 Bochum,
[2] Grönemeyer Institut für Mikrotherapie, 44799 Bochum,
[3]Orthopädische Universitätsklinik, Ruhr-Universität Bochum, 44791 Bochum
Claudia.Dekomien@neuroinformatik.rub.de

Kurzfassung. Inhalt dieser Arbeit ist die Segmentierung des Femurs aus MRT-Datensätzen mit einem Shape-based Level-Set-Ansatz. Der Algorithmus besteht aus zwei Phasen, der Modellerstellung und der Segmentierungsphase. In der Segmentierungsphase wurde ein kantenbasiertes und ein auf Intensitäten basierendes Optimierungskriterium mit einander kombiniert. Für eine lokale Verbesserung des Ergebnisses wurde zusätzlich ein Laplacian Level-Set-Verfahren angewendet. Der Femur konnte mit diesem Ansatz in drei verschiedenen MRT-Sequenzen und einem Fusionsdatensatz gut segmentiert werden.

1 Einleitung

Die automatische Segmentierung anatomischer Strukturen in medizinischen Bilddaten ist in vielen Bereichen von großem Interesse. Sie kann z.B. als Basis für weitere diagnostische Verfahren wie eine automatische Gewebeklassifikation dienen, oder aber Strukturen liefern, die zur Registrierung der Daten mit anderen Daten herangezogen werden können. Wir stellen in dieser Arbeit die modellbasierte Segmentierung des Femurs in MRT-Daten vor. Die Ergebnisse der Segmentierung sollen nachfolgend als Basis für die intraoperative Registrierung der MRT-Daten mit Ultraschalldaten dienen. Dafür ist es notwendig die Knochenoberfläche aus den Daten zu extrahieren. Während dies in CT-Daten mit schwellwertbasierten Verfahren möglich ist, erweist sich diese Aufgabe in MRT-Daten als wesentlich schwieriger. Die Registrierbarkeit von CT-Daten, sowie von MRT-Daten bei halbautomatischer Segmentierung der Knochenoberfläche konnte bereits nachgewiesen werden [1, 2].

Es existiert eine Vielzahl von Arbeiten, die sich mit MRT-Segmentierung beschäftigen [3]. Augrund von lückenhaften und fehlenden Bildinformation sowie überlappenden Intensitäten verschiederner Gewebe sind einfache, schwellwertbasierte Verfahren für die Segmentierung wenig geeignet. Die erfolgreichsten Verfahren verwenden Vorwissen in Form von Modellen für die Segmentierung [4]. Aufgrund der Flexibilität ist die Level-Set-Darstellung von Modellen besonders gut geeignet [5]. Daher haben wir uns für einen Shape-based Level-Set Ansatz [6] für die Segmentierung dreidimensionaler Knochenstrukturen entschieden. Der gewählte Algorithmus wurde bereits erfolgreich zur Segmentierung einzelner Wirbel aus CT-Daten verwendet [7].

2 Material und Methode

2.1 Daten

Von Probanden wurden dreidimensionale MRT-Daten des Knies mit verschiedenen Aufnahme Sequenzen akquiriert. Es wurden ein T1-gewichteter isotroper Datensatz (T1), ein T2-gewichteter isotroper Datensatz (T2) und ein T1-gewichteter isotroper Datensatz mit Wasseranregung (T1W) aufgenommen. Aus den beiden T1 gewichteten Daten (T1 + T1W) wurde ein fusionierter Datensatz erstellt. Hierfür wurden die Grauwerte des T1-Datensatzes zu den Grauwerten des T1W-Datensatzes addiert.

Zur Erstellung des Kniemodells standen insgesamt 16 Spiral-CT-Datensätze von Patienten und Phantomen zur Verfügung.

2.2 Datenvorverarbeitung

Alle Datensätze wurden in eine isotrope Auflösung von 0.5 mm × 0.5 mm × 0.5 mm umgerechnet. Zum Ausgleich von Helligkeitsunterschieden, unter anderem aufgrund von Sensitivitätsunterschieden der Empfangsspule, wurde ein Bias Correction-Algorithmus [8] auf die MRT-Daten angewendet.

2.3 Segmentierung

Die Segmentierung des Femurs aus MRT-Daten wurde mit einem Shape-based Level-Set-Ansatz durchgeführt. Der verwendete Algorithmus basiert auf einer Modifikation der Methode von Tsai [6, 7] und besteht aus zwei Phasen, der Modellerstellung und der Segmentierungsphase.

Um ein Femur-Shape-Modell zu erstellen, wurden verschiedene Femora, mit einem halbautomatischen Schwellwertverfahren aus CT-Datensätzen segmentiert. Alle Femurobjekte wurden binarisiert und zu einander ausgerichtet. Für jedes binäre Objekt wurde eine Signed Distance Map berechnet. Aus diesen Signed Distance Maps werden entsprechend der in [6] beschriebenen Methode ein Meanshape M und k Eigenshapes E_k gebildet. Die Level-Set-Funktion L setzt sich aus M und E wie folgt zusammen:

$$L_{w,p}(\boldsymbol{x}) = M(T_p(\boldsymbol{x})) + \sum_{i=0}^{k} w_i E_i(T_p(\boldsymbol{x})). \tag{1}$$

Hierbei stellen $w = (w_0, \ldots, w_k)$ die Gewichte für die $k\,(\leq n)$ Eigenshapes und p die Parameter für die Koordinatentransformation $T_p(\boldsymbol{x})$ eines Koordinatenpunktes dar. $T_p(\boldsymbol{x})$ beschreibt eine Rotation, eine Translation und eine Skalierung.

Die Initialisierung der Startposition für die Segmentierung wurde mit einer rigiden Landmarken-Registrierung durchgeführt. Die Level-Set-Funktion $L_{w,p}$ besteht aus zwei Regionen, einer außerhalb und einer innerhalb des Objektes. Die Objektkontur wird als Zero-Level-Set bezeichnet. Die Segmentierung erfolgt durch Optimierung der Parameter p und w. Erfolgreiche Fehlerfunktion waren das kantenbasierte Optimierungskriterium:

$$E_{\text{edge}} = \sum_{i=0}^{m} f_i \text{ ,mit } f_i = \begin{cases} g_i, L_{w,p}(\boldsymbol{x}_i) = 0 \\ 0 \ , L_{w,p}(\boldsymbol{x}_i) \neq 0 \end{cases} \text{ und } g_i = \frac{1}{1 + \nabla I(\boldsymbol{x}_i)}, \tag{2}$$

wobei $\nabla I(\boldsymbol{x}_i)$ den Gradienten des zu segmentierenden MRT-Volumen I an der Stelle $\boldsymbol{x}_i = (x_1, y_i, z_i)$ darstellt, sowie das Binary-Mean-Optimierungskriterium

$$E_{\text{mean}} = -\frac{1}{2}(\mu - v). \tag{3}$$

Hierbei stellen μ und v die mittleren Grauwertintensitäten des MRT-Volumens innerhalb und außerhalb des Zero-Level-Sets dar. Die Fehlerfunktionen E_{edge} und E_{mean} wurden gleichzeitig optimiert, indem die Fehlerfunktion $E_{multi} = E_{\text{mean}}/E_{\text{edge}}$ minimiert wurde. Zur Optimierung wurde die CMA-Evolutionsstrategie [9] verwendet. Zur lokalen Verbesserung der Segmentierung wurde zusätzlich ein Laplacian Level-Set-Verfahren aus der ITK-Libary angewendet.

3 Ergebnisse

In drei unterschiedlichen MRT-Sequenzen und einem Fusionsdatensatz eines Probanden wurde der Femur segmentiert. Abbildung 1 zeigt die Segmentierungsergebnisse in allen vier Datensätzen nach der Shape-based Level-Set-Segmentierung. In Abbildung 2 sind die Segmentierungsergebnisse mit zusätzlicher lokaler

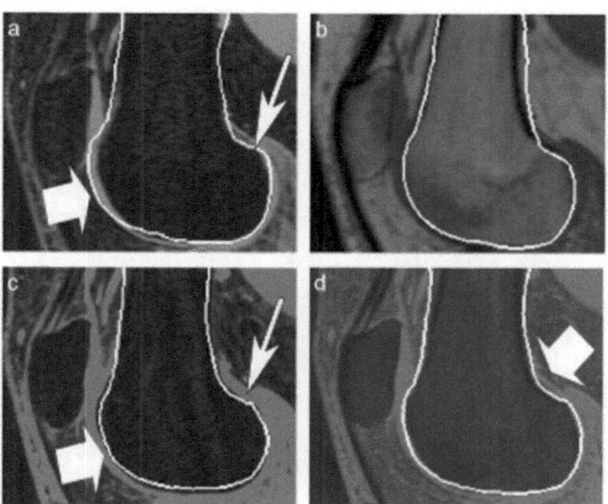

Abb. 1. Shape-based Level-Set-Segmentierung; die weiße Line repräsentiert das Segmentierungergebnis a) T2-gewichtete MRT-Sequenz b) T1-gewichtete MRT-Sequenz c) T1-gewichtete MRT-Sequenz mit Wasseranregung d) Fusionsdatensatz aus den in b) und c) dargestellten Datensätzen. Die Pfeile markieren Regionen, an denen das Segmentierungsergebnis noch nicht perfekt auf der Knochenoberfläche liegt.

Optimierung durch das Laplacian Level-Set-Verfahren dargestellt. In den Abbildungen 1 a) und c) ist deutlich zu erkennen, dass nach der Shape-based Level-Set Segmentierung der Knocherand mit dem Modell noch nicht exakt erfasst wurde. Nach der lokalen Anpassung liegt das Segmentierungsergebniss besser auf dem Knochenrand (markiert durch die dicken Pfeile) und kleine spezielle Strukturen des Knochens (markiert durch die dünnen Pfeile), die nicht im Modell enthalten sind, werden erkannt. Die Rechenzeit, auf einem Intel Core 2 Duo 2,19 GHz CPU, für die Shape-based Level-Set Segmentierung lag bei ca. 2 Minuten. Die Laplacian Level-Set Segmentierung benötigt ca. 1,5 Minuten.

4 Diskussion

Der Shape-based Level-Set-Segmentierungsalgorithmus zeigt gute Resultate bei der Segmentierung des Femurs aus allen vier MRT-Datensätzen. Mit der lokalen Anpassung der Ergebnisse durch die Laplacian Level-Set-Segmentierung konnten die Resultate noch weiter verbessert werden. Dieses lokale Verfahren führt jedoch nur zu optimalen Ergebnissen, wenn das initiale Level-Set der Form des Objektes bereits stark ähnelt. Es ist daher nich alleine einsetzbar, sondern nur als zweiter Schritt nach der modellbasierten Segmentierung.

Zusammenfassend lässt sich sagen, dass der vorgestellte Algorithmus zuverlässig den Femur aus verschiedenen Datensätzen segmentieren kann. Die Be-

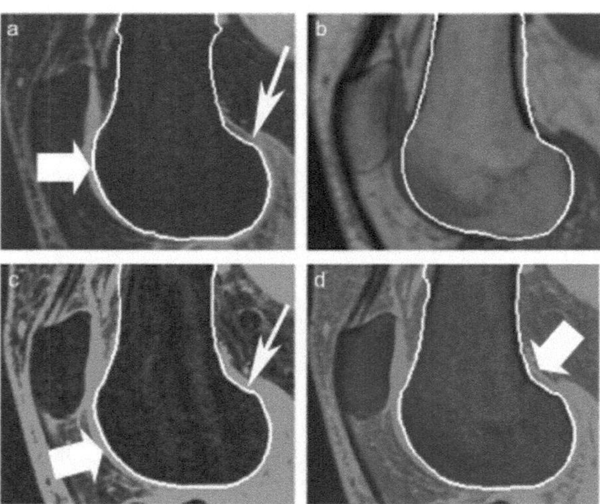

Abb. 2. Shape-based Level-Set-Segmentierung mit zusätzlicher lokaler Optimierung durch das Laplacian Level-Set-Verfahren; die weiße Line repräsentiert das Segmentierungergebnis a) T2-gewichtete MRT-Sequenz b) T1-gewichtete MRT-Sequenz c) T1-gewichtete MRT-Sequenz mit Wasseranregung d) Fusionsdatensatz aus den in b) und c) dargestellten Datensätzen. Die Pfeile markieren Stellen der Segmentierung, die sich durch die lokale Optimierung verbessert haben.

nutzerinteraktion war sehr gering und die Rechenzeit lag für präopertive Prozesse in einem vertretbaren Rahmen. Die Segmentierungsergebnisse können für MRT-Registrierungen mit verschiedenen anderen Modalitäten wie Ultraschall, CT oder auch 2D-Röntgenbildern verwendet werden. Außerdem lassen sich dreidimensionale Modelle des Femurs erstellen, die auch für eine OP-Planungen zur Verfügung stehen können.

Weitere geplante Arbeiten umfassen unter anderem eine Erweiterung des Modells um eine größere Zahl von Einzelmodellen. Dadurch können mehr Formvariationen erfasst werden. Außerdem soll im nächsten Schritt die Initialisierung der Startposition der Segmentierung mittels einer automatischen Landmarkendetektion durchgeführt werden. Das reduziert die Benutzerinteraktion weiter und trägt wesentlich zur Einsetzbarkeit des Verfahrens in der Praxis bei.

Literaturverzeichnis

1. Winter S, Brendel B, et al. Registration of CT and intraoperative 3D ultrasound images of the spine using evolutionary and gradient-based methods. IEEE Trans Evol Comput. 2008;12(3):284–296.
2. Winter S, Dekomien C, et al. Registrierung von intraoperativem 3D-Ultraschall mit präoperativen MRT-Daten für die computergestützte orthopädische Chirurgie. Z Orthopäd Unfallchir. 2007;145:586–590.
3. Fripp J, Crozier S, et al. Automatic segmentation of the bone and extraction of the bone cartilage interface from magnetic resonance images of the knee. J Comput Phys. 2007;52:1617–1631.
4. McInerney T, Terzopoulos D. Deformable models in medical image analysis: A survey. Med Image Anal. 1996;1(2):91–108.
5. Osher S, Fedkiw RP. Level set methods: An overview and some recent results. J Comput Phys. 2001;169(2):463–502.
6. Tsai A, Yezzi A, et al. A shape-based approach to the segmentation of medical imagery using level sets. IEEE Trans Med Imaging. 2003;22(2):137–154.
7. Dekomien C, Winter S. Segmentierung einzelner Wirbel in dreidimensionalen CT-Daten mit einem modelbasierten Level Set Ansatz. Biomed Tech. 2007;52.
8. Vovk U, Pernus F, et al. MRI intensity inhomogeneity correction by combining intensity and spatial information. Phys Med Biol. 2004;49(17):4119–4133.
9. Hansen N, Kern S. Evaluating the CMA evolution strategy on multimodal test functions. Parall Prob Sol Nature. 2004;3242:282–291.

Erweiterung modellbasierter Segmentierung durch lokale Deformationskriterien

Marius Erdt[1], Roman Tulchiner[1], Georgios Sakas[1,2]

[1]Abteilung Cognitive Computing & Medical Imaging, Fraunhofer IGD Darmstadt
[2]Graphisch-Interaktive Systeme, Technische Universität Darmstadt
marius.erdt@igd.fhg.de

Kurzfassung. Modellbasierte Ansätze sind heutzutage Stand der Technik zur automatischen Organsegmentierung in medizinischen Bilddatensätzen. In dieser Arbeit wird ein Verfahren vorgestellt, welches die modellbasierte Segmentierung durch lokale Deformationskriterien erweitert, um eine bessere lokale Anpassung der Oberflächenmodelle an Bildstrukturen sowohl hoher als auch niedriger Frequenz zu erreichen. Die beschriebene Methode wird anhand von Computer-Tomographie Datensätzen der Niere beschrieben und evaluiert.

1 Einleitung

Eine robuste und möglichst schnelle Segmentierung der menschlichen Organe aus Datensätzen der medizinischen Bildgebung ist nach wie vor Stand gegenwärtiger Forschung. Insbesondere in der computergestützten Strahlentherapieplanung nimmt die manuelle Konturierung von Risikoorganen und zu bestrahlenden Strukturen einen wesentlichen Zeitanteil ein. Modellbasierte Segmentierungsalgorithmen haben sich für die automatische Segmentierung von Organen bewährt, da sie durch die Verwendung eines expliziten Modells Vorwissen über die Erscheinung des Organs einbeziehen und so starke lokale Fehldeformationen verhindern können. Man unterscheidet hierbei im Wesentlichen Ansätze, die ein statistisches Formenmodell als Grundlage für die Formerhaltung verwenden (*Statistical Shape Models*, SSM), von Verfahren, welche ein einzelnes Ausgangsmodell mit explizit definierten Verformungsfunktionen einsetzen. Während SSM bspw. im Fall der Lebersegmentierung (Heimann et al. [1]) oder Herzventrikelextraktion (Zambal et al. [2], Zheng et al. [3]) erfolgreich angewendet wurden, zeigen Arbeiten von Lorenz et al. [4] und Costa et al. [5], dass sich mit explizit formbeschränkten Modellen ebenfalls gute Ergebnisse erzielen lassen. SSM haben allerdings den Nachteil, dass hochfrequente lokale Deformationen nicht trainiert werden können und somit eine Anpassung dieser Bereiche meist nicht vollständig erfolgen kann. Kainmüller et al. [6] führen daher einen free-form Segmentierungsschritt nach Anwendung der SSM aus. Das hier vorgestellte Verfahren verwendet ein einzelnes Atlasmodell als Initialisierung und kann somit auf eine Trainingsdatenbank verzichten. Zur Formerhaltung werden dabei sowohl globale als auch lokale Deformationskriterien einbezogen.

2 Material und Methoden

Als Voraussetzung für den Anpassungsalgorithmus muss zunächst ein Organmodell generiert werden. Dazu verwenden wir eine von medizinischen Experten segmentierte Version des *Male Visible Human Data Sets* [7] (s. Abb. 1(a)). Um eine möglichst gleichmäßige Gitterstruktur zu erzeugen, wird die Segmentierung resampled und anschließend mit morphologischen Operatoren geglättet (s. Abb. 1(b)). Das erzeugte Modell kann nun manuell im Datensatz platziert und bei Bedarf durch Benutzerinteraktion angepasst werden, indem das Modell durch eine 3D-Gaußfunktion in Mausbewegungsrichtung verzerrt wird. Dies verbessert insbesondere dann die Robustheit des Verfahrens, wenn die individuelle Anatomie stark vom Modell abweicht. Die Anpassung des Modells erfolgt durch Minimierung von:

$$E = E_{\text{ext}} + E_{\text{int}}, \tag{1}$$

wobei die interne Energie

$$E_{\text{int}} = \sum_i w_i \sum_{j \in N(i)} \left((p_i - p_j) - T(m_i - m_j)\right)^2 \tag{2}$$

in Anlehnung an Lorenz et al. [4] die Formähnlichkeit aller Netzpunkte p_i zu den durch die affine Transformation T registrierten Originalmodellpunkten m_i beschreibt. $N(i)$ ist die Menge aller Nachbarn von Punkt i. Wir erweitern die interne Energie durch einen Wichtungsfaktor w_i. Dadurch kann die Formerhaltung pro Netzpunkt definiert und damit unterschiedlich starke lokale Deformationen des Modells erlaubt werden. Die externe Energie

$$E_{\text{ext}} = \sum_i \alpha_i (p_i - s_i)^2 \tag{3}$$

beschreibt den Abstand zwischen Oberflächenpunkt und detektiertem Strukturpunkt s_i und wird mit dem Faktor α_i ebenfalls pro Netzpunkt gewichtet. Zur

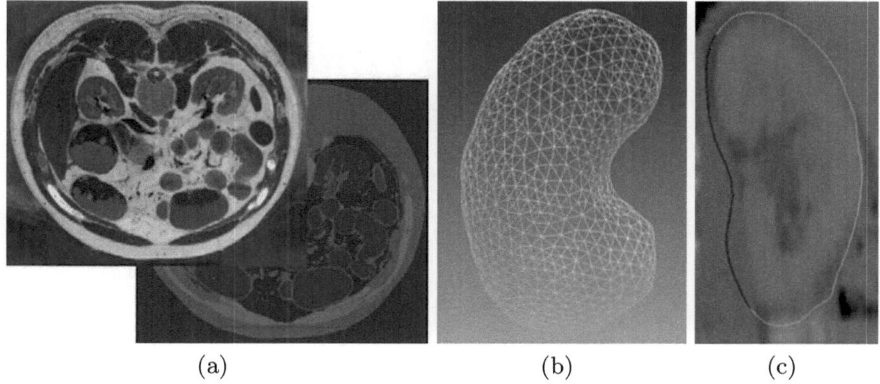

(a) (b) (c)

Abb. 1. (a) Vorsegmentierter Organatlas. (b) Erzeugtes Modell. (c) Kodierte interne Energie (Schwarz = schwache Energie, Weiß = hohe Energie).

Anpassung werden zunächst die Strukturpunkte bestimmt, indem entlang der Oberflächennormalen die stärksten Gradienten gesucht werden und der HU-Wert der Nachbarpixel überprüft wird. Kleine Abstände werden dabei bevorzugt, da die Distanz als Gewichtung in die externe Energie einfließt. Sowohl Gradientenschwelle als auch HU-Wert sind als Anpassungskriterien pro Oberflächenpunkt im Modell definiert, um das Organ von den umgebenden Nachbarsstrukturen zu unterscheiden. Gleichung (1) wird nun durch Least-Squares-Optimierung gelöst, wobei die Transformation T vorab durch Iterative-Closest-Point-Registrierung bestimmt wird.

Die Implementierung erfolgte auf Grundlage des MITK-Frameworks [8]. Zur Validierung des Verfahrens wurden insgesamt 10 CT-Datensätze der Niere mit einem Schichtabstand von 5 mm verwendet, die durch Resampling auf einen Abstand von 1 mm gebracht wurden. Bereiche hoher anatomischer Variation (Anschluss des Harnleiters, Nierenarterie/-vene) sind im Modell weniger starr definiert, als die restliche Hülle der Niere (w_i wird mit $\frac{1}{3}$ gewichtet), um eine feinere Anpassung dieser Stellen zu gewährleisten (s. Abb. 1(c)). Darüber hinaus wird die externe Energie in Bereichen geringen Kontrastes, wie dem Übergang zur Milz bzw. Leber, schwächer forciert sowie die Formerhaltungskriterien verschärft. Auf diese Weise sollen Fehldeformationen in Bereichen ähnlicher Intensität verhindert werden.

3 Ergebnisse

In Abb. 2 ist der Vorteil der lokal schwächer definierten internen Energie am Beispiel der Lunge zu sehen. Die höhere Verformbarkeit führt an diesen Stellen zu einer besseren Anpassung. Abb. 3(a) und (b) zeigen qualitativ unterschiedliche Datensätze sowie die Segmentierungsergebnisse. In Abb. 3(b) führt die lokal definierte hohe Anpassung zu einer Fehldeformation. In Tab. 1 sind die Segmentierungsergebnisse für alle getesteten Datensätze aufgeführt. Dabei wird

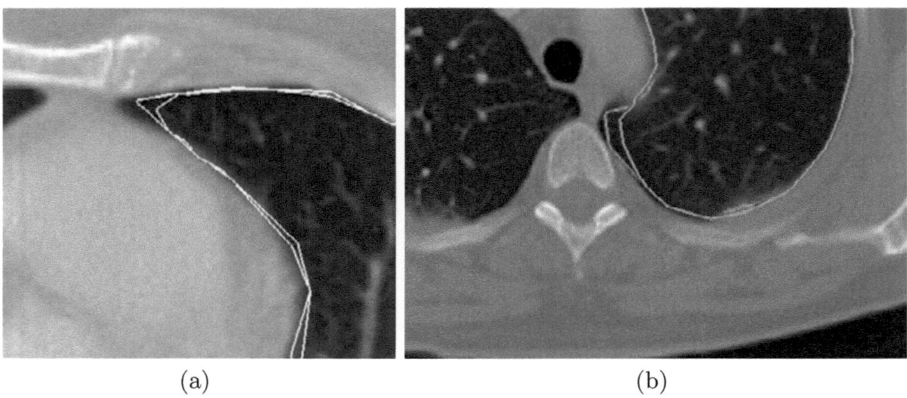

(a) (b)

Abb. 2. Anpassungsvergleich mit lokalen Deformationskriterien (äußere Kontur) und globaler Deformation (innere Kontur) am Beispiel der Lunge.

Tabelle 1. Vergleich des vorgestellten Verfahrens mit einer rein manuellen Segmentierung: Overlap, Hausdorffdistanz und Meandistanz.

Datensatz	Overlap (%)	Hausdorff distance [mm]	Directed mean distance [mm]
1	93,4128	5,91608	1
2	89,6226	4	1,44893
3	91,9572	4,24264	0,894803
4	91,6669	3,60555	1,28258
5	83,0047	4,89898	1,09193
6	93,8307	3,60555	0,640362
7	92,9281	5,38516	0,832997
8	90,9722	8,12404	1
9	94,2979	3,16228	0,545073
10	92,7521	5	0,579791

das vorgestellte Verfahren mit einer rein manuellen Segmentierung verglichen. Datensatz Nr. 5 weist eine starke Abweichung auf, da Teile des Nierenbeckens segmentiert wurden.

4 Diskussion

Die durchgeführten Tests haben gezeigt, dass eine Pro-Punkt-Definition interner und externer Energien sowie aller Anpassungskriterien die Flexibilität der Segmentierung erhöht. Der Vorteil des vorgestellten Verfahrens zeigt sich vor allem

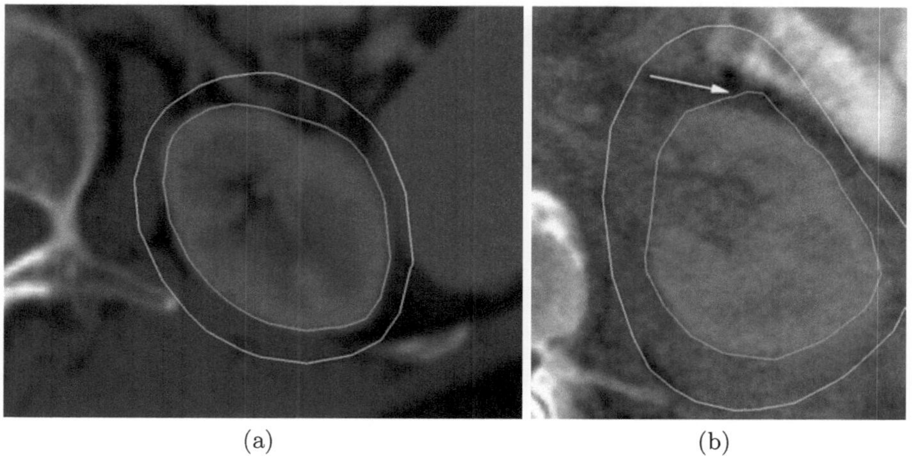

(a) (b)

Abb. 3. Initialisierung (äußere Kontur) und Endkontur (innere Kontur). (a) Anpassungsergebnis eines CT-Nierendatensatzes (3 Iterationen). (b) Zu hohe lokale Deformation zieht das Modell in Richtung eines hohen Gradienten (Pfeil) (9 Iterationen).

an anatomischen Stellen, welche erfahrungsgemäß hohe Krümmungen aufweisen. Die Anpassung kann hier genauer erfolgen und erspart somit eine manuelle Nachbesserung. Allerdings sollte das Modell insgesamt eine gewisse Starrheit behalten, da das Ergebnis sonst zu stark von der Initialisierung abhängt, was wiederum zu Fehldeformationen führen kann. Mit der erhöhten Komplexitiät, die das Verfahren mit sich bringt, steigt auch der Aufwand der Modellgenerierung an. Insbesondere im Fall der Anpassungskriterien, welche zum Teil auf den Grauwerten des Datensatzes beruhen, macht sich dies bemerkbar. Hier stellt eine automatische Bestimmung der Anpassungskriterien als Vorverarbeitung und auf Grundlage der Initialisierungsposition eine weitere Erhöhung der Robustheit des Verfahrens in Aussicht.

Literaturverzeichnis

1. Heimann T, Meinzer HP, Wolf I. A statistical deformable model for the segmentation of liver CT volumes. Procs MICCAI. 2007; p. 161–166.
2. Zambal S, Hladuvka J, Bühler K, et al. A fully automatic system for segmentation and analysis of the left and right ventricles of the heart using a bi-temporal two-component model. Int J Computer Assist Radiol Surg. 2007; p. 93–94.
3. Zhen Y, Barbu A, Georgescu B, et al. Fast automatic heart chamber segmentation from 3D CT data using marginal space learning and steerable features. Procs ICCV. 2007; p. 1–8.
4. Lorenz C, v Berg J. A comprehensive shape model of the heart. Med Image Anal. 2006;10(4):657–670.
5. Costa MJ, Delingette H, Ayache N. Automatic segmentation of the bladder using deformable models. Procs ISBI. 2007; p. 904–907.
6. Kainmüller D, Lange T, Lamecker H. Shape constrained automatic segmentation of the liver based on a heuristic intensity model. Procs MICCAI 2007 Workshop Proceedings: 3D Segmentation in the Clinic: A Grand Challenge. 2007; p. 109–116.
7. VOXEL-MAN Group. VOXEL-MAN Organ Atlas. University Medical Center Hamburg-Eppendorf.
8. Wolf I, Vetter M, Wegner I, et al. The medical imaging interaction toolkit (MITK) a toolkit facilitating the creation of interactive software by extending VTK and ITK. Procs SPIE. 2004; p. 16–27.

Individuelle Templates für Rekonstruktionen des linken Herzventrikels

Stefan Feder[1,2], Volkmar Falk[2], Matthias Gutberlet[3], Dirk Bartz[1]

[1]ICCAS, Universität Leipzig
[2]Klinik für Herzchirurgie, Herzzentrum Leipzig
[3]Abteilung für Diagnostische und Interventionelle Radiologie, Herzzentrum Leipzig
dirk.bartz@iccas.de

Kurzfassung. Bei krankhaften Vergrößerungen des linken Herzventrikels kann eine chirurgische Ventrikelrekonstruktion zur Verbesserung der Herzleistung beitragen. Die dabei erstellte Ventrikelgeometrie ist von entscheidender Bedeutung. Diese Studie befasst sich mit der computerbasierten Planung von individuellen Schablonen (Templates) für Ventrikelrekonstruktionen. Ziel ist es aus Cardio-CT-Daten, präoperativ, patientenindividuelle 3D-Modelle für Ventrikeltemplates zu erstellen. Hierfür wird aus CT-Daten der linksventrikuläre Blutpool segmentiert und daraus das Ventrikeltemplate modelliert. Dies geschieht anhand von zwei Kriterien: dem physiologischen Ventrikelfüllungsvolumen und der hämodynamisch günstigen ellipsoiden Form. Es konnten 20 3D-Templatemodelle mit einem durchschnittlichen Volumen von 144 ml erstellt werden. Die ellipsoide Form konnte durch manuelle Modellierung erreicht werden. Der Nachweis verbesserter Operationsergebnisse muss in nachfolgenden klinischen Studien erbracht werden.

1 Einleitung

Im Falle eines Myokardinfarktes oder einer strukturellen dilatativen Herzmuskelerkrankung kommt es zu Veränderungen der Geometrie des linken Herzventrikels, beispielsweise einer aneurysmatischen Erweiterung oder einer globalen Vergrößerung des Ventrikels [1]. Die Ventrikelrekonstruktion ist eine chirurgische Option, mit deren Hilfe Patienten mit vergrößertem linken Ventrikel eine verbesserte Ventrikelgeometrie und somit eine verbesserte Herzleistung gewährleistet werden soll [2]. Zur Abschätzung der entstehenden Ventrikelgeometrie werden momentan intraoperativ standardisierte Ballons im Ventrikel positioniert. Diese dienen als vereinheitlichte Schablone für die geometrische Form und das optimierte Volumen des Ventrikels. Trotz dieser Schablonen ist die postoperative Herzgeometrie häufig hämodynamisch ungünstig und erreicht daher nicht das optimale medizinische Ergebnis. Zur Verbesserung der operativ erstellten Ventrikelgeometrie sollen patientenindividuell modellierte Ventrikelschablonen, sogenannte Templates, beitragen. Ziel dieser Arbeit ist es, anhand von Cardio-CT-Daten, präoperativ, individuelle 3D-Ventrikeltemplatemodelle für den operativen Einsatz zu erstellen.

2 Material und Methoden

Es wurden enddiastolische, kontrastmittelgestützte und hochauflösende Cardio-CT-Datensätze von 20 Patienten mit Ventrikelaneurysma oder dilatativer Kardiomyopathie für die Studie ausgewählt. Im ersten Schritt wurden mit Hilfe der Segmentierungssoftware Segmeda [3] jeweils der linksventrikuläre enddiastolische Blutpool segmentiert. Dieser hebt sich aufgrund der Kontrastmittelfüllung gut von seiner Umgebung ab und kann so einfach mit einem auf Grauwerten basierenden 3D-Regiongrowing segmentiert werden. Lediglich auf Klappenebene muss hier manuell nachsegmentiert werden. Als Ergebnis erhält man einen "Ausguss" des linken Ventrikels. Das Template wird nun aus dem segmentierten Blutpool manuell und Schicht für Schicht modelliert. Hierfür wird per Hand das überschüssige Ventrikelvolumen von der Segmentierung ausgeschlossen (Abb. 1). Um eine möglichst gleichmäßige Form zu erhalten wird während der Modellierung der bearbeitete Teil jedes Schnittbildes per Maske auf die darauffolgende Schicht projiziert und dient so als Vorlage [4]. Die Templates werden anhand der Kriterien Volumen und Form modelliert. Als angestrebtes Volumen gilt das annähernd physiologische enddiastolische Ventrikelfüllungsvolumen von 152 ± 33 ml [3]. Die hämodynamisch günstigste Form ist das Ellipsoid und dient somit als Vorlage für die Templates [5]. Aufgrund der manuellen Modellierung können die individuell unterschiedlichen Ausprägungen der jeweiligen Herzmuskelerkrankung beachtet werden und im Segmentiervorgang berücksichtigt werden.

In einem weiteren Schritt wird der Herzmuskel ebenfalls per 3D-Regiongrowing segmentiert, um Herzwandbeschaffenheit und Lage der Pappilarmuskeln abschätzen zu können. Aufgrund der komplexen Struktur des Herzmuskels und der nur gering abweichenden Grauwertunterschiede zwischen Myokard und umliegendem Gewebe muss hier manuell nachsegmentiert werden um das ausgedünnte Myokard sowie die Papillarmuskeln darzustellen. Um avitales Herzmus-

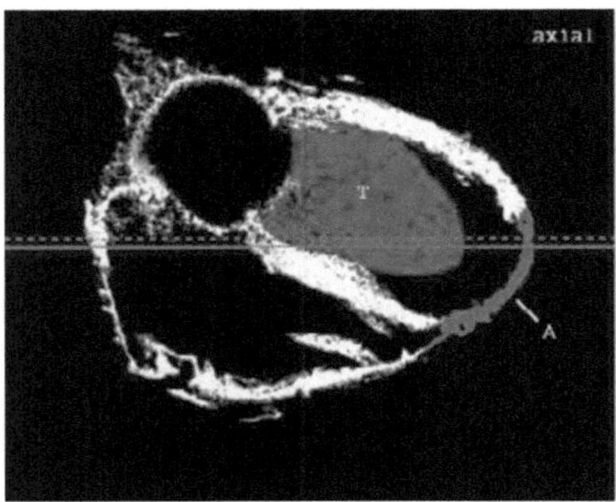

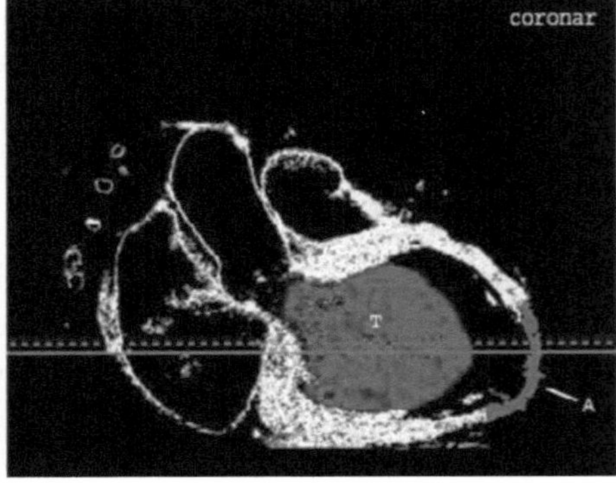

Abb. 1. Das individuell angepasste Template (T) ist in zwei Ebenen innerhalb des linken Ventrikels zu sehen. Die durchgezogenen Linien kennzeichnen die Schnittebene in der jeweils anderen Projektion. An der Herzspitze ist das akinetische Narbengewebe (A) gekennzeichnet.

kelgewebe zu verdeutlichen werden "late-enhancement" MRT-Daten [6] die der Visualisierung von Narbengewebe dienen, beurteilt. Die daraus gewonnenen Erkenntnisse über akinetisches Narbengewebe werden auf die CT-Daten projiziert und fließen so in den Segmentiervorgang ein (Abb. 1). Die Fusion der CT und MRT Daten wird zurzeit noch manuell vorgenommen.

3 Ergebnisse

Es konnten alle 20 Cardio-CT-Datensatz nach dem oben beschriebenen Schema ausgewertet werden und daraus 3D-Templatemodelle für Ventrikelrekonstruktionen erstellt werden (Abb. 2). Die erstellten Modelle haben ein durchschnittliches Volumen von 144 ml. Das durchschnittliche linksventrikuläre Volumen der segmentierten Herzdatensätze beträgt 343 ml (Abb. 2, Datensatz 21). Dies entspricht einer durchschnittlichen Ventrikelverkleinerung um 58%. Die geforderte ellipsoide Form konnte aufgrund der manuellen Modellierung entsprechend erreicht werden (Abb. 3). Die Erkenntnisse der "late-enhancement" MRT Untersuchungen konnten auf die Datensätze übertragen und farblich markiert werden.

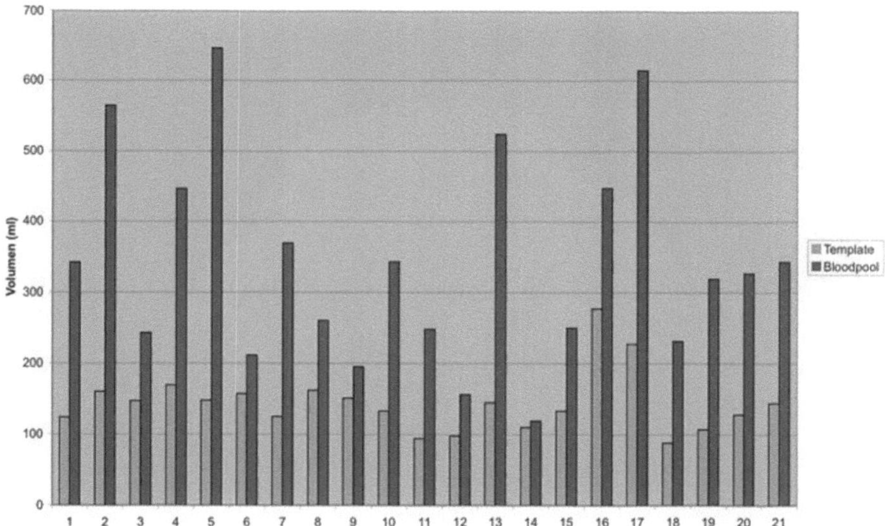

Abb. 2. Volumen der ausgewerteten Ventrikel sowie der modellierten Templates, wobei der Datensatz 21 den jeweiligen Durchschnittswert kennzeichnet.

4 Diskussion

Die Erstellung patientenindividueller Templatemodelle aus Cardio-CT-Daten ist durch die Anwendung der hier dargestellten Methode geglückt. Denkbare Vorteile der Templates sind eine verbesserte präoperative Geometrie- und Volumenplanung, die an die individuellen Unterschiede und Ausprägungen der Herzmuskelerkrankungen der Patienten angepasst werden kann. So kann ein Template für einen Patienten mit einem rein sacculären Herzmuskelaneurysma, außer im Bereich des Aneursymas, im wesentlichen dem präoperativen linksventrikulären Blutpool entsprechen, während ein global dilatierter Ventrikel einer Neumodellierung der gesamten Ventikelgeometrie bedarf. Durch diese individuelle Anpassung sollen mit Hilfe der Templates verbesserte Operationsergebnisse erreicht werden.

Das in der Studie erreichte durchschnittliche Templatevolumen von 144 ml liegt im Rahmen des von Cherniavsky et al. [7] beschriebenen gewünschten Ventrikelvolumen von 152 ± 33 ml. Das annähernd physiologische Ventrikelvolumen gewährleistet dem Patienten aufgrund der verringerten Volumenbelastung und der daraus resultierenden Abnahme der Ventrikelwandspannung eine Entlastung des Myokards und somit eine Verbesserung der Ejektionsfraktion. Lediglich zwei Templatemodelle sind größer als dieses geforderte Volumen und bedürfen einer

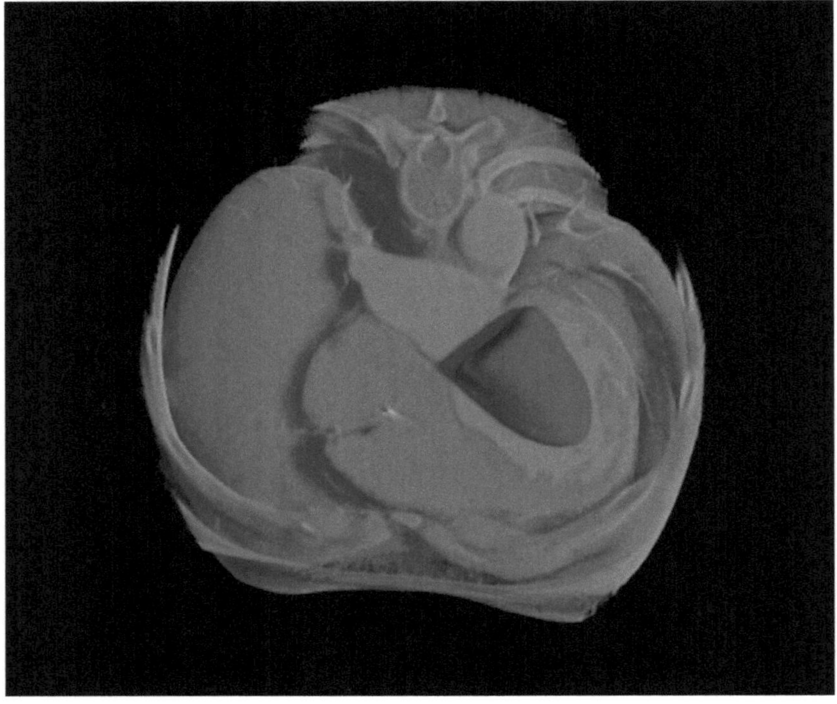

Abb. 3. 3D-Rekonstruktion eines Templates innerhalb einer Thorax Rekonstruktion

weiteren Nachsegmentierung. Fünf Templatemodelle weisen einen gering kleineren Wert auf. Bei diesen Modellen lag das präoperative Ausgangsventrikelvolumen aufgrund saccularer Ventriklelaneurysmen schon unter dem Durchschnitt. Kritisch zu diskutieren ist die noch manuelle Modellierung der Templatemodelle, die zwar individuelle Besonderheiten der Erkrankungen berücksichtigt, allerdings tendenziell ungenau ist und der persönlichen Einschätzung des Modellierers unterliegt. Hierbei soll künftig eine variable ellipsoide Schablone, anhand derer das Template aus dem segmentierten Blutpool modelliert wird, hilfreich sein. Des Weiteren birgt die rein gedankliche Fusion der CT- und Late-Enhancement-MRT-Daten Potential für Ungenauigkeiten und Inkonsistenzen. Dies soll durch eine softwaregestützte Fusion der Daten verbessert werden. Somit wäre eine präzisere übertragung der avitalen Myokardabschnitte von MRT- auf CT-Daten möglich. Diese Zusatzinformationen können dem Chirurg präoperativ ein komplexes Bild seines Operationsgebietes liefern und so zum verbesserten postoperativen Ergebnis beitragen. Neben den Verbesserungen der oben erwähnten technischen Einschränkungen sind in naher Zukunft die Erstellung und der Einsatz eines realen Templates auf Basis der Planung mittels 3D-Rapid-Prototyping [8] geplant. Im Anschluss soll insbesondere geklärt werden, ob es durch den klinischen Einsatz der individuell angepassten Templates zu tatsächlichen Verbesserungen der Operationsergebnisse gegenüber der bisherigen Vorgehensweise kommt.

Literaturverzeichnis

1. Zardini P, Marino P, Golia G, et al. Ventricular remodelling and infarct expansion. Am J Cardiol. 1993;72:96G–106G.
2. Menicanti L, Di Donato M. The dor procedure: What has changed after fifteen years of clinical practice? J Thorac Cardiovasc Surg. 2002;124:886–890.
3. Bartz D, Orman J, Gürvit O. Accurate volumetric measurements of anatomical cavities. Methods Inf Med. 2004;43(4):331–335.
4. Salah Z, Orman J, Bartz D. Live-wire revisited. Proc BVM. 2005; p. 158–162.
5. Buckberg G. Basic science review: The helix and the heart. J Thorac Cardiovasc Surg. 2002;124:863–883.
6. Gerber B, Garot J, Bluemke D, et al. Accuracy of contrast-enhanced magnetic resonance imaging in predicting improvement of regional myocardial function in patients after acute myocardial infarction. Circulation. 2002;106:1083.
7. Cherniavsky A, Karaskov A, Mechanenko A, et al. Preoperative modelling of an optimal left ventricle volume for surgical treatment of ventricular aneurysms. Eur J Card Thorac Surg. 2001;20:777–782.
8. Jacobs S, Grunert R, Mohr F, et al. 3D-imaging of cardiac structures using 3D heart models for planning in heart Surgery: A preliminary study. Interact Cardio Vasc Thorac Surg. 2008;7:6–9.

Automatische Segmentierung der Gewebegrenzen eines schlagenden embryonalen Hühnerherzens im 2D-Videobild

Jan Thommes[1], Talât Mesud Yelbuz[2]

[1]Institut für Mechatronische Systeme (ehemaliges Institut für Robotik)
Leibniz Universität Hannover
[2]Klinik für Kinderheilkunde, Padiatrische Kardiologie und Intensivmedizin
Medizinische Hochschule Hannover
thommes@imes.uni-hannover.de

Kurzfassung. Eine Klimakammer ermöglicht es, die Herzentwicklung bei Hühnerembryonen in einer schalenlosen Kultur über einen Zeitraum von etwa 50 Stunden visuell zu beobachten. Eine Hochgeschwindigkeits-Mikroskopkamera liefert eine Aufsicht auf das schlagende embryonale Herz. Da die für eine Analyse der Herzfunktion notwendige Segmentierung der Myokardgrenzen und des blutgefüllte Cavums manuell sehr zeitaufwändig ist, wird ein Ansatz zur kontinuierlichen, automatischen Segmentierung des schlagenden embryonalen Herzens mit Active Appearance Modellen präsentiert.

1 Einleitung

Die Herzentwicklung ist ein sehr dynamischer Vorgang, bei dem schon kleinste Einflüsse die strukturelle und funktionelle Entwicklung des Herzens so beeinflussen können, dass verschiedene Formen von Herzfehlbildungen resultieren. Die Bildgebung in der hierfür entwickelten Klimakammer[1] ermöglicht es, die entscheidende Phase der Herzentwicklung, das sog. Cardiac Looping kontinuierlich in vivo zu visualisieren. Über einen Zeitraum von bis zu 50 Stunden sind das Herz und dessen Funktion im Kamerabild beobachtbar, bevor der sich schließende Brustkorb detaillierte Aufnahmen unmöglich macht. In der so sichtbaren Frühphase der Herzentwicklung zeichnen sich jedoch bereits erste Abweichungen von der Normalentwicklung ab, die sich beim ausgebildeten Herzen in Form eines ausgeprägten Herzfehlers äußern[2].

Um den Prozess der Herzentwicklung zusammenhängend überwachen zu können, ist es notwendig, eine automatische Segmentierung des schlagenden Herzens vorzunehmen, um aus den ermittelten Konturen Parameter zu Funktion und Morphologie des Herzens abzuleiten.

2 Material und Methoden

Die Segmentierung der Gewebegrenzen beim schlagenden embryonalen Herzen ist aufgrund der schwach definierten Weichteilgrenzen nicht ohne die Verwendung von Vorwissen möglich. Im Folgenden soll die Bilddatenverarbeitung und der verwendete modellbasierte Segmentierungsalgorithmus vorgestellt werden.

2.1 Bilddatenverarbeitung

Als Kamerasystem kommt eine monochrome Hochgeschwindigkeitskamera (Pulnix TM-6710 CL, Jai Pulnix Inc., Sunnyvale, Ca, USA) mit entsprechender Mikroskopoptik zum Einsatz, die eine Auflösung von 640x480 Bildpunkten bei 120 Bildern/s liefert. Stand der Technik ist die Aufnahme kurzer Videosequenzen zu definierten Zeitpunkten, um daraus von Hand Endsystole und Enddiastole zu extrahieren. Anhand manuell gesetzter Landmarken in den beiden charakteristischen Herzphasen können neben Herzzeitvolumen (CO) auch andere kardiale Funktionsparameter wie Verkürzungsfraktion des Herzdurchmessers (SF) oder die systolische Flächenverkleinerung (FAC) abgeschätzt werden. Es besteht die Möglichkeit auch längere Filmsequenzen direkt zu speichern, allerdings ist der Speicherplatzbedarf einer zweitägigen Aufnahme enorm. Kontinuierliche Untersuchungen über längere Zeiträume sind aufgrund des hohen Zeitaufwandes der manuellen Segmentierung nicht möglich.

Die hier vorgestellte automatische Segmentierung des Herzens verfolgt das Ziel, einige Nachteile dieses Vorgehens zu eliminieren. Eine kontinuierliche Segmentierung jedes Herzschlages nicht nur in Endsstole und Enddiastole soll erfolgen, das Verfahren soll für einen Online-Einsatz geeigent sein, um auch ohne Videoaufnahmen wichtige Funktionsparameter des Herzens zu dokumentieren und Position und Orientierung des Herzens sollen verfolgt werden, um auf Lageänderungen des Herzens reagieren zu können.

2.2 Active Appearance Modell

Active Shape Modelle (ASM) und Active Appearance Modelle (AAM)[3] beschreiben eine formveränderliche Textur wie das Herz als auf Trainingsdaten basierendes statistisches Modell und sind bereits für die Segmentierung des Myokards in Magnetresonanztomographie- und Ultraschalldatensätzen erfolgreich eingesetzt worden. In den vorliegenden 2D-Videoaufnahmen sind die Gewebegrenzen zwischen dem blutgefüllten Innenbereich und dem Myokard, sowie zum umgebenden Gewebe aufgrund der sehr weichen Übergänge schwierig zu detektieren, zugleich ist die Formänderung während der Kontraktion beim embryonalen Herzen deutlich größer. Aus diesen Gründen wurde ein Segmentierungsansatz mit AAM gewählt, der neben Form auch die Erscheinung, d.h. Pixelintensitäten modelliert. Für die Modellbildung ist die Auswahl der Trainingsdaten von entscheidender Bedeutung, sie müssen alle später vorkommenden Variationen abdecken, das bedeutet neben Deformation aufgrund der Kontraktion auch pathologische Veränderungen sowie verschiedene Entwicklungsphasen. Zur Demonstration der Anwendbarkeit des Algorithmus wurden im Folgenden lediglich gesunde Embryonen im Alter von etwa 3 Tagen im Entwicklungsstadium HH 18, einer Einteilung der Embryonalentwicklung beim Huhn nach Hamburger und Hamilton in 46 Schritte[4], ausgewählt.

Das Formmodell umfasst 54 Landmarken, die nach einem speziellen Muster auf Innen- und Außenkontur verteilt sind. Dabei kommt eine Art Schablone zum Einsatz, die ausgehend vom Zentrum des Ausflusstraktes und des Ventrikels entlang der Kontraktionsrichtung des Gewebes eine Zuordnung der korrespondierenden Landmarken erlaubt. Eine Besonderheit stellt die starke Deformation des Herzens und das Aufteilen der Blutmenge in getrennte Bereiche des Ein- und Ausflusstraktes während des Schlages dar. Da die Anwendung der Hauptkomponentenanaylse (PCA) auf den aus den Koordinaten der 54 Landmarken bestehenden Shapevektor eine konstante Anzahl von Landmarken in jedem Trainingsbild fordert, fallen die Landmarken der Innenstruktur zusammen, wenn die Innenwände des Myokards das Blut vollständig verdrängen. Die aus den Landmarken der Trainingsbildern gewonnen Shapes werden zunächst mittels Procrustes-Analyse optimal aneinander ausgerichtet und durch Anwendung der Hauptkomponentenanalyse ins Shape-Modell überführt. Die Variation im Trainingsdatensatz lässt sich so über einen Basisshape $\boldsymbol{s}_0$ (Mittelwert der Landmarken über die Anzahl der Trainingsdaten) und eine Linearkombination aus Shapevektoren beschreiben.

$$\boldsymbol{s} = \boldsymbol{s}_0 + \sum_{i=1}^{n} p_i \boldsymbol{s}_i \tag{1}$$

Um die PCA auch auf die Textur anwenden zu können, müssen die Pixelintensitäten der verschiedenen Formen zunächst in eine Referenzform, den Basisshape transformiert werden. In diesem kann die Textur analog zur Form über eine PCA als Basisvektor A_0 und eine Linearkombination von Appearancevektoren beschrieben werden

$$A(\boldsymbol{x}) = A_0 + \sum_{i=1}^{l} c_i A_i(\boldsymbol{x}) \tag{2}$$

wobei $\boldsymbol{x}$ die Pixel innerhalb des Basisshapes beschreibt. Die Transformation geschiet durch Aufteilung in durch die Landmarken aufgespannte Dreiecke und eine stückweise affine Abbildung der Pixel in das entsprechende Dreieck im Basisshape. So kann die Variation im Trainingsdatensatz durch wenige Parameter effektiv beschrieben werden. Bei der klassischen Form der AAM reduziert eine dritte PCA auf Textur und Form die notwendigen Parameter erheblich, die so nicht mehr zu trennende Beschreibung von Form und Textur macht den Einsatz schneller Fitting-Algorithmen allerdings unmöglich. Im Hinblick auf die Anforderungen an die Segmentierung im Bezug auf die Laufzeit wurden getrennte Shape- und Appearancemodelle verwendet, so dass der Inverse-Compositional- oder Baker-Dellaert-Matthews-Algorithmus[5] für die Modellanpassung eingesetzt werden konnte. Dieser versucht die Abweichung von Modell und der in den Basisshape transformierten Bilddaten zu minimieren. Die Implementierung der Algorithmen erfolgte mit OpenCV.

3 Ergebnisse

Antrainiert wurde ein Modell mit 5 verschiedenen Embryonen für das Entwicklungsstadium HH 18, das daraufhin auf 3 weitere, dem Modell unbekannte, aber

Tabelle 1. Vergleich der Segmentierungsergebnisse bei 3 Embryonen

Embryo	Iterationen			Zeit[ms]			Anpassungsfehler
	min	max	ø	min	max	ø	ø[Pixel]
1	2	10	5,9	11	40	24,6	1,3
2	3	10	6,2	13	40	25,4	1,5
3	3	15	9,2	13	58	34,1	6,1

in der Erscheinung aber sehr ähnliche Embryonen angewandt wurde. Abbildung 1 zeigt das Einschwingverhalten des AAM auf die Herzkontur bei schlechter Initialisierung, die Abweichungen beim Verfolgen des Herzens von Bild zu Bild sind deutlich geringer. Tabelle 1 zeigt für die 3 Embryonen die erreichten Rechenzeiten und Segmentierungsgenauigkeiten. Als Anpassungsfehler ist die durchschnittliche Abweichung pro Landmarke der automatischen Segmentierung zur Expertensegmentierung zu verstehen.

Die erreichten Genauigkeiten bewegen sich annähernd im Schwankungsbereich einer manuellen Expertensegmentierung, lediglich bei Embryo 3 sind deutlich Abweichungen zu erkennen, die damit zu begründen sind, dass es sich um einen minimal jüngeren Embryo handelt, der vom Trainingsdatensatz nicht optimal wiedergegebenen werden kann. Während des Verfolgens der Herzbewegung sind im Schnitt 6 Iterationsschritte pro Bild notwendig, der inverse Fitting-Algoritmus nach Baker-Dellaert-Matthews benötigt pro Bild damit etwa eine Rechenzeit von 25 ms auf einem 2 GHz Core-2-Duo, bei dem jedoch nur ein Kern genutzt werden konnte. Die Trackingeigenschaften wurden durch eine Verschiebung des Bildausschnittes überprüft, der eine Bewegung des Embryos relativ zur Kamera simuliert. Abbildung 2 zeigt, wie der Algorithmus neben der Kontraktionsbewegung auch Rotations- und Translationsbewegungen des Embryos zuverlässig verfolgt, lediglich bei ruckartigen Bewegungen wird das schlagende Herz verloren.

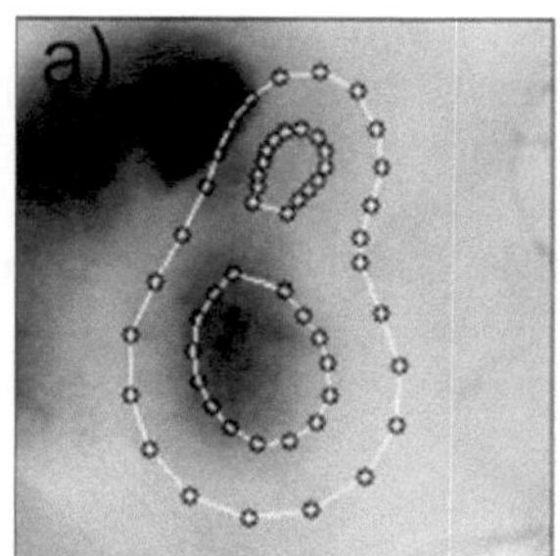

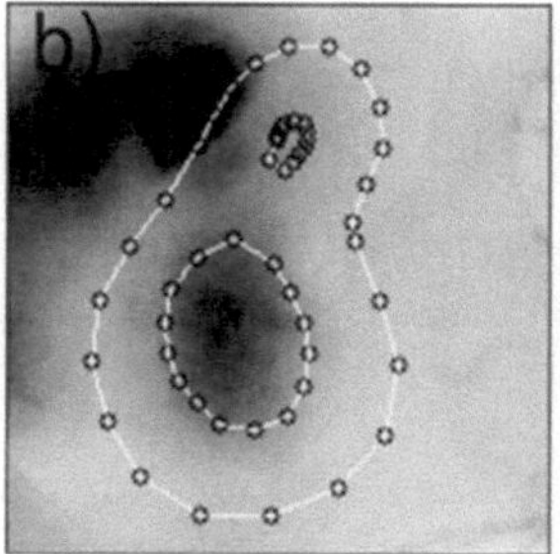

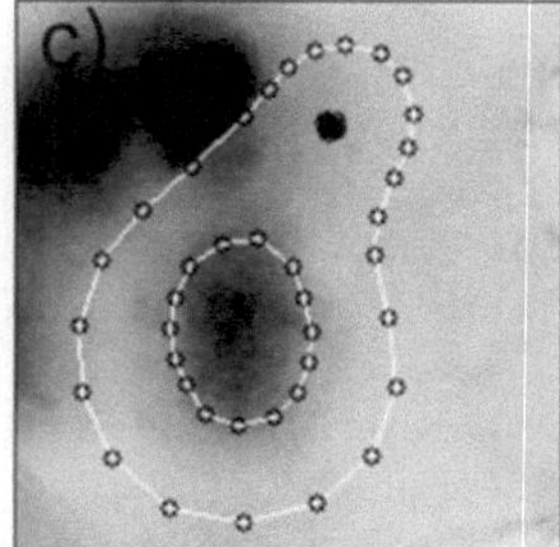

Abb. 1. Schrittweise Anpassung des Modells an den Bildinhalt. a) Initialisierung, b) nach 4 Iterationsschritten, c) nach 14 Iterationsschritten.

Abb. 2. Darstellung der Folgeeigenschaften des Algorithmus in einer Videosequenz. Rotations- und Translationsbewegungen des Embryos werden korrekt erfasst.

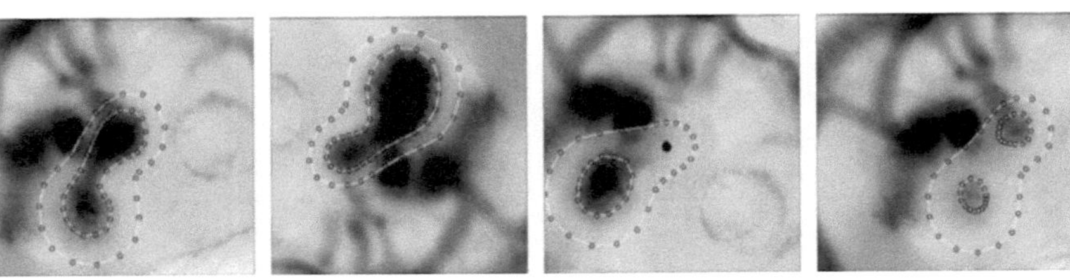

4 Diskussion

Es wurde ein Verfahren zur automatischen Segmentierung eines schlagenden embryonalen Hühnerherzens mit Active Appearance Modellen präsentiert. Das betrachtete embryonale Herz unterliegt einer starken Kontraktionsbewegung in deren Zuge aus Teilen der Herzens der komplette Blutinhalt verdrängt wird. Die beschreibenden Landmarken fallen in einem Punkt zusammen, so dass die bei der stückweise affinen Abbildung in den Basisshape transformierten Pixelwerte mit großen Unsicherheiten behaftet sind. Es zeigten sich allerdings sehr gute Segmentierungs- und Trackingergebnisse. Die erreichten Rechenzeiten pro Bild lassen auf einen Online-Einsatz des Verfahrens hoffen, was zur Vermeidung speicherintensiver Videoaufzeichnungen führen würde, so dass die Dokumentation der Herzfunktion und Herzentwicklung in Echtzeit erfolgen könnte. Die vorgestellten Algorithmen greifen kein Vorwissen zu Periodizität und somit Vorhersagbarkeit der Herzbewegung auf, es bleibt zu prüfen ob eine Genauigkeitssteigerung durch die Verwendung beispielsweise von sog. Active Appearance Motion Modellen (AAAM)[6] möglich ist, allerding stellt die dafür notwendige exakte Unterteilung der Herzschläge ohne EKG-Triggerung ein Problem dar.

Literaturverzeichnis

1. Baron S, Orhan G, Hornung O, et al. Konstruktion und Etablierung einer Klimakammer für die Untersuchung der embryonalen Herzentwicklung. Proc BVM. 2006.
2. Tutarel O, Norozi K, Hornung O, et al. Cardiac failure in the chick embryo resembles heart failure in humans. Circulation. 2005;112(24):352–353.
3. Cootes TF, Edwards GJ, Taylor CJ. Active appearance models. Proc Eur Conf Computer Vis. 1998;2:484–498.
4. Hamburger V, Hamilton H. A series of normal stages in the development of the chick embryo. In: J Morphol; 1951.
5. Matthews I, Baker S. Active Appearance Models Revisited. Robotics Institute, Carnegie Mellon University; 2003.
6. Sonka M, Mitchell SC, Lelieveldt BPF, et al. Active appearance motion model segmentation. Proc Int Workshop Digit Comput Video. 2001; p. 64.

Automatic Needle Segmentation in 3D Ultrasound Data Using a Hough Transform Approach

Philipp Hartmann[1], Matthias Baumhauer[1], Jens Rassweiler[2], Hans-Peter Meinzer[1]

[1]Division of Medical and Biological Informatics, DKFZ, Heidelberg
[2] Department of Urology, Clinic Heilbronn, University of Heidelberg, Heilbronn
p.hartmann@dkfz.de

Abstract. Segmentation in ultrasound data is a very challenging field of research in medical image processing. This article presents a method for automatic segmentation of biopsy needles and straight objects in noisy 3D image data. It uses a Hough-based segmentation approach, which has been exemplary adapted for the application on prostate biopsy data. An evaluation was performed on *in-vivo* 3D US data and shows promising results. Angular segmentation accuracy was evaluated with a mean of 2.1 degrees, which is comparable to human observers.

1 Introduction

Automatic segmentation of instruments in ultrasound (US) is a prerequisite for advancements in various diagnostic and therapeutic procedures. In this contribution, a novel method to segment needles in 3D US by means of Hough Transformation is presented. The algorithm detects straight objects in 3D images of bad quality; i.e. speckle noise bad contrast or blurry edges. Segmentation of surgical instruments on ultrasound images has to overcome certain difficulties, which are caused by ultrasound imaging itself. To those difficulties belong echo artifacts and the fact that one instrument may appear as a set of disconnected bright regions.

Exemplary, we adapted this method for the application of needle segmentation on prostate biopsy images. To test its feasibility it has been evaluated on in-vivo data sets of human prostate biopsies. The prostate biopsy is an intervention which could greatly benefit from automatic image processing. During the intervention a set of 12-16 tissue samples are taken from random positions. A major drawback is the lack of information about the exact origin. An estimation of this information based on 3D US images which are acquired during the intervention could lead to a remarkable improvement in the quality of diagnostic results. A precise determination of the tumour location could enable an accurate positioning of security margins during a resection planning and an improved conservation of surrounding healthy tissue.

Several methods have been invented to segment straight and bent needles in artificial and animal data in 2D and 3D ultrasound. Okazawa et al. [1] segmented curved needles in 2D based on a modified hough transformation technique. In 2003, Ding et al. [2] presented an early approach to 3D needle segmentation. For this purpose, binary projections of the region of interest (ROI) were made on orthogonal planes and the largest connected area was assumed as a projection of the needle. Barva et al. [3] extracted the line with the highest accumulated intensity (Parallel Integral Projection - PIP) by hierarchical mesh-grid search and classified it as the needle.

In contrast to previously presented work, we substituted iterative search methods for the generation of a global feature map with a subsequent analysis. This design concept has an increased robustness and delivers more reproducible results. Additionally, there is no risk of getting a local attractor as a result. A desirable side effect of this method is a predictable computation time. The accuracy of the analysis is flexibly scalable according to the demands of a specific task and available hardware. These key features motivate an evaluation on in-vivo data, which has -to our knowledge- not been done in previous work dealing with 3D US.

2 Methods

2.1 Automatic segmentation with Hough 3D

The basic idea of the algorithm is to find the brightest line in an image and to classify it as the needle axis. That key feature is equivalent to the highest integrated pixel value. Barva et al. [3] also used it in their PIP method and proved it to be a very robust feature. Such an approach implies that in a bent needle the longest straight part is detected and the rest neglected. However, to avoid difficulties of convergence a global approach was preferred to an iterative proceeding. Hence, the global maximum of the classification feature is robustly found and there is no risk of getting stuck at a local maximum.

In a first step, a thresholding is applied to reduce computation time. Whereas the overall brightness greatly differs among the images, a dynamic thresholding method has been used as a pre-filter. The threshold is chosen in a way that the darkest 90 % of the pixels are disregarded. This stage of preprocessing may be adjusted freely according to the actual field of application.

A second step is the generation of the so-called parameter space. To help understanding the structure of the parameter space, the mapping from source image to parameter space will be briefly introduced in the following paragraph. The aim is to find a parametrisation of lines, which is unambiguous and preserves angles. Subsequently, a bijective mapping from straight lines to the according parameters is derived. Finally, the set of coordinates which corresponds to a coordinate in the source picture is determined.

First, the set of lines running through a point in the source image has to be assigned to it. Basically, a line g in $\mathbb{R}^3$, which contains a point $\mathbf{p}$ in the source image, can be described as follows:

$$g : \mathbf{a} = \mathbf{p} + t{\cdot}\mathbf{v};\ \mathbf{a}, \mathbf{p}, \mathbf{v} \in \mathbb{R}^{\mathbf{3}};\ t \in \mathbb{R} \tag{1}$$

The direction of the line is $\mathbf{v}$ and t is a free parameter. A suitable and unambiguous parametrisation for the direction $\mathbf{v}$ is shown in eq. 2. An angular parametrisation has been chosen, in order to facilitate an implementation which provides isotropic angular resolution:

$$\mathbf{v} = \mathbf{e}_r = \begin{pmatrix} \sin\Theta\cos\Phi \\ \sin\Theta\sin\Phi \\ \cos\Theta \end{pmatrix};\ \Theta \in [0, \pi];\ \Phi \in [0, \pi] \tag{2}$$

With the chosen ranges for Θ and Φ half of the sphere (S^2) is covered. Consequently, anti parallel lines are not distinguished from each other. As it can be seen in eq. 1 and eq. 2, a line is existing for each combination of point $\mathbf{p}$ and tuple (Θ, Φ). $\mathbf{p}$ is the remaining degree of freedom in eq. 1 to completely describe the line. Since we are looking for parameters, which are unambiguous, $\mathbf{p}$ is not suitable. By examination of two points $\mathbf{p}_1$ and $\mathbf{p}_2$, there is always a tuple (Θ_0, Φ_0) with:

$$\mathbf{p}_1 - \mathbf{p}_2 = t \cdot \mathbf{v}_0;\ \mathbf{v}_0 = \mathbf{e}_r(\Theta_0, \Phi_0) \tag{3}$$

For (Θ_0, Φ_0), the line containing $\mathbf{p}_1$ and $\mathbf{p}_2$ is identical. In other words, the line, which contains both points may be described by the two angles Θ_0 and Φ_0, and *one* point on the line. From now on, this point is chosen as the intersection with the orthogonal plane containing the origin. Orthonormal vectors build up the correspondent plane for the vector $\mathbf{e}_r$; we choose

$$\mathbf{e}_\Theta = \begin{pmatrix} \cos\Theta\cos\Phi \\ \cos\Theta\sin\Phi \\ -\sin\Theta \end{pmatrix};\ \mathbf{e}_\Phi = \begin{pmatrix} -\sin\Phi \\ \cos\Phi \\ 0 \end{pmatrix}; \tag{4}$$

The plane p

$$p : \mathbf{a} = s \cdot \mathbf{e}_\Theta + t \cdot \mathbf{e}_\Phi;\ s, t \in \mathbb{R} \tag{5}$$

describes a unique set of points for each tuple (Θ, Φ) in the given range. It does not contain any line g with the corresponding direction vector $\mathbf{e}_r$, because $\mathbf{e}_r$ is perpendicular on p. Thus, the interception of line g with plane p is suitable for an explicit description of this line. The interception may be identified by the two parameters s and t from eq. 5. Due to basic geometric considerations, the tuple (s, t) may be determined as:

$$s = \mathbf{p} \cdot \mathbf{e}_\Theta;\ t = \mathbf{p} \cdot \mathbf{e}_\Phi \tag{6}$$

Whereas $\mathbf{p}$ may be *any* point on the line. With the preceding considerations we get a mapping C, which fulfils all desired requirements.

$$C : \mathbb{R}^3 \rightarrow \mathcal{P}(S^2 \times \mathbb{R}^2) \tag{7}$$

Table 1. Angle between estimated needle by the algorithm (alg) and the human observers (o1-o3) gold standard in degrees.

ds #	o1	o2	o3	alg	ds #	o1	o2	o3	alg
1	0.64	1.07	0.99	1.88	8	0.24	0.13	0.75	0.52
2	1.09	1.35	2.14	0.95	9	2.04	0.55	2.09	2.89
3	2.65	2.73	1.90	1.41	10	1.81	0.13	3.90	0.55
4	2.90	1.76	3.05	6.80	11	0.90	0.67	2.61	1.58
5	0.14	0.87	0.54	2.38	12	1.25	0.89	3.96	1.86
6	2.22	1.43	1.47	2.35	13	4.05	1.28	1.26	3.54
7	1.67	1.64	1.84	0.50	14	0.98	0.94	1.54	55.4

with

$$\mathbf{x} \mapsto \{(\Theta, \Phi, \mathbf{x} \cdot \mathbf{e}_\Theta, \mathbf{x} \cdot \mathbf{e}_\Phi) : \Theta \in [0, \pi];\ \Phi \in [0, \pi]\} \tag{8}$$

If $v(\mathbf{x}) \in \mathbb{R}$ is the pixel value at coordinate $\mathbf{x}$, the integrated pixel value of one line which is described by the tuple $(\Theta_0, \Phi_0, l_0, s_0)$ is

$$I = \int_{\text{image}} v(\mathbf{x})\delta(l_0 - \mathbf{x} \cdot \mathbf{e}_{\Theta 0}) \cdot \delta(s_0 - \mathbf{x} \cdot \mathbf{e}_{\Phi 0}) d^3x \tag{9}$$

Since I are the values in parameter space -which are being mapped on the according coordinates- the maximum of I is equivalent to the brightest line in the source image. The global maximum in the parameter space is determined and the respective parameters are transformed back into image coordinates.

The implementation of the algorithm has been done in C++ with two open source libraries; the Insight Segmentation and Registration Toolkit (ITK), and the Medical Imaging Interaction Toolkit (MITK).

2.2 Evaluation

The proposed method has been tested in fourteen in-vivo images, taken by a GE Voluson 730 US device. The size of the images is about 35 x 50 x 50 mm. The resolution is isotropic and about 4 pixels/mm. As gold standard for the evaluation, a manual segmentation of three experienced human observers has been applied. Evaluation parameter is the angle between the direction of one defined needle and the mean of the three manually segmented directions. It was calculated for each manual segmentation and compared with the automatically processed results. To reduce computation time and increase robustness, a ROI with size of 30 percent of the image volume was determined based on the known spatial relations of ultrasound transducer and biopsy needle.

3 Results

The results of the accuracy evaluation are shown in table 1. To quantify the deviation of the manual segmentation of all observers, the angle between the determined needle direction of a single observer and the mean direction was calculated. Values vary from 0.53 to 4.05 degrees.

The same parameter was calculated for the results of the automatic detection. Apart from data set 4 and 14, the values for the detection precision are of the same magnitude as the results for human observers.

The computation time varies from 45 - 200 s on a 2,4 GHz Quad Core CPU with 4GB memory. During the segmentation, about 500 MB memory were allocated. Although the algorithm is basically suitable for multithreading, the actual implementation does not feature parallel computing.

4 Discussion

To face the ambitious challenge of the automatic segmentation task on noisy 3D US data, a generic algorithm for the segmentation of straight objects in images has been implemented and adjusted for the specific purpose of prostate biopsy images. The results show a robust needle detection with a tolerable error of 2.1 ° on 3D *in-vivo* ultrasound images. Thus, the presented method emerged to be comparably accurate to the evaluated interobserver variability.

In earlier work, Heimann et al. [4] present an automated approach to segment the prostate in 3D US data by means of a statistical shape model. Combined with this method, the presented algorithm can, for instance, be the basis of a powerful support in prostate cancer diagnosis. Since there are several approaches for the localisation of the tip -Barva et al. [3] provides a promising method to deal with that issue-, a fully automated reconstruction of the extraction spot in the prostate using a single 3D US data set is feasible.

The comparison between human observer and algorithm accuracy suggests this method to be a promising approach.

The usability of the presented algorithm is not limited to biopsies or even ultrasound as imaging modality. There might be various other beneficial fields of application, such as radio frequency ablations.

Future work will address improvements in robustness and the reduction of memory demands. For this purpose, it is planned to divide the image into disjunct regions.

References

1. Okazawa SH, Ebrahimi R, Chuang J, et al. Methods for segmenting curved needles in ultrasound images. Med Image Anal. 2006.
2. Ding M, Cardinal HN, Fenster A. Automatic needle segmentation in three-dimensional ultrasound images using two orthogonal two-dimensional image projections. Med Phys. 2003;30/2.
3. Barva M. Localization of surgical instruments in biological tissue from 3D ultrasound images. 2007.
4. Heimann T, Baumhauer M, Simpfendörfer T, et al. Prostate Segmentation from 3D Transrectal Ultrasound Using Statistical Shape Models. Proc SPIE; 2008.

Texture-Based Polyp Detection in Colonoscopy

Stefan Ameling[1], Stephan Wirth[1], Dietrich Paulus[1], Gerard Lacey[2], Fernando Vilarino[2]

[1]Institute for Computational Visualistics, University of Koblenz-Landau, Germany
[2]Department of Computer Science, Trinity College Dublin, Ireland
stameling@uni-koblenz.de

Abstract. Colonoscopy is one of the best methods for screening colon cancer. A variety of research groups have proposed methods for automatic detection of polyps in colonoscopic images to support the doctors during examination. However, the problem can still not be assumed as solved. The major drawback of many approaches is the amount and quality of images used for classifier training and evaluation. Our database consists of more than four hours of high resolution video from colonoscopies which were examined and labeled by medical experts. We applied four methods of texture feature extraction based on Grey-Level-Co-occurence and Local-Binary-Patterns. Using this data, we achieved classification results with an area under the ROC-curve of up to 0.96.

1 Introduction

1.1 Medical Background

Colon cancer is one of the leading causes of cancer death worldwide [1]. Although the interest on virtual endoscopy from computed tomography images is growing, colonoscopy is still the accepted gold standard for detecting colon cancer or its precursor lesions, colorectal polyps. The removal of adenomatous polyps has been shown to prevent most cancer. Although colonoscopy has become the preferred method of screening colon cancer, several studies showed that it contains an inherent miss rate of up to 25% for the detection of polyps and cancer, depending on its size and location (e.g. [2]).

Two main causes that lead to misses can be distinguished:

1. The endoscopist does not cover all parts of the colon (parts remain "unseen" by the camera),
2. the polyp appears on the screen but remains undetected by the doctor.

Most work – as well as ours – has been done on the second problem, the computer-assisted detection. Fig. 1 shows some colonoscopic images containing polyps. Artifacts like reflexions and non-uniform illumination complicate the computer vision task.

1.2 Related work

Polyp detection methods can be classified by the types of features that are used: shape features, texture features, color, or combined approaches.

For texture-based analysis, different sets of texture features are used which are extracted from the Grey-Level Co-occurrence Matrix (GLCM), the Local Binary Pattern (LBP), the Opponent Colour-Local Binary Pattern (OC-LBP), or Wavelet Transform (WT) (e.g. [3, 4]).

Wang et al. use a two-dimensional histogram for classification which combines LBP with average intensity [5].

Reviews of polyp detection methods have shown that many research results can be called into question due to the fact that the sample sets used for testing and training were relatively small, except for a few cases [6, 7].

A reliable classification system should be based on a huge set of high-resolution images containing many different types of abnormalities. We think that a classifier trained with less than hundred images at VHS-resolution or even lower cannot detect cancer and poylps in a way that meets the requirements of a clinical system.

Apart from the video data itself, ground truth information about the abnormalities present in the images is needed for training and evaluation of a classifier. Vilariño et al. proposed a promising architecture for automatic labeling of colonoscopy video for cancer detection using eye movement of the observer, where results from gaze tracking were used to select regions in the images [8].

2 Material and methods

2.1 Database

Due to the technological progress in terms of aquisition of high-resolution images more detailed texture structures of the colon mucosa become visible that can be utilized for the detection of colororectal lesions such as polyps.

More than four hours of almost complete colonoscopies were captured in Full HD resoultion (1920 $\times$ 1080 pixels). After preselection, the videos were presented to five experts in colonoscopy to identify abnormalities. By clicking with the mouse on the relevant positions in the video, ground truth information was obtained. Afterwards, for every image a mask was created manually that labels abnormal regions (Fig. 1).

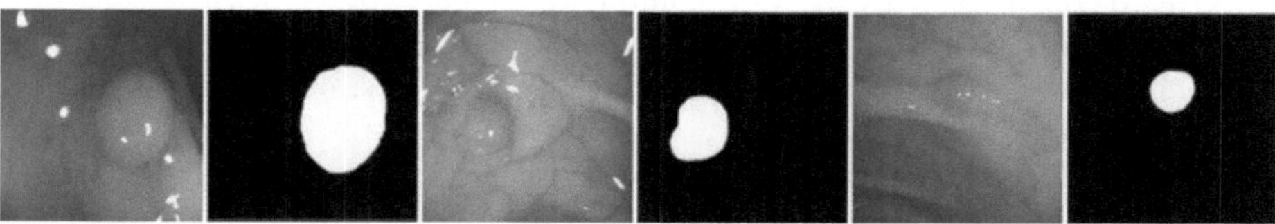

Fig. 1. Colonoscopy images with their corresponding masks labeling abnormal regions

2.2 Methods

We used two common texture analysis methods for texture feature extraction: grey-level co-occurrence matrices (GLCMs) [9] and local binary patterns (LBP) [10]. GLCMs describe how often different combinations of pixel values occure in an image. Each entry (i, j) of the matrix p represents the probability of going from one pixel value i to another pixel value j under a predefined angle α and distance d. Statistical measures on such a GLCM describe the texture and can be used as a feature vector. Some of the measures proposed in literature are: energy, homogeneity, entropy, correlation, inertia, cluster shade, and cluster prominence.

The LBP is extracted from a 3×3 neighbourhood as follows: The neighbourhood is binarised using the value of the center pixel as threshold. These values are then multiplied by certain weights and summed, leading to one single value for each neighbourhood. LBP feature vectors are formed by histogram bins of the distribution of the LBP values.

An extension of the LPB was proposed in [11], the Opponent Colour Local Binary Pattern (OC-LBP). The LPB operator is applied on each color channel separately. Additionally, each pair of colour channels is used, so that the center pixel of the neighbourhood and the neighbourhood iteself are taken from different colour channels. All the histograms are concatenated to one feature vector.

Support vector machines (SVM) [12] are a commonly used classification technique because of many attractive features, such as the ability to deal with high-dimensional feature data. At first, a model is produced with a training set containing many data instances and then the model classifies the instances from a test set.

2.3 Experiments

Four different scenes of equal length were extracted from the database, each showing a different polyp. In total we used 1736 high-resolution images and every image contains a visible polyp from varying distance, angle and illumination.

Thus, it can be found out (1) how the texture features perform in general on this large database of high-resolution images and (2) if there is a relation between particular texture features and polyp types.

Since texture is a local property, we decided to divide each image into small image patches (50^2 and 70^2 pixels were used as patch sizes). We implemented four methods based on GLCM and LBP:

- GLCM 16: Four GLCM were computed for each patch with $d = 1$ and $\alpha \in \{0°, 45°, 90°, 135°\}$. The following features have been computed on each matrix, leading to 16-dimensional feature vectors: energy, homogeneity, entropy, and correlation.
- GLCM 6: Four GLCM were computed as described above. The extracted features were: energy, homogeneity, entropy, inertia, cluster shade and cluster prominence. The means of the four values (from the four matrices) of each feature were computed leading to a 6-dimensional feature vector.

Table 1. AUC values of the different classifiers, best results are highlighted

Scene	Patch size	GLCM 6	GLCM 16	LBP	OC-LBP
1	70×70	0.83	**0.95**	0.89	0.94
2	70×70	0.70	0.75	0.76	**0.87**
3	70×70	0.89	0.88	0.95	**0.96**
4	70×70	0.65	0.68	0.80	**0.91**
1	50×50	0.80	**0.89**	0.86	**0.89**
2	50×50	0.71	0.75	0.71	**0.84**
3	50×50	0.80	0.83	0.88	**0.95**
4	50×50	0.63	0.65	0.77	**0.89**

- LBP: The LBP histogram was extracted as described in section 2.2. An amount of 64 histogram bins was used leading to a 64-dimensional feature vector.
- OC-LBP: The OC-LBP feature was extracted with an amount of 64 bins for each histogram, leading to a 576-dimensional feature vector.

With the extracted feature data an SVM-classifier was trained and tested using a radial basis function as kernel. We applied a stratified k-fold cross-validation with $k = 4$.

3 Results

Receiver Operating Characteristics (ROC) graphs were computed to analyze the performance of the classifiers based on the different texture features. To summarize the results, table 1 shows the area under the curve (AUC) values of the ROC graphs for the different scenes and patch sizes.

4 Discussion

As table 1 shows the best classification results were achieved by the OC-LBP method on almost every experiment and the GLCM 6 method performs worst.

Since the OC-LBP method is the only one of the tested methods that considers colour, colour seems to be an important feature for polyp detection in colonoscopy.

Comparing the two GLCM based methods there are two reasons for the poor results of the GLCM 6 method: (1) more features do not implicitly lead to better classification results and (2) by averaging the values from different GLCM too much information gets lost.

Another important result is, that every method itself achieves its best classification result either on scene 1 or scene 3 and its poor results either on scene 2 or scene 4. This leads to the assumption that there is no relation between one particular feature and polyp.

In general, texture seems to be a promising feature for automatic polyp detection. This reinforces results from previous works and indicates their validity for high-resolution images.

Future work with regard to an automatic polyp detection system will comprise the training of classifiers based on even more images showing different polyps, due to the high diversity of their appearences. Furthermore other methods for texture analysis will be examined.

Acknowledgement. Special thanks go to Beaumont Hospital Dublin, Ireland. This research was partly supported by Enterprise Ireland project endoview.

References

1. World Health Organization. Media Centre Fact Sheet No 297: Cancer; 2006 [cited 2008 Oct 04]. [online]. Available from: http://www.who.int/mediacentre/factsheets/fs297/en/print.html.
2. Thomson A, Ahnen D, Riopelle J. Intestinal polypoid adenomas. eMedicine, The Continually Updated Clinical Reference. 2007;Available from: http://www.emedicine.com/med/TOPIC1175.HTM.
3. Iakovidis DK, Maroulis DE, Karkanis SA. An intelligent system for automatic detection of gastrointestinal adenomas in video endoscopy. Comput Biol Med. 2006;36(10):1084–1103.
4. Karkanis SA, Iakovidis DK, Karras DA, et al. Detection of lesions in endoscopic video using textural descriptors on wavelet domain supported by artificial neural network architectures. Proc IEEE Conf Image Proc. 2001; p. 833–836.
5. Wang P, Krishnan SM, Kugean C, et al. Classification of endoscopic images based on texture and neural network. Proc IEEE EMBS. 2001;4:3691–3695.
6. Ameling S, Wirth S, Paulus D. Methods for Polyp Detection in Colonoscopy Videos: A Review. University of Koblenz-Landau; 2008. 14/2008.
7. Shevchenko N, Mühldorfer S, Wittenberg T, et al. Untersuchung von Texturanalysemethoden zur automatischen Polypenerkennung. In: 7. Jahrestagung der Deutschen Gesellschaft für Computer- und Roboterassistierte Chirugie e. V., Tagungsband; 2008. p. 205–206.
8. Vilariño F, Lacey G, Zhou J, et al. Automatic labeling of colonoscopy video for cancer detection. Proc Iberian Conf: Patt Recogn Image Anal. 2007; p. 290–297.
9. Haralick RM, Dinstein I, Shanmugam K. Textural features for image classification. IEEE Trans Syst Man Cybern. 1973;3(6):610–621.
10. Pietikainen M, Ojala T. Nonparametric texture analysis with complementary spatial operators. Texture Analysis in Machine Vision, Series in Machine Perception and Artificial Intelligence. 2000;40.
11. Mäenpää T. The local binary pattern approach to texture analysis–extensions and applications; 2003. Ph.D. thesis, University of Oulu.
12. Vapnik V. The Nature of Statistical Learning Theory. Springer; 1999.

Bildbasierte Navigationsdatenkorrektur für endoskopische Augmented Reality Anwendungen

Andreas Hussong[1], Omid Majdani[2], Tobias Ortmaier[1]

[1]Institut für Mechatronische Systeme (ehemaliges Institut für Robotik), Leibniz Universität Hannover
[2]Klinik und Poliklinik für HNO, Medizinische Hochschule Hannover
andreas.hussong@imes.uni-hannover.de

Kurzfassung. Die aktuelle Genauigkeit optischer Trackingsysteme in der Lageerkennung (Positions- und Orientierungserkennung) von Objekten führt in endoskopischen Augmented Reality Anwendungen zu deutlichen räumlichen Fehlern bei der Einblendung virtueller Objekte ins Endoskopbild. Es wird ein Verfahren präsentiert, das auf Basis der Bildinformation den Lagefehler korrigiert indem ein virtuelles Modell einer real im Bild sichtbaren Struktur optimal auf diese gematcht wird. Der hierfür verwendete Partikelfilteransatz liefert die notwendige Robustheit für das matchen und die Online-Fähigkeit des Verfahrens ermöglicht auch die Korrektur nichtstatischer Fehler. Das Leistungsfähigkeit des Verfahrens wird beispielhaft demonstriert.

1 Einleitung

Optische Navigationssysteme bieten eine nominelle Genauigkeit von ca. 0,3 mm für die Positionsbestimmung einzelner Objekte [1]. Im chirurgischen Alltag liegen auf Grund ungenauer Registrierungen oder nicht optimaler Trackingbedinungen die üblichen Genauigkeiten jedoch häufig eher im Bereich weniger Millimeter [2]. Insbesondere bei minimalinvasiven Eingriffen unter endoskopischer Kontrolle führt der unvermeidbare Abstand zwischen Endoskopspitze und Trackingtarget zu nicht vernachlässigbaren Fehlern [3]. Dies führt insbesondere bei Augmented Reality Anwendungen, bei denen aus präoperativ gewonnen Bilddaten erzeugte, virtuelle Objekte oder Zusatzinformationen positionsgenau ins Endoskopbild eingeblendet werden, zu nicht vernachlässigbaren Fehlern. Für minimalinvasive Anwendungen mit submillimetrischen Präzisionsansprüchen sind derartige Fehler nicht tolerierbar.

Werden hingegen rein bildbasierte Verfahren angewandt, um beispielsweise die Lage von Instrumentenspitzen in endoskopischen Bildern zu bestimmen [4, 5], erschwert fehlendes a-priori-Wissen über die zu erwartende Objektlage im Bild häufig das erstmalige Auffinden und sichere Verfolgen der Objekte. Zudem stellt die Generierung von 6D-Lageinformationen aus monokularen Endoskopbildern ein nicht triviales Problem dar. Im Folgenden wird daher ein Verfahren vorgestellt, das beide Konzepte effektiv verknüpft und 6D-Lageinformationen aus optischen Trackingdaten mit Mitteln der Bildverarbeitung verbessert um somit zu einer höheren Gesamtpräzision für die Ermittlung der Lage verfolgter Objekte zu gelangen.

2 Material und Methoden

2.1 Fehlermodellierung

Die relative Lage (Position und Orientierung) eines Objektes (ob) relativ zur Endoskop-Kamera (c) kann ausgedrückt werden als

$$\boldsymbol{T}^{c}_{ob} = \boldsymbol{T}^{c}_{tc}\boldsymbol{T}^{tc}_{0}\boldsymbol{T}^{0}_{to}\boldsymbol{T}^{to}_{ob} \tag{1}$$

wobei $\boldsymbol{T}^{c}_{tc}$ die Transformation zwischen Kamera (c) und Kameratarget (tc) darstellt, $\boldsymbol{T}^{tc}_{0}$ die Inverse der vom Trackingsystem gemessenen Lage des Kameratargets im Weltkoordinatensystems (0) angibt, $\boldsymbol{T}^{0}_{to}$ die ebenfalls vom Trackingsystem gemessene Lage des Objekt-Targets im Weltkoordinatensystem beschreibt und $\boldsymbol{T}^{to}_{ob}$ die Lage des Objektes relativ zum Objekt-Target definiert. Es kann angenommen werden, dass alle diese Einzeltransformationen aufgrund von Registrier- oder Messungenauigkeiten fehlerbehaftet sind. Diese Fehler können als Fehlertransformationen $\boldsymbol{E}^{a}_{b}$ aufgefasst werden, die die bekannte Transformation $\boldsymbol{T}^{a}_{b}$ von der unbekannten, realen Transformation $\hat{\boldsymbol{T}}^{a}_{b}$ unterscheidet:

$$\hat{\boldsymbol{T}}^{a}_{b} = \boldsymbol{T}^{a}_{b}\boldsymbol{E}^{a}_{b} \tag{2}$$

Somit lässt sich die exakte Position des Objektes relativ zur Kamera beschreiben als

$$\begin{aligned}\hat{\boldsymbol{T}}^{c}_{ob} &= \hat{\boldsymbol{T}}^{c}_{tc}\hat{\boldsymbol{T}}^{tc}_{0}\hat{\boldsymbol{T}}^{0}_{to}\hat{\boldsymbol{T}}^{to}_{ob} \\ &= \boldsymbol{T}^{c}_{tc}\boldsymbol{E}^{c}_{tc}\ \boldsymbol{T}^{tc}_{0}\boldsymbol{E}^{tc}_{0}\ \boldsymbol{T}^{0}_{to}\boldsymbol{E}^{0}_{to}\ \boldsymbol{T}^{to}_{ob}\boldsymbol{E}^{to}_{ob} \\ &= \boldsymbol{T}^{c}_{tc}\boldsymbol{T}^{tc}_{0}\boldsymbol{T}^{0}_{to}\boldsymbol{T}^{to}_{ob}\,{}_{ob}\boldsymbol{E}^{c}_{tc}\,{}_{ob}\boldsymbol{E}^{tc}_{0}\,{}_{ob}\boldsymbol{E}^{0}_{to}\,{}_{ob}\boldsymbol{E}^{to}_{ob} \\ &= \boldsymbol{T}^{c}_{ob}\boldsymbol{E}^{c}_{ob}\end{aligned} \tag{3}$$

wobei sämtliche Fehler zunächst in das Objektkoordinatensystem transformiert (${}_{ob}\boldsymbol{E}^{a}_{b}$) und dann in der Gesamtfehlertransformation $\boldsymbol{E}^{c}_{ob}$ zusammengefasst werden können. Ziel einer Fehlerkorrektur ist somit die Bestimmung dieser Fehlermatrix.

2.2 Algorithmus

Zur Bestimmung der Fehlertransformation wird ein Partikelfilterverfahren (siehe beispielsweise [6]) eingesetzt. Dabei wird die Wahrscheinlichkeitsfunktion für die Fehlertransformation durch eine bestimmte Anzahl an Schätzungen (sog. Partikel) diskretisiert. Diese werden in regelmäßiger Frequenz überprüft, bewertet und aktualisiert, so dass eine Mittelung des aktuellen Paritkelsatzes jeweils einen guten aktuellen Schätzwert für die Fehlertransformation liefert. Die einzelnen Schritte des Verfahrens werden im Folgenden am konkreten Problem erläutert.

Zur Überprüfung und Bewertung der Partikel wird für jedes Partikel i, das einer diskreten Schätzung der Fehlertransformation ${}_{ob}\tilde{\boldsymbol{E}}^{c}_{ob,i}$ entspricht, nach Gleichung (3) eine Schätzung für die Lage des Objektes relativ zur Kameraposition $\tilde{\boldsymbol{T}}^{c}_{ob,i}$ bestimmt und dieses entsprechend gerendert. Davon ausgehend, wird die Kontur des Objektes ermittelt und in der Umgebung dieser Kontur nach Kanten im Originalbild gesucht. Die Qualität der Schätzung und somit die Bewertung des Partikels ergibt sich aus der Nähe von Bildkanten zur geschätzten Kontur [7]. Wird das Objekt durch die Partikelschätzung somit in die Nähe der tatsächlichen Objektposition abgebildet, so ergeben sich niedrige Kantenabstände zur Kontur und somit eine hohe Bewertung der aktuellen Schätzung. Abbildung 1 zeigt beispielhaft die aus zwei Partikeln ermittelten geschätzten Konturpositionen, sowie die auf den Konturnormalen durchgeführte Suche nach Kanten im Bild. Gefundene Kanten sind mit Kreisen auf den Normalen gekennzeichnet. In jedem Iterationsschritt wird die Partikelmenge qualitätsbasiert aus der letzten Partikelmenge resampled und jeweils mit einem gauß'schen Rauschen überlagert. Mit der Zeit verdichtet sich somit die Anzahl von Partikeln in der Umgebung der wahren Fehlerkorrekturmatrix wodurch sich die aus der Mittelung über alle Partikel gewonnene Gesamtschätzung ${}_{ob}\tilde{\boldsymbol{E}}^{c}_{ob}$ verbessert. Auf Basis dieser Gesamtschätzung kann nun nach Gleichung (3) die Objektlage verbessert werden und das Objekt an der korrigierten Position im Bild dargestellt werden. Zudem liegt mit der korrigierten Transformation

$$\tilde{\boldsymbol{T}}^{c}_{ob} = \boldsymbol{T}^{c}_{ob}\tilde{\boldsymbol{E}}^{c}_{ob} \tag{4}$$

eine verbesserte Lageinformation des Objektes vor.

2.3 Setup und Versuchsdurchführung

Zur praktischen Validierung des vorgestellten Verfahrens wurde ein Versuchsstand, bestehend aus einem ARtrack2 Trackingsystem sowie einem Karl Storz

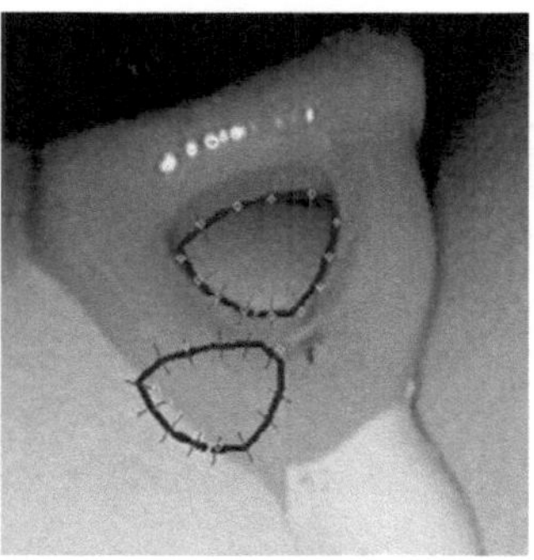

Abb. 1. Darstellung zweier ins Endoskopbild projezierter Objektkonturen mit auf Konturnormalen gefundenen Bildkanten (mit Kreisen markiert). Die jeweiligen Korrekturmatrizen werden basierend auf der Anzahl der gefundenen Kantenpunkte entlang der Normalen sowie deren Abstand zur Kontur bewertet.

Image1 S3 Endoskop mit Hopkins 1,9 mm Optik aufgebaut. Das Endoskop wurde mit einem Trackingstern ausgestatt und nach [8] die intrinsischen Parameter der Kamera ermittelt sowie die sog. Hand-Auge Kalibrierung (Registrierung der Kamera zum Trackingstern) durchgeführt. Ein Kunststoff Ohrmodell wurde als Testobjekt CT-gescannt und durch Segmentation ein 3-dimensionales STL-Objekt des Stapes erstellt. Das Modell wurde mit einem Trackingstern versehen und registriert. Die Visualisierung und Einblendung des Stapes in das Videobild des Endoskopes wurde mit Hilfe des Visualization Toolkits (VTK) realisiert.

3 Ergebnisse

Abbildung 2 zeigt die Ergebnisse des Verfahrens. In Bild *a*) ist die Einblendung auf Basis der Trackingdaten gezeigt - die Lage des virtuellen Objektes weicht deutlich von der tatsächlichen Position des Objektes im Bild ab. Bild *b*) zeigt die Innenkontur des Objektes sowie die Kontur nach Anwendung einer Partikelmenge an Korrekturmatrizen die mit leichtem Rauschen um eine Einheitsmatrix initialisiert wurde. Abbildung *c*) zeigt schließlich die korrigierte Lage des Objektes, nachdem sich eine Großzahl der Partikel an der realen Bildposition verdichtet hat (Abb. 2d).

4 Diskussion

Es wurde ein Verfahren präsentiert mit dem Kalibrier- und Messfehler eines Trackingsystems mit Hilfe von Bildinformationen korrigiert werden können. Die

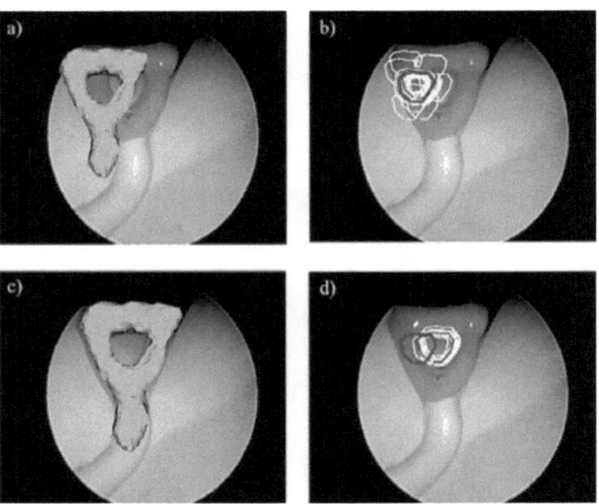

Abb. 2. Ergebnisse: a),c) Überlagerung des Modells auf Basis der Trackingdaten zu Beginn und bei erfolgreicher Korrektur; b),d) Objektkonturen auf Basis der Trackingdaten zu Beginn und bei erfolgreicher Korrektur. In rot ist die Kontur auf Basis der Trackingdaten dargestellt, in weiß die Kontur nach Korrektur durch einzelne Partikel und in blau die aus der Partikelmenge gemittelte Korrektur.

bestimmte Korrekturmatrix stellt dabei für gleichbleibende Trackingverhältnisse einen quasi konstanten Wert dar. Auf Grund anistroper, insbesondere von der Ausrichtung des Trackingtargets zur Trackingkamera abhängiger Trackingfehler, ist bei Bewegungen der getrackten Objekte eine entsprechende Adaption notwendig. Das vorgestellte Verfahren ist auf Grund seiner Online-Fähigkeit dazu in der Lage. Das System ist aktuell auf einem Standard-PC implementiert und ermöglicht bei Verwendung von 50 Partikeln eine Aktualisierungsrate der Fehlerkorrekturschätzung von ca. 1 bis 1,5 s. Der Positionsfehler kann dabei auf ca. 1 mm korrigiert werden.

Im Gegensatz zu rein auf Bilddaten basierenden Verfahren der Objektverfolgung wird die komplette räumliche Lage des Objektes bestimmt. Die durch die Trackingdaten zur Verfügung stehende a-priori-Information über die Lage des Objektes im Bild schränkt den Suchraum stark ein, was zu einer schnellen und robusten Objekterkennung führt.

Bei erfolgreicher Bestimmung der Korrekturmatrix auf Basis einer repräsentativen Struktur eines Objektes kann diese Information auch zur Einblendung anderer Strukturen des selben Objektes verwendet werden. In unserem Anwendungfall beispielsweise zur Darstellung der im Knochen eingebetteten Cochlea. Zudem kann die verbesserte Lageinformation des Objektes auch für eine Steigerung der Präzision navigierter Eingriffe dienen, bei denen definierte Zielpunkte des Objektes hoch genau angefahren werden müssen [9].

Literaturverzeichnis

1. Frantz DD, Kirsch SR, Wiles AD. Specifying 3D tracking system accuracy: One manufacturer's view. Proc BVM. 2004; p. 234–238.
2. Labadie RF, Majdani O, Fitzpatrick JM. Image-guided technique in neurotology. Otolaryngol Clin North Am. 2007;40(3):611–24.
3. Lapeer R, Chen MS, Gonzalez G, et al. Image-enhanced surgical navigation for endoscopic sinus surgery: Evaluating calibration, registration and tracking. Int J Med Robot. 2008;4(1):32–45.
4. Wei GQ, Arbter K, Hirzinger G. Real time visual servoing for laparoscopic surgery. IEEE Eng Med Biol. 1997;16:40 – 45.
5. Rilk M, Winkelbach S, Wahl F. Partikelfilter-basiertes Tracking chirurgischer Instrumente in Endoskopbildern. Proc BVM. 2006.
6. Thrun S, Burgard W, Fox D. Probalistic Robotics. MIT Press; 2005.
7. Isard M, Blake A. Active Contours. New York: Springer-Verlag; 1998.
8. Strobl KH, Hirzinger G. Optimal hand-eye calibration. Procs IEEE Int Conf: Intelligent Robots and Systems. 2006; p. 4647–4653.
9. Leinung M, Baron S, Eilers H, et al. Robotic-guided minimally-invasive cochleostomy: First results. GMS CURAC. 2007;2(1).

3D Guide Wire Navigation from Single Plane Fluoroscopic Images in Abdominal Catheterizations

Martin Groher[2], Frederik Bender[1], Ali Khamene[3], Wolfgang Wein[3], Tim Hauke Heibel[2], Nassir Navab[2]

[1]Siemens AG Healthcare Sector AX, Forchheim, Germany
[2]Computer Aided Medical Procedures (CAMP), TUM, Munich, Germany
[3]Siemens Corporate Research (SCR), Princeton, NJ, USA
groher@cs.tum.edu

Abstract. Nowadays, abdominal catheterizations are mainly guided by 2D fluoroscopic imaging from one view, which complicates this task due to missing depth information, vessel invisibility, and patient motion. We propose a new technique for 3D navigation of guide wires based on single-plane 2D fluoroscopic views and a previously extracted 3D model of the vasculature. In order to relate the guide wire, which is only visible in the fluoroscopic view, to the 3D vasculature, we comprise methods for 2D-3D registration, apparent breathing motion compensation, guide wire detection, and robust backprojection. With this 2D-to-3D transfer, the navigation can be performed from arbitrary viewing angles, disconnected from the static perspective view of the fluoroscopic sequence.

1 Introduction

Minimally invasive catheter-guided interventions are common practice in modern hospitals and are usually guided by fluoroscopic imaging from one view. A guide wire can be visualized thus, which is moving in the image sequence due to respiratory patient motion and the physician's push/pull actions. In order to visualize blood vessels, which cannot be seen in fluoroscopic X-ray views, most hospitals acquire a high-resolution 2D Digitally Subtracted Angiogram (DSA) to avoid blind navigation. Using 2D DSAs, the navigation is still difficult at vessel overlays produced by the projection, or at vessel segments that run perpendicular to the image plane. Thus, 3D angiographic data were introduced into interventional workflow. However, they must be related to the current fluoroscopic frame, which is currently done via user interactions, hampering the navigation process. In order to relate 3D high resolution data to the current 2D fluoroscopic frame, systems have been proposed based on 2D-3D registration [1], or C-arm calibration [2]. Atasoy *et al.* [3] also takes breathing motion into account, which is common in abdominal fluoroscopic sequences, by compensating for the apparent motion of the guide wire. While clearly beneficial in terms of vessel visibility, depth perception cannot be increased with these approaches.

We propose a method for 3D guide wire navigation that transfers the 2D navigational procedure to 3D by taking information about 2D guide wire tip location, apparent breathing motion, view and 3D vessel geometry into account (Fig. 1). From a vascular model extracted from a 3D scan, and a DSA, we compute the projection matrix of the C-arm device. We relate the DSA to the current fluoroscopic frame by tracking the apparent catheter motion in 2D. From possible guide wire tip locations in 2D, we determine candidate 3D locations via backprojection to the 3D vessel model. With the estimates of view geometry and motion, we derive uncertainties for all these locations and determine the most probable of all 3D candidates using a variable bandwidth kernel estimator for information fusion. With our proposed system, which has been recently presented in [4], we successfully bring abdominal guide wire navigation to 3D, thus solving the problems of blind navigation and lack of depth perception.

2 Method

2.1 Data and preprocessing

The data sets that form the basis to our method are a fluoroscopic image sequence $\mathcal{S}$, a high resolution DSA with the same projection parameters as the fluoroscopic sequence, and a 3D angiographic scan from which we extract a 3D vessel model $\mathcal{V}$ as described in [5]. To determine the 3D position $\mathbf{X}$ of the guide wire tip, we need to know its position $\mathbf{X}$ within the current 2D fluoroscopic image frame

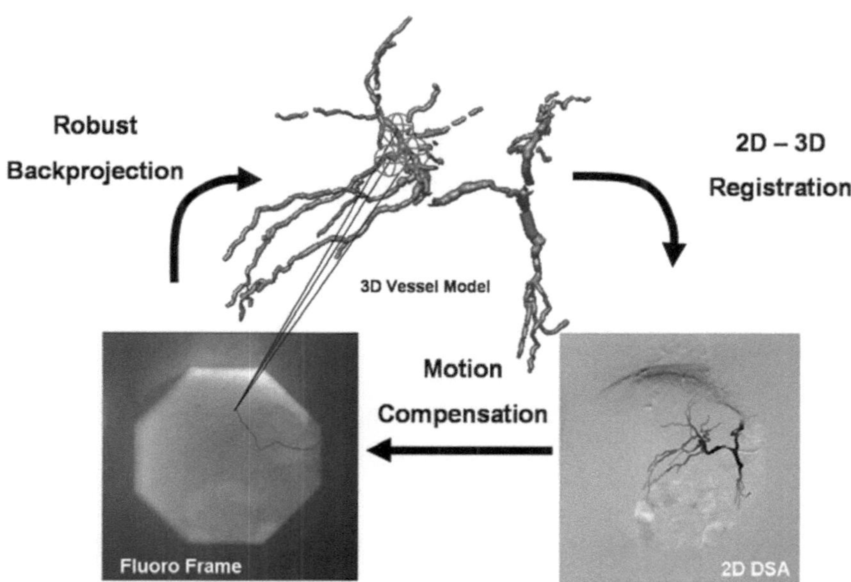

Fig. 1. 3D guide wire navigation

$\mathcal{S}_i$. To this end we employ a line detector proposed in [6]. We need a projection matrix $\mathtt{P}$, which aligns the 3D scan with the DSA image. A method, which is robust to deformation changes and different vessel contrast as proposed in [1] is used here. To countervail apparent respiratory motion, we compute the 2D motion in-between frames using the template based approach proposed in [3]. This method yields a global 2D translation, which approximates the 2D apparent breathing motion and relates each fluoroscopic frame to the initial DSA.

2.2 3D guide wire tip localization

Our method fuses all gathered information to compute the 3D correspondence of the guide wire tip location for every image frame, assuming a given uncertainty connected to each input parameter. In a first step, we subtract the respiratory motion displacement of the current image frame from the guide wire tip location to obtain the tip location $\mathbf{X}_0$ with respect to the DSA image. This is advantageous, since we can then use the pseudo-inverse of $\mathtt{P}$ to backproject the guide wire tip into 3D space. However, a simple backprojection of $\mathbf{X}_0$ will not always yield a satisfactory solution. First, ambiguities can arise if the backprojection ray intersects the vessel model multiple times. Second, the estimate of the guide wire tip location in 2D is prone to error caused by detection and motion compensation. We solve these problems with a statistical approach that is based on the creation of possible 2D guide wire tip candidates and the evaluation of their registration accuracy.

We take errors from detection and apparent motion estimation into account by randomly modifying the computed displacements in a range of $[\pm 10, \pm 10]$ pixels to generate n 2D tip candidates around $\mathbf{X}_0$, denoted by $\mathbf{X}_k$ where $k = 1..n$. We backproject each $\mathbf{X}_k$ using the pseudo-inverse of $\mathtt{P}$, compute the closest point on the vessel model $\mathcal{V}$ to the resulting ray, and define it to be a 3D correspondence candidate $\mathbf{X}_k$. Next, we compute an uncertainty connected to each $\mathbf{X}_k$ that is introduced by the uncertainty of the pose parameters Θ from $\mathtt{P}$. We randomly modify the registered pose Θ m times within an interval of $[\pm 5, \pm 5]$ mm for the translational, and $[\pm 5, \pm 5]^\circ$ for the rotational parameters. This results in m different poses Θ_j, which yield n sets of m 3D points: $\{\mathbf{X}_{k_j}\}$, $k = 1..n$, $j = 1..m$.

We assign a weight r_j to each $\mathbf{X}_{k_j}$, where r_j is computed as the reciprocal of the cost function used for 2D-3D registration [1], evaluated for pose Θ_j, and normalized such that $r_j \in [0; 1]$. The uncertainty of each $\mathbf{X}_k$ can be represented as its weighted covariance matrix (visualized by green spheres in Fig. 1)

$$C_k = \frac{1}{\sum\limits_{j=1}^{m} r_j} \sum_{j=1}^{m} r_j (\mathbf{X}_{k_j} - \overline{\mathbf{X}}_k)(\mathbf{X}_{k_j} - \overline{\mathbf{X}}_k)^T, \tag{1}$$

where $\overline{\mathbf{X}}_k = \frac{1}{\sum_{j=1}^{m} r_j} \sum_{j=1}^{m} r_j \mathbf{X}_{k_j}$ is the weighted mean.

In a final step, we fuse this uncertainty information to obtain an estimate for the 3D guide wire tip location. An approach to fuse such information is

Table 1. Results of target errors ϵ and standard deviations σ in mm

Phantom (Fig. 3(c))		ϵ_x	ϵ_y	ϵ_z	ϵ	σ_x	σ_y	σ_z	σ
Case 1	New	1.78	2.51	1.96	**3.98**	1.55	1.00	1.10	**1.44**
(light gray)	Naïve	2.70	4.97	24.39	26.59	1.38	2.94	43.41	42.58
Case 2	New	0.89	1.90	1.13	**2.66**	0.71	1.74	0.67	**1.58**
(dark gray)	Naïve	1.35	2.71	19.38	20.75	1.59	3.82	37.27	36.87

the Variable-Bandwidth Density-Based Fusion algorithm (VBDF), proposed by Comaniciu in [7]. It is robust to outliers, which occur as 3D correspondence candidates on a wrong vessel branch in our scenario, and involves the uncertainties of the measurements. In this approach, we estimate a density function from all measurement means $\overline{\mathbf{X}}_k$ and define its most significant mode to be the estimated 3D guide wire tip location $\mathbf{X}$. We involve information about the 3D location that was computed from the previous fluoroscopic image frame. The idea is to weigh the measurements $\overline{\mathbf{X}}_k$ dependent on their distance to the estimate of the previous frame. This is justified by the fact, that the guide wire will probably not move dramatically between successive image frames. To ensure the 3D guide wire to be inside a vessel, we pick the closest point on $\mathcal{V}$ to the computed $\mathbf{X}$ and define this point to be the final 3D guide wire tip position.

3 Experiments and results

To test our method, we ran a study on a realistic breathing phantom with a known ground truth. To this end we use a phantom including a vessel system, which is formed by a set of connected plastic tubes fixed in liquid wax (Fig. 3(a)). The breathing motion is simulated by an electronic pump that is attached to the phantom, yielding apparent in-plane displacements of up to 14 pixels (in 1024 $\times$ 1024 images). The image data is acquired with a Siemens AXIOM Artis dBA, a calibrated bi-plane C-arm device. It allows us to grab two fluoroscopic sequences (Fig. 3(c)) from which we can compute the guide wire tip's 3D ground truth position. The vessel model $\mathcal{V}$ is extracted from a rotational run under contrast agent. For testing our algorithm, we used only one of the projection sequences, where two particular overlay cases are evaluated (Fig. 3(b)). The DSA for registration was created from a second, contrasted sequence. 3D Euclidean errors and associated standard deviations are shown in Tab. 1. A comparison is made with a naïve approach, which does not use uncertainty information for backprojection. Please note that the error especially in ray direction (ε_z) can be reduced significantly using our method.

4 Conclusion

In this work we propose an algorithm, which robustly facilitates 3D navigation of guide wires in abdominal catheterizations using fluoroscopic images from a

Fig. 2. (a) Breathing phantom. (b) Rendered 3D volume of phantom with arrows marking the path of case 1 (light gray), case 2 (dark gray). (c) Phantom fluoroscopy showing tubes and guide wire. The circels mark the same paths as arrows in (b).

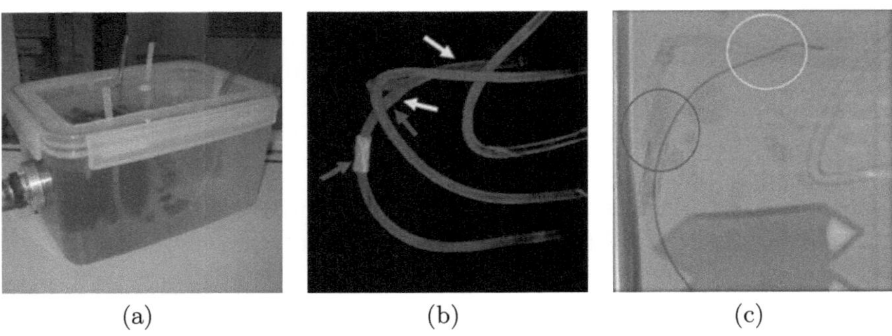

(a) (b) (c)

monoplane C-arm system. Encouraged by the good results from synthetic and phantom tests, we will proceed with an extensive patient study. Further ideas are aiming at a feedback system for physicians in cases where the C-arm configuration is not optimal in regard to the desired operation situs, or where the system's predicition is too ambiguous. The concepts and information presented in this paper are based on research and are not commercially available.

References

1. Groher M, Bender F, Hoffmann RT, et al. Segmentation-driven 2D-3D registration for abdominal catheter interventions. Procs MICCAI. 2007; p. 527–535.
2. Gorges S, Kerrien E, Berger MO, et al. Model of a vascular C-arm for 3D augmented fluoroscopy in interventional radiology. Procs MICCAI. 2005; p. 214–222.
3. Atasoy S, Groher M, Zikic D, et al. Real-Time respiratory motion tracking: Roadmap correction for hepatic artery catheterizations. Procs SPIE. 2008.
4. Bender F, Groher M, Khamene A, et al. 3D dynamic roadmapping for abdominal catheterizations. MICCAI. 2008.
5. Selle D, Preim B, Schenk A, et al. Analysis of vasculature for liver surgery planning. IEEE Tran Med Imaging. 2002;21(8):1344–1357.
6. Steger C. An unbiased detector of curvilinear structures. IEEE Trans Pattern Anal Mach Intell. 1998;20(2):113–125.
7. Comaniciu D. Nonparametric information fusion for motion estimation. Procs IEEE CVPR. 2003; p. I–59 – I–66.

A Porcine Liver Model for Validation of Registration Accuracy in Image-Guided Surgery

Matthias Peterhans[1], Benoît Dagon[2], Anne Vom Berg[3], Daniel Inderbitzin[3], Charles Baur[2], Stefan Weber[1]

[1]ARTORG Center, University of Bern, Switzerland
[2]VRAI Group, Ecole Polytechnique Fédérale de Lausanne (EPFL), Switzerland
[3]Department of Visceral and Transplantation Surgery, Inselspital, Bern, Switzerland
matthias.peterhans@artorg.unibe.ch

Abstract. Correct registration between pre-operative high-resolution images and intra-operative data of lower detail is a fundamental requirement in image-guided liver surgery. We propose a multi modality liver model for measuring the accuracy of such registration methods. A freshly explanted porcine liver is artificially perfused by a peristaltic pump and liver motion is simulated by means of inflatable objects positioned around the liver. Co-registered ultrasound and CT data sets are acquired in different deformation scenarios and allow compar-ing registration outcomes with a CT data set serving as ground truth. The pre-sent work describes the experimental setup and summarizes the results from ultrasound and CT imaging.

1 Introduction

In image-guided liver surgery, accurate registration between pre-operative image data and the intra-operative scenario is crucial for correct assistance during the surgery. Registration is either performed based on liver surface data or on information about structures inside the liver. Validation of registration is a challenging task because it is usually difficult to acquire redundant information serving as a benchmark for accuracy computation. Registration success is usually measured by means of the fitting error between corresponding structures (e.g. vessels bifurcations) in the intra-operative data and pre-operative scans [1]. This measure can lead to problems with local minima. Therefore, a measure of registration accuracy by an independent validation data set is desirable.

Related work on liver phantoms reports either synthetic models [2, 3] or an ex-vivo human liver model [4]. Bao et al. [2] create liver models with implanted fiducial markers from silicon polymer or polyurethane. Weber et al. [3] use rapid prototyping to print segmented liver structures in an elastic material and then pack the obtained structures in a tissue-mimicking material. Such models allow for multi-modality imaging of the liver (except for Doppler ultrasound) but represent a further abstraction from real liver tissue to tissue mimicking material. Müller et al. [4] propose a model based on explanted human livers which are embedded into a respiratory motion simulator for analyzing respiratory motion. Measurements are obtained by navigated needles inserted into the liver parenchyma. Multi modality imaging is mentioned but no results are shown.

In the purpose of staying close to a real surgical situation, we have developed an ex-vivo porcine liver model for multi modality imaging. The experimental setup is built on the table of a CT scanner which allows ultrasound and CT acquisition without motion between the scans. The resulting data sets will serve as ground truth for validating our non-rigid registration approach [5].

2 Materials and Methods

2.1 Methodology

Our approach to measure the registration accuracy consists of five steps (Figure 1). First, a CT-scan representing the pre-operative situation is acquired (A). Then, the liver is deformed and navigated ultrasound images representing the intra-operative situation are acquired (B). Next, a CT scan of the deformed liver is acquired (C). This CT will serve as the validation data set. Registration between the pre-operative CT and the intra-operative ultrasound is then performed (D). Finally, the accuracy is measured by calculating the differences between the registered pre-operative CT and the validation data set (E).

2.2 Liver preparation

The proposed liver model consists of an entire porcine liver specimen embedded into foam representing the abdominal organs around the liver. Blood circulation

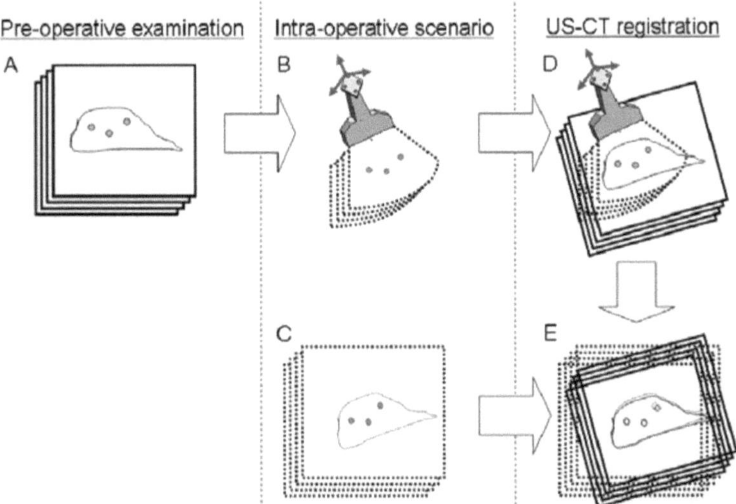

Fig. 1. Illustration of the experimental methodology

is simulated by a physiological fluid pumped through the liver by a peristaltic pump. The latter is set to provide similar flux and input pressure as observed in the circulatory system. Liver deformation is induced by means of inflatable balloons placed around the liver. Porcine livers were obtained directly from the butcher where care was taken to cut them together with the diaphragm in order not to damage the portal veins. Blood coagulation inside the liver was avoided by rinsing the specimen with Ringer saline solution directly after explantation. The livers where then transported in a cooled bath of 4°C of Ringer saline solution and experiments were performed within the same day to minimize the effects of tissue degeneration.

Liver perfusion was induced by a peristaltic pump imposing a flow of Ringer saline solution into the portal vein. Physiologic conditions are obtained when a flow of 200 ml/min is imposed at the portal vein entrance and the measured input pressure rises to 20cm H2O. The perfusion liquid was recollected at the liver veins imposing an exit pressure of 10cm H2O.

2.3 Imaging setup

The liver deformations occurring between the pre-operative CT and the surgery are simulated by means of inflatable balloons positioned around the liver. For each deformation scenario, a co-registered image pair consisting of a CT scan data set and a set of navigated ultrasound images is acquired.

Experiments were performed directly on the table of a Siemens Somatom Emotion 6 CT scanner. Liver vessels were enhanced using Gastrografin (Schering Wien, GmbH) contrast agent mixed with the Ringer saline solution used for perfusion.

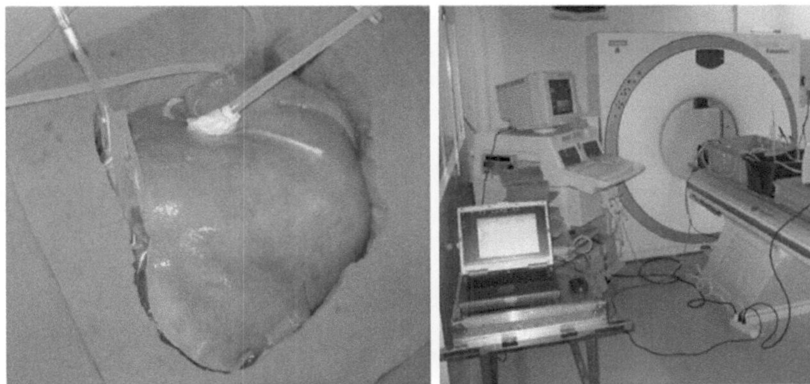

Fig. 2. (Left) Liver specimen with tubes connected to its vascular system. An inflatable bag for simulating deformation is visible on the left. (Right) Experimental setup with ultrasound and CT systems, liver model and pump on the CT table, navigation system.

After CT acquisition, ultrasound images were acquired using a calibrated and optically tracked ultrasound probe (Atracsys Easytrack 500 active optical tracking system and Philips Sonos 5500 in 2D mode with an 8MHz probe) connected to a frame grabber on a notebook computer.

Registration between the CT volume and the navigation system is obtained by pointer-based registration of radiopaque fiducial spheres mounted on the container box.

3 Results

For each of the three porcine liver specimens, several pairs of CT-ultrasound image sets were acquired at different deformation scenarios. Figure 3 shows a representative CT image slice and an ultrasound image of a vessel region. In the CT, the main vessels are clearly visible as bright regions. Smaller vessels are still visible but harder to distinguish from the liver parenchyma which also contains bright regions. The latter are due to the continuous contrast injection leading to a permanent filling of liver capillaries. Pulsatile contrast injection as used in clinics would avoid this effect and provide selective enhancement of different structures depending on the delay between contrast injection and image acquisition. However the obtained image quality is sufficient to identify the main liver vessels by semi-automatic segmentation. In the ultra-sound images, vessels are visible as ellipsoidal dark regions which indicates that per-fusion was successfully established and that the imposed pressure simulated physio-logical conditions.

Figure 4 illustrates the results of image processing on the acquired images. The figure on the left shows the superposition of results from semi-automatic segmentation of the pre-operative CT (red surface) and points extracted automatically [5] from the intra-operative ultrasound (red and green circles). On the right, two different deformation stages are visualized using rapid prototyping. Corresponding vessel branches from the pre-operative CT (red) and the validation CT (blue) are clearly visible.

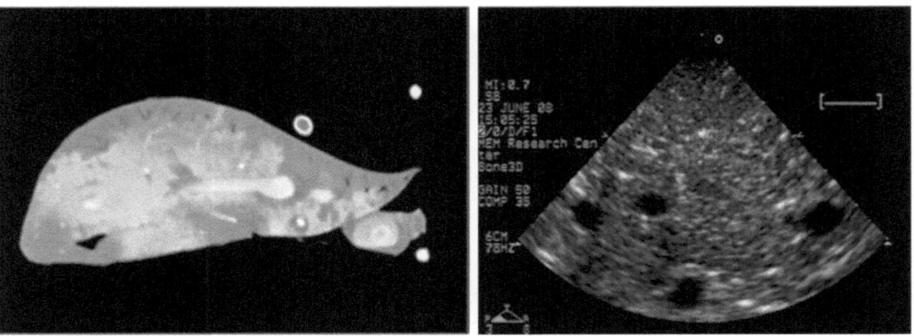

Fig. 3. Results of CT and ultrasound image acquisition on the porcine liver model

Fig. 4. (Left) Augmented reality environment combining the 3D vessel model and the ultrasound segmentation results. (Right) 3D print of liver vessels at different deformation stages.

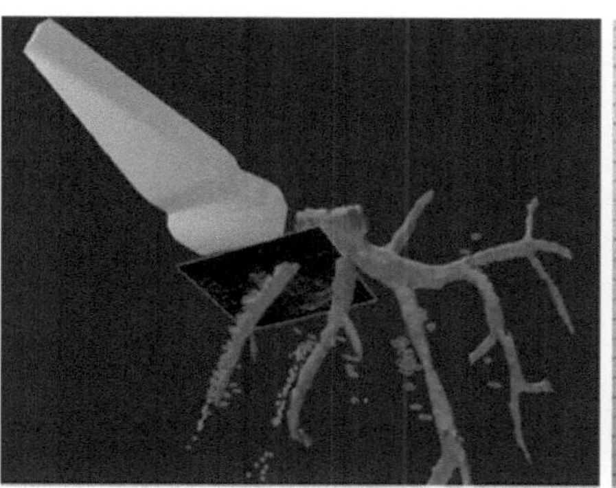

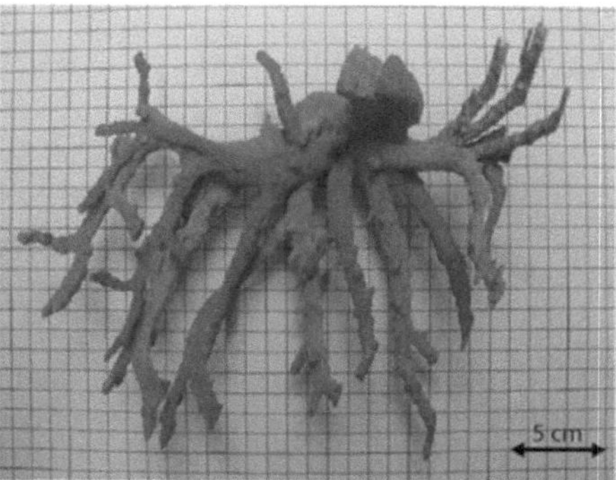

4 Discussion

Our experiments have shown the feasibility of multi modality image acquisition on an ex-vivo porcine liver under artificially induced perfusion. CT as well as ultrasound images are similar to images in a real patient scenario. Up to our knowledge, this is the first report of a multi modality imaging experiment on real liver tissue which leads to ground truth for quantitative evaluation of registration outcomes. The images resulting from these experiments will be used for the validation of a registration approach based on a mass-spring model of the liver vasculature and vessel centreline points extracted automatically from ultrasound images. The limitation of the current setup is the reduced visibility of small vessels in the contrast-enhanced CT. Future experiments will use pulsatile contrast injection in order to avoid this effect.

References

1. Lange T, Lamecker H, Hühnerbein M, et al. Validation Metrics for Non-Rigid Registration of Medical Images containing Vessel Trees. Procs BVM. 2008; p. 82–86.
2. Bao P, Warmath J, Galloway R, et al. Ultrasound-to-computer-tomography registration for image-guided laparoscopic liver surgery. Surg Endosc. 2005;19:424–429.
3. Weber S, Markert M, Lueth TC. Surface tracking of organs for registration in soft tissue surgery. In: Image Guidance and Computer Assistance for Soft-Tissue Interventions IGSTI; 2008. p. 65–74.
4. Müller SA, Maier-Hein L, Mehrabi A, et al. Creation and establishment of a respiratory liver motion simulator for liver interventions. Med Phys. 2007;34:4605–8.
5. Dagon B, Baur C, Bettschart V. Intraoperative update of liver surgery planning based on ultrasound images. In: Computer-Aided Medical Interventions: Tools and Applications. Sauramps Medical; 2007. p. 419–423.

Stereoskopische Visualisierung einer Infektion mammalischer Zellen durch pathogene Bakterien

Michael Granseier[1,2], Heike Grassmé[1], Erich Gulbins[1], Hans-Gerd Lipinski[2]

[1]Institut für Molekularbiologie, Universität Duisburg/Essen
[2]Fachbereich Informatik, Fachhochschule Dortmund
michael.granseier@arcor.de

Kurzfassung. Die Infektion mammalischer Zellen durch pathogene Bakterien ist biologisch immer noch nicht sicher geklärt. Mit Hilfe der Laserscanmikroskopie ist es mittlerweile aber möglich, räumliche Bilddaten von Zellproben zu erstellen, auf denen der Eindringvorgang der Bakterien in das Zellinnere durch verschieden leuchtende Fluoreszenzfarbstoffe visualisiert werden kann. Unter Verwendung bekannter und adaptierter 3D-Rekonstruktionsalgorithmen werden dreidimensionale Visualisierungen von Mikroskopiebildern vorgestellt, mit deren Hilfe die Analyse des Infektionsprozesses erleichtert wird. Dabei hat sich gezeigt, dass mit Oberflächenrekonstruktionsverfahren die Topografie der Zelloberfläche korrekt dargestellt werden kann, während die Darstellung der Farbstoffverteilungen besser durch ein Texture-Mapping-Verfahren gelingt. Die Rekonstruktionen konnten insbesondere durch den Einsatz von stereoskopischen Visualisierungstechniken detailgenau analysiert werden.

1 Einleitung

Infektionen gesunder mammalischer Zellen durch pathogene Bakterien werden derzeit auch mit molekularbiologischen Methoden untersucht. Im Verlauf einer solchen Infektion gelingt es den Bakterien, die Zellmembran zu durchdringen und somit die Zelle von innen zu schädigen. Das Verstehen der exakten Wechselwirkungen zwischen der Zellmembran und den Bakterien während des Eintritts des Bakteriums in das Zellinnere ist dabei für das Verständnis des Krankheitsprozesses von großem Interesse [1, 2]. Erst wenn die molekularbiologische Ursache geklärt ist, die es einem Bakterium ermöglicht, die Zellmembran zu durchdringen, kann ein effektives Medikament entwickelt werden, um die Infektion humaner Zellen mit pathogenen Bakterien zu hemmen.

Durch den Einsatz von modernen 3D-Laserscanmikroskopen lassen sich mittlerweile digitale Bilddaten von infizierten Zellproben erstellen, welche zuvor mit unterschiedlichen Fluoreszenzfarbstoffen optisch angeregt werden. Primär sind die erzeugten Bilddaten zweidimensional. Da jedoch ein Bilddatenstapel generiert wird, können die Bilddaten zu einem dreidimensionalen Bild zusammengefügt werden. Ziel dieses Artikels ist es, aus den akquirierten Mikroskopbildern unter Verwendung bekannter und modifizierter Volume-Rendering-Verfahren dreidimensionale Ansichten zu generieren, auf denen der Eintritt der Bakterien in das Zellinnere räumlich interaktiv betrachtet werden kann. Dabei ist neben der korrekten Wiedergabe der zeitlich-räumlichen Veränderungen der Membran- und Bakterienstrukturen auch auf die korrekte Wiedergabe der Intensitätsverteilung der einzelnen Fluoreszenzfarbstoffe sowie deren Kolokalisation zu achten. Zur genaueren Analyse erscheint in diesem Zusammenhang eine stereoskopische Visualisierung sinnvoll.

2 Material und Methoden

2.1 Verwendete Zellbilder

Für die Generierung der dreidimensionalen Visualisierungen standen mikroskopische Schnittbildfolgen mammalischer Zellproben (Makrophagen) zur Verfügung, die mit einem grün fluoreszierenden Mycobakterium infiziert wurden. Unter Verwendung von Fluoreszenzfarbstoffen wurden die Makrophagen so präpariert, dass in den späteren Mikroskopbildern sowohl das in der Zelle produzierte Lipid Ceramid als auch die als Signalgeber fungierenden Rab5-Proteine sichtbar gemacht werden konnten [1, 2]. Zur Unterscheidung der beiden Zellbestandteile wurde für das Ceramid ein roter und für das Rab5 ein blauer Farbstoff verwendet. Diese präparierten Makrophagen wurden dann mit einem Laserscanmikroskop der Marke Leica DMIRE 2, ausgestattet mit einem durch Öl benetzten Objektiv mit 100-facher Vergrößerung, mikroskopiert. Alle vier Proben hatten eine Größe von $150 \times 150\ \mu m^2$ in der Ebene. Die Probendicke lag zwischen 4,094 μm und 9,538 μm.

Im Laufe der Bildakquisition wurde jede Zellprobe in sechs Schichten von oben nach unten registriert, wobei durch die Laserbestrahlung die Fluoreszenzstoffe optisch angeregt wurden, so dass die oben genannten Probenbestandteile sichtbar wurden (Bakterien = grün, Ceramid = rot, Rab5 = blau). Von jeder Schicht wurde die zugehörige Bildmatrix für die drei Farbkanäle Rot, Grün und Blau gespeichert. Somit standen für die 3D-Rekonstruktion jeweils drei einzelne Bildfolgen der fluoreszierenden Bestandteile einer jeden Makrophage zur Verfügung. Die Bilder hatten eine Größe von 512×512 Bildpunkten, was einer Pixelgröße von $0,293 \times 0,293\ \mu m^2$ entspricht.

2.2 Bildvorverarbeitung und -visualisierung

Störende und nicht-relevante Bildpunkte wurden mit Hilfe eines Schwellwert-Filters entfernt. Ein solcher Filter entfernt alle Bildpunkte, die unterhalb eines manuell festgelegten Pixelwertes liegen und lässt dabei die übrigen Bildpunkte unverändert. Meist als dunkle Bildpunkte auftretendes Hintergrundrauschen konnte somit fast vollständig entfernt werden. Für die 3D-Rekonstruktion mit Hilfe des Marching-Cube-Verfahrens wurden die Zellbilder zunächst durch einen Bildkanten erhaltenden Diffusionsfilter geglättet, damit die Topografie der Zeloberfläche im Verlauf der Infektion verdeutlicht wird. Weiterhin wurden die ursprünglich sechs Schnittbilder einer jeden Probe durch lineare Interpolation von Zwischenbildern auf 21 Bilder erweitert. Erst dadurch war die Generierung brauchbarer 3D Ansichten möglich. Zur besseren räumlichen Orientierung bei der Betrachtung der dreidimensionalen Zellen wurde jeder Zelle interaktiv eine Membrankontur hinzugefügt, welche unter Verwendung einer Catmull-Rom Spline-Interpolation aus manuell festgelegten Stützstellen berechnet wurde. Die endgültigen dreidimensionalen Zellbilder wurden mit Hilfe der zwei bekannten räumlichen Rekonstruktionsverfahren „Marching-Cube“ und „Texture-Mapping“ generiert. Mit Ausnahme der Membraninterpolation wurden für die übrigen Bearbeitungsschritte Algorithmen und Methoden des Insight Toolkit (ITK) und des Visualization Toolkit (VTK) verwendet [3]. Als Entwicklungsumgebungen dienten der Borland C++ Builder 5 sowie das Microsoft Visual Studio .NET 2003.

2.3 Stereoskopische Darstellung

Die Möglichkeit des stereoskopischen Sehens basiert auf den etwas unterschiedlichen Perspektiven, mit denen die Augen ein Objekt erkennen. Linkes und rechtes Auge nehmen dabei leicht voneinander abweichende Bilder wahr, aus denen das Gehirn die räumliche Ansicht bildet. Dieses Prinzip kann mit Hilfe spezieller Stereoskopie-Monitore künstlich umgesetzt werden, wobei auf dem Display ein verschachteltes Gesamtbild mit jeweils verschiedenen Informationen für beide Augen dargestellt wird. Es existieren eine Reihe von Darstellungsverfahren, für die u.U. auch eine spezielle Sehhilfe benötigt wird, um jedem Auge das ihm zugeordnete Bild sichtbar zu machen. Es kamen die bekannten Stereoskopie-Verfahren „Dresden“ und „Crystal-Eyes“ zum Einsatz. Die verwendete Hardware bestand aus einem 20 Zoll SeeReal Cn 3D Display und einem 20 Zoll Planar SD2020 Display.

3 Ergebnisse

Die Abbildung 1 auf Seite 369 zeigt die dreidimensionalen Visualisierungen der unterschiedlichen Makrophagen unter Verwendung des Texture-Mapping Verfahrens. Dargestellt ist jeweils der relevante Ausschnitt der Zelle, innerhalb dessen die Bakterien in das Zellinnere eindringen. Jede Bildserie beinhaltet im Original 20 3D-Schnittbilder, die ein Eindringen von oben nach unten in die Zelle zeigen. Von jeder Zellprobe wurden beispielhaft fünf Abbildungen ausgewählt. Die verwendeten Fluoreszenzfarbstoffe zeigen die Verteilung des Ceramid, des Rab5 sowie der Bakterien während des Infektionsvorgangs. Gut erkennbar sind in allen Abbildungen auch die Intensitätsunterschiede der einzelnen Farbstoffe, bedingt durch unterschiedlich starke Ansammlungen der an die Farben gekoppelten Zellprobenbestandteile. Die Kolokalisationen zwischen Bakterien und Rab5 sowie zwischen Rab5 und Ceramid werden durch die additive Überlagerung der entsprechenden Fluoreszenzfarbstoffe als cyan- bzw. violettfarbene Bereiche wiedergegeben. In der Abbildung 2 auf Seite 370 sind die gleichen Schnittbilder unter Verwendung des Marching-Cube-Verfahrens dargestellt. Die Topografie der Zeloberfläche ist hier deutlich erkennbar. Zur besseren Visualisierung der zeitlichen

Abb. 1. Dreidimensionale Texture-Mapping-Rekonstruktion der Makrophagen. Ceramid ist rot eingefärbt, Rab5-Proteine blau und pathogene Bakterien grün. Von links nach rechts sieht man jeweils den zeitlichen Verlauf des Infektionsprozesses durch Abtragung der jeweils obersten Schnittebene. Die Nummerierung steht für die Position des Bildes in der vollständigen 3D-Schnittbildfolge.

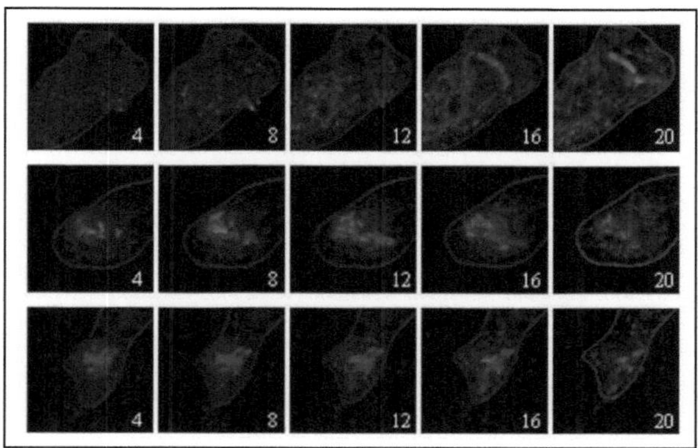

Veränderungen der Bakterien- und Rab5-Strukturen wurden diese durch zweidimensionale Isolinien dargestellt. Die nachträglich hinzugefügte Zellmembran ist in den Bildern ebenfalls rot dargestellt. Sie dient allerdings nur der besseren Abgrenzung der Zelle gegenüber dem Hintergrund und ist nicht als Ceramid-Aggregation zu betrachten. Bei allen Abbildungen handelt es sich aus drucktechnischen Gründen nicht um stereoskopische Darstellungen, da dieser Effekt nur mit entsprechenden Hilfsmitteln (Monitor, Brille etc.) erzielt werden kann.

4 Diskussion

Mit Hilfe des räumlichen Rekonstruktionsverfahrens „Marching-Cube" konnte die Topografie der Zelloberfläche im Verlauf der Bakterieninfektion deutlich dargestellt werden. Da es sich hierbei um ein Oberflächen-Rendering-Verfahren handelt, lassen sich durch die Bakterienaktivität bedingte Deformationen der Zellmembran besonders gut räumlich visualisieren, wobei vor allem Einbuchtungen, die das Eindringen der Bakterien ermöglichen, von besonderem Interesse sind. Um die Oberflächentopografie eindeutig analysieren zu können, mußten die Zellbilder zunächst mit einem Diffusionsfilter geglättet werden. Diese Glättung führt jedoch zu dem Problem, dass die biologisch wichtige Granularität der Ceramid-Aggregationen verloren geht. Des Weiteren können die unterschiedlichen Farbintensitäten der Fluoreszenzstoffe über das Marching-Cube-Verfahren nicht wiedergegeben werden. Somit stellen die 3D-Rekonstruktionen des Marching-Cube keine biologisch korrekten Abbildungen dar.

Durch den Einsatz des Texture-Mapping-Verfahrens lassen sich solche Defizite beheben. Diese Visualisierungstechnik bildet die Konzentrationsunterschiede des Ceramid und des Rab5 in den einzelnen Zellebenen korrekt ab, wodurch z.B. Rückschlüsse auf Aktivitätsschwerpunkte innerhalb der Bakterienansammlung

Abb. 2. Dreidimensionale Marching-Cube-Rekonstruktion der geglätteten Makrophagenbilder. Ceramid ist rot eingefärbt, Rab5-Proteine blau und pathogene Bakterien grün. Von links nach rechts sieht man jeweils den zeitlichen Verlauf des Infektionsprozesses durch Abtragung der jeweils obersten Schnittebene. Die Nummerierung steht für die Position des Bildes in der vollständigen 3D-Schnittbildfolge.

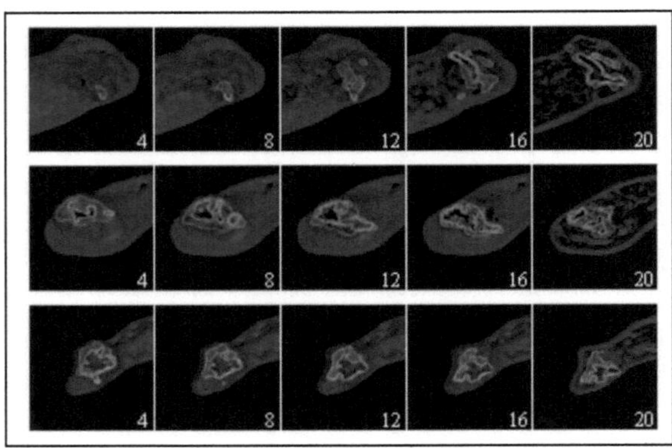

gezogen werden können. In den Bildern 8 bis 16 der Abbildungen 1 und 2 zeigen sich in allen drei Proben schlauchartige Ausformungen der grünen Bakterienansammlungen. Diese Ausformungen deuten darauf hin, dass in diesem Moment das tatsächliche Eindringen der Bakterien in das Zellinnere stattfindet. Im Bereich dieser Aktivität werden signalgebende Rab5-Proteine in den Zellen aktiviert, die sich deutlich durch den blauen Fluoreszenzfarbstoff von den restlichen Bestandteilen der Zellprobe abheben.

Insgesamt können mit beiden räumlichen Rekonstruktionen die genauen Wechselwirkungen zwischen der Zellmembran und den Bakterien untersucht werden. Insbesondere durch die Möglichkeit der stereoskopischen Visualisierung lassen sich die genannten Details des Infektionsvorgangs in fast greifbarer räumlicher Virtualität noch exakter analysieren. Hierbei steht auch die Rolle des Ceramid im Vordergrund [4, 5]. Es eröffnet sich somit ein neuer Ansatz zur adäquaten Analyse von Infektionsvorgängen mammalischer Zellen.

Literaturverzeichnis

1. Grassmé H, Jendrossek V, Riehle A, et al. Host defense against Pseudomonas aeruginosa requires ceramid-rich membrane rafts. Nat Med. 2003;9(3):322–330.
2. Grassmé H, Riethmüller J, Gulbins E. Biological aspects of ceramide-enriched membrane domains. Prog Lipid Res. 2007;46:161–170.
3. Schroeder W, Martin K, Lorensen B. The Visualization Toolkit (3rd Edition). United States of America: Kitware Inc.; 2004.
4. Cremesti A, François P, Grassmé H, et al. Ceramide enables fas to cap and kill. J Biol Chem. 2001;267(26):23954–23961.
5. Gulbins E, Kolesnick R. Raft ceramide in molecular medicine. Oncogene. 2003;22:7070–7077.

Interactive Boundary Detection for Automatic Definition of 2D Opacity Transfer Function

Martin Rauberger, Heinrich Martin Overhoff

Medical Engineering Laboratory, University of Applied Sciences Gelsenkirchen, Gelsenkirchen, Germany
martin.rauberger@fh-gelsenkirchen.de

Abstract. In computer assisted diagnostics nowadays, high-value 3-D visualization intake a supporting role to the traditional 2-D slice wise visualization. 3-D visualization may create intuitive visual appearances of the spatial relations of anatomical structures, based upon transfer functions mapping data values to visual parameters, e.g. color or opacity. Manual definition of these transfer functions however requires expert knowledge and can be tedious. In this paper an approach to automatizing 2-D opacity transfer function definition is presented. Upon few parameters characterizing the image volume and an user-depicted area of interest, the procedure detects organ surfaces automatically, upon which transfer functions may automatically be defined. Parameter setting still requires experience about the imaging properties of modalities, and improper setting can cause falsely detected organ surfaces. Procedure tests with CT and MRI image volumes show, that real time structure detection is even possible for noisy image volumes.

1 Introduction

Direct volume rendering (DVR) of medical image volumes from modalities, like X-ray CT, MRI, 3-D ultrasound, or PET can often give a clear hint to morphologic, physiologic and/or functional pathologies. With the technological progress of imaging modalities producing image volumes of steadily increasing quality, 3-D visualization techniques take in a viable supportive function to the traditional 2-D slice-wise finding in clinical routine.

DVR relies on opacity transfer functions (OTFs) to define the transparency (transparency t, opacity $\alpha = 1-t$) of each voxel [1], and thus to visually separate the diagnostically relevant anatomical structures (structures of interest) from the dispensable structures. OTFs are however to be defined for every finding and image volume, requiring a definition process to be flexible for varying application purposes and time saving, in order to reach clinical acceptance.

1.1 The projected histogram

Kindlmann and Durkin [2] introduced that material boundaries are distinguishable as arches in a greyscale encoded frequency distribution in the domain of data value (voxel $\mathbf{x}$, data value $f(\mathbf{x})$) versus first order gradient magnitude ($|f'(\mathbf{x})|$), further referred to as projected histogram. Different types of homogeneous material (v_n) appear as clotted regions (dark), whereas boundaries between these materials occur as regions of continuous data value change, and thus of higher gradient magnitude as seen in Fig. 1. In present medical imaging these curves are however not infinitely thin and regular, but blurred and distorted due to material inhomogeneities and characteristics of the imaging modality. By defining 2-D OTFs assigning highest opacity values to one boundary arch in the projected histogram, materials can be visually separated.

1.2 Related work

The topic of defining OTFs has been increasingly discussed in recent years. As the approach presented in this paper focuses on material boundaries and for 2-D OTF definition, only related work for visualizing material boundaries using 2-D OTFs is discussed.

Kniss et al. [3] proposed interaction widgets, with which to select peaks of the arches for 2-D OTF definition. Upon these widgets, a higher level of abstraction to alleviate user interaction is proposed by Salama et al. [4], where the number of freely definable parameters is cleverly reduced. But however to the cost of flexibility due to the specialization on one certain application.

Šereda et al. [5] address remaining insufficiency in the visual separation of 2-D OTFs using data value and gradient, introducing the L-H-histograms for improved separation of materials and their boundaries.

These approaches all succeed visual separation acceptable for clinical finding, but do however require the user to interact with additional elements to those of slice-by-slice viewing. Moreover do some propose direct interaction in an abstract projected histogram, requiring expert knowledge for OTF definition.

In order to avoid intense interaction with images and image-related parameters, a method for boundary detection based solely on interaction with the visualized image volume is presented. It exploits scatter plots and calculates

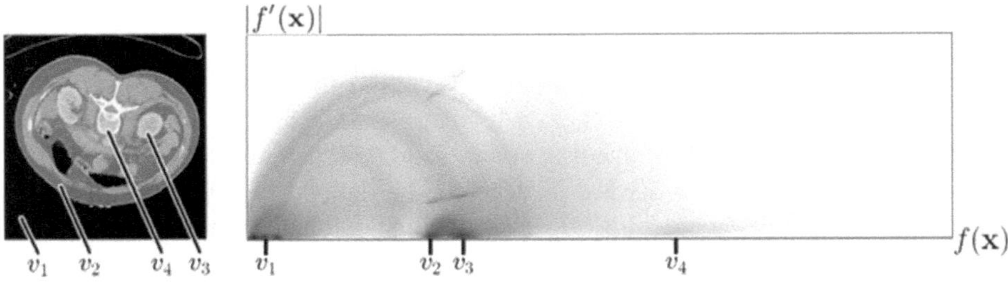

Fig. 1. Example of a projected histogram with first order gradient magnitude $|f'(\mathbf{x})|$ versus grey-scale $f(\mathbf{x})$ (right) shown together with a slice of CT image volume of human torso (left).

mathematical arch representations for later automatic 2-D OTF definition. Its performance is investigated with the focus on clinical application.

2 Materials and methods

Using a standard 2-D mouse as input device, the user can specify a structure of interest in the visualized image volume by e.g. clicking, resulting in a vector describing a straight path throughout the volume. By summing-up the data values and gradients of passed voxels, a scatter plot is calculated. Four examples of scatter plots are seen in Fig. 2, where four straight sampling paths visualize material boundary arches between aorta and mediastinum in a CT image of the human thorax. It is seen, that scatter plots of the same anatomical structure (aorta) vary throughout the image volume, due to the material inhomogeneities and imaging characteristics mentioned in chapter 1.1.

In order to receive the best fitting geometric representation of the boundary arch within reasonable time, approximations of skewed circles are preferred due to their calculatory simplicity (in opposition to e.g. ellipses or splines). Approximations are performed upon numerous scatter plots collected by incorporating the local neighborhood of the passed voxels. For this instance the method of least squares is applied and its sum is compared to a predefined maximum value.

The approximation routine is initiated when a material boundary is supposed passed, by evaluating the gradient magnitudes mean value ($\overline{|f'|}$) and data value standard deviation (σ_f) of every passed voxel and local neighborhood. For this

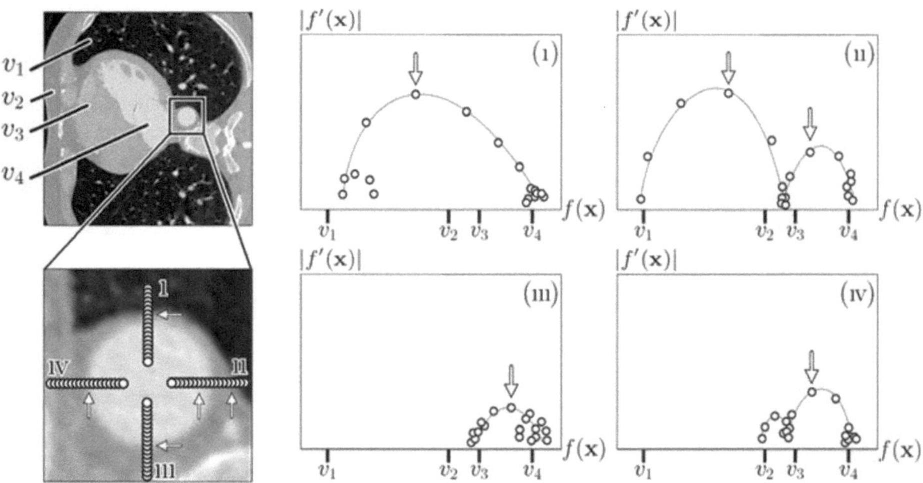

Fig. 2. Four examples of scatter plots calculated from straight sampling paths. Thin spline approximated arches depict material boundaries between aorta and mediastinum in a CT image of the human thorax. Thick lines depict the simple geometric representations of skewed circle approximations.

instance, $\overline{|f'|}$ and σ_f are compared to predefined parameters determining the image volume.

After validating the relative position of the geometric representation to a predefined minimum gradient value ($|f'|_{\min}$), the resulting mathematical descriptions of material boundary arches in the projected histogram may then serve as background for automatic 2-D OTF definition.

3 Results

The presented approach succeeds in finding even subtle material boundaries, needing the user to simply click on the structure of interest while interacting with nothing more than the visualized 3-D image volume (Fig. 3). The approach saves time in clinical finding, as the time from user clicking to calculated mathematical representation of the boundary arch is below 0.5 seconds. The testing platform was a standard PC with Intel Pentium™Core 2 Duo CPU 2×2.40 GHz, 2048 GB DDR2-RAM, a GeForce 8800 graphics card and Windows XP™Professional. The testing image volume was a DICOM MRI image volume with $576 \times 576 \times 96$ voxels.

4 Discussion

The approach provides the user with a fast tool for finding material boundaries intuitively, and to calculate mathematical representations for later automatic 2D OTF definition. As the boundary detection relies on predefined reference parameters (for gradient magnitudes mean value $\overline{f'}$, data value standard deviation σ_fs), improper setting of these parameters may result in detecting only the most prominent material boundaries, or in falsely detecting material inhomogeneities as material boundaries. The process of finding representative values

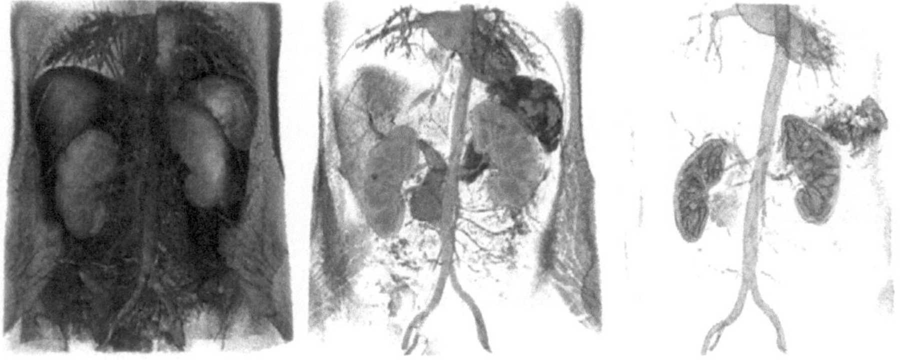

Fig. 3. Three examples of high-quality rendering results based upon a MRI image volume of the human abdomen. Through sequential clicking on an anatomical structure of interest (e.g. a kidney), the rendering becomes clearer from left to right.

for these parameters may tedious and thus future research will focus on their automatic definition, through analysis and evaluation of the overall data value and gradient magnitude distribution.

Regardless of imaging modality, the data value ranges of anatomical structures vary throughout the image volume. As the mathematical representation calculated from a spatially narrowed region (scatter plot), the OTF may thus lack in visualizing the full extent of the structure of interest. The final rendering may thus only partially visualize anatomical structures, which can be misleading to interpret. Moreover may interfering structures be visualized, that share the same data value range, requiring expert knowledge in order to determine faulty and misleading visualization results. Solutions to this problem may be considered in applying a neighboring algorithm, only visualizing voxels within a solid structure around a seed point, or utilizing local transfer functions [6] applying several OTFs spatially separated throughout the image volume and thus compensating the spatial variances of the structure of interest. Also, introducing additional data value dimensions (e.g. L and H values [5]) may provide improved visual separation.

References

1. Levoy M. Display of surfaces from volume data. IEEE Computer Graph Appl. 1988;8(3):29–37.
2. Kindlmann GL, Durkin JW. Semi-automatic generation of transfer functions for direct volume rendering [Master's thesis]. Proc IEEE Symp Vol Vis. 1998; p. 79–86.
3. Kniss J, Kindlmann GL, Hansen CD. Multi-dimensional transfer functions for volume rendering. In: Johnson CR, Hansen CD, editors. The Visualization Handbook. Academic Press; 2004. p. 181–201.
4. Salama CR, Keller M, Kohlmann P. High-level user interfaces for transfer function design with semantics. IEEE Trans Vis Computer Graph. 2006;12(5):1021–1028.
5. Šereda P, Bartrolí AV, Serlie IWO, et al. Visualization of Boundaries in Volumetric Data Sets Using lh Histograms. In: IEEE Trans Vis Computer Graph. vol. 12; 2006.
6. Šereda P. Facilitating the Design of Multidimensional and Local Transfer Functions for Volume Visualization. Advanced School for Computing and Imaging. Delft, The Netherlands; 2007.

Towards Projector-Based Visualization for Computer-Assisted CABG at the Open Heart

Christine Hartung[1], Claudia Gnahm[1], Stefan Sailer[1], Marcel Schenderlein[1], Reinhard Friedl[2], Martin Hoffmann[3], Klaus Dietmayer[1]

[1]Institute of Measurement, Control and Microtechnology, University of Ulm
[2]Department of Cardiac Surgery, University Hospitals of Ulm and Lübeck
[3]Department of Diagnostic Radiology, University Hospital of Ulm
christine.hartung@uni-ulm.de

Abstract. Computer-assistance in coronary artery bypass grafting at the open heart with intraoperative navigation enables accurate placement of a bypass graft to a preoperatively planned anastomosis site. So far, navigation information were displayed on a monitor, requiring the operating surgeon to change focus from the monitor to the surgical site and vice versa during the navigation process. In this work, a mechanism is presented which is intended to enable the projection of registered preprocedural information directly onto the surface of the open heart. The method was tested on a heart phantom yielding good results.

1 Introduction

Open heart coronary artery bypass grafting (CABG) is the standard treatment in advanced coronary artery diseases. For effective revascularization, optimal placement of the bypass graft is very important. Enhancing current clinical practice with a concept for computer-assistance comprising preoperative planning and intraoperative navigation helps the surgeon with the fast and accurate localization of the optimal anastomosis site for bypass grafting. For the left anterior descending coronary artery (LAD), intraoperative navigation is possible both at the beating [1] and at the arrested heart [2] yielding mean accuracies of approximately 2.5 mm. For navigation at the beating heart, preprocedural information extracted from a multi-slice computed tomography (MSCT), i.e. the paths of the LAD vessel tree and the planned anastomosis site, are registered with intraoperative stereo video data of the open, beating heart [3], acquired with a stereo camera system mounted on a robotic arm above the patient, see fig. 1 (a). Visualization for the surgeon is currently being performed by overlaying this information on a live video stream and displaying it on a monitor, see fig. 1 (b). In consequence, the operating surgeon has to change focus from the monitor to the surgical site and vice versa during the navigation process. This can be avoided by projecting the registered planning data directly onto the surface of the open heart. In this work, a two-step calibration method is presented which aims at enabling projector-based visualization during computer-assisted CABG surgery at the open heart.

2 Methods

To enable the projection of navigation information onto the surface of the heart, it has to be determined which projector pixel has to be switched on to illuminate a specific point of the surface. One possibility is to project patterns on the surface while observing it with one or more cameras. This way, point correspondences can be established between the features in the projected image and the features recorded in the camera image, and a non-linear mapping between the camera pixels and the projector pixels can be calculated. Since except for occlusions unique correspondences exists between camera pixels and surface points, this mapping also implicitely describes the correspondences between projector pixels and surface points. The standard method for generating point correspondences between camera and projector image is projecting a sequence of binary stripe patterns on the surface for binary encoding of the projector pixels. Another possibility is to project and detect a sequence of single points [4]. In both cases, a series of images has to be projected and recorded with the camera. Such methods are usually applied for using multiple projectors in the context of immersive displays [5]. In the clinical field, projectors have been proposed for displaying general information in the surgeon's field of view [6], and have already been used for navigation tasks in maxillofacial surgery [7]. While these methods work well for the described applications, they cannot directly be employed at the open heart. Novel methods have to be developed in order to consider the following additional points:

1. The heart is exposed only during the procedure, after opening the chest, and moved several times relatively to the projector before navigation. Therefore, at least part of the calibration has to be performed intraoperatively. This part must be performable fast in order to avoid prolongation of the operation.
2. The open heart is set lower than the surrounding opened chest, therefore the surface illuminated by the projector exhibits pronounced discontinuities.
3. For future usage at the beating heart, it has to be possible to perform the calibration for a specified phase point of the heart cycle. To avoid synchronizing the projector with the ECG signal over several heart cycles, it is desirable to perform the calibration process with a single projected image instead of a sequence of images.

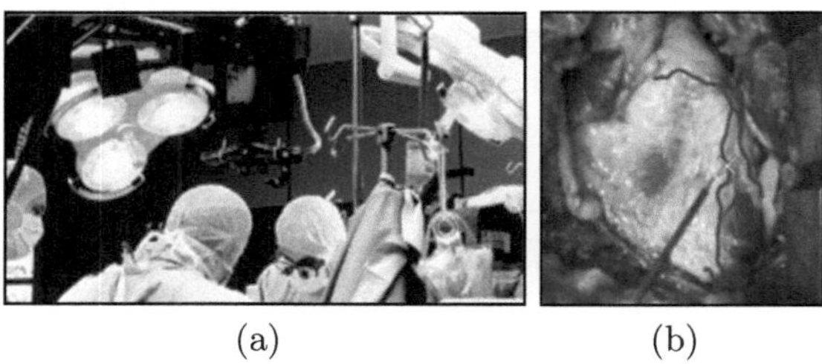

(a) (b)

Fig. 1. (a) Stereo camera system on robotic arm, (b) registered planning data overlayed on intraoperative video images, as displayed on a monitor during surgery.

In order to satisfy these requirements, a region of interest (ROI) based two-step method was developed for enabling the projection of planning data on the surface of the open heart during CABG procedures. It is assumed that the planning data are already registered with stereo video data of the open heart. In the first step, the paths of light rays emitted by the projector are determined. In the second step, the mapping between camera and projector for correct projection onto the surface is determined.

Step 1: A regular point grid is projected to an even surface which is positioned within the measurement volume at different distances from the stereo-camera projector system. For each position, a stereo image pair is recorded. The projected points are automatically detected in the image pairs by means of a scale space approach [8] and the corresponding 3D positions are reconstructed. Points reconstructed from different image pairs that belong to one point in the projector image, i.e. to one ray emitted by the projector are grouped and the 3D paths of the projector rays are reconstructed.

Step 2: The starting point of the second step of the calibration are the registered planning data, i.e. the vessel paths and a planned anastomosis site that were extracted from the MSCT data and intraoperatively registered with the coordinate system (CS) of the stereo camera system. The goal is to transform the planning data from the camera CS to the projector CS in such a way that they are projected to the correct sites on the surface of the heart. For this purpose, the point grid from calibration step 1 is projected to the heart surface and an image pair is recorded. Additionally, a disparity map of the surface is generated. The further workflow is illustrated in fig. 2. With the 2D image coordinates of the planning data in the camera CS, a ROI is defined by dilating the convex region around the vessel tree by a margin of fixed size. Within the ROI, points are automatically detected with a scale space blob detection approach [8]. Performing the calibration only for this ROI on the one hand makes the process faster, on the other hand avoids most problems with surface discontinuities. Additionally, a validity check is applied to each detected point by evaluating the disparity map for a small window around the point. If the window can be devided into two regions of significantly different disparity values by analyzing the histogram, it is assumed that the point is close to a discontinuity and it is discarded. For the valid points, 3D positions are reconstructed and compared to the paths of the projector rays from calibration step one. By determining the projector ray passing closest to each point, each valid point in the camera image is associated with one point in the projector image. Points for which the distance to the closest projector ray is too large are discarded. The

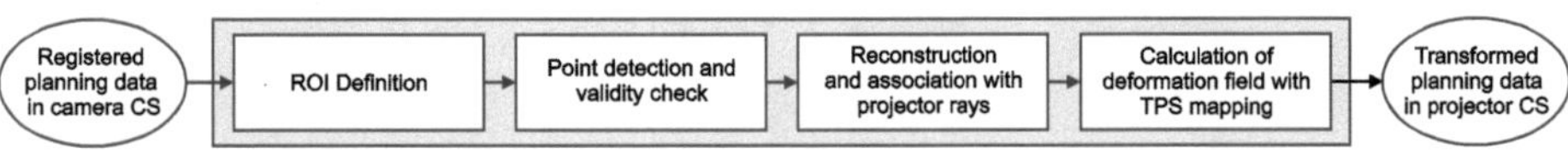

Fig. 2. Workflow of the second calibration step for projecting navigation information onto the surface of the heart.

validity checks reduce the risk of false associations between image points and projector rays. After performing the association step, point correspondences between the image coordinate system of the camera, which is the coordinate system of the registered planning data, and the image coordinate system of the projector are available. Based on these correspondences, a smooth deformation field can be calculated using a thin-plate-spline (TPS) interpolation approach in order to describe how the planning data have to be warped to the projector image for correct projection to the surface of the heart.

A commodity projector was used in the experiment presented here. Lenses were introduced into the light path of the projector to narrow the beam width and thus reduce the size of the illuminated area, as the target area is usually smaller than 20 cm by 20 cm. The method was tested on a heart phantom. To emulate the real heart in the opened chest during surgery, the heart phantom was embedded in a model of an open thorax. The ROI, i.e. the area around the vessel tree on the surface of the heart, usually does not contain surface discontinuities. However, as some of the vessels may run close to the edges between the visible part of the heart surface and the thorax, surface discontinuities might sometimes occur close to the borders of the ROI. The heart phantom and the thorax model were arranged accordingly to take this case into account.

3 Results

To evaluate the accuracy of the projection, an image pair of the heart phantom was acquired with the stereo camera system and the vessel tree was labeled in the left video image. Additionally a point on the LAD vessel was marked as the planned anastomosis site. The resulting 2D coordinates in the camera image CS simulate the registered planning data, see fig. 3 (a). These data were then transformed to the projector image coordinate system according to the method proposed above. Fig. 3 (b) shows the point grid that is projected to the heart phantom and the ROI with detected points. Fig. 3 (c) depicts the transformed planning data in the projector image and the TPS deformation field. Fig. 3 (d) shows the back projection to the heart phantom. As can be seen, the projected vessels are well aligned with the original paths of the vessels on the surface of the heart phantom, showing the viability of the proposed method. The first step of the calibration, which could be carried out before surgery in a clinical application, can be performed within in a few minutes. The second step takes less than 20 seconds and therefore could be carried out during a procedure.

4 Discussion

A two-step mechanism was developed which is intended to enable the projection of preprocedural information registered with intraoperative stereo video data onto the surface of the open heart during bypass grafting procedures. Evaluation of the method on a heart phantom showed accurate results. The method

Fig. 3. (a) The vessel tree of the heart phantom is labeled in the video image, a point on the LAD is marked to simulate the planned anastomosis site, the resulting ROI is indicated. (b) The point grid is projected to the surface. Projected points are detected in the ROI (marked with circles), several points (marked with crosses) at the edge of the ROI are discarded because they are close to surface discontinuities. (c) With the determined point correspondences a TPS deformation field (represented by grid lines) from camera image to projector image is calculated and used to transform the planning data accordingly. (d) The transformed planning data are projected back to the heart phantom, showing good accordance.

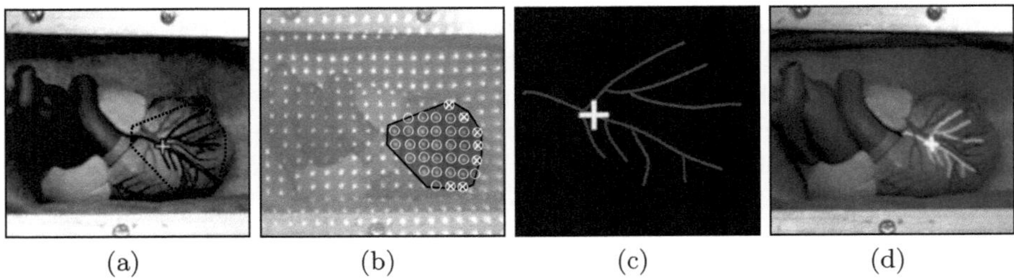

(a) (b) (c) (d)

presented here differs from previous approaches to calibration methods for projection on arbitrary surfaces in the following points: (1) Instead of projecting a series of patterns to the surface, only one pattern is projected, which can be helpful for calibration at a specified heart cycle phase point. (2) A ROI is automatically determined for the calibration, which makes the process faster and avoids problems with surface discontinuities. For using the proposed mechanism in a computer-assisted open heart CABG procedure, the first calibration step should be carried out before the procedure. Since the second step takes less than 20 seconds, it could be performed intraoperatively after registration and before navigation starts without causing significant prolongation of the procedure.

References

1. Hartung, C et al. Computer-assisted LAD bypass grafting at the open heart. Procs SPIE. 2009.
2. Gnahm, C et al. Computer assisted navigation on the LAD during open heart CABG. Procs CURAC. 2008; p. 247–250.
3. Hartung, C et al. Image guidance for coronary artery bypass grafting. Int J CARS. 2008;3:505–510.
4. Raskar, R et al. Multi-Projector Displays Using Camera-Based Registration. Procs IEEE Vis. 1999; p. 161–168.
5. Brown, M et al. Camera-Based Calibration Techniques for Seamless Multiprojector Displays. IEEE Trans Vis Comput Graph. 2005;11(2):193–206.
6. Tardif, J -P et al. Projector-Based Augmented Reality in Surgery without Calibration. Procs IEEE EMBS. 2003;1:548–551.
7. Hoppe H. Projektorbasierte Erweiterte Realität in der rechnergestützten Chirurgie. GCA; 2004.
8. Lindeberg T. Scale-space Theory in Computer Vision. Kluwer Academic Publishers; 1994.

Interaktive Visualisierung von Abständen und Ausdehnungen anatomischer Strukturen für die Interventionsplanung

Ivo Rössling[1,2], Christian Cyrus[1], Lars Dornheim[1,2], Peter Hahn[2], Bernhard Preim[1], Andreas Boehm[3]

[1]Otto-von-Guericke-Universität Magdeburg
[2]Dornheim Medical Images*
[3]Universitäts-Klinikum Leipzig
iroess@isg.cs.uni-magdeburg.de

Kurzfassung. Im Rahmen der Interventionsplanung muss der Chirurg therapierelevante Entscheidungen auf Basis räumlicher Relationen anatomischer Strukturen treffen. Interaktive 3D-Visualisierungen unterstützen diesen Prozess qualitativ. Quantitative Fragestellungen (Tumorausdehnung, Infiltrationstiefe, etc.) erfordern die Integration einer Bemaßung, deren Nutzen wesentlich von einer geeigneten Darstellung abhängt. In dieser Arbeit haben wir allgemeine Kriterien für die Eignung von Visualisierungen von Bemaßungen in interaktiven 3D-Szenen erarbeitet. Daran orientierend haben wir verschiedene Varianten der Darstellung von Abständen und Ausdehnungen anatomischer Strukturen betrachtet und ihr Erscheinungsbild hierzu zweckmäßig parametrisiert. Die Ausprägungen dieser Darstellungsparameter wurden in einer Studie auf ihre visuellen Wirkung hin an Chirurgen evaluiert. Es zeigte sich, dass die befragten Mediziner höchsten Wert auf Kohärenz und klare Zuordnung der Bemaßung setzten und überraschenderweise dafür sogar Abstriche in der direkten Lesbarkeit in Kauf nahmen.

1 Einleitung

Für die chirurgische Diagnostik und Therapieplanung spielt die Beurteilung anatomischer und pathologischer Strukturen eine tragende Rolle. Bildgebende Verfahren unterstützen den Arzt, sich ein umfassendes Bild des vorliegenden Falles zu verschaffen. Neben dem rein qualitativen visuellen Eindruck ist die quantitative Bewertung von zentraler Relevanz. Kennwerte zur räumlichen Konstitution relevanter Strukturen haben sich hierfür als äußerst wichtig herausgestellt.

Diese Maße müssen aus Gründen klinischer Sicherheit und Effizienz dem Chirurgen in einer Form präsentiert werden, die ihm auf intuitive Weise eine leichte und korrekte Ablesung erlaubt. Trotz der Relevanz dieser Thematik lässt sich kaum Literatur zur Visualisierung spatialer Kennwerte in medizinischen 3D-Szenen finden. Einen Abriss zu den üblichsten Anwendungsfällen gibt [1].

* Gefördert durch EXIST, BMWi und ESF

Veranschaulicht wird jeder Fall dabei anhand einer medizinischen 3D-Szene und einer möglichen Visualisierung. Für räumliche Punktabstände und Längenskalen werden Distance Lines und Interactive Rulers aus [2] beispielhaft angeführt. Auch eine Vermessung von Winkeln und Volumina wird illustriert. In [3] werden Abstände und Abmaße von Strukturen interaktiv bestimmt. Es wird eine etwas simplere Darstellung gewählt, bei der Bemaßung und Maßzahl visuell voneinander getrennt sind. [2] präsentiert abschließend noch ein Beispiel für die Darstellung automatisch berechneter Abmaße anatomischer Strukturen. Ansonsten wird in den genannten Quellen ein klarer Fokus auf die interaktive manuelle Vermessung gesetzt, bei der Anwender direkt mit den Maßen selbst interagiert.

Allen Quellen ist gemein, dass sie zwar jeweils eine konkrete Darstellungsvariante vorstellen, jedoch keine denkbaren Alternativen diskutieren. Vor diesem Hintergrund haben wir für ausgewählte Maße verschiedene Visualisierungsformen entwickelt und in einer Nutzerstudie evaluiert. Drei Anwendungsfälle wurden dabei betrachtet, die sich aus wichtigen medizinischen Fragestellungen für die Interventionsplanung ableiten lassen: Die Visualisierung von kürzesten Abständen, von größten Ausdehnungen und von Abmaßen anatomischer Strukturen.

2 Material und Methoden

Wie eine Bemaßung letztlich vom Betrachter wahrgenommen wird, hängt von einer Reihe von Präsentationsparametern ab. Für gute visuelle Wirkung haben wir in Anlehnung an [4] die folgenden qualitativen Kriterien postuliert:

- *Klare Zuordnung:* Sowohl die Zuordnung von Bemaßungen zu ihren Objektreferenzen als auch die von Maßzahlen zu ihren Maßlinien muss jeweils eindeutig und klar erkennbar sein [4].
- *Lesbarkeit:* Die Maßzahlen müssen eine leichte und korrekte Ablesung erlauben und dürfen insbesondere nicht verdeckt werden.
- *Kohärenz:* Im Rahmen der Interaktion mit der 3D-Szene sollten weder Maßlinien noch Maßzahlen den Betrachter durch auffällige (z.B. sprunghafte) Änderungen ablenken.

An diesen Kriterien orientierend haben wir verschiedene Darstellungsvarianten entwickelt. Auf eine Betrachtung visueller Details wie Farbe, Font oder Linienstil wurde dabei bewusst verzichtet.

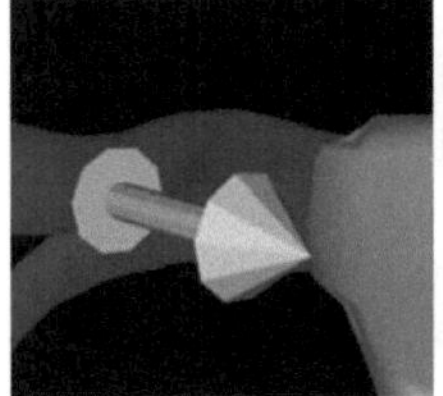 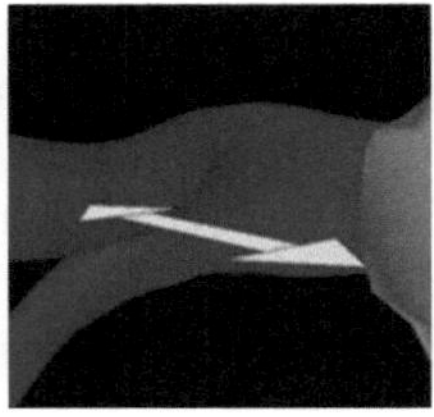 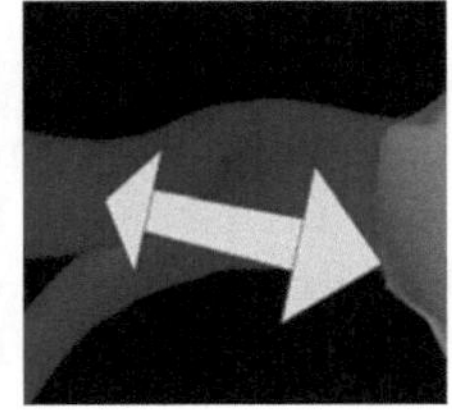 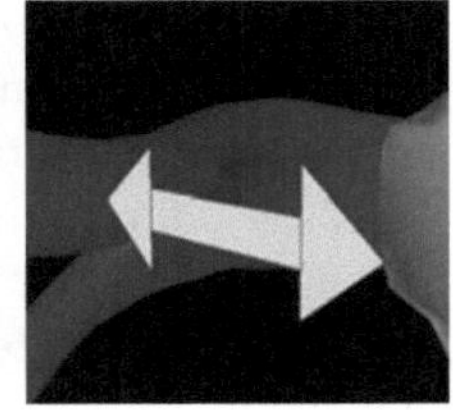

Abb. 1. Dimensionalität und Ausrichtungskorrektur: 3D-Pfeil, sowie 2D-Pfeil in den Varianten statisch, sicht-optimal, und *(smooth-)flip*.

Abb. 2. Verdeckung: Behebung des Problems durch Objekttransparenz, Überstand oder Außenansetzung der Maßpfeile sowie durch Hilfslinien.

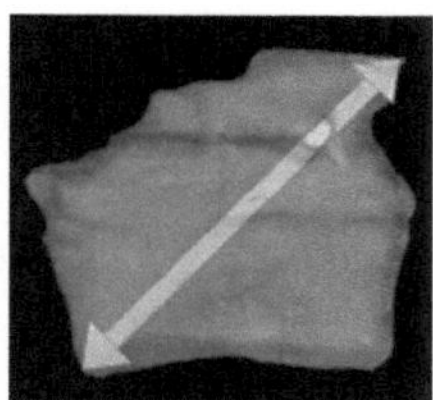
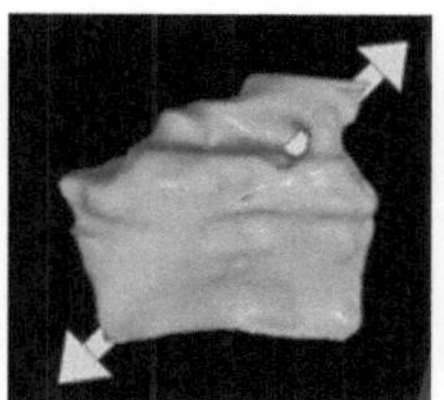
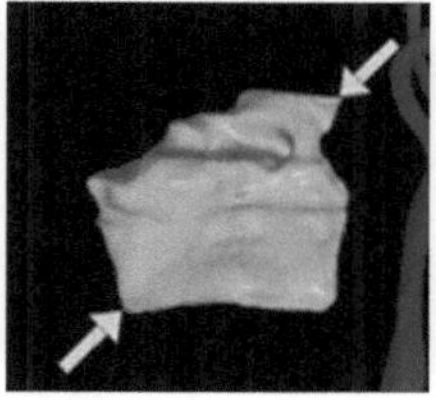
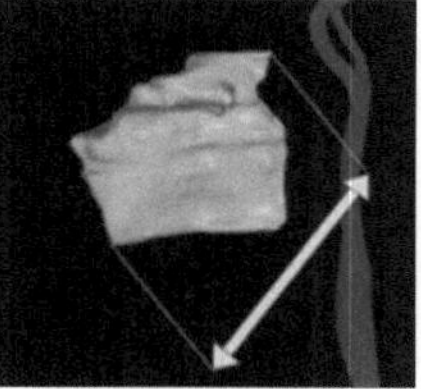

Für die Visualisierung der Maßlinien wurden zunächst zwei allgemeine Darstellungsparameter herausgearbeitet (Abb. 1):

– *Dimensionalität:* Für den 3D-Pfeil mit zylindrischem Schaft und Kegelspitze aus [4] wurde als schlichtere Alternative ein planares Gegenstück eingeführt.
– *Ausrichtungskorrektur:* Beim 2D-Pfeil ergibt sich aufgrund der Planarität das Problem, dass eine feste Ausrichtung (statisch) zu extrem flachen Blickwinkeln führen kann. Dies kann durch eine Neuausrichtung der Pfeilebene korrigiert werden. Drei Lösungen wurden erarbeitet: Der Pfeil wird beim Winkel von 45° einfach umgeklappt (*flip*), immerfort zum Betrachter hin gedreht (sicht-optimal) oder behält seine feste Ausrichtung zunächst bei und wird in einem Grenzbereich dann kontinuierlich übergeblendet (*smooth-flip*).

Im Anwendungsfall der größten Ausdehnung verläuft das Referenzmaß meist innerhalb des Objektes. Vier Parameter werden dann zusätzlich relevant: Objekttransparenz, Pfeilüberstand, Außenansetzung und Hilfslinien (Abb. 2). Im Anwendungsfall der Abmaße treffen drei Maße orthogonal aufeinander. Dies führt zu zwei letzten Parametern für die Darstellung von Maßlinien (Abb. 3):

– *Anordnung:* Im einfachsten Falle schneiden sich die Pfeile im Schwerpunkt des Objektes oder im Mittelpunkt der Bounding-Box. Alternativ können sie sich in einem gut sichtbaren Eckpunkt selbiger treffen. Ferner ließen sich ähnlich einer technischen Zeichnung Silhouettenkanten der Bounding-Box dynamisch bestimmen, die eine Überlagerung des Objektes vermeiden.
– *Bounding-Box:* Als potentielle visuelle Unterstützung kann zusätzlich die zugehörige Bounding-Box der Struktur angezeigt werden.

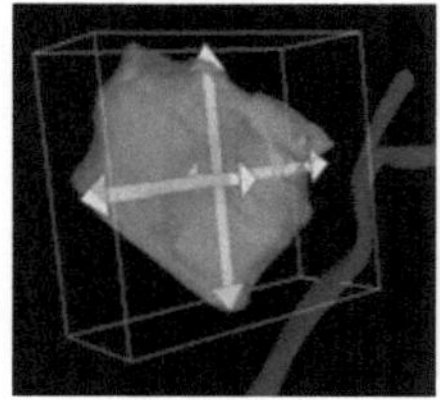
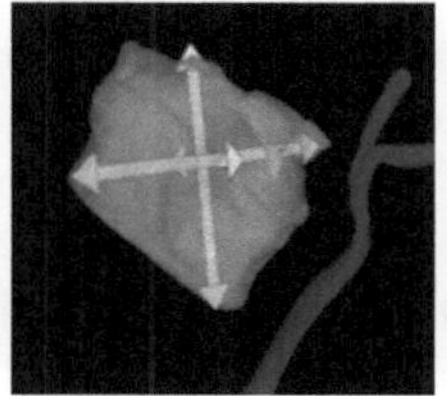
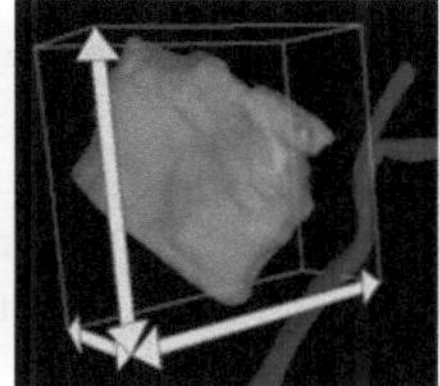
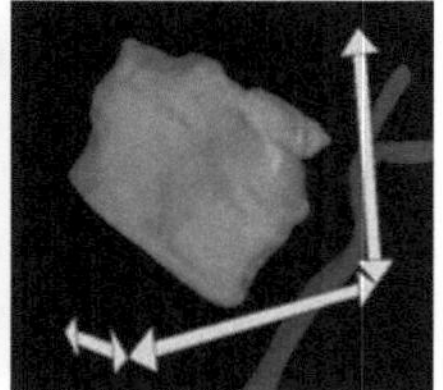

Abb. 3. Anordnung orthogonaler Maße: Mittelpunkt*, Schwerpunkt, Eckpunkt* und Silhouettenkanten (* = mit zusätzlicher Bounding-Box).

Abb. 4. Anordnung der Beschriftungen: An der Spitze, neben, auf oder als Unterbrechung zum Pfeil, davon zweimal in Pfeilrichtung ausgerichtet.

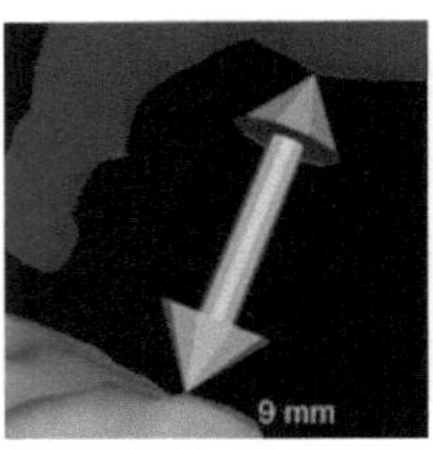

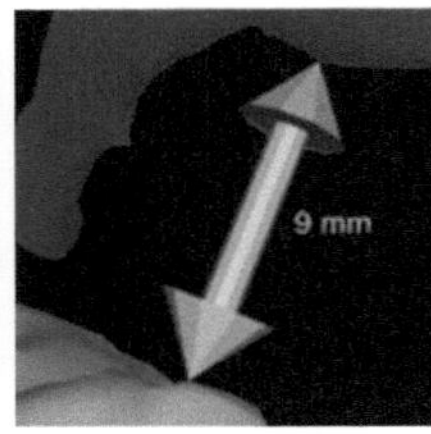

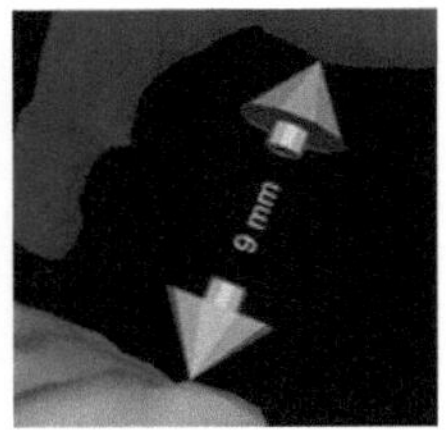

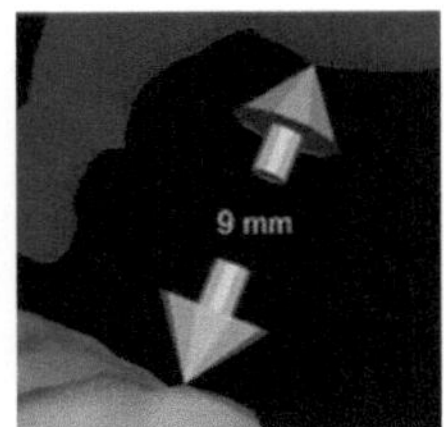

Neben der Maßlinie selbst lässt sich auch ihre Beschriftung visuell parametrisieren. Für diesen Aspekt haben wir folgende Varianten berücksichtigt (Abb. 4):

- *Ausrichtung:* Die Maßzahlen können waagerecht in der Kameraebene oder perspektivisch in Pfeilrichtung ausgerichtet sein.
- *Positionierung:* Die Maßzahlen können an der Pfeilspitze, neben, auf oder als Unterbrechung zum Pfeilschaft positioniert werden.

Zur Evaluierung der beschriebenen Aspekte wurde eine Test-Suite entwickelt. In Form einer Simultan-Ansicht wurden dabei in jedem Schritt die verschiedenen Ausprägungen des jeweiligen Parameters einander gegenübergestellt, wobei jede Nutzerinteraktion stets synchron auf alle Viewports angewandt wurde.

Um der Nutzerbefragung ein möglichst realistisches Test-Szenario zugrunde zu legen, wurde eine 3D-Szene segmentierter anatomischer Strukturen des Halses gewählt. Die Darstellungsparameter wurden unabhängig evaluiert. Tabelle 1 zeigt die in den drei Anwendungsfällen jeweils getesteten Parameter.

Die Nutzergruppe bestand aus Angehörigen unserer Forschungseinrichtung sowie Mitarbeitern des klinischen Partners (Chirurgen), darunter ein Oberarzt.

3 Ergebnisse

Beim Großteil der Fragen herrschte Einigkeit unter den Testpersonen. So wurde Transparenz bei objektinternen Maßen generell als hilfreich empfunden. Von außen angesetzte Maßlinien wurden dagegen als nur bedingt geeignet bewertet, da der korrekte Eindruck der bemaßten Strecke darunter leidet. Überstehende Pfeilenden wurden als verwirrend abgelehnt. Hilfslinien fanden zwar Akzeptanz, doch eine innenliegende Bemaßung mit Transparenz wurde durchweg bevorzugt.

Unterschiedlicher fielen die Antworten zu Dimensionalität und Ausrichtungskorrektur sowie Anordnung dreier Pfeile aus. Während Nicht-Mediziner sich teils durchaus für den 2D-Pfeil aussprachen und dabei sicht-optimal für Abstände und *smooth-flip* für Abmaße klar bevorzugten, äußerten die Ärzte eine absolute Präferenz für den 3D-Pfeil und lehnten neben *flip* auch *smooth-flip* (nicht aber statisch) als störend ab. Bei der Anordnung dreier Pfeile gab es bei den Nicht-Medizinern unterschiedliche Präferenzen. Seitens der Ärzte wurden äußere Bemaßungslinien als weniger geeignet eingestuft. Sie empfanden die Variante Schwerpunkt am ansprechendsten, eine Bounding-Box dagegen irreführend.

Tabelle 1. Übersicht der in den drei Anwendungsfällen evaluierten Parameter

	Dimens.	Ausrtg.-korrektur	Transpz.	Überstand	Außen-ansetzg.	Hilfslinien	Anordng.	BBox	Richtung	Position
(kürzester) Abstand	×	×							×	×
(größte) Ausdehnung			×	×	×	×				
räumliche Abmaße	×		×	×	×		×	×	×	×

Bei den Maßzahlen herrschte Einigkeit, dass die Beschriftung mit Unterbrechung des Pfeils präferiert wurde. Im Gegensatz zu den Nicht-Medizinern bevorzugten die Ärzte aber die perspektivische Variante.

4 Diskussion

Die Ergebnisse der Studie waren zum Teil überraschend. Es bestätigte sich die Annahme, dass schlechte Kohärenz in der Interaktion als besonders störend empfunden würde. Erstaunlich war jedoch, dass neben der Variante *flip* auch *smoothflip* von den Ärzten als sehr ablenkend eingestuft wurde.

Der vermutete Zuspruch für 2D-Pfeile blieb aus. Seitens der Mediziner wurde diese Dimensionsreduktion als störende visuelle Hervorhebung empfunden.

Eine positive Bewertung der Transparenz und die konsequente Ablehnung der überstehenden Pfeile entsprach unseren Annahmen. Auch die Präferenz der Platzierung der Maßzahl in Unterbrechung zur Maßlinie hatten wir vermutet.

Unerwartet war jedoch die Reaktion der Mediziner auf Anordnung der Pfeile und Ausrichtung der Beschriftungen. Hinsichtlich der eingangs aufgestellten Kriterien gingen wir von einem hohen Stellenwert der Lesbarkeit aus. Gerade hier waren die Mediziner jedoch bereit, beschränkt Einschnitte in Kauf zu nehmen, wenn dafür ein Maximum an klarer Zuordnung, Kohärenz erreicht würde.

Wir kommen zu dem Schluss, dass für die medizinische Visualisierung 3D-Pfeile, die der transparenten Struktur inneliegen und deren Maßzahl perspektivisch als Unterbrechung in den Pfeil gesetzt ist, eine geeignete Wahl sind.

Literaturverzeichnis

1. Preim B, Bartz D. Chapter 13 - Measurements in Medical Visualization. In: Visualization in Medicine. Morgan Kaufmann Publishers Inc.; 2007. p. 313–339.
2. Preim B, Tietjen C, Spindler W, et al. Integration of measurement tools in medical 3d visualizations. Procs IEEE Vis. 2002; p. 21–28.
3. Hastreiter P, Rezk-Salama C, Tomandl B, et al. Fast analysis of intracranial aneurysms based on interactive direct volume rendering and CTA. Proc MICCAI. 1998; p. 660–669.
4. Preim B, Sonnet H, Spindler W, et al. Interaktive und automatische Vermessung von 3D-Visualisierungen für die Planung chirurgischer Eingriffe. Proc BVM. 2001; p. 19–23.

Triple-Modality Normalized Mutual Information Based Medical Image Registration of Cardiac PET/CT and SPECT Images

Comparison with Triple MI and Dual NMI Methods

Laszlo Papp[1], Maaz Zuhayra[1], Reinhard Koch[2]

[1]Department of Radiology and Nuclear Medicine, UK-SH Campus Kiel
[2]Inst. of Informatics and Applied Mathematics, Christian Albrechts University, Kiel
lpapp@nuc-med.uni-kiel.de

Abstract. An extension of the normalized mutual information similarity measurement was proposed to register cardiac PET/CT and SPECT images representing coronary artery disease in the heart. 23 PET/CT images obtained by a hybrid camera, and their corresponding SPECT were processed. The SPECT was registered to the PET/CT image pairs by a triple NMI based auto-registration. For validation and comparison an triple MI based registration among the PET-SPECT-CT images was performed. Two further dual NMI based auto-registrations between the SPECT-CT and SPECT-PET were performed as well. Based on the comparative results gained by a medical expert, our triple NMI method gave the best transformation parameters with a minimal number of iterations to superimpose the images.

1 Introduction

Nuclear heart scans based on SPECT and PET help diagnosing heart diseases such as coronary artery disease by providing different information about the stage of the heart, while CT provides anatomical information for better localization. Examining all the three images indicates the necessity of a registration step, since one of the functional images is performed with a stand alone camera. In our cases PET/CT heart image pairs obtained by a hybrid camera and their corresponding stand alone SPECT were collected and processed. Previous works have shown that involving three images to an extended mutual information based registration increases the accuracy of superimposing them even if the images are quite different [1, 2]. It is known that dual MI methods might fail the registration due to their sensitivity in overlap changing, while dual NMI methods are proven to be overlap invariant [3]. Although the same negative behaviour of the triple MI methods has not been recorded yet, the unknown overlap ratio of our images might bring uncertainty in triple MI based results. Due to this uncertainty we superimposed the SPECT image with a higher dimensional normalized mutual information based auto-registration to avoid possible overlap related misregistrations. Comparison with the triple MI [1] and classic dual NMI methods [3] was done. A program was implemented in IDL 7.0 to validate the registration methods mentioned above with the triple fusion of our patient data.

2 Materials and methods

2.1 Patient data

23 PET/CT and SPECT heart images were collected representing possible coronary artery disease. The PET/CT images were already superimposed, since they were obtained by a hybrid camera. During the PET/CT acquisitions the patients were not moved to avoid additional misalignments. The SPECT images were obtained in a different time with a SPECT camera.

2.2 Registrations

All images were resampled to (1 x 1 x 1) mm voxel size and their grey values were stretched between 0 and 255 to decrease the size of their joint histogram [4]. Downhill-Simplex method [5] was performed for function minimization with functional tolerance 0.0001. The cost function of the registration was a triple normalized mutual information similarity measurement (triple NMI) based on equation 1. In the triple NMI measurement the PET and the CT images were both reference of the registration, while the SPECT was the reslice image.

$$\frac{H(A)+H(B)+H(C)}{H(A,B,C)} \tag{1}$$

Where $H(A)$ is the Shannon entropy of the image A and $H(A,B,C)$ is the Shannon entropy of the joint probabilities of images A, B and C [4].

To compare our method a triple MI [1] similarity measurement (equation 2) and a dual NMI [3] similarity measurement (equation 3) was also implemented. The triple MI included all the three images in the registration, while the dual NMI method registered both CT - SPECT and the PET - SPECT image pairs one-by-one.

$$H(A)+H(B)+H(C)-H(A,B,C) \tag{2}$$

$$\frac{H(A)+H(B)}{H(A,B)} \tag{3}$$

Where $H(A,B)$ is the Shannon entropy of the joint probabilities of images A and B.

2.3 Fusion and validation

All the PET/CT and the superimposed SPECT images were fused in a triple fusion window to represent the result of the registration methods (Fig. 1). Validation of the registrations was done manually based on visual assessment by a medical physician in the fusion window. The additional manual modifications of the automatic registration parameters were recorded to determine the errors for each registration methods. The number of iterations, the shifting and rotation errors were calculated for all registration methods.

Table 1. Comparative results of our triple NMI method with the triple MI and the two dual NMI registrations. Values represent the means and the standard deviations respectively.

Registration method	Shift error (mm)	Rotation error (degrees)	No. iterations
Triple NMI	2.20 ± 0.65	0.54 ± 0.22	177 ± 45
Triple MI	2.89 ± 0.97	0.46 ± 0.46	192 ± 75
Dual NMI (CT-SPECT)	4.71 ± 1.23	5.12 ± 2.14	218 ± 68
Dual NMI (PET-SPECT)	3.56 ± 9.86	1.98 ± 1.65	202 ± 72

3 Results

Comparative results of the registration methods on our patient data are represented by Table 1.

4 Discussion

Although the dual modality fusion and registration is the most common method to visualize and superimpose multimodality data, the necessity of registering and fusing three modalities becomes essential when a patient has three different images to investigate a given disease. In our case three different modalities - SPECT, PET and CT - were needed for better diagnosis related with coronary artery disease of the heart. Since heart SPECT has poor anatomical information, registering it to the CT by a dual mutual information similarity measurement is a challenging task, and often additional processing is needed to provide an acceptable auto-registration [6]. The similarity ratio of PET and SPECT is higher, since they are both functional images, but due to their low spatial resolution a dual registration between them might not be effective enough. Building on the

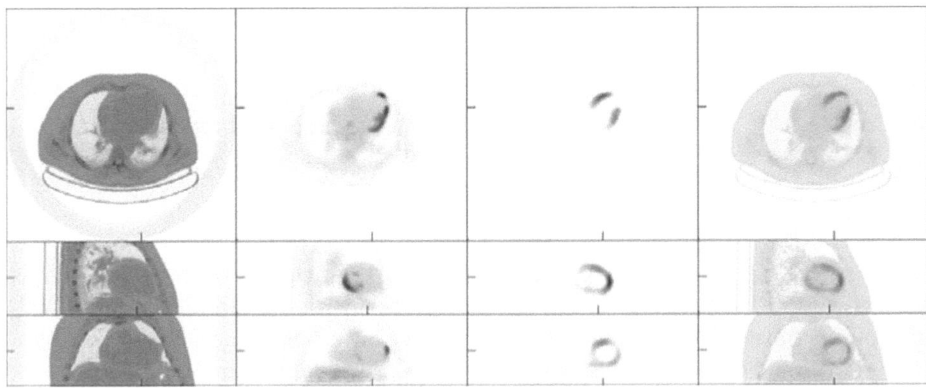

Fig. 1. Validation window based on the superimposed CT , PET, SPECT cardiac study and their triple fusion.

fact that the hybrid camera-made PET/CT images are already superimposed, it is a logical step to involve both of them to an extended mutual information based auto-registration next to the stand alone SPECT. Table 1 represents that if all the three images are involved in a triple NMI registration the shift and rotation error as well as the number of iterations can be minimized, since the presence of two reference images increases the certainty of the auto-registration. Although the triple MI registration did not fail because of overlap changing, our triple NMI measurement produced better registration parameters. The next step of our work will be the evaluation of our method on a higher number of clinical data.

References

1. Boes JL, Meyer CR. Multi-variate mutual information for registration. Med Image Comput Computer Ass Interven. 1999;1679:606–612.
2. Andersson JLR, Thurfjell L. A multivariate approach to registration of dissimilar tomographic images. Eur J Nucl Med. 1999;26(7):718–733.
3. Studholme C, Hill DLG, Hawkes DJ, et al. An overlap invariant entropy measure of 3D medical image alignment. Pattern Recogn. 1999;32(1):71–86.
4. Pluim JPW, Maintz JBA, Viergever MA. Mutual-information-based registration of medical images: A survey. IEEE Trans Med Imaging. 2003;22(8):986–1004.
5. Bernon JL, Mariano-Goulart D, Zanca A. A comparative study of Powell's and Downhill simplex algorithms for a fast multimodal surface matching in brain imaging. Comput Med Imaging Graph. 2001;25(4):287–297.
6. Guetter C, Wacker M, Xu C, et al. Registration of cardiac SPECT/CT data through weighted intensity co-occurrence priors. Proc MICCAI. 2007;4791:725–733.

Modellbasierte interindividuelle Registrierung an der lateralen Schädelbasis

M. Riechmann[1], P. U. Lohnstein[2], J. Raczkowsky[1], T. Klenzner[2], J. Schipper[2], H. Wörn[1]

[1]Institut für Prozessrechentechnik, Automation und Robotik, Universität Karlsruhe (TH)
[2]Hals-Nasen-Ohren-Klinik, Universitätsklinikum Düsseldorf
matthias.riechmann@kit.edu

Kurzfassung. Bei chirurgischen Eingriffen an der lateralen Schädelbasis wird in der zur Zeit gängigen Praxis das Knochengewebe unter optischer Kontrolle großflächig ablativ entfernt, um den Operationssitus freizulegen und konventionell operieren zu können. Prinzipiell soll dabei die Schonung vital und funktional bedeutender Strukturen berücksichtigt werden. Zur weiteren Minimierung der Traumatisierung und zur Erhaltung der strukturellen anatomischen Integrität soll eine alternative endoskopische Operationstechnik entwickelt werden, bei der der Situs durch dünne im Knochen liegende Bohrkanäle erreicht wird. Im Rahmen der Evaluierung der generellen Eignung der geometrischen Ausprägungen der humanen lateralen Schädelbasis wurden Methoden entwickelt, die anhand virtueller Modelle die Zugänglichkeit der anatomischen Zielstrukturen bestimmen können. Ein dabei auftretendes Problem ist die interindividuelle Vergleichbarkeit der Ergebnisse, da aufgrund der anatomischen Variationen eine zuverlässige interindividuelle Registrierung nicht trivial ist. Diese Arbeit beschreibt ein modellbasiertes Verfahren zur automatischen Registrierung mehrerer Felsenbeine zu einander über die prägnante Geometrie der Cochlea.

1 Einleitung

Chirurgische Eingriffe an der lateralen Schädelbasis bringen beim heutigen Stand der Operationstechnik Traumatisierungen des Patienten mit sich. Die Einführung endoskopischer Operationstechniken bei solchen Eingriffen (Minimal Traumatische Chirurgie) verspricht die Erhaltung der strukturellen anatomischen Integrität durch eine gezielte Verringerung des Knochenabtrags: Der Zugang zum Situs muss nicht mehr durch umfangreiches Abtragen von Knochengewebe mit Hilfe einer Fräse geschaffen werden. Statt dessen wird dieser durch wenige Millimeter durchmessende lineare Bohrkanäle, die im Vorfeld roboterassistiert unter Schonung der physiologisch-funktionell kritischen Strukturen[1, 2] angelegt werden, hergestellt. Dabei können keine natürlichen Kavitäten genutzt und auch kein Gewebe verdrängt werden. Angestrebte Einsatzgebiete für diese Technik sind die Dekompression des Saccus endolymphaticus und die transmastoidale Tumorexstirpation am inneren Gehörgang.

Im Rahnen von Voruntersuchungen, wurde eine Reihe von Simulationen zur Untersuchung der Machbarkeit der Eingriffe an mehreren virtuellen Felsenbeinmodellen durchgeführt[3]. Dies ist erforderlich, da die Anatomie der lateralen Schädelbasis erheblichen interindividuellen Variationen unterliegt[4] und einfache schematische Vorgehensweise somit ausgeschlossen sind. Ein immer wiederkehrendes Problem ist die interindividuelle Vergleichbarkeit der Ergebnisse von Simulationen, da die besagten Variationen auch Auswirkungen auf die Platzierung der verwendeten Landmarken haben und zu Fehlern führen. Als Alternative wird in dieser Arbeit eine ICP-Registrierung zwischen der Geometrie der Bogengänge mit Cochlea und eines Modells vorgeschlagen. Aufgrund der prägnanten Form der untersuchten anatomischen Struktur kann zudem ein einheitliches Koordinatensystem über aus den Bogengängen hervorgehende Ebenen definiert werden.

2 Material und Methoden

Das Ausgangsmaterial der Untersuchung besteht aus 16 zufällig ausgewählten, anonymisierten und normalbefundeten rechtseitigen Fel sen bein-Dünn schicht-CTs, die im Rahmen regulärer medizinischer Untersuchungen aufgenommen wurden. Die axiale Auflösung beträgt zwischen 0,2 und 0,6 mm, der Schichtabstand, zwischen 0,4 und 2 mm. In den Datensätzen wurden mit Hilfe des DICOM-Viewers OsiriX und eines Grafiktabletts die Cochlea mit den Bogengängen und eine Reihe weiterer anatomischer Strukturen manuell segmentiert. Zu Registrierungszwecken wurden 6 Landmarken identifiziert. Drei davon liegen zentral in der Nähe der Cochlea, die anderen weiter in der Peripherie: Hammerkopf, Ductus endolymphaticus, Facialiskanal am Ganglion geniculi, Anfang innerer Gehörgang, Anfang äußerer Gehörgang, Mastoidspitze.

Aus den so attribuierten Volumendatensätzen wurden anschließend mit Hilfe einer auf Algorithmen aus dem Insight Toolkit (ITK) und dem Visualization Toolkit (VTK) basierenden Bildverarbeitungsfilterkette (Weichzeichner, Marching Cubes[5], Dezimierung[6], größengetreuer Polygonweichzeichner[7]) dreidimensionale Polygondatensätze berechnet. Ein wichtiger Aspekt dieser Verarbeitungskette ist neben einer möglichst guten Übereinstimmung mit den segmentierten Volumina die Reduzierung der Komplexität der Oberflächenmodelle, da diese einen großen Einfluss auf die Laufzeit von Berechnungen auf den Modellen hat. Die Anatomiepräsentationen können in einer Planungssoftware dargestellt und in einer triplanaren Ansicht auf ihre Übereinstimmung mit den originalen medizinischen Bilddatensätzen verglichen werden.

Das Referenzmodell zur Registrierung der Bogengänge und der Cochlea besteht aus der orthogonalen Anordnung dreier Tori und einer Kugel, die jeweils die drei Bogengänge und die Cochlea repräsentieren. Die Anordnung ist prototypisch, das heißt, sie wurde manuell anhand eines segmentierten Datensatzes erstellt. Es zeigte sich, daß dies ohne große Fehler auf andere Cochleamodelle übertragbar war. Auf Abb. 1 sind die geometrische Konfiguration des Modells und die verwendeten Bemaßungen zu sehen.

Abb. 1. Das prototypische Modell der Cochlea. Bemaßungen in mm

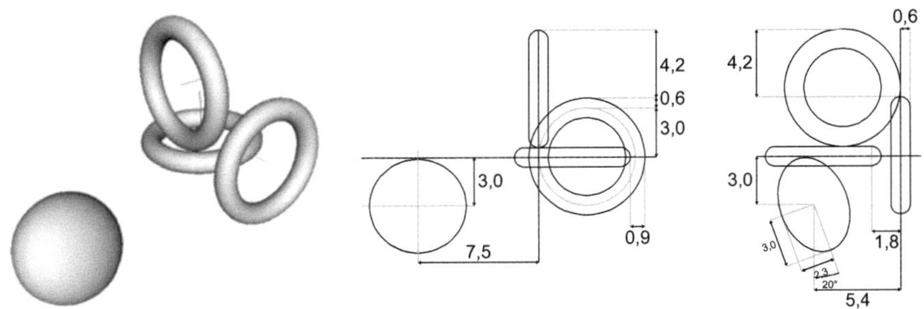

(a) 3D-Darstellung des Modells (b) Bemaßungen des Modells - Links: Profunde Ansicht, rechts: anterior

Das Modell wird mit Hilfe der Landmarken einer Vorregistrierung nach der Methode von Horn[8] unterzogen und anschließend durch eine Iterative Closest Point Registrierung[9] in die Geometrie der Bogengänge und der Cochlea eingepasst. Die verwendeten Registrierungsimplementierungen entstammen dem VTK.

3 Ergebnisse

Nach Tests an den zwölf zur Verfügung stehenden virtuellen Felsenbeinen zeigte sich eine hohe Robustheit des gewählten Ansatzes: Das Referenzmodell lässt sich ohne manuelle Anpassungen bei allen Datensätzen in die Geometrie einpassen und nach optischer Kontrolle können alle vier geometrischen Primitive als am korrekten Ort befindlich befunden werden. Abb. 2 zeigt eine exemplarische Cochlearepräsentation mit darauf registriertem Referenzmodell.

Da die Dimensionen und Ausrichtungen der Teilkomponenten des Modells bekannt sind, können die Tori zur Definition eines Koordinatensystems herangezogen werden: Die X-Achse steht orthogonal auf dem superioren Bogengang, die

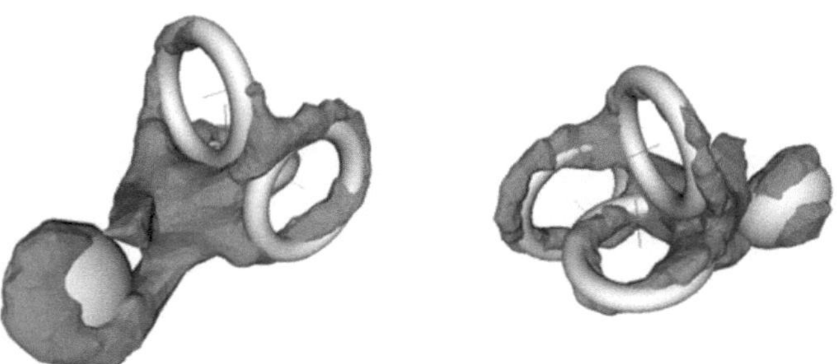

Abb. 2. Zwei verschiedene Ansichten des registrierten Referenzmodells (weiß) und der Cochleageometrie (grün).

Y-Achse auf dem posterioren Bogengang und die Z-Achse auf dem horizontalen. Analog liegen die YZ-Ebene in der vom superioren Bogengang aufgespannten Grundebene, die XZ-Ebene im posterioren Bogengang und die XY-Ebene am horizontalen Bogengang. Abb. 3 zeigt die Ausrichtung des Koordinatensystems relativ zur Cochlea und den in Abschnitt 1 beschriebenen anatomischen Strukturen. Zur Verbesserung der Übersicht sind die Pfeile entlang der X-Achse verschoben, der Ursprung liegt auf der Höhe des superioren Bogengangs.

4 Diskussion

In dieser Arbeit ist es mit Hilfe eines modellbasierten Ansatzes gelungen die Cochlea und die Bogengänge als Registrierkörper zur Definition eines einheitlichen Koordinatensystems an der lateralen Schädelbasis heranzuziehen. Durch die Verwendung parametrischer geometrischer Primitive ist es theoretisch sogar möglich über wenige Parameter Koordinaten auf der Oberfläche der Cochlea und den Bogengängen eindeutig zu definieren. Zusätzlich können die Öffnungen der Bogengänge ohne eine aufwändige Formanalyse der Oberflächenmodelle lokalisiert werden. Aufgrund der Achsensymmetrie des Kopfes ist das Koordinatensystem nicht ohne weiteres auf die linke Schädelseite übertragbar. Das Modell muß zuvor gespiegelt werden, was auch die Umkehrung einer der definierten Achsen nach sich zieht.

Für die Minimal Traumatische Chirurgie sind mindestens zwei Einsatzgebiete für das entwickelte Verfahren denkbar: Zum einen ermöglicht ein einheitliches Koordinatensystem in der lateralen Schädelbasis die Vergleichbarkeit der Analysen von Zugangswegen verschiedener Patienten. Zum anderen können Standard-Zugangswege definiert werden, die bei patientenindividuellen Operationsplanungen zur automatischen Berechnung sinnvoller Trajektorienvorschläge herangezogen werden können.

Derzeit ist eine manuelle Vorsegmentierung der Cochlea notwendig. Wünschenswert sind an dieser Stelle Verfahren zur semi- oder vollautomatischen Segmentierung. Interessante Ansätze hierzu, die langfristig auf eine automatische Segmentierung des Felsenbeins abzielen, finden sich in [10, 11].

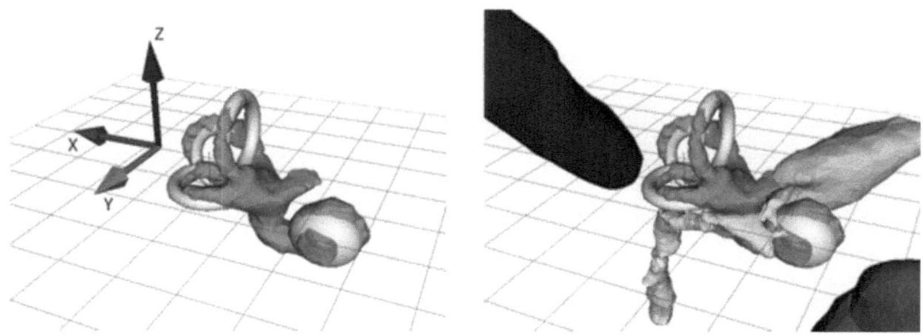

Abb. 3. Die Cochlea in dem vom Referenzmodell definierten Koordinatensystem

Literaturverzeichnis

1. Knapp FB, Ngan CC, Schipper J, et al. Hexapod-gestützte Bohrerführung für eine navigierte Cochleostomie. In: 77. Jahresversammlung der Deutschen Gesellschaft für Hals-Nasen-Ohren-Heilkunde, Kopf- und Hals-Chirurgie; 2006.
2. Chan LL, Manolidis S, Taber KH, et al. Surgical anatomy of the temporal bone: An atlas. Neuroradiology. 2001;43:797–808.
3. Riechmann M, Lohnstein PU, Raczkowsky J, et al. Identifying access paths for endoscopic interventions at the lateral skull base; 2008.
4. Riechmann M, Lohnstein PU, Raczkowsky J, et al. Ein probabilistisches dreidimensionales computermodell des felsenbeins. In: Tagungsband der 6. Jahrestagung der Deutschen Gesellschaft für Computer- und Roboterassistierte Chirurgie; 2007. p. 223–226.
5. Lorensen WE, Cline HE. Marching cubes: A high resolution 3D surface construction algorithm. SIGGRAPH Comput Graph. 1987;21(4):163–169.
6. Schroeder WJ, Zarge JA, Lorensen WE. Decimation of triangle meshes. Procs SIGGRAPH. 1992; p. 65–70.
7. Taubin G, Zhang T, Golub GH. Optimal surface smoothing as filter design. Procs ECCV. 1996;I:283–292.
8. Horn BKP. Closed-form solution of absolute orientation using unit quaternions. JOSA A. 1987;4(4):629–642.
9. Zhang Z. Iterative point matching for registration of free-form curves and surfaces. Int J Computer Vis. 1994;13(2):119–152.
10. Noble JH, Warren FM, Labadie RF, et al. Automatic segmentation of the facial nerve and chorda tympani using image registration and statistical priors. Proc SPIE. 2008.
11. Xianfen D, Siping C, Changhong L, et al. 3D Semi-automatic Segmentation of the cochlea and inner ear. Proc IEEE EMB Ann Conf. 2005.

Quantifizierung der Darmperistaltik mittels deformierbarer Registrierung

Detektion von Bewegungsstörungen

Daniel Stein[1], Tobias Heye[2], Hans-Ulrich Kauczor[2], Hans-Peter Meinzer[1]

[1]Abteilung für Medizinische und Biologische Informatik, DKFZ Heidelberg
[2]Abteilung für Diagnostische und Interventionelle Radiologie
Universitätsklinikum Heidelberg
D.Stein@dkfz.de

Kurzfassung. In diesem Beitrag werden zwei neuartige Methoden zur Detektion von Bewegungsstörungen des Darms vorgestellt und evaluiert. Dazu werden aus dynamischen 3D MRT Datensätzen jeweils ein geeigneter koronarer 2D+t Datensatz ausgewählt und über mehrere Zeitschritte registriert. Aus den entstehenden einzelnen Bewegungskarten wird in der ersten Methode ein neues Bild generiert, das für jeden Bildpunkt alle dazugehörigen Vektorbeträge addiert. Für die zweite Methode werden die Beträge nur aus den lateralen Vektorkomponenten der Verschiebungsvektoren berechnet und somit überwiegend die Atembewegung künstlich entfernt. In einer ersten Evaluation werden für beide Methoden 5 Probanden mit 5 Patienten mit nachgewiesener eingeschränkter Darmperistaltik verglichen. Es wurde festgestellt, dass für die erste Methode mit Atmung eine Klassifizierung zwischen Probanden und Patienten nur bedingt möglich ist. Für die zweite Methode konnte jedoch gezeigt werden, dass die mittlere Bewegung in den Bewegungskarten mit Krankheitsbild ungefähr 35% geringer ist und somit erstmals eine Klassifizierung zwischen normaler und eingeschränkter Darmperistaltik ermöglicht wird.

1 Einleitung

Einschränkung der Darmperistaltik durch Verwachsungen nach chirurgischen Eingriffen oder bei chronisch entzündlichen Darmerkrankungen stellen für die Medizin und speziell für die diagnostische Bildgebung ein schwer quantifizierbares Problem dar. Dynamische MRT Daten ermöglichen es, Bewegungen des Darms festzustellen und aufzuzeichnen [1]. Untersuchungen der Darmbeweglichkeit werden bisher vom behandelnden Arzt durch visuelle Analyse der dynamischen MRT Daten durchgeführt. Glocker et al. [2] und Kutter et al. [3] haben bereits ein Verfahren zur Bewegungsanalyse des Dickdarms vorgestellt. Allerdings gibt es unseres Wissens nach noch keine computergestützten Verfahren zur Bewegungsanalyse, die den gesamten Darmtrakt berücksichtigen.

In der hier vorgestellten Arbeit werden zwei Methoden zur Bewegungsanalyse des gesamten Darmtrakts unter Verwendung von deformierbarer Registrierung entwickelt. Ihre Einsatzfähigkeit wird im Folgenden anhand von 10 Datensätzen (5 Probanden und 5 Patienten) untersucht.

2 Methoden

Beide entwickelten Methoden sehen es vor, dynamische MRT Datensätzen zu nutzen, um die Bewegung des Darms patientenspezifisch über die Zeit zu quantifizieren. Die Daten wurden mit einem 1,5 Tesla MRT Scanner (Symphony, Siemens, Deutschland) unter Normalatmung als 3D+t Datensätze aufgenommen. Dabei erfolgte die Aufnahme in 10 koronaren Schichten mit je 30 Zeitschritten, da in den koronaren Schichten der Darm und dessen Bewegung am besten dargestellt wird. Die Aufnahmezeit beträgt 3-4 Minuten.

Um die Bewegung des Darmes mit Hilfe von deformierbarer Registrierung in angemessener Zeit zu bewerten ist es sinnvoll, die Registrierung nicht auf dem gesamten 3D+t MR Datensatz durchzuführen, sondern lediglich eine koronare Schicht zu extrahieren, die möglichst den gesamten Darmbereich beinhaltet. Hierzu wurde zunächst für jede der 10 koronaren Schichten aus dem 3D+t Datensatz ein eigener 2D+t Datensatz erstellt. Aus diesen neuen Datensätzen wurde dann manuell ein geeigneter Datensatz ausgesucht, der dann weiter verarbeitet wurde (Abb. 1(a)).

Mittels deformierbarer Registrierung aller 30 Zeitschritte der ausgewählten 2D+t Datensätze wurden Bewegungskarten zwischen den einzelnen Zeitschritten berechnet. Dazu wurde die Implementierung des Demons-Algorithmus [4] von ITK [5] angewendet und die Ergebnisse mit MITK [6] visualisiert.

Der Demons-Algorithmus liefert als Ergebnis ein Deformationsfeld zwischen den einzelnen Zeitschritten, dass die Verschiebung für jeden Bildpunkt des Ausgangsbildes in Form eines Vektors enthält. Um eine Quantifizierung der Darmbe-

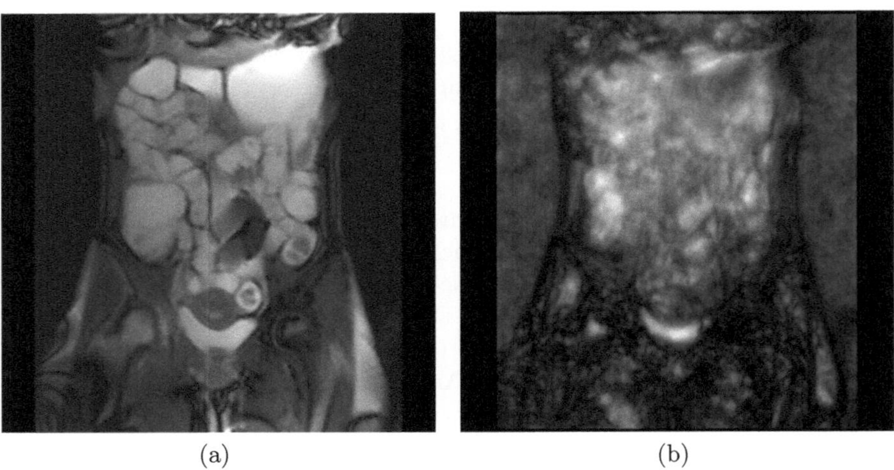

(a) (b)

Abb. 1. (a): ausgewählte koronare Schicht einer MRT Aufnahme des Abdomens eines Probanden zu einem Zeitpunkt, die den Darmtrakt gut darstellt; (b): Vektorbetragsbild der Bewegung über alle 30 Zeitschritte mit künstlich entfernter Atmung: je heller der Bildpunkt, desto größer ist die Bewegung. Der größte Teil der Bewegung liegt innerhalb des Darmtraktes.

wegung über die Zeit zu erhalten, wurde ein neues Bild generiert, dass für jedes Pixel des Ausgangsbildes die Summe der dazugehörigen Vektorbeträge aus den Deformationsfeldern der einzelnen Zeitschritte enthält und somit die gesamte Bewegung des Darmes darstellt.

Da bedingt durch die 3-4 Minuten dauernde Aufnahmezeit für die dynamischen MR Daten nur eine Aufnahme unter Normalatmung möglich ist, wird davon ausgegangen, dass ein großer Anteil der Bewegung zwischen den Zeitschritten durch Atmung entsteht. Deshalb wird das oben beschriebene Verfahren zur Generierung des Vektorbetragsbildes derart geändert, dass nur noch die laterale Bewegungskomponente aus den einzelnen Vektoren berücksichtigt wird. Hierzu wurde in jedem Vektor der Teil, der für die koronare Richtungsverschiebung steht, gelöscht und anschließend erneut das Betragsbild aus den Summen der Vektorbeträge aus den Deformationsfeldern der einzelnen Zeitschritte berechnet.

Für die automatische Klassifikation innerhalb eines CAD-Systems ist ein einzelner Wert von Vorteil. Deswegen erfolgt die Bewertung einer eingeschränkten Darmperistaltik anhand der mittleren Bewegung, also dem Mittelwert des Betragsbildes. In einer Vorstudie wurden die Ergebnisse der 5 Probanden mit denen der 5 Patienten mit diagnostizierter eingeschränkter Darmperistaltik verglichen. Dieser Vergleich erfolgte sowohl für die Ergebnisse mit Atmung, als auch für die Ergebnisse mit künstlich entfernter Atmung.

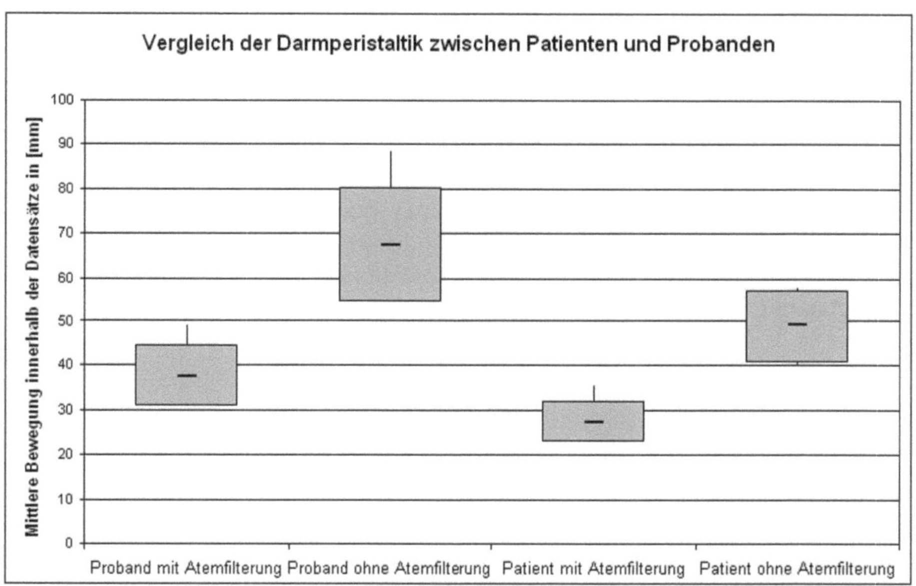

Abb. 2. Vergleich der Darmperistaltik zwischen 5 Patienten und 5 Probanden sowohl mit Atemfilterung als auch ohne Atemfilterung. Das Boxplot-Diagramm zeigt den Mittelwert, die obere und untere Standardabweichung sowie das Minimum und das Maximum der über jeweils 30 Zeitschritte gemittelten Bewegungen.

Tabelle 1. Mittlere Bewegung innerhalb eines Datensatzes in [mm], berechnet aus der gemittelten Summe aller Vektorbeträge der Deformationsfelder von 30 Zeitschritten.

	Mittlere Bewegung mit Atmung [mm]	Mittlere Bewegung ohne Atmung [mm]
Proband 1	57,7	35,5
Proband 2	68,4	38,5
Proband 3	56,7	31,4
Proband 4	66,0	33,4
Proband 5	88,4	48,9
Patient 1	56,6	25,6
Patient 2	41,7	26
Patient 3	58	35,4
Patient 4	40	24,1
Patient 5	48,8	26,1

3 Ergebnisse

Das Vektorbetragsbild eines Probanden in Abbildung 1(b) zeigt, dass die Bewegungen innerhalb einer Zeitserie hauptsächlich im Darmbereich auftreten und deshalb ein globales Verfahren zur Berechnung und zum Vergleich der Darmperistaltik zwischen Patienten und Probanden verwendet werden kann.

Tabelle 1 zeigt, dass die mittlere Bewegung in den Datensätzen der Probanden über 30 Zeitschritte mit künstlich entfernter Atmung ca. 5-10 mm höher ist als bei den Datensätzen mit eingeschränkter Darmperistaltik. Die Unterschiede der mittleren Bewegung der Probanden zur mittleren Bewegung der Patienten sind mit Atmung nicht immer eindeutig.

In dem Boxplot-Diagramm in Abbildung 2 wird der Vergleich der Darmperistaltik zwischen Patienten und Probanden dargestellt. Der Mittelwert der Darmbewegung bei den Probanden liegt sowohl mit Atmung als auch mit gefilterter Atmung höher als bei den Patienten.

4 Diskussion

Mit dem hier vorgestellten Verfahren mit künstlich entfernter Atmung ist es möglich festzustellen, ob eine eingeschränkte Darmperistaltik vorliegt. Aus den Ergebnissen kann man schließen, dass sich Probanden mit normaler Darmperistaltik hinsichtlich der Stärke der Bewegung innerhalb des Datensatzes über die einzelnen Zeitschritte von Patienten mit eingeschränkter Darmperistaltik unterscheiden.

Besonders durch unterschiedlich starke Atmung zwischen den einzelnen Patienten und Probanden kann es zu stärkeren oder schwächeren Summen der Bewegung aus den einzelnen Zeitschritten kommen. Deshalb konnte durch das künstliche Entfernen der Atmung eine deutliche Verbesserung in der Bewegungsdifferenz zwischen den Probanden und den Patienten erzielt werden. Allerdings wurde mit diesem Vorgehen nicht nur Atembewegung entfernt, sondern auch Anteile von Darmbewegung. Zukünftige Analysen werden untersuchen, ob tiefe Atemzüge automatisch über einen Schwellwert für die koronare Bewegung detektiert werden können. Ist dies der Fall, so können die stark veratmeten Zeitschritte automatisch entfernt und aus benachbarten Zeitschritten interpoliert werden. Hierdurch könnte mehr Darmbewegung berücksichtigt werden.

Es wird angemerkt, dass mit den Beträgen der Bewegungsvektoren gerechnet wird. Ansonsten würde sich die Bewegung anteilsmäßig aufheben, da sich der Darm über die Zeit in alle Richtungen bewegt.

Eine zusätzliche Verbesserung des Verfahrens kann darin bestehen, nicht mehr global die mittlere Bewegung über den gesamten Datensatz zu berechnen, sondern diesen in kleinere, interessantere Bereiche zu unterteilen und diese getrennt von einander zu beurteilen. Dadurch wäre auch gleichzeitig eine Lokalisation der eingeschränkten Darmperistaltik möglich.

Das vorgestellte Verfahren mit künstlich entfernter Atmung vereinfacht die Befundung für den behandelnden Arzt, da nicht mehr sämtliche Zeitschritte betrachtet werden müssen, sondern direkt auf dem Bewegungsdatensatz nach Auffälligkeiten gesucht werden kann. Dies kann durch das Verwenden einer geeigneten Look-Up-Tabelle zusätzlich farblich verdeutlicht werden. Hierfür müssen aber noch weitere Studien mit einem größeren Probanden- und Patientenkollektiv durchgeführt werden.

Literaturverzeichnis

1. Froehlich JM, Patak MA, von Weymarn C, et al. Small bowel motility assessment with magnetic resonance imaging. J Magn Res Imaging. 2005;21(4):370–375.
2. Glocker B, Buhmann S, Kirchhoff C, et al. Towards a computer-aided diagnosis system for colon motility dysfunctions. Proc SPIE. 2007;6514.
3. Kutter O, Kirchhoff S, Berkovich M, et al. Spatio-temporal registration in multiplane MRI acquisitions for 3D colon motiliy analysis. Proc SPIE. 2008;6915.
4. Thirion JP. Image matching as a diffusion process: An analogy with Maxwell's demons. Med Image Anal. 1998;2(3):243–260.
5. Ibanez L, Schroeder W, Ng L, et al. The ITK Software Guide. Insight Software Consortium; 2003. Available from: http://www.itk.org/ItkSoftwareGuide.pdf.
6. Wolf I, Vetter M, Wegner I, et al. The medical imaging interaction toolkit (MITK). Proc SPIE. 2004;5367:16–27.

Vector Extrapolation-Based Acceleration of Regularized Richardson Lucy Image Deblurring

Steffen Remmele[1], Jürgen Hesser[1,2]

[1]Institute for Computational Medicine, University of Heidelberg
[2]Experimental Radiooncology, Medical Centre Mannheim, University of Heidelberg
steffen.remmele@ziti.uni-heidelberg.de

Abstract. Confocal fluorescence microscopy has become an important tool in biological and medical sciences for imaging thin specimen, even living ones. Due to out-of-focus blurring and noise the acquired images are degraded and thus it is necessary to restore them. One of the most popular methods is an iterative Richardson-Lucy algorithm with total variation regularization. This algorithm while improving the image quality is converging slowly whereas with a constantly increasing amount of image data fast methods are required. In this paper, we present an accelerated version of the algorithm and investigate the achieved speed up. The acceleration method is based on a vector extrapolation technique and avoids a computational intensive evaluation of the underlying cost function. To evaluate the acceleration two synthetic test images are used. The accelerated algorithm reaches an acceptable result within 30% to 40% less computational time.

1 Introduction

1.1 Image formation model

Confocal fluorescence microscopy images suffer from both blurring and Poisson noise. The images are blurred due to the optical aperture and the physical resolution of light itself. This blurring is described by a convolution with a point spread function (PSF) [1]. In this paper, the PSF is noted as h and we assume that it is known. In addition, since confocal microscopy is a low-photon imaging technique the acquired images are degraded by Poisson noise $\phi(.)$. Thus a suitable image formation model, where i is the observed image, o the original image and $\otimes$ represents the convolution operator is given by:

$$i = \phi(o \otimes h) \tag{1}$$

The likelihood of an original image o for a recorded image i is given by the following equation due to the Poisson process describing the low-photon imaging nature of the confocal fluorescence microscopy. In this distribution, it is assumed that the noise is statistically uncorrelated.

$$P(i|o) = \prod_{x \in \Omega} \frac{[(o \otimes h)(x)]^{i(x)}\, e^{-(o \otimes h)(x)}}{i(x)!} \tag{2}$$

1.2 Deblurring methods

Maximizing the probability $P(i|o)$ with respect to o using a multiplicative gradient-based algorithm (expectation-maximization) leads to the Richardson-Lucy (RL) algorithm [2], [3]:

$$o_{k+1}(x) = \left\{ \left[\frac{i(x)}{(o_k \otimes h)(x)} \right] \otimes h(-x) \right\} o_k(x) \tag{3}$$

The RL algorithm improves the image quality first but after several iterations noise is amplified and the algorithm does not converge. In order to overcome this problem a priori knowledge $P(o)$ about the image is added and the a posteriori distribution $P(o|i) = P(i|o)P(o)$ is then maximized (MAP). The a priori model is included by adding a regularization term and in the last decade several regularization terms have been introduced. In [4] a Total Variation (TV) regularization suppresses noise amplification by smoothing the image while at the same time preserving the edges. Introduced in [5], TV was used to denoise images. A TV regularized multiplicative RL algorithm (RLTV) with λ being the regularization parameter and ∇ being the gradient is given by:

$$o_{k+1}(x) = \left\{ \left[\frac{i(x)}{(o_k \otimes h)(x)} \right] \otimes h(-x) \right\} \frac{o_k(x)}{1 - \lambda \nabla \frac{\nabla o_k(x)}{|\nabla o_k(x)|}} \tag{4}$$

1.3 Acceleration of RL algorithm

In [6], an adaptive accelerated Richardson-Lucy method is presented. The main objective of this work is the acceleration of the convergence speed of the standard multiplicative RL algorithm presented in (3) by adding an exponent to the multiplicative correction ratio. This exponenet is computed adaptively by using the deblurred images from previous iteration steps. Since there is no regularization in this method, noise amplification is a problem. Supervising the root mean square error (RMSE) shows a considerable noise amplification after few iterations. Thus, the authors suggest stopping the algorithm at the minimum RMSE. In case of noise-free images, it is shown that the new accelerated methods is able to obtain better results regarding the RMSE after less iterations.

2 Materials and methods

2.1 Acceleration of RLTV

In order to accelerate the multiplicative RLTV (accRLTV) algorithm (4), we use a method introduced by Biggs and Andrews [7]. This acceleration method is based on vector extrapolation and does not require an evaluation of the cost function. In general, the method can be applied to various techniques as long as the basic iterative algorithm contains a known independent functional ψ that can be used to calculate the next iteration step (5). The multiplicative RLTV fulfills this requirement.

$$o_{k+1} = \psi(o_k) \tag{5}$$

In the original algorithm the current iteration o_k is used in the functional ψ in order to get the next iteration o_{k+1}. In the accelerated version, a virtual point g_k is calculated and this point is used in the functional ψ to determine the next iteration $o_{k+1} = \psi(g_k)$. In order to determine the virtual point g_k, the direction $d_k = o_k - o_{k-1}$ being the difference between the current and the previous iteration is used. In addition, an acceleration parameter α_k is needed to weight the direction d_k when calculating the virtual point g_k:

$$g_k = o_k + \alpha_k \cdot d_k \tag{6}$$

In the used method, α_k is estimated by using the results of previous iteration steps. A more accurate solution could be obtained by a line search but this is no option because of the computational effort. In order to estimate α_k, the differences l_k between the virtual point g_{k-1} and the respectively next iteration o_k are used $l_k = o_k - g_{k-1}$. These differences describe the actual changes made by the functional ψ. α_k is then calculated using following formula where $\odot$ denotes an element-wise multipication and $\sum$ sums all elements in the data.

$$\alpha_k = \frac{\sum_{\Omega} (l_{k-1} \odot l_{k-2})}{\sum_{\Omega} (l_{k-1} \odot l_{k-1})} \tag{7}$$

In addition, each α has to fulfill the condition $0 \leq \alpha \leq 1$ and is modified after the estimation accordingly in case this condition is not fulfilled. Figure 1 shows graphically how the acceleration influences the calculation. It can be seen that instead of the original step size much larger changes can be achieved in each iteration step by using the virtual points.

2.2 Numerical stability

The values in the fluorescence images are positive or zero since they represent a photon count. The RLTV (4), however, is not well defined for zero values and thus a modified version of the TV regularization is applied [8]. Additionally, the values used for λ are restricted in order to avoid negative or zero values in the denominator and we thus use 0.002 as suggested in [4].

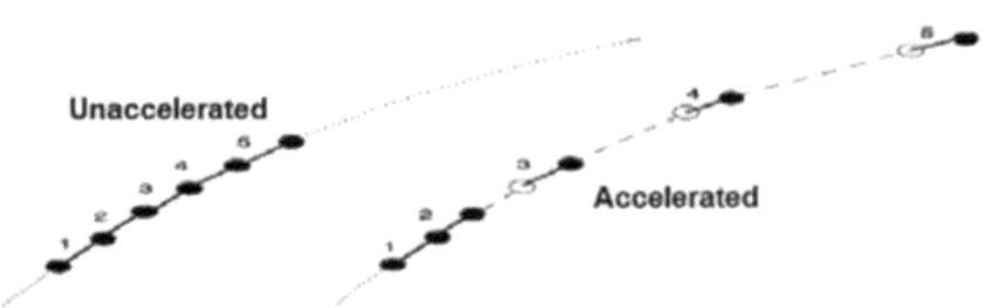

Fig. 1. Illustration of acceleration

Fig. 2. left to right: original image, blurred and noisy image, RLTV, accRLTV

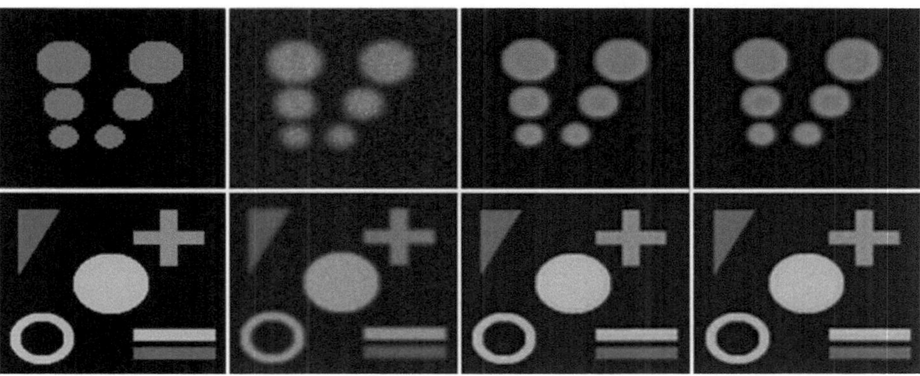

2.3 Quality of the results

To quantify the quality of the restored images, it is usual to use the I-divergence (IDiv) being equivalent to the likelihood distribution of the Poisson noise (2). IDiv compares the recorded image i with the reblurred reconstructed image $o \otimes h$. Since the original image $\tilde{o}$ is known for our synthetic test images, we use the mean square error (MSE) to compare $\tilde{o}$ with the reconstructed image o as well.

$$Idiv_{A,B} = \sum_{x \in \Omega} \left\{ A(x) ln(\frac{A(x)}{B(x)}) - (A(x) - B(x)) \right\} \tag{8}$$

3 Results

For our evaluation, we use two synthetic test images (3D) sized $100 \times 100 \times 60$ voxels and $200 \times 200 \times 50$ voxels. The images are blurred with a Gaussian PSF of size $9 \times 9 \times 9$ voxels with a variance of 1.8 voxel size and corrupted by Poisson noise. One slice of each test image together with their degraded versions are shown in figure (2). Furthermore, the results of the deblurring for the RLTV and accRLTV are displayed.

In average, one iteration of the accRLTV algorithm takes 5% longer than the RLTV (Average time for one iteration image 1: RLTV 1.38 seconds and

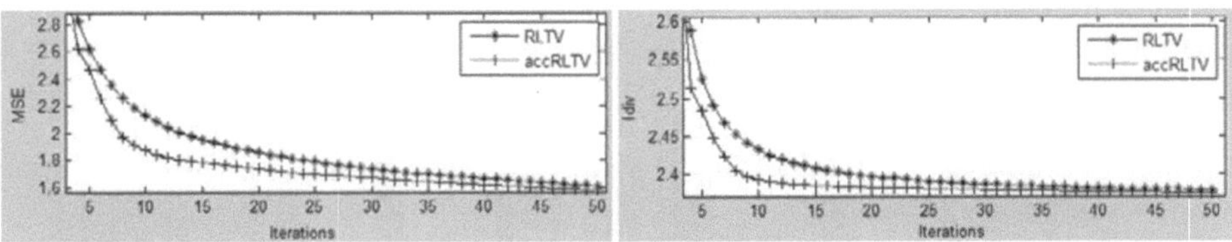

Fig. 3. a) MSE b) IDiv

Table 1. Amount of iterations to deblur the images

	RLTV(1)	accRLTV(1)	RLTV(2)	accRLTV(2)	RLTV(3)	accRLTV(3)
first test image	29	18	31	21	30	19
second test image	25	15	25	14	26	16

accRLTV 1.45 seconds with a 2.6 GHz Quad Core CPU). Each test image was degraded three times and restored with both the RLTV and the accRLTV. The deblurring is stopped when a certain MSE is reached and the amount of necessary iterations is shown in Table 1. The progress of both the MSE and the IDiv are shown in Figure 3 for one test image.

4 Discussion

In Figure 2, it can be seen that the result images of both algorithms are nearly identical. Since the differences in the computational time for both algorithms are quite small the computational time can be neglected in the further evaluation. For the first test image the desired MSE is reached by the accRLTV within 30% less iterations compared with the RLTV. In case of the second test image the improvement is even higher: it takes 40% less iterations to reach the specified MSE for the accRLTV. The progress of the MSE and Idiv in figure 3 shows graphically that the accRLTV reconstructs the image faster than the original algorithm. In summary, the accRLTV produces acceptable results and requires considerably less computational time than the RLTV.

References

1. Yoo H, Song I, Gweon DG. Measurement and restoration of the point spread function of fluorescence confocal microscopy. J Microscopy. 2005;221:172–176.
2. Lucy LB. An iterative technique for rectification of observed distributions. Astronom J. 1974;79:745–765.
3. Richardson WH. Bayesian-based iterative method of image restoration. JOSA. 1972;62:55–59.
4. Dey N, Blanc-Féraud L, Zimmer C, et al. Richardson-Lucy algorithm with total variation regularization for 3D microscope deconvolution. Microscope Res Techn. 2006;69:260–266.
5. Rudin LI, Osher S, Fatemi E. Nonlinear total variation based noise removal algorithms. Physica D. 1992;60:259–268.
6. Singh MK, Tiwary US, Kim YH. An adaptively accelerated Lucy-Richardson method for image deblurring. EURASIP J Adv Signal Process. 2008;8:1–10.
7. Biggs D, Andrews M. Acceleration of iterative image restoration algorithms. Appl Optics. 1997;36:123–145.
8. Chan T, Marquina A, Mulet P. High-order total variation-based image restoration. SIAM J Sci Comput. 2000;22:503–516.

Towards an Estimation of Acoustic Impedance from Multiple Ultrasound Images

Christian Wachinger[1], Ramtin Shams[2], Nassir Navab[1]

[1]Computer Aided Medical Procedures (CAMP), Technische Universität München
[2]Research School of Information Sciences and Eng., The Australian National Univ.
wachinge@in.tum.de

Abstract. Reflection of sound waves, due to acoustic impedance mismatch at the interface of two media, is the principal physical property which allows visualization with ultrasound. In this paper, we investigate reconstruction of the acoustic impedance from ultrasound images for the first time. Similar to spatial compounding, we combine multiple images to improve the estimation. We use phase information to determine regions of high reflection from an ultrasound image. We model the physical imaging process with an emphasis on the reflection of sound waves. The model is used in computing the acoustic impedance (up to a scale) from areas of high reflectivity. The acoustic impedance image can either be directly visualized or be used in simulation of ultrasound images from an arbitrary point of view. The experiments performed on in-vitro and in-vivo data show promising results.

1 Introduction

Ultrasound (US) has many advantages in comparison to other imaging modalities which has lead to its widespread use in clinical practice; it is (i) harmless at low power, (ii) portable, (iii) a real-time modality, and (iv) most importantly, cost effective. The recent introduction of 2D array US transducers in the market makes further applications possible, due to the instantaneous acquisition of ultrasound volumes. Furthermore, the next generation of transducers with capacitive micromachined ultrasound transducer (CMUT) technology offers superior and efficient volumetric imaging at a lower cost. However, ultrasound has a number of disadvantages including: (i) a limited field-of-view (FOV), (ii) occlusions behind structures with high acoustic impedance, and (iii) a low singal-to-noise ratio (SNR). Spatial compounding of several views, acquired from different positions, helps to reduce these shortcomings.

The prerequisite for spatial compounding is to know the relative positions of the acquired images. This can either be obtained by tracking the ultrasound transducer or by image registration. When working with 2D US images compounding from different positions poses a problem, because all the scans have to be in one plane. Therefore, multi-angle compounding with beam steering is typically performed, where the probe remains fixed [1]. Moving to 3D imaging, compounding from different positions offers much more flexibility, inspiring several groups to work on this subject e.g. [2, 3]. In the following, we assume that we know the alignment of the images, and focus on how to combine their intensity information. As we will discuss later in this report, combining ultrasound images is non-trivial due to the highly view-dependent nature of the ultrasound. We will introduce a novel approach, which is based on the estimation of the acoustic impedance of the imaged scene [4]. From each image, we will reconstruct an acoustic impedance image, which we subsequently average to get an estimation for the whole imaged area. These images can either be directly presented to the physician or can be used in simulation of ultrasound images from an arbitrary point of view.

2 Acoustic impedance estimation

Core to our method is the estimation of the acoustic impedance of the region depicted in the ultrasound image. As we will see, acoustic impedance images are related to CT attenuation values expressed in Hounsfield units and no longer exhibit view-dependent artifacts and emphasized interface boundaries as in ultrasound images. Having the acoustic impedance images z_i from all views, the creation of a global acoustic impedance image z for the whole imaging scenario is possible.

We first reduce speckle in the images by median filtering them, and further identify regions of high reflectivity by calculating the local phase. Third, we use these regions to reconstruct the impedance for each image, and finally we find the global impedance estimation by averaging acoustic images obtained from each ultrasound image.

2.1 Phase calculation

Essential for the acoustic impedance estimation is the identification of regions with high reflectivity, indicating a change in acoustic impedance. We use phase information for this purpose because it provides us with structural information independent of the brightness and contrast [2]. For 1-D signals the phase is constructed from the original signal and its Hilbert transform. There are different approaches to extend this concept to N-D. Here we will use the recently introduced monogenic signal approach [5]. It uses a generalization of the Hilbert transform, the Riesz transform, to calculate phase information in N-D. The image is filtered by N filters, which are given in the Fourier domain by

$$R_i(f_1, \ldots, f_N) = \frac{f_i}{\sqrt{\sum_{j=1}^{N} f_j^2}} \tag{1}$$

with $f_1, \ldots, f_N$ the Fourier domain coordinates. We follow [2] in applying log-Gabor filters prior to the calculation of the monogenic signal of the image to extract frequency and spatial localization. The monogenic signal provides us with information about the phase and orientation of each pixel (Fig. 1). We threshold the phase image to get a mask (Fig. 1) to extract the reflectivity part from the ultrasound image.

2.2 Acoustic impedance calculation

We estimate for each US image u_i an acoustic impedance z_i

$$\arg\min_{z_i} \left(u_i(\mathbf{x}) - \frac{\log\left(1 + a \cdot (\cos\varphi(\mathbf{x}))^m \cdot \rho_{z_i}(\mathbf{x})\right)}{\log(1+a)} \right)^2 \tag{2}$$

with a paramterizing the log-compression, $\varphi(\mathbf{x})$ the incidence angle at position $\mathbf{x}$, m modeling the heterogeneity of the interface, and the reflection coefficient

$$\rho_z(\mathbf{x}) = \left(\frac{z(\mathbf{x}) - z(\mathbf{x} - \Delta\mathbf{d})}{z(\mathbf{x}) + z(\mathbf{x} - \Delta\mathbf{d})} \right)^2 . \tag{3}$$

In order to perform the optimization, we make the assumption that the incidence angle for the impedance and ultrasound image are roughly the same

$$\cos\varphi(x) = \left| \mathbf{d}. \frac{\nabla z(\mathbf{x})}{|\nabla z(\mathbf{x})|} \right| \approx \left| \mathbf{d}. \frac{\nabla u(\mathbf{x})}{|\nabla u(\mathbf{x})|} \right| . \tag{4}$$

Since the orientation of the interfaces in impedance and ultrasound image should be the same, this approximation is reasonable.

The only term in Equation (2) that is still dependent on the acoustic impedance is the reflection coefficient $\rho_{z_i}(\mathbf{x})$. Since this term is recursively defined, depending on the previous estimation $z(\mathbf{x} - \Delta\mathbf{d})$, we need an initial value to make the calculation along the scanline. When taking *e.g.* acquisitions in a water bath, we can directly use the acoustic impedance of water. But it is not always possible to acquire a proper initialization and as such, in general, a reconstruction up to a scale is possible. This is sufficient for visualization and US simulation. In the future, further information from the US image such as tissue estimation from RF data or speckle could be integrated to make the estimation more precise.

Having the acoustic estimates z_i, we get the global acoustic impedance image z by calculating the mean.

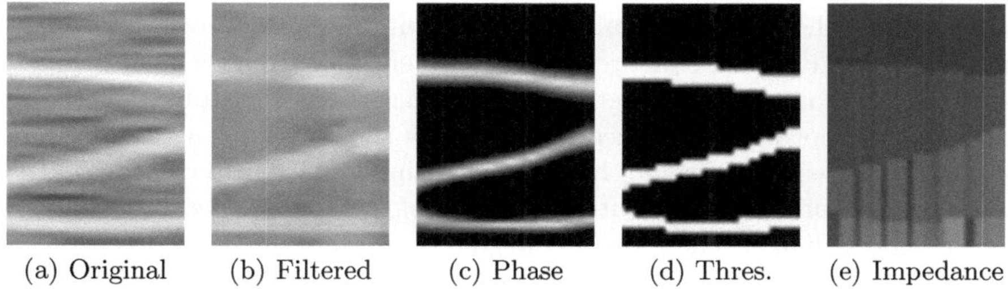

(a) Original (b) Filtered (c) Phase (d) Thres. (e) Impedance

Fig. 1. Processing steps for acoustic impedance estimation of simulated ultrasound

3 Visualization

Once the global acoustic impedance image z is estimated, we have to find ways to visualize it for the physician. One possibility would be to directly present the acoustic impedance image, but this may be of limited clinical value, because physicians are not used to these images and may have problems interpreting them. A better way may be to create artificial ultrasound views [6], see Figure 3(h). The simulation of US from the acoustic impedance image is feasible because it is the acoustic impedance that determines the structure of the US images. It has the advantage, that US views can be simulated that were initially not recorded, and from positions that are physically not possible.

4 Results

We perform experiments on simulations of ultrasound from CT [6] producing realistic test images. The images are acquired from different viewing angles varying from $-20°$ to $20°$ to create a realistic spatial compounding scenario. We show as an example the processing steps for the estimation of the simulated US images acquired at $0°$ in Figure 1, with a wavelength of 60mm, $a = 83$, and $m = 0.1$. After doing the same with the four remaining images and mapping them back to the reference frame at $0°$, see Figures 3(a) - 3(e), we can calculate the global acoustic impedance image, see Figure 3(f). It is the average of the separate estimations and one clearly sees the improved quality. When comparing it to the original CT image, which can to some respect be seen as ground truth, the good quality of the reconstruction becomes apparent. Finally, we use the global impedance image to simulate an ultrasound image, see Figure 3(h), with the same method we originally used to simulate the US images from CT.

5 Conclusion

We have presented a method to estimate acoustic impedance from multiple ultrasound images. The key to the acoustic impedance calculation is to have a model from the physical imaging process to be able to analyze US images. We have presented such a model and adapted it to the specific needs of acoustic impedance estimation, where we focused on modeling reflections. This allows us to estimate the impedance values at tissue interfaces. We proposed a phase-based image analysis to extract regions of high reflection from the image. Similar to spatial compounding, we average several images to get a robust estimation of the global acoustic impedance. Our results show that acoustic impedance estimation is feasible. It would, however, be helpful to integrate further data in the estimation process coming from RF, elastography, and speckle analysis, to make it more reliable. The acoustic impedance image would play a central role for combining these different data sources. For a more detailed version of this article, we refer the reader to [4].

Fig. 2. Acoustic impedance estimation in the overlap area from the 5 simulated US images, transformed in reference coordinate system. Mean of estimations, and in comparison the original CT. (h): Simulation of US image from the global acoustic impedance image (f).

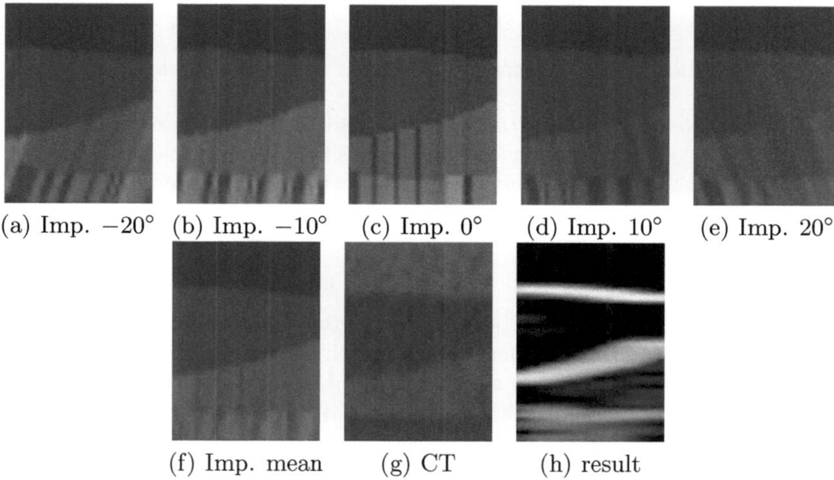

(a) Imp. −20° (b) Imp. −10° (c) Imp. 0° (d) Imp. 10° (e) Imp. 20°

(f) Imp. mean (g) CT (h) result

References

1. Wilhjelm JE, Jensen MS, Jespersen SK, et al. Visual and quantitative evaluation of selected image combination schemes in ultrasound spatial compound scanning. IEEE Trans Med Imaging. 2004;23(2):181–190.
2. Grau V, Becher H, Noble JA. Registration of multiview real-time 3-D echocardiographic sequences. IEEE Trans Med Imaging. Sept 2007;26(9):1154–1165.
3. Wachinger C, Wein W, Navab N. Three-dimensional ultrasound mosaicing. Proc MICCAI. 2007.
4. Wachinger C, Shams R, Navab N. Estimation of acoustic impedance from multiple ultrasound images with application to spatial compounding. In: Procs IEEE Workshop: Mathematical Methods in Biomedical Image Analysis. Anchorage, Alaska; 2008.
5. Felsberg M, Sommer G. The monogenic signal. IEEE Trans Sign Process. 2001;49(12):3136–3144.
6. Shams R, Hartley R, Navab N. Real-time simulation of medical ultrasound from CT images. Proc MICCAI. 2008.

Reduktion von Rissartefakten durch nicht-lineare Registrierung in histologischen Schnittbildern

Nicole Schubert[1], Uwe Pietrzyk[1,2], Martin Reißel[3], Christoph Palm[1,2]

[1]Institut für Neurowissenschaften und Biophysik 3, Forschungszentrum Jülich
[2]Abteilung für Physik, Universität Wuppertal
[3]Fachbereich Technomathematik, Fachhochschule Aachen
ch.palm@fz-juelich.de

Kurzfassung. In dieser Arbeit wird ein Verfahren vorgestellt, das Rissartefakte, die in histologischen Rattenhirnschnitten vorkommen können, durch nicht-lineare Registrierung reduziert. Um die Optimierung in der Rissregion zu leiten, wird der Curvature Registrierungsansatz um eine Metrik basierend auf der Segmentierung der Bilder erweitert. Dabei erzielten Registrierungen mit der ausschließlichen Segmentierung des Risses bessere Ergebnisse als Registrierungen mit einer Segmentierung des gesamten Hirnschnitts. Insgesamt zeigt sich eine deutliche Verbesserung in der Rissregion, wobei der verbleibende reduzierte Riss auf die Glattheitsbedingungen des Regularisierers zurückzuführen ist.

1 Einleitung

Histologische Rattenhirnschnitte sind hochaufgelöste 2D Aufnahmen einzelner Gehirnschichten. Für die gute Ortsauflösung von 6×6 μm wird jedoch der Bezug der Schichten untereinander eingebüßt. Das Ziel eines konsistenten 3D Datensatzes kann mit affiner und nicht-linearer Registrierung erreicht werden [1, 2]. Die Registrierung bringt zwei Bilder mit korrespondierenden Strukturen durch eine Transformation in räumliche Übereinstimmung. Ein Templatebild wird dabei einem Referenzbild angeglichen.

Während des Schneide- und Präparationsprozesses der Histologie können jedoch Artefakte des Schnittgewebes auftreten, die die Zuordnung der Objektstrukturen erschweren. In dieser Arbeit liegt das Augenmerk auf Rissartefakte. Das Problem hierbei ist, dass bei auftretenden Artefakten im Bild die korrespondierenden Rissstrukturen im Referenzbild fehlen, um die Optimierung des Registrierungsprozesses leiten zu können. Außerdem widersprechen die Glattheitsbedingungen an das Verschiebungsfeld im nicht-linearen Registrierungsansatz notwendigen lokalen Transformationen zum Schließen von Rissen.

Die nicht-lineare Registrierung in ihrer bekannten Form führt also nicht zur Reduktion von Rissartefakten, die in histologischen Schnitten auftreten können.

Daher wird der bekannte Curvature Registrierungsansatz [3, 4] um eine Metrik erweitert, die den Abstand zwischen den Distanzbildern der segmentierten

Bilder misst. Als Grundlage dient dazu die Arbeit von Han et al. [5], wobei wir keine Landmarken verwenden. Als Ersatz für den fehlenden Riss im Referenzbild wird eine künstliche Risslinie im Referenzbild erzeugt. Ein weiteres nicht-rigides Registrierungsverfahren mit Distanztransformationen wird in [6] vorgestellt.

2 Material und Methoden

2.1 Nicht-lineare Registrierung

Die zu registrierenden d-dimensionalen Bilder seien $R, T : \Omega \to \mathfrak{R}$ mit $\Omega \subset \mathfrak{R}^d$. Gesucht wird ein Verschiebungsfeld $u : \mathfrak{R}^d \to \mathfrak{R}^d$, so dass die Distanz D zwischen $R(x)$ und $T(x - u(x))$ minimal wird. Für die Glattheit von u wird ein Regularisierer S eingeführt, der durch den Regularisierungsparameter α gesteuert wird. Daraus ergibt sich ein Funktional, das zur Lösung des nicht-linearen Registrierungsproblems minimiert wird:

$$\mathfrak{J}[u] := D[R, T; u] + \alpha S[u]. \tag{1}$$

Für monomodale Bilder wird üblicherweise ein einfaches, grauwert-basiertes Distanzmaß wie *sum of squared differences* (SSD) verwendet:

$$D^{\mathrm{SSD}}[R, T; u] = \frac{1}{2} \int_{\Omega} (T(x - u(x)) - R(x))^2 dx. \tag{2}$$

Der Curvature Regularisierer lautet [4]:

$$S^{\mathrm{curv}}[u](x) = \frac{1}{2} \sum_{l=1}^{d} \int_{\Omega} (\Delta u_l(x))^2 dx. \tag{3}$$

2.2 Erweiterte nicht-lineare Registrierung

Für die Regulierung der Optimierung in der Rissregion wird ein zusätzliches Abstandsmaß definiert. Dafür werden die Bilder segmentiert, d.h. das Bildobjekt wird vom Hintergrund separiert. Die Segmentierung erfolgt hier manuell. In Frage kommende Segmente sind der gesamte Hirnschnitt und der Riss allein. Es ist zu beachten, dass im Referenzbild kein Rissartefakt auftritt. Das Äquivalent eines geschlossenen Risses muss künstlich erzeugt werden, da die Registrierung nur ähnliche Strukturen aus Referenz- und Templatebild angleicht. Deshalb wird entlang der Skelettlinie des Risssegments des Templatebildes ein Pseudo-Riss in das segmentierte Referenzbild eingefügt.

Alle Punkte des Segments gehören zum Gebiet $\Omega_O \subset \Omega$, die Außenkontur des Segments ist dann $\partial\Omega_O$. Aus den segmentierten Bilder werden mit der *signed distance function* [5] die Distanzbilder berechnet:

$$\phi(x) = \begin{cases} -d^{\mathrm{eukl}}(x, \Gamma) & : \ x \in \Omega_O \\ 0 & : \ x \in \partial\Omega_O = \Gamma \\ d^{\mathrm{eukl}}(x, \Gamma) & : \ \text{sonst} \end{cases} \tag{4}$$

wobei $d^{\text{eukl}}(x, \Gamma)$ der minimale euklidische Abstand eines Pixels $x \in \Omega$ von der Objektkontur Γ ist.

Aus den Distanzbildern wird ein konturbasiertes Abstandsmaß definiert [5], das wie das intensitätsbasierte Distanzmaß den Unterschied der beiden Bilder misst:

$$D^{\text{con}}[\phi^R, \phi^T; u] = \frac{1}{2} \int_\Omega (\phi^T(x - u(x)) - \phi^R(x))^2 dx. \tag{5}$$

Das Energiefunktional (1) wird durch D^{con}, gewichtet mit einem Faktor β, erweitert. Somit ergibt sich ein neues zu minimierendes Energiefunktional:

$$\mathfrak{J}[u] = (1 - \beta) D^{\text{SSD}}[R, T; u] + \beta D^{\text{con}}[\phi^R, \phi^T; u] + \alpha S^{\text{curv}}[u]. \tag{6}$$

Anders als Han et al. [5] verwenden wir in unserem Ansatz keine Landmarken.

Das Minimierungsproblem wird durch die zugehörige partielle Differentialgleichung, die Euler-Lagrange Gleichung, gelöst. Damit u das Funktional minimiert, muss es die Euler-Lagrange-Gleichung erfüllen:

$$(1 - \beta) f^{\text{SSD}}(x, u(x)) + \beta f^{\text{con}}(x, u(x)) + \alpha \Delta^2 u(x) = 0 \tag{7}$$

mit

$$f^{\text{SSD}}(x, u(x)) = (R(x) - T(x - u(x))) \nabla T(x - u(x)) \tag{8}$$

$$f^{\text{con}}(x, u(x)) = (\phi^R(x) - \phi^T(x - u(x))) \nabla \phi^T(x - u(x)). \tag{9}$$

Die Implementierung dieser Registrierung basiert auf der Klassenbibliothek ITK.

3 Ergebnisse

Als Bildmaterial dienen zwei histologische Rattenhirnschnitte mit einer Dicke von 20 μm und einer Auflösung von 6×6 μm. Zwischen den Schnitten ist eine Lücke von 380 μm, was neben dem deutlichen Rissartefakt des Templatebildes zu erheblichen anatomischen Unterschieden führt. Vor der nicht-linearen Registrierung erfolgte eine rigide Vorregistrierung des artefaktfreien Referenzbildes (Abb.1(a)) und des rissbehafteten Templatebildes (Abb.1(b)). Die manuell erstellten Konturen sind in Abbildung 1(c) und (d) zu sehen. Für verschiedene Parameter α und β aus (7) werden die Bilder miteinander registriert.

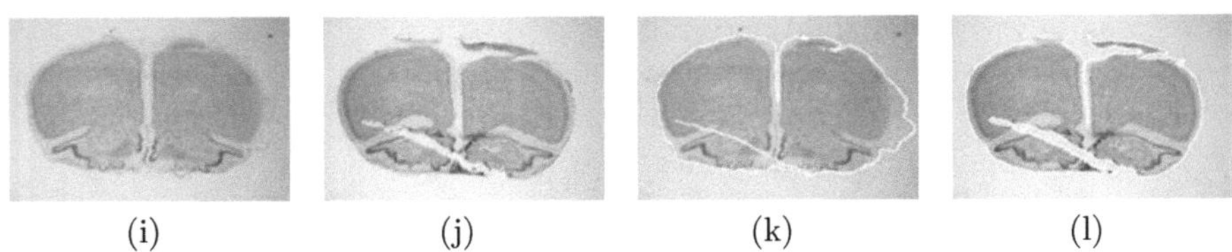

(i) (j) (k) (l)

Abb. 1. (a): Referenzbild R, (b): Templatebild T, (c): Referenzbild mit Kontur (weiß), (d): Templatebild mit Kontur (weiß).

Es zeigte sich, dass Registrierungen basierend auf einer Segmentierung des gesamten Hirnschnitts ungenügende Ergebnisse liefern. Ein Deformationsfeld einer solchen Registrierung ist in Abbildung 2(a) dargestellt. Es ist zu erkennen, dass in der Rissregion kaum Verschiebungen stattfinden, sie aber am Objektrand verstärkt auftreten. Das Deformationsfeld aus Abbildung 2(b) ist das Ergebnis einer Registrierung, bei der nur der Riss segmentiert und in der Metrik berücksichtigt wurde. Die Konzentration auf die Rissregion ist deutlich zu sehen.

Die Abbildung 3(a) zeigt das Resultat der Registrierung ohne Einfluss der Segmentierung. Die Ergebnisse der Registrierung basierend auf der Segmentierung wurden mit dem Referenzbild verglichen, indem die summierten Abstandsquadrate der Intensitäten berechnet werden. Daraus ergab sich für die Registrierung mit der gesamten Hirnkontur das beste Ergebnis für $\alpha = 0.03$ und $\beta = 0.00005$ (Abb.3(b)). Mit der Registrierung basierend auf der Segmentierung des Risses kann der Riss weiter geschlossen werden. Das beste Ergebnis liefert die Registrierung für $\alpha = 0.03$ und $\beta = 0.0002$ (Abb.3(c)).

4 Diskussion

Wir haben eine Methode vorgestellt, die die Reduzierung von Geweberissen ermöglicht. Dabei zeigt die Beschränkung des konturbasierten Abstandsmaßes auf die Rissregion bessere Ergebnisse und einen nahezu vollständigen Rissschluss.

Im Ergebnis der reinen Curvature Registrierung ist deutlich erkennbar, dass in der Rissregion keine Verbesserung stattfindet und ungewünschte Verschiebungen am Objektrand entstehen (Abb.3(a)). Sie sind auf die sehr unterschiedlichen Objektränder zurückzuführen. Der Objektrand im Referenzbild ist teilweise stark ausgefranst, während der Rand des Templatebildes eine klare Struktur aufweist, jedoch an einigen Stellen unterbrochen wird.

Das Ergebnis der Registrierung mit Segmentierung des gesamten Hirns zeigt eine Rissbewegung, jedoch entlang der Außenkontur vermehrt ungewünschte Auswüchse und Verschiebungen (Abb.3(b)). Diese lassen sich aus der zusätzlichen Konturinformation aus der Segmentierung ableiten. Durch die gravierenden

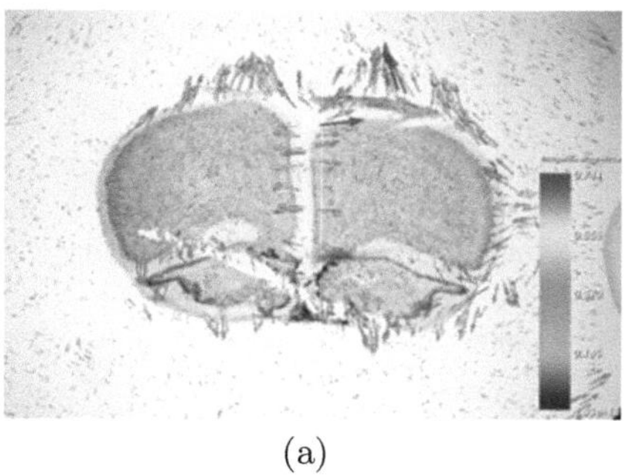

(a)

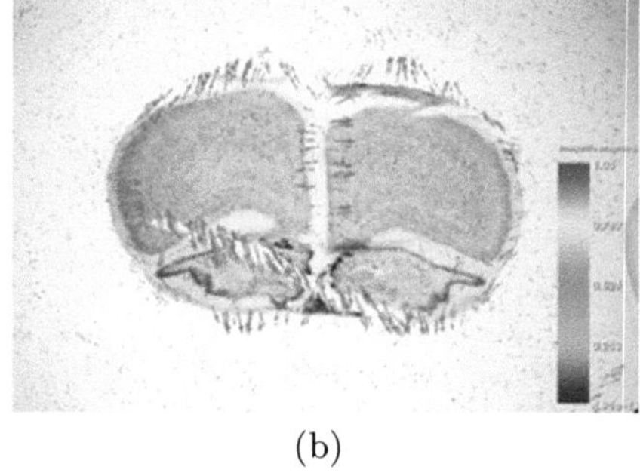

(b)

Abb. 2. Verschiebungsfelder von Registrierung: (a): mit Segmentierung der gesamten Kontur, (b): mit Segmentierung des Risses.

Abb. 3. Registrierungsergebnisse für Registrierung: (a) ohne Segmentierung, $\alpha = 0.03$, $\beta = 0$ (b): mit Segmentierung der gesamten Kontur, $\alpha = 0.03$, $\beta = 0.00005$, (c): mit Segmentierung des Risses $\alpha = 0.03$, $\beta = 0.0002$.

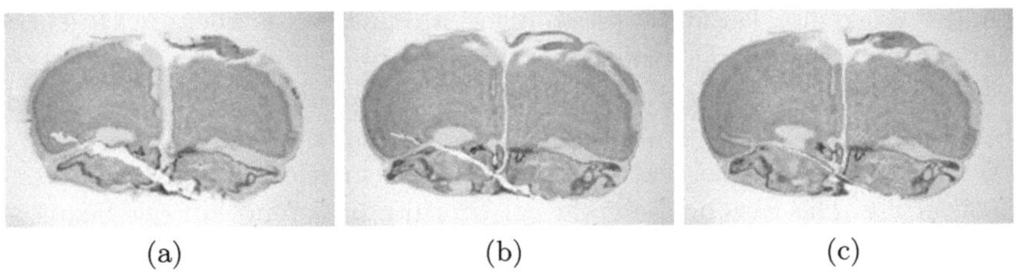

(a) (b) (c)

Unterschiede in der Kontur werden die Verschiebungen am Objektrand zu groß, bevor sich der Riss genügend schließen kann.

Indem nur der segmentierte Riss in der Registrierung verarbeitet wird, werden diese Randbewegungen wieder vermindert. Allerdings treten gleichzeitig ungewollte Verzerrungen in der Rissregion auf (Abb.3(c)). Diese lassen sich dadurch erklären, dass in der Risszone nur das konturbasierte Abstandsmaß greift, da im Grauwert-Referenzbild keine Rissstruktur existiert und die anatomischen Unterschiede groß sind. Das steht im Gegensatz zur Arbeit von Han et al. [5], die korrespondierende Konturen in Referenz- und Templatebild betrachten.

Unser Verfahren beruht auf der Annahme, dass die Position des geschlossenen Risses in Form der Skelettlinie des Risssegments bekannt ist. Das Fehlen eines Goldstandards macht die Überprüfung dieser Annahme unmöglich. Erschwert wird die Registrierung durch erhebliche anatomische Unterschiede. Um den Interaktionsaufwand des Verfahrens zu verringern, bedarf es einer automatisierten Segmentierung, die mit Standardverfahren durchgeführt werden kann. Die künstliche Risserzeugung ist anhand des segmentierten Risses leicht erstellbar.

Literaturverzeichnis

1. Schmitt O, Modersitzki J, Heldmann S, et al. Image registration of sectioned brains. Int J Computer Vis. 2007;73:5–39.
2. Wirtz S, Fischer B, Modersitzki J, et al. Vollständige Rekonstruktion eines Rattenhirns aus hochaufgelösten Bildern von histologischen Serienschnitten. Proc BVM. 2004; p. 204–208.
3. Fischer B, Modersitzki J. Curvature based image registration. J Math Imaging Vis. 2003;18:81–85.
4. Modersitzki J. Numerical Methods for Image Registration. Oxford University Press; 2004.
5. Han J, Hornegger J, Kuwert T, et al. Feature constrained non-rigid image registration. Front Sim. 2005; p. 638–643.
6. Paragios N, Rousson M, Ramesh V. Non-rigid registration using distance functions. Computer Vis Image Underst. 2003;18:142–165.

Automatic Classification of Embryonic Fruit Fly Gene Expression Patterns

Andreas Heffel[1], Sonja J. Prohaska[1,2], Peter F. Stadler[1−5], Gerhard Kauer[6], Jens-Peer Kuska[1]

[1]Interdisciplinary Centre for Bioinformatics, University of Leipzig,
[2]Department of Computer Science, University of Leipzig,
[3]RNomics Group, Fraunhofer Institute for Cell Therapy and Immunology, Leipzig;
[4]Institut for Theoretical Chemistry, University of Vienna; [5]Santa Fe Institute;
[6]Faculty Technical Sciences, University of Applied Sciences O/O/W, Emden
heffel@izbi.uni-leipzig.de

Abstract. Carefully studied in-situ hybridization Gene expression patterns (GEP) can provide a first glance at possible relationships among genes. Automatic comparative analysis tools are an indispensable requirement to manage the constantly growing amount of such GEP images. We present here an automated processing pipeline for Segmenting, Classification, and Clustering large-scale sets of Drosophila melanogaster GEP images that facilitates automatic GEP analysis.

1 Introduction

With the advent of large-scale automated whole-mount in-situ hybridization (ISH), the boom in high throughput techniques has also seized modern developmental biology [1, 2, 3, 4]. The spatio-temporal expression patterns of genes often provide rapid direct insight in the potential functional roles of novel or poorly studied genes and allows at least a first glance at possible relationships among genes. This can be exploited to develop new diagnostic methods. Where single genetic markers are not sufficient to distinguish healthy tissue from a diseased phenotype, combinations of genes can enhance diagnostic strength [5]. Microscopy and comparative analysis of images is therefore becoming an important tool to study the spatio-temporal distribution of multiple gene products. For Drosophila, gene expression patterns for all (about 13,500) genes across a set of developmental stages are being generated systematically, leading to the accumulation of a wealth of high dimensional data with complex encoding. Bioinformatics currently helps with data management, storage, access, and integration (e.g. BDGP [6, 4, 7, 8] and FlyBase [9]), but could also assist in data processing, data analysis and provide an observation tool for researchers in the field. Such an attempt has been made by Fly Express [10]. With 57,083 images mapping the expression patterns of 3,366 genes (April 30, 2008), it is currently the largest database that computes and holds standardized images. It offers the Basic Expression Search Tool, BEST, [11], to retrieve genes with expression patters similar to a given query pattern. An alternative and more robust set of algorithms was proposed by Peng et al. [12, 13]. Here, we describe a processing pipeline for automatic segmentation, classification and clustering of ISH images, which is based on the representation of expression patterns by means of Bessel eigenfunctions. This spectral representation facilitates a faster and easier pattern classification once the coefficients are calculated. We apply our approach to a subset of 681 genes for which images are available in Fly Express for all 6 developmental stages.

2 Materials and methods

As previously explained in our recent publication [14] the elaborated processing pipeline include six basic steps. The preprocessing (i) consists of a shading correction and a contrast optimization method resulting in a "‘clean image"’. The shape segmentation (ii) is executed on the clean image by computing the magnitude of the gradient followed by a fragmentation of the gradient feature space with the Gaussian Mixture Model [15, 16] instead of using a static threshold. The result is a probability map describing the probability for the membership to one of the classes (background, embryo). After filtering with a total variation filter, a smoothed mask is obtained with an unpredictable count of holes in it, because some areas in the embryo have feature values similar to the background. We close the holes and obtain the binary Segmentation Result. Gradient vector field snakes are used in case of several touching embryos, to isolate the embryo (iii) [17, 18]. The binary images are rigidly registered onto an ellipse prior to the snake segmentation, to allow an automatic placement of the initial contour.

The registration (iv) of the extracted embryo outline onto an ellipse is a necessary step to align the shapes and hence the patterns consequently. This is done in two steps: first, we apply a rigid registration [19] and second, a nonlinear registration onto the ellipse [20, 21]. The found transformations onto an ellipse, computed from the registration of the embryo outlines, are then applied to the masked embryo images to obtain the expression pattern mapped onto an ellipse. Due to the fact that the orthonormal system that we have chosen for the pattern representation is defined on a circle, the ellipse is finally stretched to circular shape.

The GEP extraction (v) step has been modified from the GMM method described in [14] to a HSV color space transformation. The pattern is extracted by taking the color intensity information from the V-channel and setting all values smaller than 20 percent to zero (denoising).

Finally the pattern classification (vi) step can be computed on the extracted GEP sets. Thereby the patterns $\mathcal{P}(r,\phi)$ are described by a set of Fourier coefficients:

$$\mathcal{P}(r,\phi) = \sum_{j=1}^{\infty}\sum_{k=0}^{\infty} a_{j,k}\, \psi_{j,k}(r,\phi) \tag{1}$$

As basis, the eigenfunctions of the Laplace operator on a circle of radius ℓ,

$$\psi_{j,k}(r,\phi) = N_{j,k}\, e^{ik\phi} J_k\left(\frac{r j_{k,j}}{\ell}\right), \tag{2}$$

are used, where ℓ is the radius of the circle, $J_k(z)$ are the k-th Bessel function, $j_{k,j}$ is the j zero of the k-th Bessel function and $N_{j,k}$ is a normalization factor.

3 Results

The gradient based GMM shape segmentation (ii) produces a reliable and accurate separation of the embryos on the border of the focal plane. About 30 percent of the examined images contain several touching embryos. In this case additional knowledge about the expected shape must be included to obtain the mask of a single embryo. This is accomplished by using the active contour approach (iii). The subsequently application of the rigid and nonlinear registration steps (iv) minimizes the distortions produced by the nonlinear registration. The pattern extraction step (v) using the HSV color space transformation is a simple but effective method. In cases of different staining colors or very dark (black) staining regions the HSV extraction method provides robust results.

The reason for choosing the Bessel base functions for the pattern representation is that they form a complete orthonormal system. Our empirical studies and reflections about the possible complexity of the GEP shows that every pattern can be adequately expressed by a set of 420 eigenfunctions ($k \in [0, \ldots, 20]$, $j \in [1, \ldots, 20]$). Fig. 1 summarizes the processing pipeline using the example of one image showing several coherent embryos.

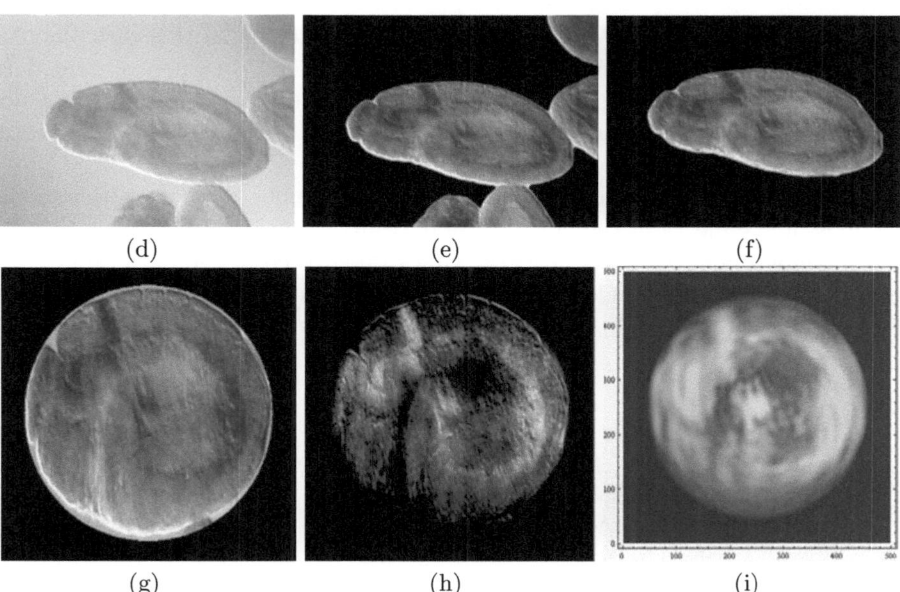

Fig. 1. Illustration of the process flow steps. (a) original image showing several coherent embryos. (b) preprocessing and shape segmentation result (c) isolation of the embryo by snake segmentation (d) registration to circular shape (e) GEP extraction (f) reconstructed GEP from the 420 Fourier coefficients.

Fig. 2. Hierarchical clustering on a set of 8 images that demonstrates that images representing the same genes (CG5690, rg, knrl) in the same developmental stage (Stage 5) are correctly grouped together.

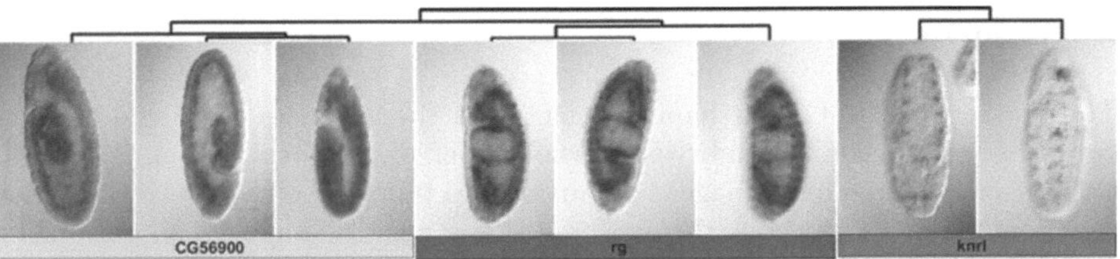

4 Discussion

Naturally, the pictures of Drosophila embryos are much simpler in structure than many other ISH data, which show expression patterns superimposed on complex morphologies (such as mouse or zebrafish embryos). However, the examined images show a lot of difficulties such as blurred contours, background shading, coherent partial embryos, and different staining colors. Our approach is capable of dealing with such complications and achieve a considerable reduction of the data amount needed to represent the patterns. The Euclidean distance in the truncated 420 dimensional space of Fourier coefficients can be used for hierarchical clustering. This allows a classification of expression patterns. As an example, Fig. 2 shows that similar expression patterns, in this case different image representing the same gene, are indeed clustered together. Larger data sets of images show a similar agreement with the visual expectation (data not shown). In particular, images showing the same gene in the same developmental stage are most often grouped together.

In practical applications, the orientation of the embryo with respect to the two axis of symmetry of the ellipse is important. At present, the correct orientation is not generated automatically. Unless annotated in the initial image, all four orientations are included in the clustering and in the end an expert control [6] is inevitable.

References

1. Gawantka V, Pollet N, Delius H, et al. Gene expression screening in Xenopus identifies molecular pathways, predicts gene function and provides a global view of embryonic patterning. Mech Dev. 1998;77:95–141.
2. Neidhardt L, Gasca S, Wertz K, et al. Large-scale screen for genes controlling mammalian embryogenesis, using high-throughput gene expression analysis in mouse embryos. Mech Dev. 2000;98:77–93.
3. Kudoh T, Tsang M, Hukriede NA, et al. A gene expression screen in zebrafish embryogenesis. Genome Res. 2001;11:1979–1987.
4. Tomancak P, Beaton A, Weiszmann R, et al. Systematic determination of patterns of gene expression during Drosophila embryogenesis. Genome Biology. 2002;3:0088.

5. Schubert W, Bonnekoh B, Pommer AJ, et al. Analyzing proteome topology and function by automated multidimensional fluorescence microscopy. Nat Biotechnol. 2006;24:1270–1278.
6. BDGP: Berkeley Drosophila Genome Project. http://www.fruitfly.org/.
7. Tomancak P, Berman BP, Beaton A, et al. Global analysis of patterns of gene expression during Drosophila embryogenesis. Genome Biology. 2007;8:R145.
8. Montalta-He H, Reichert H. Impressive expressions: Developing a systematic database of gene-expression patterns in Drosophila embryogenesis. Genome Biology. 2003; p. 205–205.
9. FlyBase: A Database of Drosophila Genes and Genomes. http://flybase.bio.indiana.edu/.
10. Van Emden B, Ramos H, Panchanathan S, et al. FlyExpress: An image-matching web-tool for finding genes with overlapping patterns of expression in Drosophila embryos; 2006. www.flyexpress.net.
11. Kumar S, Jayaraman K, Panchanathan S, et al. BEST: A novel computational approach for comparing gene expression patterns from early stages of Drosophila melanogaster development. Genetics. 2002;162:2037–2047.
12. Peng H, Myers EW. Comparing in situ mRNA expression patterns of Drosophila embryos. In: Proc Int Conf Res Comput Mol Biol; 2004. p. 157–166.
13. Peng H, Long F, Zhou J, et al. Automatic image analysis for gene expression patterns of fly embryos. BMC Cell Biology. 2007;8 (Suppl 1):S7.
14. Heffel A, Stadler PF, Prohaska SJ, et al. Process flow for classification and clustering of fruit fly gene expression patterns. Proc IEEE ICIP. 2008; p. 721. http://www-video.eecs.berkeley.edu/Proceedings/ICIP2008/ICIP2008.html.
15. Pernkopf F, Bouchaffra D. Genetic-based EM algorithm for learning Gaussian mixture models. IEEE Trans Pattern Anal Mach Intell. 2005;27:1344–1348.
16. Moon TK. The expectation-maximization algorithm. IEEE Signal Processing Magazine. 1996;(6):47–60.
17. Xu C, Prince JL. Snakes, shapes, and gradient vector flow. IEEE Trans Image Process. 1998;7:359–369.
18. Kass M, Witkin A, Terzopoulos D. Snakes: Active contour models. Int J Computer Vis. 2004;1:321–331.
19. Gottesfeld Brown L. A survey of image registration techniques. ACM Computing Surveys. 1992;24:325–376.
20. Braumann UD, Kuska JP. A new equation for nonlinear image registration with control over the vortex structure in the displacement field. Proc IEEE Int Conf Image Process. 2006; p. 329–332.
21. Braumann UD, Kuska JP. Influence of the boundary conditions on the result of non-linear image registration. Proc IEEE Int Conf Image Process. 2005; p. I-1129–I-1132.

MRI Composing for Whole Body Imaging

B. Glocker[1,3], C. Wachinger[1], J. Zeltner[2], N. Paragios[3], N. Komodakis[4], M. Hansen[5], N. Navab[1]

[1]Computer Aided Medical Procedures (CAMP), TU München, Germany
[2]Siemens Healthcare, Erlangen, Germany
[3]Mathématiques Appliquées aux Systèmes (MAS), Ecole Centrale Paris, France
[4]Computer Science Department, University of Crete, Greece
[5]Technical University of Denmark
glocker@in.tum.de

Abstract. Whole-body magnetic resonance imaging is an emerging application gaining vast clinical interest during the last years. Although recent technological advances shortened the longish acquisition time, this is still the limiting factor avoiding its wide-spread clinical usage. The acquisition of images with large field-of-view helps to relieve this drawback, but leads to significantly distorted images. In this paper, a novel scheme for MRI composing is presented. The approach is based on simultaneous registration of two MRI volumes to their linear weighted average. The method successfully compensates for the distortions and allows to generate high-resolution whole body images. Results on several in-vivo data sets are presented.

1 Introduction

Whole-body (WB) magnetic resonance imaging (MRI) is becoming a popular clinical tool due to the recent technological advances in MRI, making faster acquisitions possible. Unlike computed tomography (CT), the acquisition of high-resolution MR images is not feasible during continuous table movement, making a multi-station scanning necessary to cover larger body regions. The compounding of the partially overlapping volumes is straightforward, since the MR scanner keeps track of their exact spatial locations.

The creation of WB images further increases the number of clinical applications for MRI, so far reserved for other modalities. From a current perspective, the major disadvantage using MRI for WB imaging in comparison to CT is the longer scanning time. In this report, we use MR acquisitions with a large field-of-view (FOV), enabling to cover with the same number of scans larger parts of the body. This, however, leads to a degradation of the images by geometrical distortion artefacts towards the boundaries, further described in [1, 2]. We propose a novel method, originating from the field of brain atlas construction, to correct for the geometrical distortion in the overlapping area (Sect. 2). Our experiments show the good results on in-vivo data (Sect. 3).

2 Method

In order to introduce our approach of deformable composing recently proposed [3], we define the two volumes to be stitched as $I_1 : \Omega_1 \subset \mathbb{R}^3 \to \mathbb{R}$ and $I_2 : \Omega_2 \subset \mathbb{R}^3 \to \mathbb{R}$. The overlapping domain is denoted as $\Omega_o = \Omega_1 \cap \Omega_2$. Since the overlap Ω_o is the only part where the two images share any information, a naive approach for the composing could be defined as a minimization problem with respect to a certain distance/similarity measure $\rho(\cdot)$, or

$$\hat{\mathcal{T}}_{1,2} = \arg\min_{\mathcal{T}_{1,2}} \int_{\Omega_o} \rho(I_1(\mathcal{T}_1(\mathbf{x})) - I_2(\mathcal{T}_2(\mathbf{x})))d\mathbf{x} \tag{1}$$

where $\mathbf{x} = (x, y, z)$ denotes a voxel position, and $\mathcal{T}_{1,2}$ are the parameters of the transformations $\mathcal{T}_1$ and $\mathcal{T}_2$ relating the two volumes in the spatial domain. The most common approach in pairwise registration is to assume that one of the two transformations is equal to the identity transformation. In our case, such an approach would lead to several problems: (i) through the selection of a moving and a fixed image, we would introduce a certain bias on the registration result, (ii) since both volumes are distorted due to the inhomogeneous magnetic field in the overlap volume, none of them is actually representing a good reference frame, and (iii) a registration performed only within the overlap may result in discontinuities with respect to the rest of the volumes. In order to overcome these problems, we propose an iterative simultaneous registration using a *linear weighted average*. The idea of the weighted average is to account for the underlying physical properties of increasing distortions towards the volume boundaries. Assuming that the boundary information is less reliable, we would like to reduce its influence to the registration.

2.1 Simultaneous registration to linear weighted average

Let us define another volume $S : \Omega_s$ on the union of the two volume domains $\Omega_s = \Omega_1 \cup \Omega_2$. The intensities of S are set using our average model, or

$$S(\mathbf{x}) = \begin{cases} f(\mathbf{x}), & \text{if } \mathbf{x} \in \Omega_o \\ I_1(\mathcal{T}_1(\mathbf{x})), & \text{if } \mathbf{x} \in \Omega_1 \setminus \Omega_2 \\ I_2(\mathcal{T}_2(\mathbf{x})), & \text{if } \mathbf{x} \in \Omega_2 \setminus \Omega_1 \end{cases} \tag{2}$$

where $f(\cdot)$ is a function computing the linear weighting in the overlap volume, or

$$f(\mathbf{x}) = (1 - h(\mathbf{x})) \cdot I_1(\mathcal{T}_1(\mathbf{x})) + h(\mathbf{x}) \cdot I_2(\mathcal{T}_2(\mathbf{x})). \tag{3}$$

The linear function $h(\cdot)$ has a range of $(0, 1)$ and is defined for the overlap domain Ω_o with respect to the composing direction. In our application, this direction is usually along the head-feet axis which corresponds to the y-axis of our common 3D coordinate system for all the MRI volumes.

The setup for the deformable composing and the initialization of the linear weighted average is illustrated in Fig. 1. We can reformulate the naive registration in Eq. 1 in order to pose a simultaneous registration based on the linear weighted average S. In terms of an energy function (which is to be minimized), we define

$$E_{\text{data}}(\mathcal{T}_{1,2}) = \sum_{i=1}^{2} \int_{\Omega_o} \rho(S(\mathbf{x}) - I_i(\mathcal{T}_i(\mathbf{x})))d\mathbf{x}. \tag{4}$$

In order to reduce the dimensionality of the problem, we consider Free Form Deformations as the transformation model for the two images. A deformation grid $G : [1, K] \times [1, L] \times [1, M]$ is superimposed onto the volume domain Ω_s. By deforming the grid (with a 3D displacement vector $\mathbf{d_p}$ for each control point) the underlying structures are aligned. The transformation of a voxel $\mathbf{x}$ can be expressed using a combination of basis functions, or

$$\mathcal{T}(\mathbf{x}) = \mathbf{x} + \mathcal{D}(\mathbf{x}) \quad \text{with} \quad \mathcal{D}(\mathbf{x}) = \sum_{\mathbf{p} \in G} \eta(|\mathbf{x} - \mathbf{p}|)\, \mathbf{d_p} \tag{5}$$

where $\eta(\cdot)$ is the weighting function (based on cubic B-Splines) measuring the contribution of the control point $\mathbf{p}$ to the displacement field $\mathcal{D}$.

Now, we can rewrite the objective function defined in Eq. 4 based on the two deformation grids G_1 and G_2, or

$$E_{\text{data}}(\mathcal{T}_{1,2}) = \sum_{i=1}^{2} \frac{1}{|G_i|} \sum_{\mathbf{p} \in G_i} \int_{\Omega_o} \hat{\eta}(|\mathbf{x} - \mathbf{p}|) \cdot \rho(S(\mathbf{x}) - I_i(\mathcal{T}_i(\mathbf{x})))d\mathbf{x}. \tag{6}$$

where $\hat{\eta}(\cdot)$ computes the influence of a voxel $\mathbf{x}$ to a control point $\mathbf{p}$. Such a function acts as a *projection* of the distance/similarity measure computed from the volume domain back to the coarser level of control points. Different definitions of the $\hat{\eta}(\cdot)$ have to be considered with respect to the used similarity measure. We use the normalized cross correlation (NCC) which is robust to intensity variations common in MRI. For statistical measures such as NCC, we define

$$\hat{\eta}(|\mathbf{x} - \mathbf{p}|) = \begin{cases} 1, & \text{if } \eta(|\mathbf{x} - \mathbf{p}|) > 0 \\ 0 & \text{otherwise} \end{cases}. \tag{7}$$

Basically, this function masks voxels influenced by a control point $\mathbf{p}$ resulting in a local image patch centered at the control point. From this patch, a *local* similarity measure can then be computed.

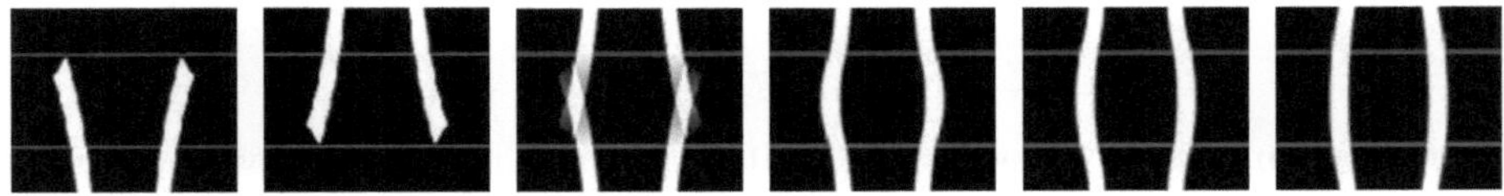

Fig. 1. Synthetic example of a deformable composing. The first and second image are to be composed where both are significantly distorted. The initialization of our linear weighted average is shown in the third image. The horizontal gray lines indicate the borders of the overlap area. Fourth to sixth image is an illustration of the registration progress and the iterative improvement of the linear weighted average.

The simultaneous registration to an average should overcome the problems for the reference selection, mentioned before. This is very similar to atlas construction approaches where the average is used as the reference image in order to achieve an unbiased coordinate frame (e.g. for shape models) [4]. In addition, we try to account for the increasing distortions using a linear weighted average. For optimization of the proposed method we make use of discrete framework for image registration presented [5].

3 Experimental validation

We evaluate our method on 8 whole-body T1- and T2-weighted data sets from three different Siemens MR scanners: Avanto 1.5T, Trio 3T, and Espree 1.5T. The overlaps vary between 5 and 27 cm. An example mosaic is shown in Fig. 2, consisting of three volumes having a FOV of $50 \times 50 \times 28$ cm^3, a resolution of $448 \times 448 \times 35$ voxels, and an overlap of 5 cm. The resolution for the final stitching is $448 \times 1256 \times 35$ where the computation of the two composings take together approximately 25 min. To illustrate that the proposed method also works for varying overlaps, we show the stitching of 3 volumes for whole-spine MR, see Fig. 3. The first overlap is with 15.2 cm very large and our method arrives at producing a sharper average. The second one, with only 1.4 cm,

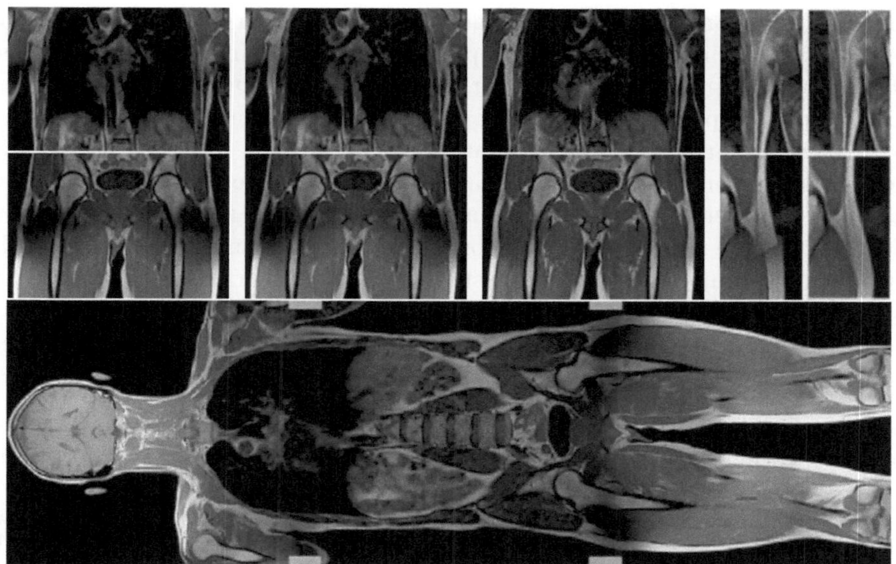

Fig. 2. Top from left to right: Initial average, final composing after 3 optimization cycles, reference scan where the overlap volume is centered within the MR scanner, and magnification of initialization and final composing. Our method is able to reproduce similar smooth and continuous transitions as present in the reference images. Bottom: Resulting whole body image after composing of all three stations.

Fig. 3. Composing of 3 spine volumes. Top: initial average. Bottom: result. Gray bars indicate overlap.

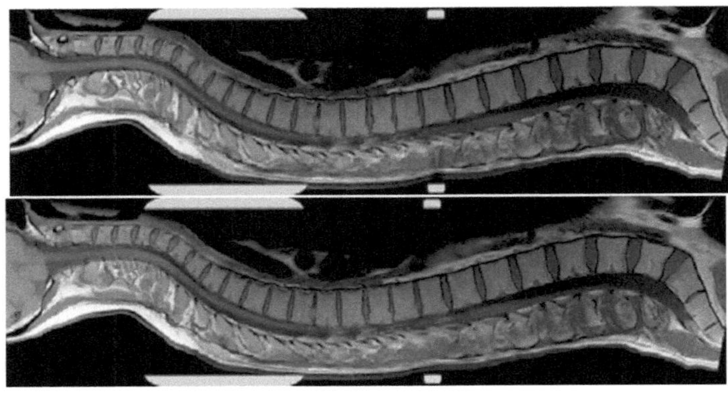

shows discontinuities in the initial average, which are removed after deformable composing.

4 Conclusion

Speeding up the acquisition for WB-MRI with large FOV images leads to significant distortions towards the boundaries. Methods for distortion correction proposed in the literature are not applicable to the WB imaging setup because they either elongate the workflow or only correct for specific system-induced distortions. We propose the usage of simultaneous deformable registration in a composing scenario, which has not yet been done before. Key for the simultaneous registration is the creation of a linear weighted average, each of the two images is registered to. Our experiments on synthetic and in-vivo data show the ability of the method to correct for distortions. The unaltered clinical workflow makes our approach very interesting for being integrated into further MR scanner generations.

References

1. Chang H, Fitzpatrick J. A technique for accurate magnetic resonance imaging in the presence of field inhomogeneities. IEEE Trans MI. 1992;11(3):319–329.
2. Doran SJ, Charles-Edwards L, Reinsberg SA, et al. A complete distortion correction for MR images: I. gradient warp correction. Phys Med Biol. 2005;50(7):1343–1361.
3. Wachinger C, Glocker B, Zeltner J, et al. Deformable mosaicing for whole-body MRI. Proc MICCAI. 2008.
4. Joshi S, Davis B, Jomier M, et al. Unbiased diffeomorphic atlas construction for computational anatomy. NeuroImage. 2004;23:151–160.
5. Glocker B, Komodakis N, Tziritas G, et al. Dense image registration through MRFs and efficient linear programming. Med Image Anal. 2008;12(6):731–741.

Analysis of 2D Phase Contrast MRI in Renal Arteries by Self Organizing Maps
Initial Experiences

Frank G. Zöllner, Lothar R. Schad

Computer Assisted Clinical Medicine, University of Heidelberg, Germany
frank.zoellner@medma.uni-heidelberg.de

Abstract. We present an approach based on self organizing maps to segment renal arteries from 2D PC Cine MR images to measure blood velocity and flow. Such information are important in grading renal artery stenosis and support the decision on surgical interventions like percutan transluminal angioplasty. Results show that the renal arteries could be extracted automatically. The corresponding velocity profiles show high correlation (r=0.99) compared those from manual delineated vessels. Furthermore, the method could detect possible blood flow patterns within the vessel.

1 Introduction

Renal artery stenosis (RAS) is the leading cause of secondary hypertension caused by the reduced flow triggering the auto-regulation (renin-angiotesin) of the systemic circulation including the contralateral kidney. By time this may lead to loss of renal parenchyma in the stenosed kidney and microangiopathy in the glomeruli of the non-stenosed contralateral kidney. To be successful, a percutan transluminal angioplasty (PTA) should be performed before these changes have developed past certain limits in flow-reduction, flow velocity, kidney-size and the overall- and split-renal function. Ignoring these measures may lead to a wrong selection of patients treated with PTA and might be a reason why improvement after PTA has shown to be rather low [1]. Thereby, MRI provides a good tool for measuring these processes [2]. Cine Phase-Contrast MR (PC-MRI) blood flow measurements can be used for non-invasive quantification of renal artery blood flow. During acquisition two images are generated, a magnitude image and a phase image, encoding blood velocity and direction. From these images the blood flow within the vessel can be quantified and abnormalities in the flow or velocity profiles over the cardiac cycle can be assessed and RAS can be graded.

Blood flow quantification from PC-MRI acquisition is usually performed by manual delineations of the vessel area [3]. This is time consuming and subject to operator dependent variability. Kozerke et al. [4] proposed an active contour approach for vessel segmentation from PC-MRI. A segmentation approach taking the waveform of the velocities into account and applying correlation and thresholding has been proposed in [5] and segmentation by k-means clustering has been presented in [6]. However, all these approaches still involve manual interaction during the initialization and thus, operator dependent variability. In the present approach we utilize self organizing maps (SOM)[7] for the segmentation task. This technique provides a model free and unsupervised approach to the segmentation task. Similar to [6] it further allows for a functional segmentation, i.e. to take the velocity profiles into account.

2 Materials and methods

2.1 Data acquisition

Ten subjects (3 healthy volunteers, 7 patients) underwent renal blood flow measurements on a 1.5 T scanner as described in [8]. We used a ECG gated 2D cine PC-MR sequence with TR=37ms, TE=4ms, FA=30°, VENC=100 cm/s. Within the cardiac cycle between 20 and 25 images with matrix 256x192 and spatial resolution 0.9x0.9x6 mm^3 were acquired.

2.2 Self organizing maps for PC-MRI analysis

Self organizing maps generate nodes on a two-dimensional grid. The distribution of these nodes on the grid corresponds to the distribution of the associated node patterns in feature space. Thereby, a mapping of a high dimensional feature space onto a 2D grid is reached maintaining the underlying topology of the feature space. Briefly, each node n on a $N \times N$ regular grid a prototype vector $u^{(k)}$, $k = 1, \ldots, N^2$ is assigned and initialized randomly. Then, a data sample $x^{(i)}$is presented and the best matching or winning node $n^{(\kappa)}$ (BMU) on the grid is searched:

$$\kappa = \arg\min_k\{|u^{(k)} - x^{(i)}|^2\} \tag{1}$$

The $u^{(\kappa)}$'s prototype vector is then updated according to its distance to the training sample. In addition, the neighbors' prototype vectors on the grid are updated, too. This update process is controlled by a iteratively decreasing learning rate $\epsilon(t)$ and is described by the Kohonen's learning rule [7]

$$u^{(k)}(t+1) = u^{(k)}(t) + \epsilon(t)\exp(-\frac{d_{ij}}{\sigma^2})(x^{(i)}(t) - u^{(k)}(t)) \tag{2}$$

where d_{ij} is the distance between nodes i and j determined by the neighborhood relation. σ^2 is an operating parameter, $\epsilon(t)\exp(-\frac{d_{ij}}{\sigma^2})$ is one for $i = j$, namely the BMU, and decreases when the distance becomes large. For flow analysis, the sequence of phase images were transformed into a 2D matrix of size # pixels $\times$ time points and then processed using the SOM toolbox [9]. Critical parameters of the SOM are the number of node $N \times N$, the initial and final neighborhood size (σ_i, σ_f) and the number of iterations ν. Following [10] we set $\nu = 10^3 * N^2$, a linear decrease of $\sigma_i = N$ to $\sigma_f = 0.2 * N$, and a linear decrease of $\epsilon(t)$. The size of the grid was varied from N=2 to N=8.

2.3 Evaluation

To evaluate the influence of the grid size on the segmentation of the vessel within the phase images the quantization error and the topology error derived from the trained maps was calculated. The quantization error depicts the average distance between each data vector and its BMU. The topology error describes the proportion of all data vectors for which first and second BMUs are not adjacent units. Furthermore, to evaluate the clustering, our approach has been compared to the k-means segmentation presented in [6] and to available manual delineated vessel lumen. Here, the correlation between the velocity profiles derived by the different methods was investigated.

3 Results

Twenty data sets (10 subjects) were analyzed by the SOM. Fig. 1 shows the results of varying the number of nodes, i.e. grid size. Whereas the quantization error steadily decreases, the topology error mainly keeps constant for different values of N.

Fig. 2, as an example, depicts the results of the SOM algorithm for one data set. Each node on the grid subsumes a certain amount of pixels with similar velocity time profiles (VTP). The prototypes are given in Fig. 2c. Similar colors represent close nodes, i.e. possible super cluster structures (Fig. 2 a, b). Here, the yellow color node represents the vessel lumen (white round region in Fig. 2 d). From the analysis, four clusters could be identified (yellow, red, blue, and green). Figure 3 depicts the comparison of the derived VTP from the segmentations of the same data set depicted in Fig. 2. The k-means has been initialized by four classes. The manual delineation however could only provide two classes. The correlation between the VTP of the clusters representing the vessel lumen by each method is high (r=0.99).

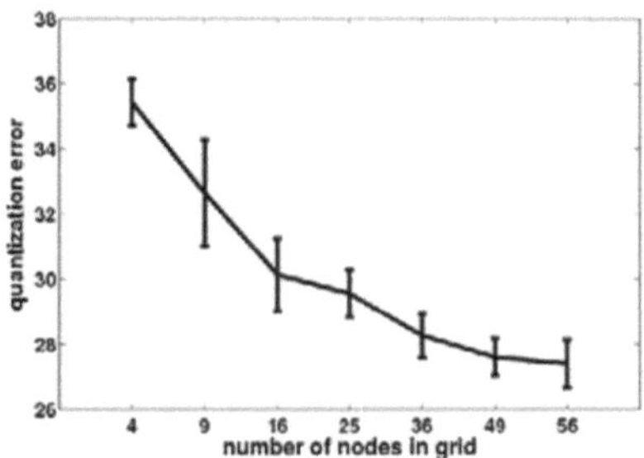

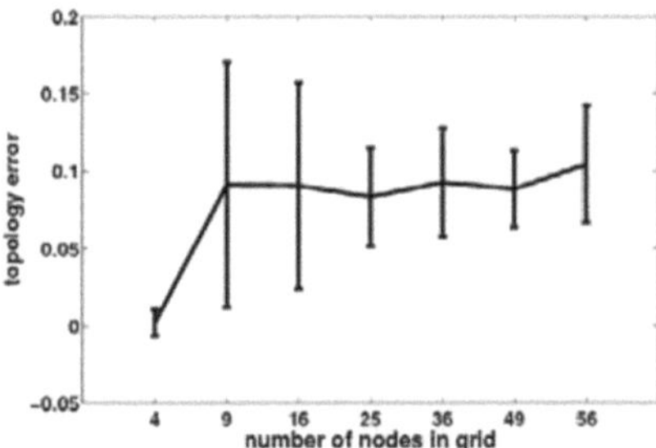

Fig. 1. Quantization and topology error for all subjects for the given range of grid sizes. Error bars depict the standard deviations within the 20 data sets.

4 Discussion

In this contribution an approach to segment and analyze 2D PC-MRI examinations using SOMs was presented. The SOM method could automatically segment the vessel from the images. From Fig. 1 a grid size of $N = 2-5$ seems reasonable. For a lower N the topology of the underlying feature space is more preserved, however, the quantization error is higher since also feature vectors that are more far away from the BMU are subsumed. For larger N the topology error increases because data samples with lower similarity are assigned to different (probably nearby) nodes. Thus, the quantization error is reduced while the topology error increases. However, for higher N, the beneficial property of the SOM to form super clusters could be exploited. By visualizing the similarities within nodes on the grid (here via color coding) the relation between sub and super cluster could be assessed (Fig. 2). Such merging could also be automatized, e.g. by applying hierarchical clustering of the SOM. In contrast to other proposed techniques like k-means [6] or to Alperin's work [5], no operator given initialization is needed. Comparing the velocity profiles derived from SOM, k-means, and manual delineation a high correlation is yielded suggesting a valid segmentation. In summary, by using SOM as a tool to analyze PC-MRI flow and velocity data a flexible and automated approach is available.

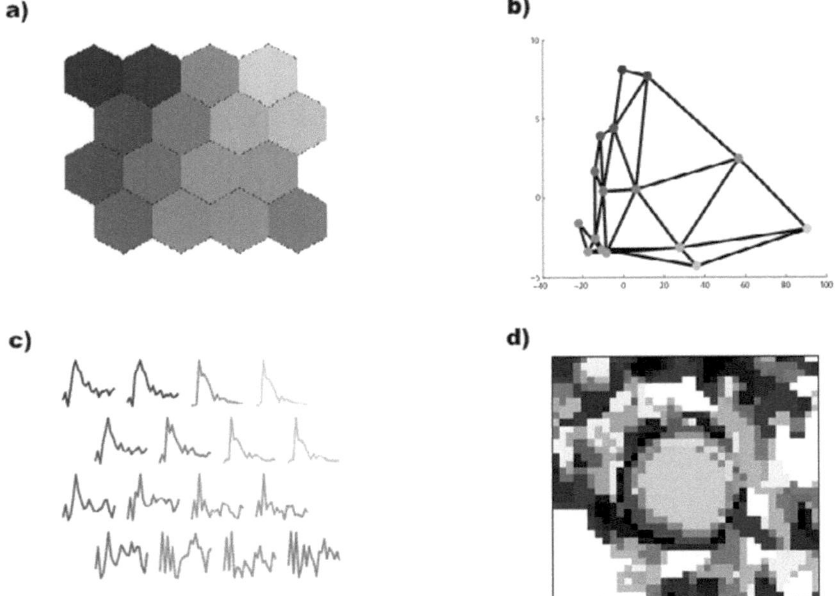

Fig. 2. Results of SOM analysis. Here a 4×4 hexagonal lattice has been used. a) depicts the similarity between neighboring nodes, b) shows a 2D projection of the prototypes onto the grid, c) prototypes associated by the nodes, and d) labeled image according to the best matching node. In a)- c) colors are corresponding.

Fig. 3. Comparison of velocity profiles by different methods for one data set. Solid black curve: derived by k-means clustering, gray curve: derived by manual delineation of vessel lumen, dashed curve: results by SOM algorithm.

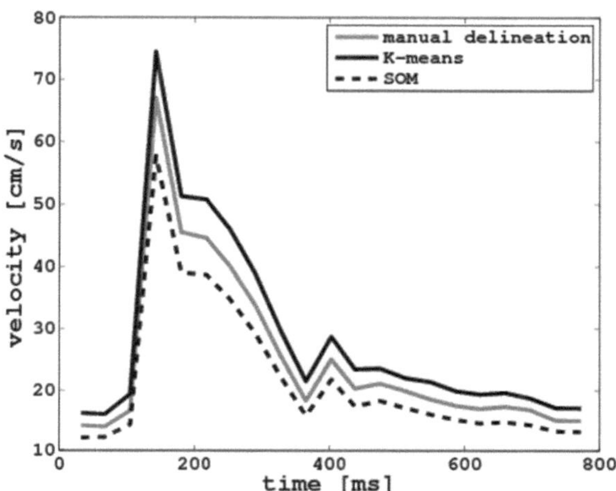

References

1. Krijnen P, van Jaarsveld BC, Deinum J, et al. Which patients with hypertension and atherosclerotic renal artery stenosis benefit from immediate intervention? J Hum Hypertens. 2004;18(2):91–96.
2. Michaely HJ, Schoenberg SO, Oesingmann N, et al. Renal artery stenosis: Functional assessment with dynamic MR perfusion measurements–feasibility study. Radiology. 2006;238(2):586–596.
3. Florez YN, Moratal D, Forner J, et al. Semiautomatic analysis of phase contrast magnetic resonance imaging of cerebrospinal fluid flow through the aqueduct of Sylvius. MAGMA. 2006;19(2):78–87.
4. Kozerke S, Botnar R, Oyre S, et al. Automatic vessel segmentation using active contours in cine phase contrast flow measurements. J Magn Reson Imaging. 1999;10(1):41–51.
5. Alperin N, Lee SH. PUBS: Pulsatility-based segmentation of lumens conducting non-steady flow. Magn Reson Med. 2003;49(5):934–944.
6. Zöllner FG, Monssen JA, Rørvik J, et al. Blood flow quantification from 2D phase contrast MRI in renal arteries using an unsupervised data driven approach. Z Med Phys. 2008;In press.
7. Kohonen T. Self-organizing maps. Berlin: Springer; 2001.
8. Schoenberg SO, Knopp MV, Bock M, et al. Renal artery stenosis: Grading of hemodynamic changes with cine phase-contrast MR blood flow measurements. Radiology. 1997;203(1):45–53.
9. Vesanto J. Neural network tool for data mining: SOM toolbox. Proc TOOLMET). 2000; p. 184–196.
10. Nattkemper TW, Wismüller A. Tumor feature visualization with unsupervised learning. Med Image Anal. 2005;9(4):344–351.

Concurrent Particle Tracking Using an Iterative Kalman Filter Approach

Benny Bürger[1], Jürgen Hesser[1]

[1]Institut for Computational Medicine, University of Heidelberg
benny.buerger@ziti.uni-heidelberg.de

Abstract. Particle tracking is a widespread research question for quantitative biology. In contrast to other approaches, we developed a local greedy technique based on the Kalman filter. To overcome the problem of guessing the first state of a particle, the algorithm runs iteratively in forward and backward direction. The algorithm was successfully tested with simulated and real data.

1 Introduction

Main tasks for analyzing particles in microscopic images are segmentation and tracking. While there is a vast quantity of segmentation algorithms that can be successfully used, tracking algorithms often fail on difficult data. Our goal is to develop an algorithm, which can be applied to a wide range of tracking problems, especially on difficult data.

Cheezum et al. [1] compared different tracking algorithms and found that a Gaussian fit is the best algorithm when tracking single fluorophores. Godinez et al. figured out, that a probablilistic approach based on a particle filter outperforms deterministic algorithms [2] and that independant particle filters outperforms those using a mixture of particle filters [3]. Genovesio et al. [4] propose a method to track multiple moving biological spot-like particles using Bayesian filtering. Wu et al. [5] implemented their Bayesian framework using the Kalman filter [6]. While their approach handles only a single trajectory each run, our algorithm estimates all trajectories at once and additional has some improvements in the Kalman filter. To overcome the problem of invisible particles Li et al. [7] introduced a compiler linker which connects two tracks segments belonging together.

In our approach, the Kalman filter determines the individual transition probabilities between particle locations in two subsequent frames given a motion model. Starting from an initial guess of the first track position, the forward model finds, after a while a consistent track tail. In order to compensate an eventual incorrect starting position, a backward tracking is applied. Further, our method pays attention to all particle trajectories at once to obtain better results on images with lots of particles. Last but not least, it is able to introduce faked particles, to overcome the problem of missing particles.

2 Materials and methods

The particles visible in the microscopy images are first located using a local maxima selection followed by a Gaussian fit to get the intensity. While this is not an optimal method, it is sufficient for testing the algorithm with real data.

Thus, the information about every particle in each frame is its position and intensity. Based on these information, for each particle in a time-frame t, the most likely corresponding particle is chosen from the next timeframe $t+1$ using the Kalman filter. This filter estimates the next state of a particle using the prior state like position, velocity and intensity, of the particle, and a mathematical model for the dynamics of the process to be estimated. All relevant parameters for the filter are set manual by the user.

If no corresponding particle is found, a fake particle is created to overcome the problem, that in some cases particles may not be visible due to image acquisition or segmentation issues. The state of the fake particle is estimated using the Kalman filter. When the estimation error is getting too high, the fake particle is destroyed and the trajectory ends at the point with the last real particle.

Our simulation data consists of an area with 500x500 pixels with two particle streams. The streams are crossing and each stream has 50 particles with different speed from 1.5 to 3 Pixels per frame. Since segmentation is not the emphasis of this paper the simulated data is made up of already segemented data. To take failures in segmentation into account, several parameters define the quality of the segmentation. The parameters μ and σ define the Gaussian noise, adding a small localization error to each particle position. α describes the percentage of non-segmented particles in a frame and β the ratio between false particles and real particles.

Eq (1) shows the calculation for the estimation error, where N is the total number of particles, *est* is an estimated particle and p the corresponding real particle. Several simulations were done, each with different simulation parameters, which simulate potential failures from image acquisition and segmentation.

$$err = \sqrt{\frac{1}{N}\sum_{k=1}^{N} \|est_k - p_k\|^2} \tag{1}$$

Each measurement was created using the average of 50 simulations with 100 timeframes each. The different versions of the algorithm are quoted with the abbreviations *F* for faked particles and *I* for the iterative version.

3 Results

The following table (Tab. 1) shows the results for the simulations. Each row represents one measurement. The values in the first three columns indicate the parameters used for the measurements and are expressed as percentages. In the next four columns the localization error *err* is shown for each different version

Table 1. Tracking errors for several measurements using different algorithms: (-) Standard approach, (F)aked particles, (I)terative approach, (F,I) faked particles and iterative approach.

Parameters			Localization error				Correctly
Noise N(μ,σ)	Inv. part. α	Seg. error β	-	F	I	F, I	assigned particles
0/0.1	0.01	0.01	0.33	0.33	0.16	0.13	99
0/0.5	0.05	0.05	0.77	0.77	0.74	0.62	94
0/0.1	0.1	0.1	0.77	0.77	0.53	0.41	87
0/1	0.1	0.1	1.15	1.16	1.08	1.00	87
0/0.5	0.01	0.1	1.21	1.21	1.18	0.94	99
0/0.5	0.1	0.01	0.65	0.65	0.51	0.46	87

of the algorithm. The last column indicates the percentage of correctly assigned particles.

We tested the image using an image stack from a cell obtained from a Zeiss Axiovert 200 M. The results showed a good agreement with anticipated trajectories.

4 Discussion

Our algorithm performs visually correct on real microscopy images. For an evaluation of the robustness of the approach, simulated test cases were considered. According to the results the advantage of the additional forward and backward iteration of the algorithm can be clearly seen. While the amount of correct assigned particles changed only marginal (below one percentage), the estimation error *err* decreased significantly. It showed that the introduction of faked particles alone had no benefits, compared to the standard algorithm, but using the faked particles in addition to the iterative version of the algorithm the estimation error could be further decreased.

In the future the tracking algorithm shall be compared to manually tracked data. In order to ease setting up the parameters for the kalman filter a semi-automatic approach like in [7] using the expectation maximizating algorithm [8] could be used. Further the segmentation algorithm could be exchanged in order to take advantage of the characteristics of the specific microscopy images.

We have presented a robust method to track particles in microscopic images. The main advantage of this method over methods from state of the art, especially from Wu et al. [5] is the iterative processing and the use of faked particles. This way, the algorithm is more robust against failures in segmentation and noisy data.

References

1. Cheezum M, Walker WF, Guildford WH. Quantitative comparison of algorithms for tracking single fluorescent particles. Biophy J. 2001;81:2378–2388.
2. Godinez WJ, Lampe M, Worz S, et al. Tracking of Virus Particles in time-lapse Fluorescence Microscopy Image Sequences. Procs ISBI. 2007; p. 256–259.
3. Godinez WJ, Lampe M, Worz S, et al. Probabilistic tracking of virus particles in fluorescence microscopy image sequences. Procs BVM. 2008; p. 448–452.
4. Genovesio A, Liedl T. Multiple particle tracking in 3-D+t microscopy: Method and application to the tracking of endocytosed quantum dots. IEEE Trans Image Process. 2006;15.
5. Wu X, Li J, Xu Y, et al. Three-dimensional tracking of GLUT4 vesicles in TIRF microscopy. J Zhejiang Univ Sci A. 2008.
6. Kalman RE. A new approach to linear filtering and prediction problems. Trans ASME-J Basic Eng. 1960;82.
7. Li K, Miller ED, Chen M, et al. Cell population tracking and lineage construction with spatiotemporal context. Med Image Anal. 2008;12(5):546 – 566.
8. Shumway R, Stoffer D. An approach to time series smoothing and forecasting using the EM algorithm. Med Image Anal. 2008;12(5):546 – 566.

Finite Elemente Modell des Beckens zur Simulation komplexer ligamentärer Instabilitätsszenarien

Roland Hülse[1], Niels Hammer[2], Hanno Steinke[2], Jörg Stadler[3], Kathrin Hülse[1], Volker Slowik[4], Peter Vaitl[1], Christoph Josten[1], Jörg Böhme[1]

[1]Universitätsklinikum Leipzig, Klinik für Unfall- und Wiederherstellungschirurgie
[2]Universität Leipzig, Medizinische Fakultät, Institut für Anatomie
[3]Leibniz Institut für Neurobiologie (IfN), Magdeburg
[4]Hochschule für Technik, Wirtschaft & Kultur, Institut für Materialprüfung, Leipzig
c.roland.hue@web.de

Kurzfassung. Die Klassifikation als eine Grundlage des operativen Vorgehens nach instabilen Beckenringfrakturen stellt sich als ausgesprochen schwierig dar. Insbesondere ligamentäre Begleitverletzungen können nur ungenügend diagnostiziert und damit berücksichtigt werden. Um die funktionellen Auswirkungen einer solchen ligamentären Begleitverletzung zu konkretisieren, wurde ein biomechanisches Finite Elemente Modell (FE) des menschlichen Beckens generiert. Erstmals wurden Bandstrukturen unter Verwendung von 7 Tesla MR-Tomographie sowie Dünnschichtplastinationstechnik beschrieben und anschließend in das FE-Modell integriert. Dafür wurden die Bänder in ihrer Geometrie exakt vermessen, digitalisiert und katalogisiert. Unser neues Modell stellt ein validiertes, anatomisch exaktes FE-Modell des Beckens, der Wirbelkörper L4-5 sowie 18 pelviner Ligamenta dar.

1 Einleitung

Die funktionellen Langzeitergebnisse nach schweren instabilen Beckenringfrakturen vom Typ B und C in der auf Tile und Pennal basierenden Klassifikation von Beckenringfrakturen [1] sind nach wie vor unbefriedigend [2]. Insbesondere besteht eine auffällige, statistisch signifikante Diskrepanz zwischen radiologisch diagnostiziertem Ergebnis einerseits und dem funktionellen Ergebnis auf der anderen Seite [3]. Eine Erklärung hierfür konnte noch nicht gefunden werden. Dabei stellt die Schwierigkeit ligamentäre Begleitverletzungen sicher zu diagnostizieren einen Mangel dar, der die derzeit gängige Klassifikation als fehlerbehaftet erscheinen lässt [4]. Die Fragestellung inwieweit ligamentäre Begleitverletzungen pathognomonisch für das schlechte Outcome sind, lässt sich mittels experimenteller Versuchsreihen am Kadaverbecken aufgrund einer Vielzahl offener Problemkonstellationen nur schwer beantworten. In solchen Fällen stellen numerische Simulationen eine methodische Alternative dar, welche die Beantwortung komplexer pelviner und spinopelviner Fragestellungen erlaubt. Frühere Arbeiten klammerten dabei den Bandapparat meist vollends aus. In dieser Arbeit präsentieren wir somit erstmals ein biomechanisch validiertes Finite Elemente Computermodell (FEC) des knöchernen Beckens mit integriertem Bandapparat sowie der Wirbelkörper L4 und L5. Dieses FEC erlaubt dabei die Beschreibung und Beantwortung komplexer Fragestellungen zum menschlichen Beckenring.

2 Material und Methode

Primär wurde ein FE-Grundmodell des knöchernen Beckens basierend auf einem CT-Datensatz (64-Zeilen CT Brilliance, Philips; 120 kV, 100 mAs, Pitch 0.983, Tischvorschub 39.32 mm, Kollimation 64×0,625 mm) des humanen Beckens inklusive Wirbelkörpern L4-L5 generiert. Hierbei wurden die individuellen mechanischen Eigenschaften von Spongionsa und Kortikalis differenziert voneinander mittels schalenartiger und tetraedaler Elementtypen modelliert. Bandscheiben, der Discus interpubicus und Gelenke wurden über das Mooney-Rivlin Stoffgesetz analog der Arbeiten von Zuoping Li [5] als Tetraederelemente implementiert.

Zur anatomisch und mechanisch korrekten Integration des Bandapparates war eine exakte digitale Vermessung und Katalogisierung der ligamentären Strukturen und die Ermittlung der genauen Materialeigenschaften notwendig (siehe Tabellen 1 und 2). Dafür wurden die Becken mittels MR-Tomographie visualisiert. Verwendet wurde ein 7 Tesla Magnet (90 cm Bohrung, Magnex, Oxford, UK) mit einer Avanto Gradienten Spule mit Sonata Gradientenverstärker (31 mT/m, 150 μs/(mT/m)). Die besten Ergebnisse wurden in einer DESS Sequenz erzielt. Anschließend wurden die Becken durch Dünnschichtplastination in 400μm dicke Scheiben geschnitten. Die Plastination bietet die Möglichkeit mittels modifizierter Giemsa Färbung ligamentäre Strukturen farb zu kodieren und in submakroskopischer Auflösung darzustellen. Die Ligamenta konnten so nach Digitalisierung mit dem MRT-Datensatz koregistriert werden. Neben der exakten Vermessung der Beckenbänder wurden beckenspezifische Materialeigen-

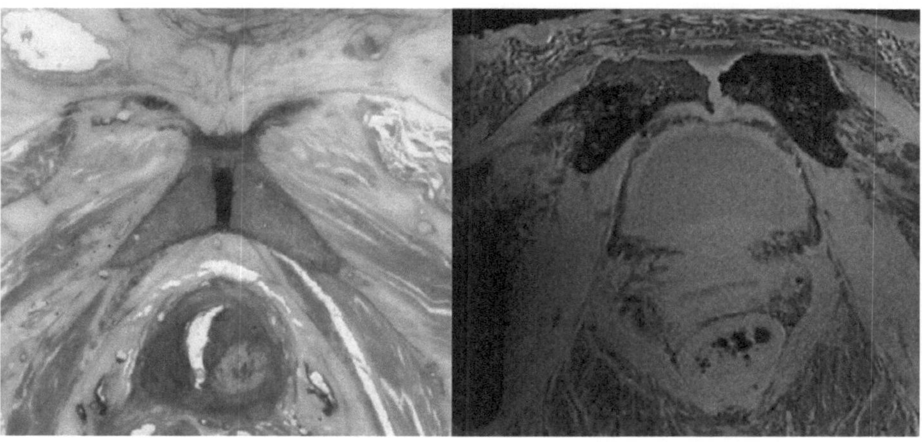

Abb. 1. Symphyse im 400 μm Dünnschichtplastinat (*links*), als 7T-MRT (*rechts*)

Tabelle 1. Zudefinierte Materialeigenschaften

Bestandteil	E-Modul [N/mm^2]	Querdehnzahl [–]
Knochen Spongiosa	150	0.20
Knochen Kortikalis	18000	0.29
Disci und Gelenke	500	0.30
Ligamenta	26.35	0.45

schaften, wie das Elastizitätmodul, ermittelt, welche zur validen numerischen Analyse benötigt werden. Hierfür wurden Sacrotuberal- und Sacrospinalbänder in einer Materialprüfmaschine unter Berücksichtigung des Hysteresisphänomens mehrzyklisch [6] belastet. Dabei zeigen die ermittelten Materialeigenschaften eine deutliche intra- als auch interindividuelle Varianz und sowohl die E-Module als auch die Dehnsteifigkeiten pelviner Ligamenta weichten signifikant von denen extrapelviner ab.

Nach Integration der genauen Ligamentgeometrie in das FEC durch Stabelemente und der Zuordnung der materialspezifischen Kennwerte wurden verschiedene Instabilitätsszenarien numerisch simuliert. Angenommen wurde das Gewicht eines 80kg schweren Mannes im Zweibeinstand. Für die Berechnung der daraus resultierenden Kraftvektoren wurde der im CT-Datensatz gemessene Caput-Collum-Diaphysen-Winkel von 121.12 Grad verwendet. Zur genauen Analyse des Lastfalles wurde ein lokales Koordinatensystem angenommen, welches Translation und Rotationen erlaubt. Über die Variation der zudefinierten Ligamentdehnsteifigkeiten wurden die funktionellen Auswirkungen einer ligamentären Partialruptur konkretisiert und die Genese pelviner Instabilitäten eruiert. Zur Validierung der simulierten Ergebnisse wurde eine experimentelle Versuchs-

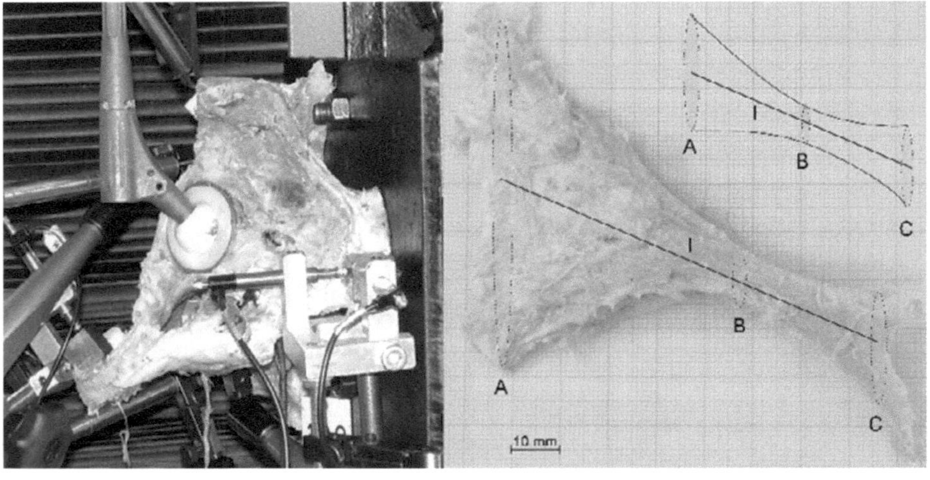

Abb. 2. Experimentelle Validierung (*links*), vermessenes Sakrotuberalband (*rechts*)

Tabelle 2. Exakte Querschnittsflächen

Bandbezeichnung	Querschnittsfläche [mm^2]
Lig. iliolumbale	21
Ligg. sacro-iliaca anteriora	96
Ligg. sacro-iliaca posteriora	17
Ligg. sacro-iliaca interossea	7
Lig. pubica anteriores	22
Lig. pubicum superius	7
Lig. arcuatum pubis	28
Lig. sacrotuberale	45
Lig. sacrospinale	35

reihe am humanen Semipelvis durchgeführt. Das in eine Materialprüfmaschine eingespannte Semipelvis wurde über die Ableitung einer Vielstellenmessanlage beruhend auf 12 induktiven Wegaufnehmern Typ „W 10TK“ (Hottinger Baldwin Messtechnik GmbH) auf räumliche Verschiebungen und Rotationen analog der FE-Simulation untersucht.

3 Ergebnisse

Das vorgestellte FE-Modell stellt ein anatomisch exaktes, experimentell validiertes Modell zur Ausarbeitung verschiedenster Fragestellungen in der Beckenmechanik unter besonderer Berücksichtigung des Bandapparates dar. Durch die Auswertung der numerischen und experimentellen Ergebnisse konnte die Bedeutung der pelvinen Ligamenta spezifiziert werden. Insbesondere die Ligg. sacrotuberalia et sacrospinalia zeigen stärkeren Einfluss auf den elastischen Lastabtrag des Beckens als in der Literatur angegeben. Neben der Restriktion der Nutationsbewegung sind sie maßgeblich am transartikulären Lastabtrag beteiligt. Eine

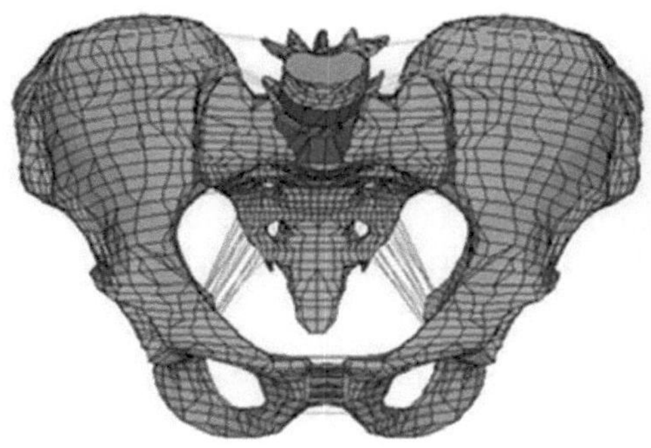

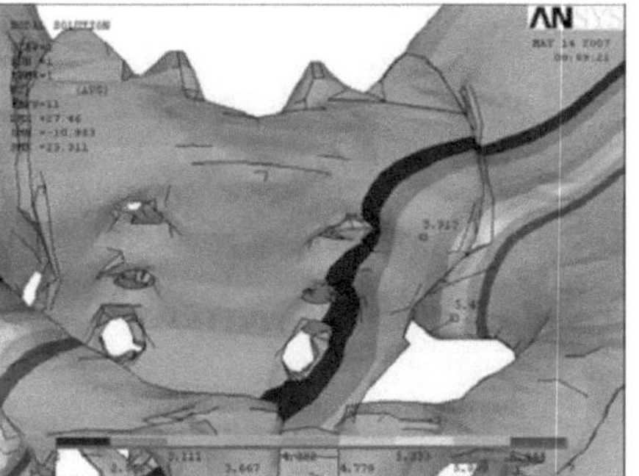

Abb. 3. FE-Modell: Becken von ventral (*links*), unter Belastung (*rechts*)

Verletzung beider Bänder bedingt eine Zunahme der intraartikulären Beweglichkeit um 2,23 mm. Die Genese iliosakraler Mikroinstabilitäten konnte nummerisch aufgezeigt werden. Dabei fiel auf, dass schon geringen Dehnsteifigkeitsvariationen im Modell von weniger als 20% alterierende Belastungsachsen innerhalb des Sakroiliakalgelenkes bedingen und ein differierender transpelviner Kraftfluß entsteht.

4 Diskussion

Die gewonnenen Daten verdeutlichen die Problematik der derzeit gängigen Klassifikation instabiler Beckenringverletzungen. Obwohl die ligamentäre Begleitverletzung für die pelvine Stabilität und Mechanik entscheidend ist, kann sie mit der standardmäßig eingesetzten Diagnostik wie Röntgen und Spiral-CT nicht direkt erfasst werden. Somit ist die als Grundlage der Klassifikation eingesetzte Diagnostik nicht ausreichend. Klinisch interessant war auch das frühzeitige Auftreten sakroiliakaler Mikroinstabilitäten und damit verbunden die Genese alterierender iliosakraler Belastungsachsen. Diese können eine Ursache persistierender SI-Schmerzsyndrome und arthrotischer Veränderungen innerhalb des SI-Gelenkes darstellen [7]. Perspektivisch wird die Praktikabilität des Modells als Hilfestellung für die Klassifikation und damit für die präoperative Entscheidungsfindung des behandelnden Chirurgen ermittelt. Die Erstellung eines modifizierten Modells mit variierenden probabilistischen Geometrien wird angestrebt. Ein derart modifiziertes Modell könnte die Integration patientenspezifischer Geometrien in die präoperative Planung ermöglichen und damit Rückschlüsse auf ligamentäre Begleitverletzungen, zum Beispiel beim polytraumatisierten Patienten, zulassen.

Literaturverzeichnis

1. Pennal G. Fractures of the pelvis (motion picture). American Acadamy of Orthopedic Surgeons (AAOS). Film Libary: Park Tidge IL; 1961.
2. Suzuki T, Shindo M, Soma K. Long-term functional outcome after unstable pelvic fracture. J Trauma. 2007;63:884–888.
3. Polemann T, Gänsslen A, Schellwald O. Outcome after pelvic ring injuries. Injury. 1996;27(Suppl 2):B31–8.
4. Attias N, Arzani S, Duncan G. Sectional imaging anatomy: Pelvic ring ligaments. J Comput Assist Tomogr. 2001;25(6):975–979.
5. Li Z, Kim J, Davidson J. Biomechanical response of the pubic symphysis in lateral pelvic impacts: a finite element study. J Biomech. 2007;40(12):2758–2766.
6. Schatzmann L, Brunner P, Stäubli H. Effect of cyclic preconditioning on the tensile properties of human quadriceps tendons and patellar ligaments. Knee Surg Sports Traumatol Arthrosc. 1998;6(Suppl.1):556–561.
7. Dujardin F, Roussignol X, Hossenbaccus M. Experimental study of the sacroiliac joint micromotion in pelvic disruption. J Orthop Trauma. 2002;16(2):99–103.

3D-Meshes aus medizinischen Volumendaten

Eine Methode zur Generierung von konformen Hexaeder-Meshes aus gelabelten Volumendaten

Sascha Zelzer, Hans-Peter Meinzer

Abteilung für Medizinische und Biologische Informatik, DKFZ Heidelberg
s.zelzer@dkfz.de

Kurzfassung. Diese Arbeit beschreibt eine template-basierte Methode zur Erzeugung von adaptiven Hexaeder-Meshes aus Volumendaten, welche komplizierte konkave Strukturen aufweisen können. Es wird ein vollständiger Satz von Templates generiert der es erlaubt, die Ränder konkaver Regionen feiner zu zerlegen als angrenzende Bereiche und somit die Gesamtzahl an Hexaeder verringert. Der Algorithmus arbeitet mit beliebigen gelabelten Volumendaten und erzeugt ein adaptives, konformes, reines Hexaeder-Mesh.

1 Einleitung

Simulationen von physikalischen Vorgängen aller Art wurden in letzter Zeit durch die rasant steigenden Rechnerkapazitäten immer realistischer bzw. erst machbar. Letzeres trifft vor allem auf die Medizin zu, die aufgrund der komplexen physikalischen Prozesse oft entweder stark vereinfachte Modelle erstellen, oder extrem lange Rechenzeiten in Kauf nehmen muss. Viele Methoden zur numerischen Behandlung dieser Modelle beruhen auf einer Diskretisierung der räumlichen Strukturen, welche in der Medizin (Gefäßbäume, Hirngewebe, ...) oft hoch komplex sind. Ein direkter Weg, den Rechenaufwand zu minimieren, liegt in der Minimierung der Anzahl von Zellen, die eine solche Diskretisierung bilden.

Die drei am häufigsten benutzen Mesh-Typen in $\mathbb{R}^3$ sind Tetraeder-, Hexaeder- und Hybrid-Meshes. Die Anforderungen an solche Gitter sind normalerweise derart, dass sie wichtige geometrische Merkmale erhalten, indem sie in diesen Bereichen fein genug sind. Gleichzeitig sollen sie aber in homogenen Bereichen nicht unnötig fein sein, um die Zellenanzahl nicht zu erhöhen. Zur Zeit bieten Tetraeder-Meshes die größte Flexibilität um komplexe Daten vollautomatisch zu modellieren [1]. Sie benötigen aber meist eine große Anzahl an Zellen.

Eine Schwierigkeit bei der Erzeugung eines adaptiven Hexaeder-Meshes aus komplexen Strukturen besteht in der Verfeinerung konkaver Regionen. In [2, 3] wurde die Directional Refinement Methode vorgestellt, die konkave Bereiche verfeinern kann, ohne eine große Zahl neuer Zellen einzuführen. Der Nachteil dieser Methode ist allerdings deren schlechte Skalierbarkeit. In unserem Ansatz verwenden wir die Methode in [2], um einen vollständigen Satz von Templates zu erstellen, welcher die Vorteile der directional refinement Methode besitzt und in template-basierten Algorithmen verwendet werden kann.

2 Methoden

2.1 Der Algorithmus

Unser Algorithmus gehört zur Klasse der Octree-basierten Template-Techniken und besteht aus den folgenden drei Schritten:

1. Erzeuge einen initialen Octree mit den gewünschten Eigenschaften
2. Identifiziere die zu verfeinernden Oktanten
3. Ersetze die Oktanten aus Schritt 2 durch passende Templates

Die Eingabe für den Algorithmus kann als Abbildung $f : D \rightarrow L$ beschrieben werden, mit D eine nicht-leere beschränkte Teilmenge von $\mathbb{R}^3$ und L eine endliche Menge, die die verschiedenen Labels (Strukturen) repräsentiert. Die Ausgabe ist ein konformes Hexaeder-Mesh.

Um den initialen Octree in Schritt 1 zu erzeugen, benutzen wir eine Kombination von vorhandenen Methoden. Die Identifizierung der Oktanten in Schritt 2 und der neue Satz von Templates bilden unseren neuen Beitrag.

Schritt 1: Erzeugung des initialen Octrees Zuerst erzeugen wir ausgehend von f einen uniformen, signierten Octree. Wenn D unendlich ist, müssen wir den tiefsten Octree-Level vorgeben. Ist D endlich (normalerweise besteht D aus den Punkten eines homogenen, rechtlinigen Gitters), dann wird der tiefste Octree-Level so gewählt, dass alle geometrischen Merkmale von D erhalten bleiben.

Wir benutzen nun den Vereinfachungsalgorithmus in [4], um den Octree so weit wie möglich zu vergröbern, ohne die Topologie der Grenzflächen zu verändern. Um das directional refinement Verfahren später anwenden zu können, muss der Octree streng 1-balanciert sein:

Definition 1. *Ein d-dimensionaler Baum heißt k-balanciert, $k \in [0, d)$, dann und nur dann wenn sich kein Blatt q mit Level $l(q)$ eine m-dimensionale Fläche, $m \in [k, d)$, mit einem anderen Blatt q' mit $l(q') > l(q) + 1$ teilt.*

Mit dieser Definition ist ein 2-balancierter Octree also ausbalanciert an den Flächen, ein 1-balancierter Octree ausbalanciert an den Flächen und Kanten und ein 0-balancierter Octree ausbalanciert an den Flächen, Kanten und Ecken.

Definition 2. *Ein d-dimensionaler Baum heißt streng k-balanciert, $k \in [0, d)$, dann und nur dann wenn (i) für alle Knoten gilt, dass entweder alle oder keines der Kinder wiederum Kinder hat und (ii) Definition 1 gilt.*

Schritt 2: Verfeinerungskonfiguration Wir müssen nun diejenigen Oktanten des streng 1-balancierten Octrees finden, die in Schritt 3 durch passende Templates ersetzt werden. Dazu betrachten wir die Oktanten mit Blättern als Kinder und nennen sie Pseudoblätter. Diese Pseudoblätter werden in Schritt 3 ersetzt, daher bestimmen wir für jedes Pseudoblatt q eine eindeutige Verfeinerungskonfiguration wie folgt:

Betrachte alle Flächen-, Kanten- und Ecken-Nachbarn von q im selben Octree-Level. Ein solcher Nachbar q' ist entweder ein Blatt, ein Pseudoblatt oder ein Oktant, dessen Kinder alle wieder Kinder besitzen (siehe Definition 2). Nur im letzten Fall markieren wir die Ecken von q, die auch gleichzeitig Ecken von q' sind. Sei nun M_q die Menge der markierten Ecken von q. Die Verfeinerungskonfiguration von q ist dann durch

$$T_q = \{m \in M_q \mid \exists m' \in M_q, m' \neq m\,, \text{sodass}\, \overline{m\,m'}\, \text{eine Kante von}\, q\, \text{ist}\,\}$$

gegeben. Wir streichen also alle markierten Ecken, die nicht mit einer anderen markierten Ecke durch eine Kante von q verbunden werden können (der Grund liegt in der directional refinement Methode, welche nur Flächen und Kanten verfeinert). Die Menge T_q identifiziert dann in eindeutiger Weise das passende Template, siehe Tabelle 1.

Schritt 3: Templates Das Problem mit existierenden Templates besteht in deren Inflexibilität bezüglich der Verfeinerung von konkaven Bereichen (siehe Abb. 1 (a) und (b)). In medizinischen Datensätzen mit komplexen Strukturen resultiert dies in eine enorme Steigerung der Zellenanzahl.

Wir konstruieren nun unseren neuen Satz von Templates mit Hilfe des directional refinement Verfahrens. Für jede mögliche Verfeinerungskonfiguration eines Pseudoblattes (siehe Tabelle 1, Spalte 1) verfeinern wir die Kinder wie in [2] beschrieben. Die Resultate sind unsere neuen Templates (Tabelle 1, Spalte 2), welche den Vorteil haben keine hängenden Flächen zu besitzen. Diese neuen Templates können nun verwendet werden um die Pseudoblätter aus Schritt 2 zu ersetzen und ein konformes Gitter zu erzeugen.

2.2 Evaluierung

Um unsere Templates zu evaluieren, haben wir sie mit zwei anderen Sätzen von gängigen Templates aus [5] und [6] verglichen. Als Datensätze verwendeten

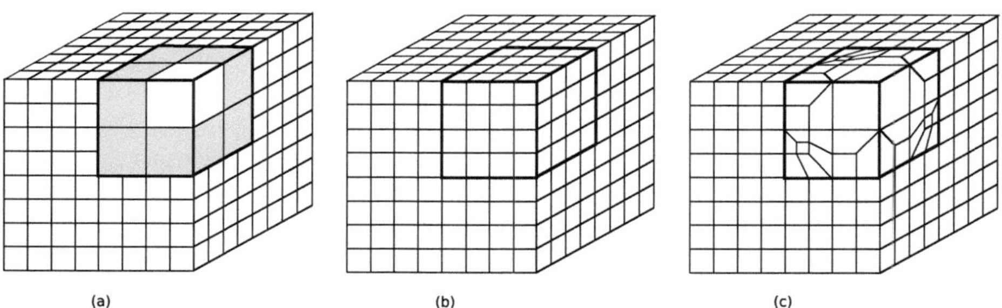

Abb. 1. Konkave Verfeinerung. (a) Die grauen Oktanten müssen verfeinert werden, um ein konformes Gitter zu erzeugen (b) Die Verwendung bestehender Templates führt zu übermäßiger Verfeinerung (c) Verfeinerung der Kinder des Pseudoblatts mit passenden Templates.

Tabelle 1. Links, mögliche Verfeinerungskonfigurationen für Pseudoblätter. Mitte, die dazugehörigen Templates, konstruiert mit dem directional refinement Verfahren (die inneren Ecken und Kanten wurden nicht visualisiert).

Verfeinerungskonfiguration (T_q)	Template	# Vertices / # Hexaeder
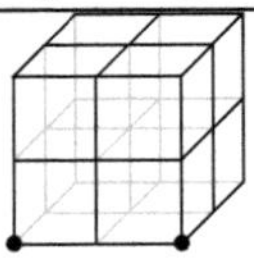	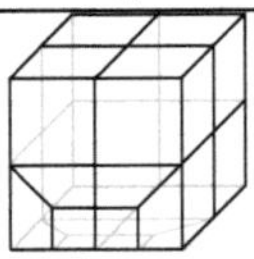	38 / 14
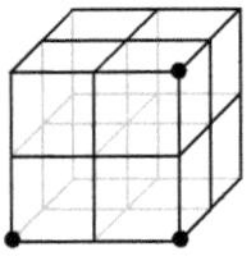	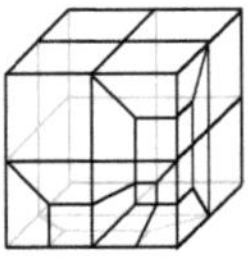	54 / 24
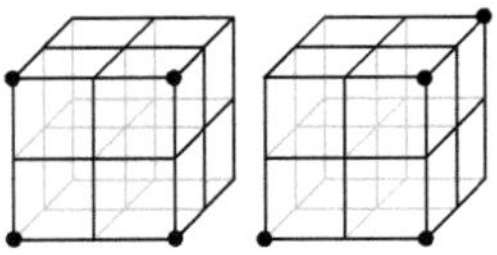	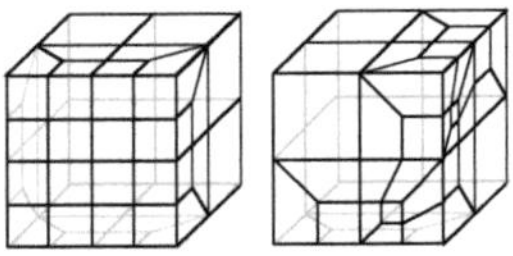	67 / 32 70 / 34
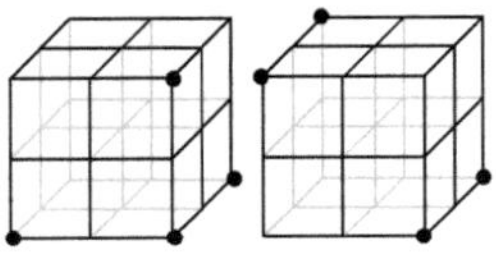	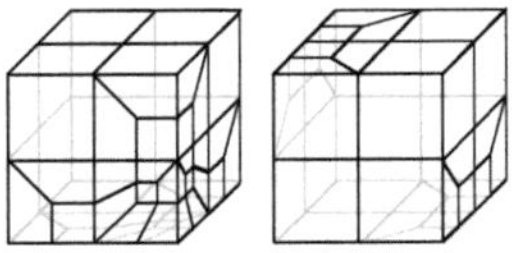	77 / 40 49 / 20
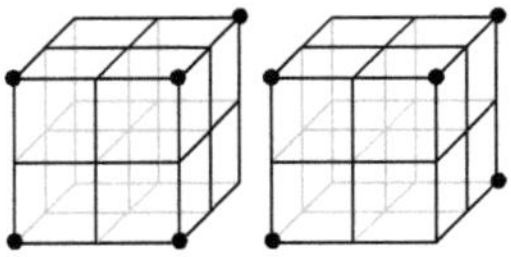	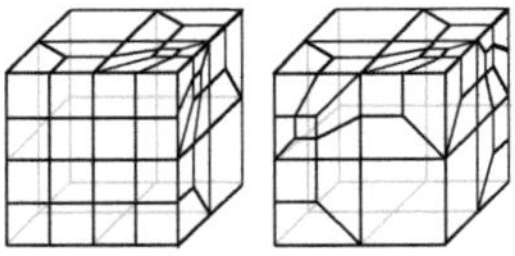	90 / 48 86 / 44
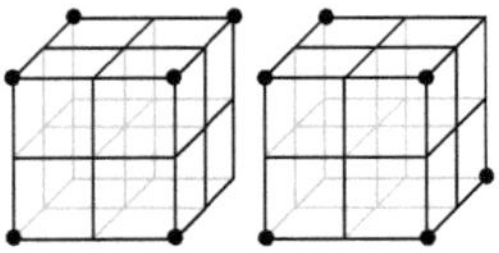	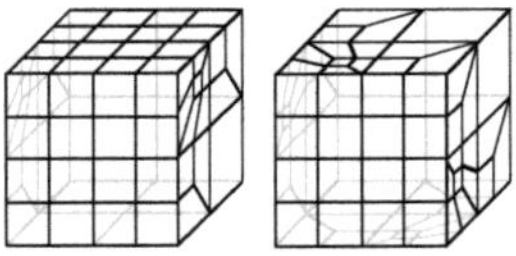	110 / 62 113 / 64
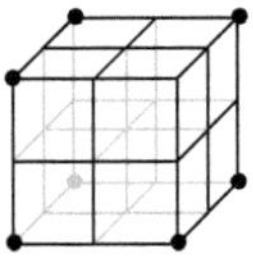	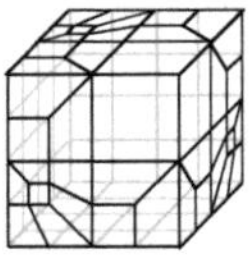	129 / 74

wir eine segmentierte Leber mit einem Gefäß und Tumor (65x41x27 Voxel), ein segmentiertes Herz (Perikard und die vier Kammern, 286x261x158 Voxel) und ein segmentiertes Gehirn (15 Strukturen, 181x217x181 Voxel).

3 Resultate

Tabelle 2 gibt eine Übersicht über die Anzahl der Punkte und Hexaeder in den erzeugten Meshes für die drei Datensätze. Die Verfahren in [5] und [6] erzeugen für die ersten beiden Datensätze (Leber und Herz) neunmal bzw. ca. fünfmal so

Tabelle 2. Die Anzahl der Vertices und Zellen eines Hexaeder-Meshes erzeugt aus gelabelten Datensätzen mit drei verschiedenen Methoden.

# Vert/# Zellen	Unsere Methode	Methode von [5]	Methode von [6]
Leber	14000 / 12000	112000 / 112000	49000 / 49000
Herz	498000 / 494000	4504000 / 4503000	2882000 / 2880000
Gehirn	1532000 / 1526000	4384000 / 4383000	3798000 / 3798000

viele Zellen im Vergleich zu unserem Verfahren. Im letzten Datensatz sind es 2.9 bzw. 2.5 mal so viele.

4 Diskussion

Mit der Einführung unserer neuen Templates sind wir in der Lage, beliebige konkave Strukturen am Rand feiner aufzulösen und gleichzeitig die Anzahl der neuen Zellen gering zu halten. Vergleicht man die Zahlen in Tabelle 2 wird klar, dass die zuvor vorhandenen Templates nicht ausreichten, um medizinische Strukturen mit einer vertretbaren Anzahl von Zellen zu diskretisieren. Insbesondere ist das Verfahren in [5] überhaupt nicht - und das Verfahren in [6] nur eingeschränkt - in der Lage, konkave Regionen lokal zu verfeinern. Mit zunehmender Komplexität der geometrischen Strukturen erzeugen die bisherigen Ansätze fast homogene Gitter, die bis auf Voxelgröße verfeinert wurden. Unser Ansatz hingegen reduziert in solchen Fällen die Anzahl der Zellen und Vertices auf weniger als die Hälfte.

Zukünftige Arbeiten umfassen eine systematische Untersuchung der Mesh-Qualität, eine Anpassung der Knoten des Meshes an die internen Grenzflächen und die Anwendung eines Glättungsverfahrens. Eine solche Glättung würde die Qualität der Diskretisierung weiter erhöhen und somit zu einer erhöhten numerischen Genauigkeit bei Simulation führen.

Literaturverzeichnis

1. Pons JP, Ségonne E, et al JDB. High-quality consistent meshing of multi-label datasets. Inf Process Med Imaging. 2007;20:198–210.
2. Schneiders R. Octree-based hexahedral mesh generation. Int J Comput Geom Appl. 2000;10(4):383–398.
3. Tchon KF, Dompierre J, Camarero R. Automated refinement of conformal quadrilateral and hexahedral meshes. Int J Numer Methods Eng. 2004;59:1539–1562.
4. Ju T, Losasso F, Schaefer S, et al. Dual contouring of hermite data. Procs SIGGRAPH. 2002; p. 339–346.
5. Schneiders R. Refining quadrilateral and hexahedral element meshes. Procs Int Conf Numerical Grid Generation in Computational Field Simulations. 1996; p. 699–708. Available from: citeseer.ist.psu.edu/schneiders96refining.html.
6. Zhang H, Zhao G. Adaptive hexahedral mesh generation based on local domain curvature and thickness using a modified grid-based method. Finite Elem Anal Des. 2007;43(9):691–704.

High Quality Image Magnification Using Cross-Scale Self-Similarity

André Gooßen[1], Arne Ehlers[1], Thomas Pralow[2], Rolf-Rainer Grigat[1]

[1]Vision Systems, Hamburg University of Technology, D-21079 Hamburg
[2]General X-Ray, Philips Medical Systems, D-22335 Hamburg
andre.goossen@tu-harburg.de

Abstract. In medical imaging there is a frequent need to magnify a certain region of interest (ROI) of an image. However many modalities suffer from severe noise and traditional upscaling methods produce poor enlargement results. We present an approach based on cross-scale similarity of an image extendable to sequences using time domain information without explicit motion compensation. It combines noise suppression and upscaling and hence yields superior image quality compared to standard zooming algorithms. We evaluated our algorithm using artificial and clinical fluoroscopy acquisitions.

1 Introduction

Image magnification is the process of computing a high-resolved image from an observed low-resolution image. In the field of medical X-ray image processing the observation is provided by the X-ray detector. Because of the limited resolution of image sensors and the influence of noise during image acquisition, especially in X-ray fluoroscopy, the observation is a degraded version of the captured scene. Using traditional upscaling techniques [1, 2] such as cubic interpolation, Lanczos, etc. that incorporate neighboring pixel to interpolate the high-resolved image tend to smooth structures and do not perform well in the presence of noise. The recently proposed non-local means filter [3] besides denoising shows potential for image magnification [4].

2 Methods and materials

In this section we first briefly introduce the problem of image zooming that has to be solved and derive the technique of incorporating self-similarity from the general non-local means filtering approach [3].

2.1 Image zooming problem

For the image zooming problem we assume a simple degradation model in which the relation between the observation and the high-resolution image is given by

$$u = \mathcal{H}v + \eta \tag{1}$$

with u denoting the low resolution observation and v is the high-resolved image, that should be reconstructed. η is additive white Gaussian noise with zero mean and variance σ^2. Besides we assume that the resolution of the image v is z-times higher than the resolution of the observation with $z \in \mathbb{N}$ being a positive integer.

The operator $\mathcal{H}$ is a composition of blurring and downsampling and has to be inverted when solving the ill-posed problem of reconstructing v from u.

2.2 Non-local means filtering

Let $u : \Omega \to \mathbb{R}$ be an image with $\Omega \subset \mathbb{R}^2$ and let $\mathcal{N}_u^r(\boldsymbol{x}) \subset \Omega$ denote a quadratic neighborhood of size $R \times R$, $R = 2r + 1$ within u around the center $\boldsymbol{x} \in \Omega$. Then the weighting function

$$w(\boldsymbol{x}, \boldsymbol{y}) = e^{-\frac{1}{h^2}\|(\mathcal{N}_u^r(\boldsymbol{x}) - \mathcal{N}_u^r(\boldsymbol{y}))\|^2} \tag{2}$$

maps similarity of neighborhoods around $\boldsymbol{x}$ and $\boldsymbol{y}$ to the interval $[0, 1]$. The parameter h controls the steepness of this mapping function. Exploiting this measure it is possible to average information according to its similarity:

$$v(\boldsymbol{x}) = \frac{1}{W(\boldsymbol{x})} \int_\Omega w(\boldsymbol{x}, \boldsymbol{y}) \cdot u(\boldsymbol{y}) d\boldsymbol{y}, \quad \boldsymbol{x}, \boldsymbol{y} \in \Omega \ . \tag{3}$$

The similarity weights are normalized by $W(\boldsymbol{x}) = \int_\Omega w(\boldsymbol{x}, \boldsymbol{y}) d\boldsymbol{y}$. The result $v(\boldsymbol{x})$ contains a filtered version of $u(\boldsymbol{x})$ based on similarity of neighborhoods in u.

With N denoting the number of pixels in each dimension, i.e. $|\Omega| = N^2$, this method has a complexity of $O\left(N^4 \cdot R^2\right)$. The algorithm can be simplified by reducing the search space for similar neighborhoods to $\mathcal{N}_u^s(\boldsymbol{x})$ of size $S \times S$, $S = 2s + 1$ which corresponds to updating the weights $w(\boldsymbol{x}, \boldsymbol{y})$ to

$$\widetilde{w}(\boldsymbol{x}, \boldsymbol{y}) = w(\boldsymbol{x}, \boldsymbol{y}) \cdot \sigma\left(\|\boldsymbol{x} - \boldsymbol{y}\|_\infty\right), \quad \sigma\left(\|\boldsymbol{x} - \boldsymbol{y}\|_\infty\right) = \begin{cases} 1 & \|\boldsymbol{x} - \boldsymbol{y}\|_\infty < s \\ 0 & else \end{cases} . \tag{4}$$

2.3 Image zooming using self-similarity

The algorithm introduced in this section allows to up-scale a single low-resolution image by a factor $z \in \mathbb{N}$. A method similar to the Non-local means filter is used which works on neighborhoods of different scales exploiting cross-scale similarity [4] within an image.

Let u denote the image to zoom and v denote the result of the magnification. The initial estimation v' is computed by upscaling u with a Lanczos interpolation. Then for a certain position $\boldsymbol{x}$ we compare the neighboring pixels on a z-spaced grid, i.e. $\boldsymbol{y} = \boldsymbol{x} + (m \cdot z, n \cdot z)^T$ with $n, m \in \mathbb{Z}$. Hence we derive the weights by

$$w(\boldsymbol{x}, \boldsymbol{y}) = e^{-\frac{1}{h^2}\|(\mathcal{N}_{v'}^r(\boldsymbol{x}) - \mathcal{N}_{v'}^r(\boldsymbol{y}))\|^2} \ . \tag{5}$$

Now instead of replacing the pixel at $\boldsymbol{x}$ with samples from v' we extract the information from the corresponding pixel of the low resolution image u. Inverting the decimation, we insert the averaged pixel only at $\boldsymbol{x}$ avoiding the blurring effect of interpolating methods. Hence we derive the high-resolved magnified image by

$$v(\boldsymbol{x}) = \frac{1}{W(\boldsymbol{x})} \sum_{\Omega} w(\boldsymbol{x}, \boldsymbol{y}) \cdot u\left(\frac{1}{z}\boldsymbol{y}\right) d\boldsymbol{y}, \quad \boldsymbol{x}, \boldsymbol{y} \in \Omega . \tag{6}$$

This can be enhanced by not only using the image itself but also the recent frames within the sequence of acquisitions. In [5] we propose a temporal extension of the NLM filter based on a multi-scale motion estimation

$$v_{\bar{t}}[\boldsymbol{x}] = \frac{1}{W[\boldsymbol{x}]} \sum_{t=\bar{t}}^{\bar{t}-\tau} \sum_{\Omega} w_t[\boldsymbol{x}, \boldsymbol{y}] \cdot u_t\left[\frac{1}{z}\boldsymbol{y}\right], \quad W[\boldsymbol{x}] = \sum_{t=\bar{t}}^{\bar{t}-\tau} \sum_{\Omega} w_t[\boldsymbol{x}, \boldsymbol{y}] \tag{7}$$

with $t \in \mathbb{N}$ denoting the index of a certain frame within the sequence history and τ determining the number of frames to consider for filtering the current frame at $t = \bar{t}$.

For the motion estimation we decompose the image into a Gaussian pyramid representation and compute the sum of squared difference (SSD) for each level i. Thus the estimated position of the block center within u_t for a given block $\mathcal{N}^b_{u_{\bar{t}}}(\boldsymbol{x})$ of size $B \times B$, $B = 2b + 1$ is calculated by

$$\boldsymbol{y}_i = \underset{\boldsymbol{y} \in \Omega}{\operatorname{argmax}} \left\| \mathcal{N}^b_{\mathcal{G}_i(u_{\bar{t}})}(\boldsymbol{x}) - \mathcal{N}^b_{\mathcal{G}_i(u_t)}(\boldsymbol{y}) \right\|, \quad i = 0, 1, \cdots, n \tag{8}$$

$$\|\boldsymbol{y}_i - \boldsymbol{y}_{i+1}\| < B, \quad \boldsymbol{y}_{n+1} = \mathbf{0} \tag{9}$$

with $\mathcal{G}_i(\cdot)$ denoting the Gaussian level i and $\mathcal{G}_0(u) = u$.

The restriction of higher level estimations $\boldsymbol{y}_i$ to the vicinity of the lower level estimation introduces a natural regularization compared to matching only full resolution blocks and prevents outliers. However the proposed approach does not depend on accurate motion detection. A rough estimation is sufficient to select the correct neighborhood and even outliers do not spoil the algorithm as the contained neighborhoods will have very low weights and hence will not influence the reconstructed value.

To achieve best results v' can be assigned the result v and the method may be iterated l times. Experiments have shown that $l = 2$ iterations are usually sufficient and further loops do not yield significant enhancements. Incorporating the simplification shown in Equation (4) the total complexity of the proposed method is $O\left(N^2 \cdot S^2 \cdot R^2 \cdot \tau \cdot l\right)$.

2.4 Test set

To evaluate the proposed method we used clinical fluoroscopy sequences containing continuous navigation frames acquired at low X-ray doses and single exposures at higher doses of the same anatomy. Thus we were able to compare impression of sharpness and noise with traditional upsampling as well as the high dose image serving as ground truth. In addition we processed a sequence containing an artificial rotating phantom and evaluated the noise suppression capability and resolution of our method.

3 Results

We visualize the results for two test sequences. The first one is a frame taken from a clinical angiography. Fig. 1 shows a part of the cranium magnified by traditional Lanczos interpolation compared to the proposed method.

As one can see, Lanczos interpolation significantly suffers from the inherent noise in low dose frames. The proposed method achieves a noise impression that is comparable to a high dose exposure and preserves sharpness but is not able to reconstruct all details contained in the high dose exposure from multiple low dose frames. The difference image between both methods contains only noise and the histogram shows an almost ideal Gaussian distribution.

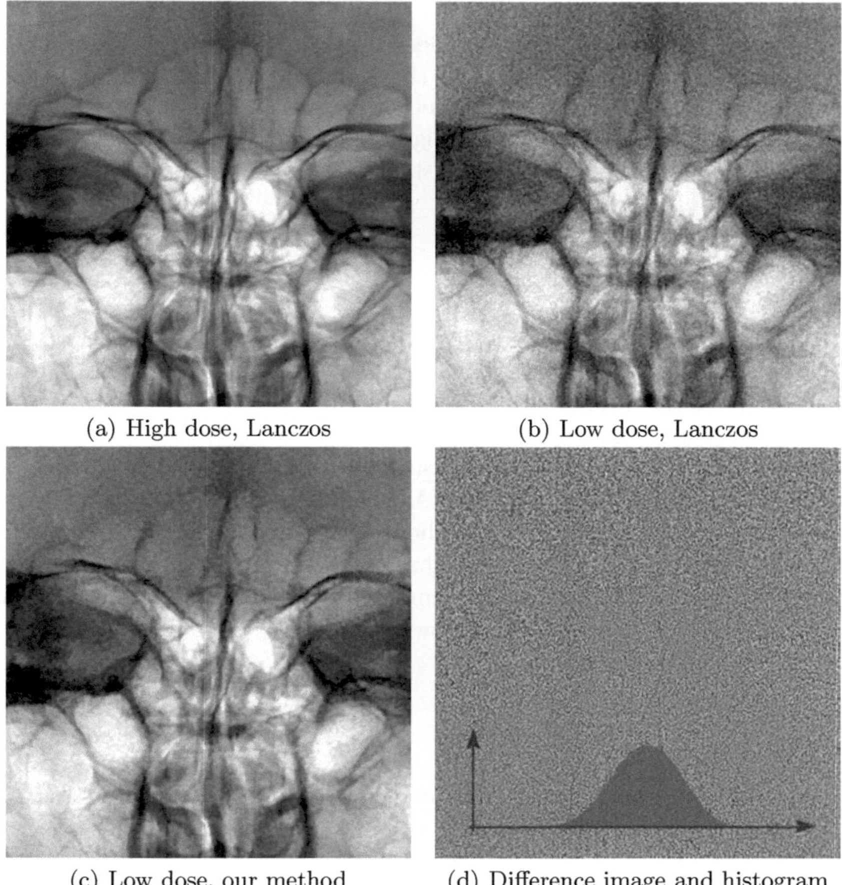

(a) High dose, Lanczos (b) Low dose, Lanczos

(c) Low dose, our method (d) Difference image and histogram

Fig. 1. Magnifying a cranial angiography: (a) Single frame acquired with high X-ray dose enlarged with Lanczos interpolation, (b) same anatomy acquired with low dose enlarged with Lanczos filter and (c) from $\tau = 10$ frames with the proposed magnification method, (d) contains the difference between Lanczos filtered and proposed image.

Fig. 2. Comparison of magnification techniques: The part marked by the red rectangle is upsampled for enhanced visibility. The complete detail view is magnified using (a) Lanczos interpolation and (b) the proposed method. (c) and (d) contain contrast enhanced detail views respectively.

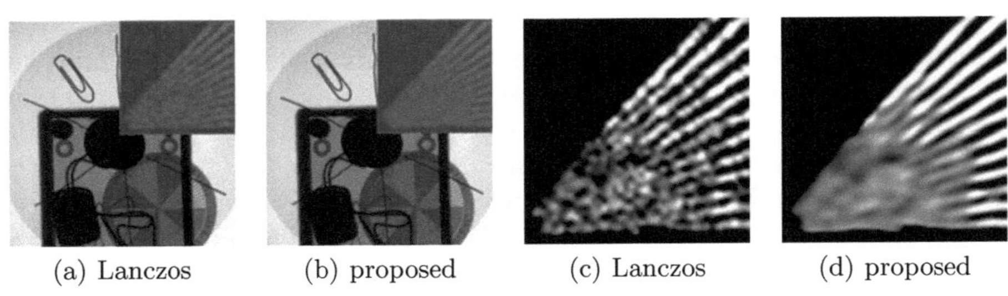

(a) Lanczos (b) proposed (c) Lanczos (d) proposed

The second sequence (Fig. 2) has been chosen to evaluate the spatial resolution. The Siemens star contained in this sequence is corrupted by noise and Lanczos as well as other interpolation methods even amplify this noise upon magnification. The proposed method though slightly degrading contrast achieves superior magnification and even reconstructs the corrupted pattern. Noise is heavily reduced and lines are better recognizable.

4 Discussion

In direct comparison to simple interpolation the proposed magnification shows superior quality. Evaluation of difference images indicates that no relevant structure is lost due to the filtering operation. Hence it is possible to achieve enhanced magnification of noisy image data without tampering the diagnostic information. As a rule of thumb the X-ray dose of a single high dose exposure corresponds to 30 seconds of navigation at low dose. As this technique might render some of the exposures unnecessary, we reduce the overall dose for patients and staff.

The high complexity yet prevents the algorithm from being executed interactively, however we have successfully implemented a real-time similarity based denoising [5] and as computational power grows it will be possible to do the same for the proposed method.

References

1. Keys R. Cubic convolution interpolation for digital image processing. IEEE Trans ASSP. 1981;29(6):1153–60.
2. Turkowski K. Filters for common resampling tasks. Apple Computer; 1990.
3. Buades A, Coll B, Morel JM. A non-local algorithm for image denoising. Proc IEEE CVPR. 2005;2:60–5.
4. Ebrahimi M, Vrscay ER. Examining the role of rcale in the context of the non-local-means filter. LNCS. 2008;5112:170–81.
5. Gooßen A, Pralow T, Grigat RR. Medical X-ray image enhancement by intra-image and inter-image similarity. Proc SPIE. 2009.

Quantitative Analyse und Visualisierung der Herzfunktionen

Anne Sauer[1], Tobias Schwarz[1], Nicole Engel[1], Mathias Seitel[1], Hannes Kenngott[1], Carsten Mohrhardt[2], Dirk Loßnitzer[2], Evangelos Giannitsis[2], Hugo A. Katus[2], Hans-Peter Meinzer[1]

[1]Abteilung für Medizinische und Biologische Informatik, DKFZ Heidelberg
[2]Abteilung für Innere Medizin III, Universitätsklinikum Heidelberg
a.sauer@dkfz-heidelberg.de

Kurzfassung. Die computergestützte bildbasierte Analyse der Herzfunktionen ist mittlerweile Standard in der Kardiologie. Die verfügbaren Produkte erfordern meist ein hohes Maß an Benutzerinteraktion und somit einen erhöhten Zeitaufwand. In dieser Arbeit wird ein Ansatz vorgestellt, der dem Kardiologen eine größtenteils automatische Analyse der Herzfunktionen mittels MRT-Bilddaten ermöglicht und damit Zeitersparnis schafft. Hierbei werden alle relevanten herzphysiologsichen Parameter berechnet und mithilfe von Diagrammen und Graphen visualisiert. Diese Berechnungen werden evaluiert, indem die ermittelten Werte mit manuell vermessenen verglichen werden. Der hierbei berechnete mittlere Fehler liegt mit 2,85 mm für die Wanddicke und 1,61 mm für die Wanddickenzunahme immer noch im Bereich einer Pixelgrösse der verwendeten Bilder.

1 Einleitung

Herzkreislauferkrankungen, insbesondere der Herzinfarkt, führten in Deutschland im Jahr 2007 zu über 350.000 Sterbefällen. Sie ist damit die häufigste Todesursache in Deutschland [1]. Aus diesem Grund ist die frühzeitige Diagnose von Herzkreislauferkrankungen bzw. die Ermittlung des Schweregrads von Erstinfarkten umso wichtiger, um bessere Präventionen, Nachuntersuchungen und Therapien bzw. chirurgische Eingriffe zu ermöglichen.

In der Kardiologie gibt es wichtige Kenngrößen 2.2, die aus nicht invasiven Methoden, wie der medizinischen Bildgebung, gewonnen werden können. Diese herzphysiologischen Parameter helfen den Kardiologen bei der Diagnosefindung. Anhand von rechnergestützen Anwendungen können diese Parameter extrahiert und visualisiert werden, was zur Beschleunigung und Erhöhung der Reproduzierbarkeit der Diagnosefindung führt. Verschiedene kommerzielle Anbieter sowie verschiedene Forschungseinrichtungen haben bereits Lösungsansätze hierzu entwickelt. Dabei wurden verschiedene Schwerpunkte gesetzt, beispielsweise die Narbendetektion [2] und Analyse des rechten Ventrikels [3], sowie die myokardiale Perfusion [4].

Die genannten Lösungsansätze erfordern meist jedoch hohe Benutzerinteraktion (wie zum Beispiel die Eingabe von Parametern oder das Setzen einer Region), um eine möglichst fehlerfreie Segmentierung zu erreichen. Die hohe Benutzerinteraktion verlangt eine erhöhte Aufmerksamkeit des Benutzers über einen längeren Zeitraum. Des Weiteren kann die erhöhte Interaktion zu einer schlechteren Reproduzierbarkeit führen.

Um die geschilderte Problematik zu umgehen, werden in diesem Ansatz statistische Formmodelle (Shape Models) [5] [6] zur Segmentierung eingesetzt. Basierend auf dieser Segmentierung wird eine größtenteils automatische Auswertung erstellt. Die Benutzerinteraktion wird dadurch auf ein Minimum reduziert, wodurch die Arbeitsabläufe des Kardiologen beschleunigt werden. Zusätzlich ist es erstmals möglich longitudinale Ausmessungen des Herzventrikels automatisch zu erstellen.

2 Material und Methoden

Die Methoden wurden auf Basis der Software-Bibliotheken Medical Imaging Interaction Toolkit (MITK), Insight Segmentation and Registration Toolkit (ITK) und Visualization Toolkit (VTK) implementiert. Damit war es möglich auf bereits etablierte Algorithmen aufzubauen.

Der Workflow führt den Kardiologen in wenigen Schritten durch die Analyse des Herzens bis hin zur Ausgabe der in 2.2 beschriebenen herzphysiologischen Parameter. Um den Benutzer die Möglichkeit der Manipulation zu geben, wird momentan ein Wizardkonzept eingesetzt.

Der erste Schritt hierbei ist die Segmentierung des Endokards (Herzinnenwand) und des Epikards (äusserste Schicht der Herzwand). Dabei werden Shape Models, die auf einer grossen Anzahl von 3D+T MRT-Trainingsdaten basieren, zur automatischen Segmentierung eingesetzt. Hierbei wurden MRT-Bilddaten des Herzens mit einer räumlichen Auflösung von 1,84 x 1,84 x 5,0 mm und einer zeitlichen Auflösung von 25 Zeitschritten verwendet, die einen kompletten Herzzyklus abbilden. Das Ergebnis ist eine zeitaufgelöste Oberfläche mit ihren zugehörigen Binärdaten.

Beim zweiten Schritt wird automatisch der Zeitpunkt der Endsystole und der Enddiastole aus der Oberfläche über volumetrische Unterschiede ermittelt. Diese beiden Zeitschritte sind für die meisten kardiologischen Parameter von zentraler Bedeutung, da es sich bei der Endsystole um die maximale Kontraktion und bei der Enddiastole um die maximale Entspannung des Ventrikels handelt. Daher bezieht sich die Auswertung im Normalfall auf diese beiden Zeitschritte. Es kann aber zusätzlich auch zeitlich weiter aufgelöst werden.

Der dritte Schritt beinhaltet die Ausrichtung der Herzachsen nach dem American Heart Association-Standard (AHA). Diese Ausrichtung ist wichtig für die räumliche Einteilung der Oberfläche in Segmente, wodurch die Projektion der Parameter auf eine etablierte Visualisierung (Bull's Eye 2.1) ermöglicht wird.

Der letzte Schritt ist die Auswertung. Dabei werden die in 2.2 beschriebenen herzphysiologischen Parameter berechnet und in standardisierten Diagrammen und Graphen ausgegeben.

2.1 Bull's Eye Plot

Das Bull's Eye ist ein kardiologisches Auswertungsdiagramm und wird für die Visualisierung kardiologischer Parameter eingesetzt. Die Standardeinteilung besteht aus 17 Segmenten (Abb. 1(f)). Das Ventrikel wird dabei in vier räumliche Bereiche eingeteilt: basal, mid, apical sowie den Apex [7].

Die Projektion der Oberfläche auf das Bull's Eye erfolgt anhand von Schnitten durch die Ergebnisoberfläche. Die Schnittebenen werden entlang der sagitalen Ventrikelachse ermittelt(Abb .1(e)). Aus den einzelnen Schnitten resultieren kreisähnliche Polygone. Die Werte, die aus den Punkten der Polygone gewonnen werden, werden auf die Punkte innerhalb der Bull's Eye Segmente projiziert. Die Ausrichtung des Polygons erfolgt momentan noch durch eine Richtungsangabe des Benutzers.

2.2 Kardiologische Parameter

Bei der hier beschriebenen Analyse der Herzfunktionen gibt es folgende Standardparameter: Volumen des Ventrikels in Endsys- und Enddiastole, Schlagvolumen (stroke volume), Auswurffraktion (ejection fraction), Herzminutenvolumen (cardiac output), Wandmasse (wall mass) und Herzindex (cardiac index). Des Weiteren gibt es die Wandbewegung (Wall Motion), Wanddicke (Wall Thickness) und Wanddickenzunahme (Wall Thickening), die sowohl global als auch lokal berechnet werden [9]. Sie werden im Bull's Eye visualisiert. Da diese Arbeit auf Shape Models basiert, konnten die zuletzt genannten Parameter wie folgt berechnet werden.

– *Wandbewegung:* Die Wall Motion beschreibt die Bewegung des Herzmuskels innerhalb eines Herzzyklus. Hierbei wird ein Verschiebungsvektorfeld

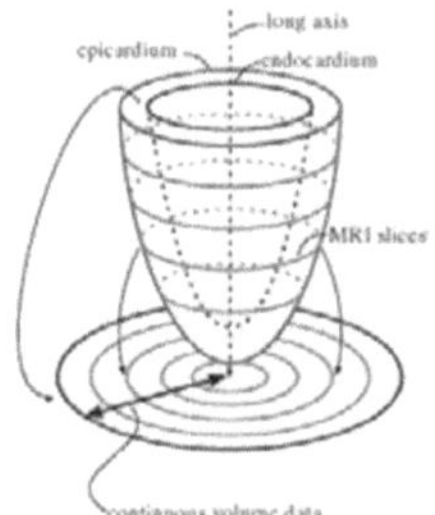

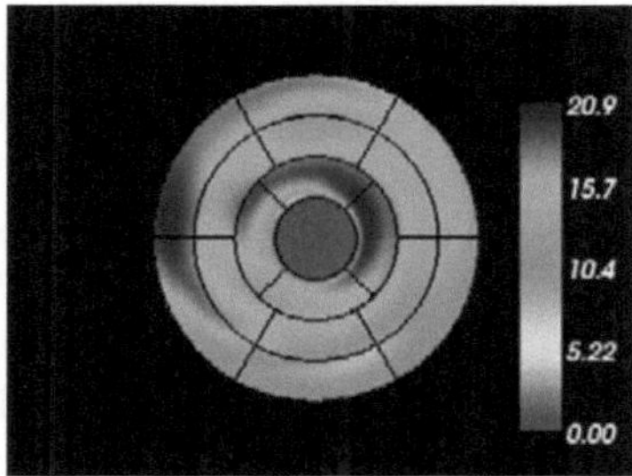

Abb. 1. Projektion der Oberfläche auf das Bull's Eye [8] (links); ein Bull's Eye der Wandbewegung (rechts)

Tabelle 1. Mittlerer Fehler der Wanddicke und Wanddickenzunahme gegenüber der Messung durch einen Experten.

	Mittelwert (mm)	Standardabweichung (mm)
Wanddicke	2,85	2,68
Wanddickenzunahme	1,61	1,93

zwischen den Stützpunkten (Landmarken) der Endokardoberfläche des endsystolischen und des enddiastolischen Zeitschritts berechnet. Shape Models geben hier die Möglichkeit Landmarken-Korrespondenzen zu bilden. Dies wird erreicht durch die Verwendung eines Verfahrens zur Optimierung der Landmarken[10]. Anhand der Beträge der Vektoren kann die zurückgelegte Distanz berechnet werden.
- *Wanddicke:* Die Myokardwanddicke wird während der Enddiastole anhand des Abstands zwischen Endokardoberfläche und Epikardoberfläche bestimmt.
- *Wanddickenzunahme:* Die Wanddickenzunahme wird anhand der Differenz der Wanddicke zur Zeit der Endsystole und Enddiastole für jeden Punkt (lokal) berechnet.

Aufgrund der bereits erstellten Oberfläche können erstmals verschiedene longitudinale Ausmessungen automatisch berechnet werden, insbesondere die Ausmessung des Ventrikels vom Apex zur Mitralklappe zum Zeitpunkt der Enddiastole (mitral annular plane systolic excursion, MAPSE).

3 Ergebnisse

Zur Evaluation der Anwendung wurden verschiedene Parameter betrachtet. Zum einen von klinischem Interesse ist der benötigte Zeitaufwand für die Analyse eines kompletten Datensatzes. Der Hauptzeitaufwand entfällt hierbei auf die Segmentierung der zeitaufgelösten Daten. Diese kann je nach Bildmaterial und Anzahl der Zeitschritte bis zu vier bis fünf Minuten dauern. Da der Segmentierungsschritt automatisch abläuft, kann die Berechnung im Hintergrund geschehen. Die eigentliche Auswertung der herzphysiologischen Parameter beträgt anschliessend lediglich eine Minute bei minimal benötigter Benutzerinteraktion.

Zum anderen wurde zur quantitativen Validierung der Parameterbestimmung die minimalen, maximalen und mittleren Werte der Wanddicke und Wanddickenzunahme auf fünf Datensätzen mit der Anwendung im 3D-Raum bestimmt. Diese wurden mit den von Hand vermessenen Daten eines kardiologischen Experten verglichen. Dabei bezog sich der Experte auf drei Segmente jedes Datensatzes, die er besonders gut ausmessen konnte. Die manuellen Daten wurden gemäß des Standards wie in [9] beschrieben im 2D-Raum erhoben. Die bisherigen Ergebnisse sind in Tabelle 1 zusammengefasst.

4 Diskussion

In dieser Arbeit wurde eine größtenteils automatische Anwendung zur Analyse von herzphysiologischen Parametern vorgestellt. Diese basiert auf einer Segmentierung mithilfe von statistischen Formmodellen, anhand derer schnell und intuitiv eine Auswertung und Visualisierung erstellt werden kann.

Die Evaluation hat gezeigt, dass zwischen den Ergebnissen einer manuellen Vermessung und der automatischen noch Differenzen bestehen. Man sieht jedoch im Vergleich der Daten, dass dieser Fehler überwiegend auf die lokal ungenaue Segmentierung zurückzuführen ist. Zu beachten ist hierbei, dass der Fehler in der Größenordnung der räumlichen Bildauflösung liegt und deshalb im Mittel nur eine Abweichung von einem Pixel darstellt.

Um eine segmentierungsunabhängige Evaluation zu erhalten, ist eine umfangreiche Studie an einem Phantom geplant. Hierbei soll die automatische und manuelle Vermessung eines adaptierten Lungenbeatmungsphantoms verglichen werden. Des Weiteren soll die Applikation als Basis für weitere kardiologische Auswertungsmöglichkeiten dienen. Beispielweise sollen eine automatische Reportererstellung sowie erweiterte Visualisierungsmöglichkeiten hinzugefügt werden. Wir hoffen, dass unsere Ergebnisse zu einer besseren Akzeptanz computergestützter Methoden in der kardiologischen Diagnostik und einer besseren Integration in den klinischen Workflow führen.

Literaturverzeichnis

1. Bundesamt S. Gesundheitsberichterstattung des Bundes; 2008. www.gbe-bund.de.
2. Säring D, Stork A, Juchheim S, et al. HeAT: A software assistant for the analysis of LV remodeling after myocardial infarction in 4D MR follow-up studies. LNCS. 2006; p. 537–543.
3. Wesarg S. Automatisierte Analyse und Visualisierung der Koronaraterien und grossen Kavitäten des Herzens für die klinische Anwendung. TU Darmstadt, Fachbereich Informatik; 2007.
4. Oeltze S, Kuss A, Hennemuth A, et al. Integrierte Visualisierung von Anatomie und Perfusion des Myokards zur Früherkennung der Koronaren Herzkrankheit. BVM. 2006.
5. Heimann T. Statistical shape models for 3D medical image segmentation. University of Heidelberg; 2008.
6. Schwarz T, Heimann T, Wolf I, et al. 3D heart segmentation and volumetry using deformable shape models. Proc Comp Cardiol. 2007.
7. Cerqueira MD, Weissmann NJ, Dilsizian V. Standardized myocardial segmentation and nomenclature for tomographic imaging of the heart. Circulation. 2002; p. 5.
8. Termeer M, Bescos JO, Breeuwer M, et al. CoVICAD: Comprehensive visualization of coronary artery disease. IEEE Trans Vis Comput Graph. 2007;13:1632–1639.
9. Schulte B, Bolt A, Beyer D. MRT des Herzens und der Gefässe. Springer Berlin Heidelberg; 2005. 978-3-540-22209-5.
10. Heimann T, Wolf I, Williams TG, et al. 3D active shape models using gradient descent optimization of description length. Inf Process Med Imaging. 2005;19:566–577.

MITK-IGT: Eine Navigationskomponente für das Medical Imaging Interaction Toolkit

Jochen Neuhaus, Ingmar Wegner, Johannes Kast, Matthias Baumhauer, Alexander Seitel, Ingmar Gergel, Marco Nolden, Daniel Maleike, Ivo Wolf, H.-P. Meinzer, Lena Maier-Hein

Abteilung für Medizinische und Biologische Informatik, DKFZ Heidelberg
j.neuhaus@dkfz-heidelberg.de

Kurzfassung. MITK-IGT ist eine Erweiterung des Medical Imaging Interaction Toolkits, die es ermöglicht Softwareprogramme im Bereich bildgestützte Therapie zu erstellen. Dieser Beitrag stellt die Architektur und Designprinzipien von MITK-IGT vor und vergleicht sie mit anderen Open Source Lösungen. Neben der Ansteuerung von Trackingsystemen und Visualisierungsmodulen liegt der Fokus von MITK-IGT auf einer Filterarchitektur, die das schrittweise Verarbeiten von Trackingdaten erlaubt. Zur BVM 2009 wird die erste Version von MITK-IGT als Open Source veröffentlicht.

1 Einleitung

Das Medical Imaging Interaction Toolkit (MITK) ist ein Open Source C++ Toolkit für medizinische Bildverarbeitung [1]. Es basiert auf dem Insight Segmentation and Registration Toolkit (ITK) und dem Visualization Toolkit (VTK) und erweitert diese um anwendungsspezifische Aspekte. Viele verschiedene Anwendungen im Bereich computerunterstützte Diagnose und Therapieplanung basieren auf MITK. Dieser Beitrag stellt eine Erweiterung für MITK vor, die es ermöglicht, mit Hilfe von MITK auch Anwendungen im Bereich bildgestützte Therapie (Image Guided Therapy, IGT) zu erstellen. Obwohl medizinische Navigationssysteme für rigide Strukturen seit mehreren Jahren kommerziell erhältlich sind, ist IGT immer noch ein aktives Forschungsgebiet, vor allem im Bereich von Weichgewebeeingriffen [2].

Es existieren mehrere Open Source Softwarebibliotheken, die das Erstellen von IGT-Anwendungen erlauben. Gemeinsam ist allen, dass sie verschiedene im medizinischen Umfeld gebräuchliche Trackingsysteme ansteuern, eine Registrierung der Trackingdaten mit Bilddaten erlauben und Module für eine Visualisierung der registrierten Daten beinhalten. Das Image Guided Surgery Toolkit (IGSTK) [3] legt den Fokus auf Softwarequalität, vor allem Robustheit. Das CISST package (Computer Integrated Surgical Systems and Technology) [4] besteht aus mehreren Low-Level Bibliotheken zur Hardwareabstraktion von medizinischen Sensoren und Robotern. Darauf baut die Surgical Assistant Workstation (SAW) [5] auf. Ihr Fokus liegt auf roboterassistierter Chirurgie und 3D

Benutzerinteraktion mit speziellen Eingabegeräten. Das Image Guided Therapy Toolkit (IGT:Toolkit, www.na-mic.org/Wiki/index.php/IGT:ToolKit) kombiniert die weit verbreitete Software 3D Slicer (www.slicer.org) über das Netzwerkprotokoll OpenIGTLink (www.na-mic.org/Wiki/index.php/OpenIGTLink) mit IGSTK.

Außer dem IGT:Toolkit, das 3D Slicer mit einer Trackingsystemansteuerung verbinden, beschränken sich alle anderen Bibliotheken auf den Image Guided Therapy Bereich. Komplett integrierte Anwendungen, die Bildanalyse, Therapieplanung und Navigation unterstützen, lassen sich damit nicht oder nur umständlich erstellen. Im Bereich intrainterventioneller Bildgebung ist die Kombination aus Bildanalyse und Navigation jedoch essentiell. Deswegen haben wir den Ansatz gewählt, das weit entwickelte MITK Framework um die MITK-IGT Komponente zu erweitern, so dass damit erstellte Navigationsanwendungen von allen Vorteilen und Features von MITK profitieren können.

2 Material und Methoden

Bei dem Entwurf von MITK-IGT konnten wir auf Erfahrungen aus der Entwicklung mehrerer Navigationssysteme zurückgreifen. Eine Analyse existierender IGT-Projekte zeigte viele Bereiche, die als wiederverwendbare Komponenten modelliert werden können. Ein Ziel beim Entwurf war, einen Schritt weiter zu gehen als andere Toolkits. MITK-IGT soll nicht nur grundlegende Komponenten zur Hardwareabstraktion und Visualisierung bereitstellen sondern zusätzlich eine Architektur definieren, mit der sich auch komplexe Navigationsanwendungen durch Kombination einfacherer Verarbeitungsschritte modellieren lassen.

Die MITK-IGT Komponente ist in zwei Bereiche aufgeteilt. Eine Tracking Komponente bietet Klassen zur Interaktion mit Trackingsystemen. Darauf baut eine Navigationskomponente auf, die weitreichende Verarbeitungsmöglichkeiten der Trackingdaten erlaubt.

2.1 Trackingkomponente

Die Trackingkomponente erlaubt die Ansteuerung verbreiteter Trackingsysteme wie Polaris, Aurora (beide NDI Inc., Waterloo, Kanada), MicronTracker (Claron Technology Inc., Toronto, Kanada) aber auch speziellerer Systeme wie beispielsweise des Space Navigators (3DConnexion, Fremont, USA) oder der Wiimote (Nintendo, Kyoto, Japan). Das Auslesen der Daten aus den Trackingsystemen geschieht in einem eigenen Thread, so dass die Trackingdaten ohne weitere Latenz zur Verfügung stehen, wenn sie benötigt werden. Die Trackingkomponente stellt eine einheitliche Schnittstelle für die verschiedenen Trackingsysteme bereit, so dass eine Navigationssoftware mit geringen Anpassungen mit verschiedenen Trackingsystemen verwendet werden kann.

2.2 Navigationskomponente

In allen untersuchten Anwendungsszenarien wurden die Daten der Trackingsysteme mehrstufig verarbeitet. Dies führte zu dem Entschluss, das in der Bildverarbeitung verbreitete Architekturprinzip einer Filterpipeline auf Trackingdaten zu übertragen. Mit diesem Ansatz lassen sich viele Verarbeitungsschritte als wiederverwendbare Filter kapseln. Die MITK-IGT Filterpipeline basiert auf der ITK Data Processing Pipeline [6]. Abbildung 1 zeigt ein Beispiel für eine MITK-IGT Filterpipeline. Jedes Filterobjekt kann mehrere Trackingdaten als Eingabe haben, verarbeitet sie und stellt sie anderen Filterobjekten als seine Ausgabe bereit. Indem man die Ausgabe eines Filters als Eingabe eines anderen Filters verwendet, wird eine Verarbeitungspipeline aufgebaut. Am Anfang einer solchen Pipeline stehen Filter, die Trackingdaten entweder direkt von der Trackingkomponente, aus einer Datei mit aufgezeichneten Trackingdaten oder über eine Netzwerkschnittstelle erhalten. Ein Filterobjekt kann Trackingdaten unterschiedlicher Filterobjekte als Eingabe bekommen und seine Ausgabe auch wieder mehreren Filtern bereitstellen. Die Filterpipeline funktioniert nach dem Pull-Prinzip. Wenn die Ausgabe eines Filters abgefragt wird, veranlasst er zuerst eine Aktualisierung seiner Eingabefilter, bevor er mit deren Ergebnissen seine eigenen Berechnungen durchführt. In der Regel wird eine Filteraktualisierung zeitgesteuert in einer festen Frequenz durchgeführt. Alternativ erzeugen die Quellfilter immer, wenn sie von Trackingsystem, Logdatei oder Netzwerk neue Trackingdaten bekommen, ein Event, das mit der Aktualisierungsmethode der

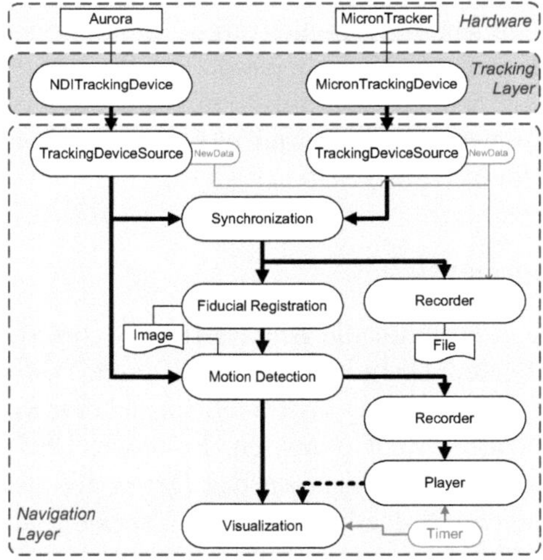

Abb. 1. Beispiel einer MITK-IGT Filterpipeline. Der TrackingDeviceSource - Synchronization - Recorder Teil der Pipeline wird über Events mit der Frequenz der Trackingsysteme betrieben. Der Rest der Pipeline wird von einem Timer mit niedrigerer Frequenz aktualisiert. Die Visualisierung kann zwischen den Trackingsystemen und einem Recorder/Player Paar umgeschaltet werden, um die Visualisierung während einer Intervention „zurück zu spulen“.

Filter gekoppelt werden kann. Dadurch kann mit MITK-IGT neben dem Pull-Mechanismus auch ein eventgesteuerter Push-Mechanismus realisiert werden.

Ein wichtiger Aspekt bei der Pipelineaktualisierung ist, dass nicht alle Teile einer Verarbeitungspipeline in der gleichen Frequenz aktualisiert werden müssen. Da für jeden Filter einer Pipeline getrennt eine Aktualisierung veranlasst werden kann, können einzelne Teile von verschiedenen Threads in verschiedenen Frequenzen aktualisiert werden. Redundante Berechnungen werden mit Hilfe von Zeitstempeln und einer Pufferung der Ausgabedaten vermieden. Mit Hilfe dieser Filterarchitektur können viele Anforderungen erfüllt werden, indem passende Filterobjekte erstellt und miteinander kombiniert werden. Es existieren beispielsweise Filter für folgende Features:

- *Senden und Empfangen von Trackingdaten über ein Netzwerk.* Trackingdaten können über eine Netzwerkschnittstelle gesendet und empfangen werden. Dies erlaubt das Entkoppeln der Trackingsystemansteuerung, der Verarbeitung und der Visualisierung auf mehrere Computer. Beispielsweise können unterschiedliche Visualisierungen einer Intervention parallel auf mehreren Computern erzeugt werden.
- *Speichern und Wiedergabe von Trackingdaten.* Dies erlaubt das Auszeichnen von Interventionen. Bei der Wiedergabe lässt sich die Wiedergabegeschwindigkeit variieren, so dass sowohl Zeitraffer- als auch Zeitlupenfunktionen möglich sind.
- *Synchronisation mehrerer Trackingsysteme.* Ein Synchronisierungsfilter kann Trackingdaten mehrerer Trackingsysteme zeitlich synchronisieren, um unterschiedliche Latenzzeiten auszugleichen. Zusammen mit einem Registrierungsfilter, der die Trackingdaten in ein gemeinsames Koordinatensystem transformiert, können mehrere Trackingsysteme zu einem virtuellen Trackingsystem kombiniert werden.
- *Koordinatensystemtransformation.* Über verschiedene Registrierungsfilter können Trackingdaten in andere Koordinatensysteme transformiert werden.
- *Visualisierungsfilter.* Es existieren Filter für Instrumenten- und Kameravisualisierung, Virtual- und Augmented Reality und spezielle Zielführungsdarstellungen.
- *Particle- und Kalmanfilter.* Diese Filter erlauben die räumliche und zeitliche Filterung von Trackingdaten, um einzelne Messfehler und Aussetzer zu überbrücken.

Die Trackingdaten enthalten neben Position, Orientierung und Zeitstempel auch eine Datenstruktur zur Fehlerpropagierung, so dass sowohl die Trackingsysteme als auch einzelne Filter eine Fehlerabschätzung für die Trackingdaten abgeben können. Da für eine Intervention meist mehrere Objekte getrackt werden müssen, können Toolkonfigurationen zusammen mit allen weiteren benötigten Daten wie Oberflächenmodellen, Geometriebeschreibungen, Tooltypen, Toolaufgaben und anderen Metadaten in einer gemeinsamen Beschreibungsdatei gespeichert und geladen werden.

Für jeden Filter existieren GUI Widgets, die dazu verwendet werden können, die Parameter des Filters einzustellen. Ein Filter kann mehrere GUI Widgets besitzen, etwa ein User-, ein Experten- und ein Debug-Widget.

3 Ergebnisse

Eine interne Version von MITK-IGT wird bereits für mehrere Navigationssysteme verwendet [7]. Eine Open Source Version ist momentan in Entwicklung. Zur BVM 2009 wird eine erste Version auf www.mitk.org unter einer BSD-kompatiblen Lizenz veröffentlicht.

4 Diskussion

Softwaresysteme, die während einer Intervention eingesetzt werden, müssen höchste Qualitätsanforderungen erfüllen. Zuverlässigkeit ist dabei der wichtigste Qualitätsfaktor. IGSTK versucht, Zuverlässigkeit einerseits durch explizite Modellierung und Kontrolle der Objektzustände mit Zustandsmaschinen, andererseits durch Minimierung der Schnittstellen und Features zu erreichen. Die dahinter stehende Idee ist, dass einfache Software weniger Fehler enthält als komplexe Software. Im Forschungsbereich halten wir diesen Ansatz für zu einschränkend. MITK-IGT soll es gerade ermöglichenauch komplexe Navigationssoftware zu entwickeln. Es soll eine Umgebung bieten, die es erlaubt sich auf neue Aspekte zu konzentrieren, in dem es eine erweiterbare Sammlung von wiederverwendbaren Grundfunktionalitäten und ein flexibles Framework, um diese zu einem Gesamtsystem zu kombinieren, bereit stellt.

Literaturverzeichnis

1. Wolf I, Nolden M, Böttger T, et al. The MITK approach. Proc MICCAI Workshop: Open-Source Software. 2005.
2. Baumhauer M, Feuerstein M, Meinzer HP, et al. Navigation in endoscopic soft tissue surgery: Perspectives and limitations. J Endourol. 2008;22(4):751–766.
3. Gary K, Ibáñez L, Aylward S, et al. IGSTK: An open source software toolkit for image-guided surgery. IEEE Computer. 2006;39(4):46–53.
4. Deguet A, Kumar R, Taylor R, et al. The cisst libraries for computer assisted intervention systems. Proc MICCAI Workshop: Systems and Architectures for Computer Assisted Interventions. 2008;Http://hdl.handle.net/10380/1465.
5. Vagvolgyi B, DiMaio SP, Deguet A, et al. The surgical assistant workstation. Proc MICCAI Workshop: Systems and Architectures for Computer Assisted Interventions. 2008;Http://hdl.handle.net/10380/1466.
6. Ibáñez L, Schroeder W, Ng L, et al. The ITK Software Guide. Kitware Inc.; 2003.
7. Meinzer HP, Maier-Hein L, Wegner I, et al. Computer-assisted soft tissue interventions. Proc IEEE ISBI. 2008.

Haptische Modellierung und Deformation einer Kugelzelle

Darius Schippritt[1], Martin Wiemann[2,3], Hans-Gerd Lipinski[1]

[1]Fachhochschule Dortmund, Fachbereich Informatik
[2]Physiologisches Institut, Universität Duisburg-Essen
[3]Institut für Biologische Emissionsbewertung (IBE) Marl
d.schippritt@stud.fh-dortmund.de

Kurzfassung. Haptische Simulationsmodelle dienen in der Medizin in erster Linie dem Training operativer Eingriffe. Sie basieren zumeist auf physikalischen Gewebemodellen, welche eine sehr genaue Simulation der biomechanischen Eigenschaften des betreffenden Gewebes erlauben, aber gleichzeitig sehr rechenintensiv und damit zeitaufwändig in der Ausführung sind. Die menschliche Wahrnehmung kann allerdings auch eine ungenaue haptische Modellierung psychooptisch ausgleichen. Daher kann es sinnvoll sein, haptische Simulationen auch mit nicht vollständig physikalisch definierten Deformationsmodellen durchzuführen. Am Beispiel der haptischer Simulation einer in-vitro Fertilisation wird gezeigt, dass durch die Anwendung eines geometrischen Deformationsmodells eine künstliche Befruchtung unter realistischen experimentellen Bedingungen in Echtzeit haptisch simuliert und damit trainiert werden kann.

1 Einleitung

Im Rahmen molekularbiologischer oder genetischer in-vitro Experimente, einschließlich der in-vitro Fertilisation (ISCI), werden Substrate bzw. genetisches Material mit Hilfe einer Mikropipette, im Folgenden als „Kanüle“ bezeichnet, gezielt in das Zellinnere gebracht, um dort bestimmte biochemische Prozesse auszulösen. Dazu wird eine mit der in die Zelle zu verbringenden Substanz gefüllte Kanüle mit Hilfe einer Steuerungsmechanik unter mikroskopischer Kontrolle an die Zelle herangeführt, durch definierte Kraftanwendung die Zellwand mit der Kanüle durchstoßen und das Material aus dem Kanüleninneren in die Zelle verbracht.

Um einen solchen experimentellen Eingriff erfolgreich durchzuführen, ist ein entsprechendes Training notwendig. Unter realen Bedingungen bedeutet das den Einsatz von möglicherweise teurem Zellkultur-Material nur für Übungszwecke. Bei einer virtuellen Zellpenetration mit einem haptischen System sollte der gleiche Übungszweck ohne den Verbrauch von lebendem Material erreichbar sein. Allerdings sind die Kosten für das haptische System mit 2000 EUR zu kalkulieren. Aus diesem Grunde wurde ein haptisches Modell entwickelt, das einen virtuellen Eingriff in eine kugelförmige Zelle ermöglicht.

2 Material und Methoden

2.1 Biomechanische Modellierung

Betrachtet werden kugelförmige Zellen, welche mit Zytoplasma gefüllt sind, das einen gleichmäßigen hydrostatischen Druck auf die Zellmembran ausübt. Bei einer Deformation bleibt das Volumen der Zelle konstant während die Biomembran gedehnt wird und dabei linear elastische Eigenschaften besitzt. Die Kanüle mit dem Radius c wird senkrecht zur Membran in die Zelle eingeschoben, wodurch eine radialsymmetrische Deformation der Membran mit dem Radius r entsteht. Abhängig von der einwirkenden Kraft dringt die Kanüle mit der Tiefe $z(r)$ in die Zelle ein. Auf der gegenüberliegenden Seite erfolgt eine an die Oberflächenform der Fixierung angepasste Deformation (i.a. ebene Form) mit dem Radius x_0. Die Zelle nimmt wegen der auftretenden Verformung allerdings einen neuen Radius R an (Abb. 1B). Der Kraftaufwand ist im Wesentlichen nur für die Penetration der Zellmembran erforderlich. Im Zellinneren treten so gut wie keine Gegenkräfte für die Kanüle auf. Weiterhin gilt die Annahme, dass sich die Zelle wie ein lineares elastisches System verhält. Die von außen an der Zellmembran wirkende Deformationskraft F ist gleich der Summe von interner Kraft und Rückstellkraft. Im radial-symmetrischen Fall lässt sich daraus das von Sun et al. [2] entwickelte Deformationsmodell ableiten. Dabei ist r der Abstand vom Rand der Kanüle, δ die Membrandicke, c der Kanülenradius und σ_d ein Elastizitätsparameter. Für das erzeugte radialsymmetrische Deformationsprofil gilt:

$$z(r) = \frac{F}{4\pi \cdot \sigma_d \cdot \delta} \cdot \left[1 - \left(\frac{r}{x_0} \right)^2 + ln \left(\frac{r}{x_0} \right)^2 \right] \quad \text{mit} \quad c \leq r \leq r_0 \tag{1}$$

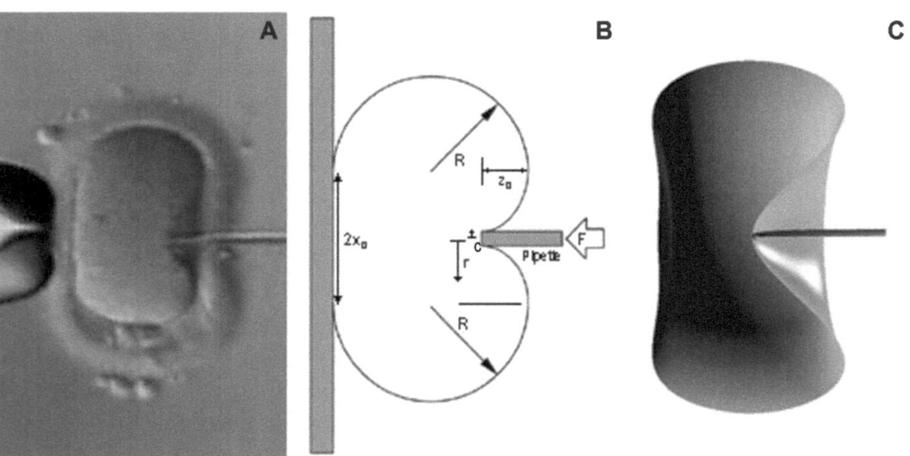

Abb. 1. Deformationsverläufe an einer sphärischen Zelle. A: Beobachtete Zellpenetration [1]; B: Modell nach Sun et al. [2]; C: entwickeltes haptisches Modell.

Der Gradient von z ist nach diesem Modell unmittelbar an der Kanülenspitze maximal und nimmt mit zunehmendem r fortlaufend ab. Eine solche Deformationsgeometrie lässt sich durchaus bei zahlreichen Zellpenetrationsexperimenten beobachten [3]. Gleichwohl gibt es zahlreiche Fälle, in denen am Rand der Kanüle zunächst eine Zunahme des Gradienten zu beobachten ist [1, 4]. Erst nach einem gewissen Abstand von der Kanüle wird dann der Übergang zu einem abnehmenden Gradienten beobachtet. Die Abbildung 1A zeigt ein solches typisches Deformationsverhalten, das durch das Modell von Sun et al. [2] nicht vollständig erklärt werden kann. Um auch solche Deformationsprofile erzeugen zu können, lässt sich eine „Morphing"-Funktion definieren, womit durch die Wahl des Parameterwertes von p auch das Modell von Sun et al. simulierbar ist. Dieses allgemeine Deformationsprofil z_M wird durch folgende Funktion beschrieben:

$$z_M(r) = \frac{z_{M,0}}{2} \cdot \left[1 + cos\left(\pi \cdot a \cdot \left(\frac{r}{x_0}\right)^p\right)\right] \quad \text{mit} \quad a, b > 0 \tag{2}$$

wobei $z_{M,0}$ die Eindringtiefe der Kanüle ist, die aufgrund einer deformierenden Kraft F erzeugt wird. Der Parameter z_M ist daher eine Funktion der Kraft F, deren Zusammenhang aus experimentell gewonnenen Daten bestimmt werden kann [2]. Die Parameter a und p repräsentieren die elastomechanischen Eigenschaften der Membran. Mit der Wahl des Parameters p lässt sich zudem graphisch die Steilheit des Deformationsprofils beeinflussen, so dass sowohl das Modell von Sun et al. als auch andere, im Experiment beobachtbare Deformationsprofilverläufe simuliert werden können, wie die Abbildung 1C exemplarisch zeigt.

2.2 Haptische Modellierung

Als haptisches System kommt das SensAble PHANTOM®Omni™ zum Einsatz, welches durch seine sechs Freiheitsgrade alle Bewegungen, die bei einer intrazytoplasmatischen In-Vitro-Fertilisation mit der Kanüle durchgeführt werden, ermöglicht. Darüber hinaus werden keine besonderen Anforderungen an das verwendete Computersystem gestellt. Für die Systementwicklung wird die Programmiersprache C++ unter der Entwicklungsumgebung Microsoft Visual C++ 6.0 benutzt. Die Visualisierung des Prozesses erfolgt mit Hilfe von OpenGL unter Verwendung von „Blending" und „Texturing", um eine möglichst realistische Darstellung zu erzielen. Als Datenmodell wird ein dem Masse-Feder-Modell ähnlicher Ansatz gewählt, wobei lediglich die Knoten (Nodes) berücksichtigt werden. Für jeden Knoten werden aktuelle Position, Ausgangsposition und Status gespeichert. Aus der Literatur ist bekannt, dass die für eine Perforation der Zellmembran notwendige Kraft etwa 10-50 μN beträgt [2]. Bei einem Kraftübertragungsfaktor von 1000 ist am haptischen Gerät eine Kraft von ca. 10-50 mN aufzuwenden. Damit können die auftretenden Kräfte gut wahrgenommen werden, ohne dass durch erhöhten Kraftaufwand eine rasche Ermüdung des Benutzers eintritt. Die zur Berechnung der Deformation benötigte Zeit beträgt auf einem Intel Core 2 Duo 6600 (1 Core-Nutzung) für 2500 Knoten weniger als 1 ms, so dass die Zelldeformation faktisch in Echtzeit erfolgt.

2.3 Praktische Anwendung

Als praktische Anwendung des haptischen Zellmodells wird eine in-vitro Fertilisation (ISCI) gewählt. Zur Anpassung des Deformations- und Perforationsverhaltens der simulierten Eizelle werden Bildreihen von realen in-vitro Fertilisationen verwendet, um das biomechanische Verhalten der simulierten Eizelle an der realen Eizelle anzupassen [1, 4]. Um das dynamische Verhalten realer ISCI im Vergleich zur Simulation untersuchen zu können, werden zusätzlich zu den Bildreihen auch Videos von intrazytoplasmatischen Spermieninjektionen herangezogen.

3 Ergebnisse

Mit Hilfe der vorgestellten Modelle lässt sich die Deformation einer kugelförmigen Zelle durch eine Kanüle am Beispiel einer in-vitro Fertilisation realitätsnah

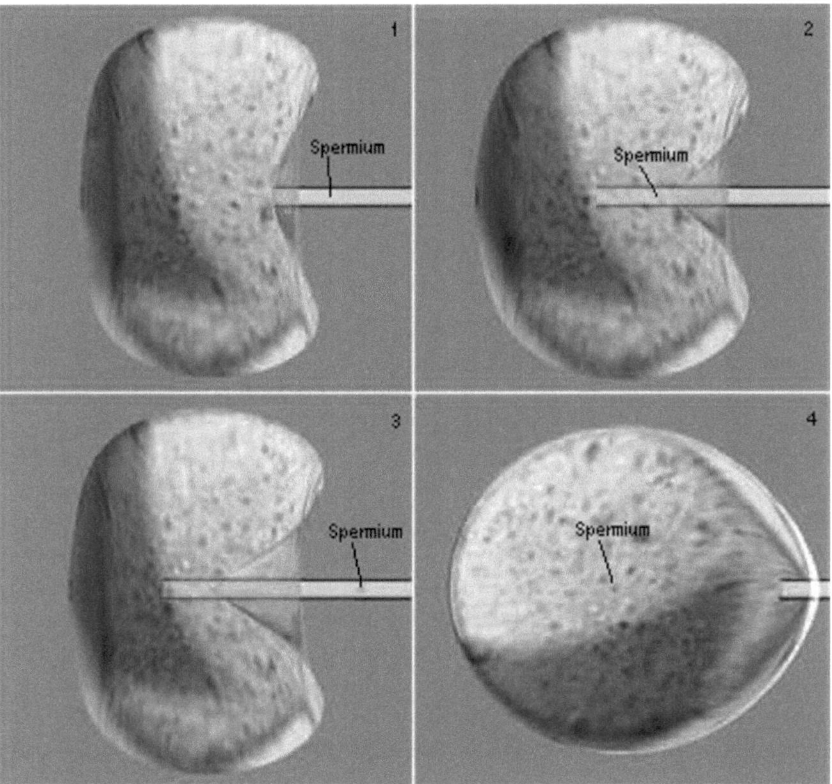

Abb. 2. Bildreihe der simulierten ICSI; 1. Deformation der Membran durch die Mikropipette; 2. Eizelle nach Perforation; 3. Aspiration des Zytoplasmas; 4. Eizelle nach erfolgter Spermieninjektion.

simulieren. Abbildung 2 zeigt einige Bilder einer solchen simulierten in-vitro-Fertilisation. Zunächst erfolgt die Heranführung der Kanüle an die modellierte Eizelle und die Erzeugung des Deformationsprofils (Bildteil 1). Danach wird die Membran durchstoßen und die Kanüle befindet sich im Zellinneren (Bildteil 2). Anschließend erfolgt eine Aspiration des Zytoplasmas mit anschließender Ausschwemmung der Spermien (Bildteil 3). Nach Beendigung dieser Prozedur wird die Kanüle wieder aus der Zelle herausgezogen (Bildteil 4). Dabei erfolgt eine typische Umkehr des Deformationsprofils, welches sich ebenfalls mit den Modellen (1) und (2) erreichen lässt.

4 Diskussion

Die Ergebnisse verdeutlichen, dass mit einfachen haptischen Deformationsmodellen durchaus realistische Szenen von Zellpenetrationen in Echtzeit erzeugt werden können. Durch die Skalierung der für die Durchstoßung der Membran notwendigen Kraft wird auch das Trainieren solcher Eingriffe möglich. Eine vollständige biomechanische Modellierung unter Einbeziehung sämtlicher mechanischer Parameter würde zweifelsohne die Form der Deformationen noch realistischer machen, was jedoch zu einem Performanzproblem führen würde. In diesem Fall müssten die biomechanischen Differentialgleichungen, die die Deformation vollständig beschreiben, für jede Kanülenbewegung neu gelöst werden, was so rechenintensiv ist, dass eine Echtzeit-Simulation kaum erreicht werden kann.

Da die gesamte Wahrnehmung eines Übenden bei der Benutzung eines haptischen Systems zum größten Teil aus dem visuellen Eindruck besteht, erscheinen kleinere Abweichungen bei der Darstellung der Deformation durchaus tolerabel, wie auch andere Untersuchen zeigen [5]. Vor diesem Hintergrund erscheint der vorgestellte Ansatz mit seiner visuell realitätsnahen Simulation als interessante und performante Alternative zu vollständig physikalisch basierten Modellen.

Bevor dieses System in der Praxis eingesetzt werden kann, bedarf es einer Evaluation durch erfahrene Praktiker. Darüber hinaus sollte zur Erhöhung der Performance eine Multi-Core Nutzung und ggf. GPU-Nutzung moderner Grafikkarten erwogen werden.

Literaturverzeichnis

1. Zentrum für Reproduktionsmedizin Kriobank, Video einer ICSI [Online]. [2005?] [cited 2008 Jun 18]. Available from: http://www.kriobank.pl.
2. Sun Y, Wan KT, Roberts K, et al. Mechanical property characterization of mouse zona pellucida. IEEE Tran Nano Biosci. 2003;2(4):279–286.
3. Pillarisetti A, Pekarev M, Brooks AD, et al. Evaluating the role of force feedback for biomanipulation tasks. Proc IEEE Symp: Haptic Interfaces Virtual Environment Teleoperator Systems. 2006.
4. De PESE/ICSI behandeling, Punctie bij ICSI [Online]. [2006?] [cited 2008 Jun 18]. Available from: http://mencoengeraldien.wordpress.com/de-behandeling/.
5. Yamamoto T, Okamura AM. Evaluation of human performance with kinematic and haptic errors. Proc IEEE EuroHaptics Conference. 2007; p. 78–83.

Mehrstufige zeit- und bewegungsabhängige Rauschreduktion in Echtzeit mittels CUDA

Elmar Bührle[1], Benjamin Keck[1,2], Stefan Böhm[3], Joachim Hornegger[1]

[1]Lehrstuhl für Mustererkennung, Martensstraße 3, 91058 Erlangen
[2]Siemens Healthcare, CV, Medical Electronics & Imaging Solutions, Postfach 3260, 91050 Erlangen
[3]Siemens Healthcare, Imaging & IT, Angiography, Siemensstr. 1, 91301 Forchheim
elmar@buehrle.org

Kurzfassung. Dieser Beitrag beschäftigt sich mit der Echtzeit 2D-Bildverarbeitung mittels NVIDIAs CUDA-Schnittstelle anhand des gewählten komplexen Filters. Es werden verschiedene Optimierungsdetails hevorgehoben und erläutert, die für CUDA-Implementierungen verallgemeinert werden können. Dabei erzielt unsere Umsetzung eine Beschleunigung um den Faktor 45 gegenüber der Referenzimplementierung auf CPU-Basis und ist damit zu aktueller Spezialhardware konkurrenzfähig.

1 Einleitung

Die Bildgebung interventionell genutzter Angiographieanlagen mittels Röntgentechnologie stellt heute sehr hohe Anforderungen an die Bildqualität. Die Bildqualität wird durch verschiedenste Faktoren beeinflusst und ist für den Echtzeitbetrieb sicherzustellen, d.h. typischerweise sind die Algorithmen zur Bildverbesserung für einen maximalen Datenstrom von 480-600MBits/s (monoplan-System) bei einer maximalen Latenz von ca. 100 ms auszuführen. Für unsere Untersuchung haben wir einen mehrstufigen zeit- und bewegungsabhängigen Rauschreduktionsalgorithmus gewählt, der in kommerziellen Angiographiegeräten verwendet wird. Die Berechnungsgeschwindigkeit von Bildverarbeitungsalgorithmen ist sowohl von der Komplexität der Algorithmen als auch von der verwendeten Hardware abhängig. Um die Echtzeitfähigkeit des Systems bei der Verarbeitung der akquirierten Bildfolge zu garantieren, muss bei vielen Produkten auf Spezialhardware, wie z.B. DSPs oder FPGAs, zurückgegriffen werden. Die Konsequenz ist ein erhöhter Aufwand für die Hardware-Entwicklung und für die Implementierung der Algorithmen auf der Spezialhardware.

Im Jahre 2007 stellte der Grafikprozessorhersteller NVIDIA gemeinsam mit einer neuen Generation von Grafikprozessoren (GPUs) eine Programmierschnittstelle namens "Common Unified Device Architecture"(CUDA) vor. Mithilfe einfacher Erweiterungen der Programmiersprache C kann eine CUDA-fähige Grafikkarte zur Berechnung verschiedenster Algorithmen verwendet werden. Die erste Generation entsprechender GPUs (G80) erreichte durch die extreme Parallelität bereits eine Leistung von mehr als 300 Gigaflops.

In unserer Untersuchung gehen wir auf die Eignung der im Vergleich zu Spezialhardware günstigeren, sowohl leicht integrierbaren als auch vergleichsweise einfach programmierbaren Hardware am Beispiel des gewählten Algorithmus ein.

2 Stand der Forschung und Beitrag

Die Eignung von Grafikkarten zur Beschleunigung von Berechnungen im Bereich der Medizinischen Bildverarbeitung wird bereits seit über einem Jahrzehnt erforscht [1]. Mack et. al. zeigten 2004 [2] die Verwendbarkeit von Grafikkarten im Bereich der "Echtzeit-Röntgenbildverarbeitung", wobei die verwendeten Algorithmen mittels Direct3D auf die bisherige Rendering Pipeline abgebildet wurden. Algorithmen werden dabei mittels Shader-Programmiersprachen wie GLSL oder HLSL in die spezialisierte Grafikwelt abgebildet. Die effiziente Umsetzung von Algorithmen auf GPUs mittels CUDA konnte bereits 2007 im Bereich der 3D-Rekonstruktion gezeigt werden [3]. In unserem Beitrag möchten wir die Eignung von GPUs zur Echtzeit 2D-Bildverarbeitung mittels CUDA und die dabei zu beachtenden Programmiertechniken anhand eines Beispielalgorithmus erläutern.

3 Methoden und Algorithmen

Bei dem beschriebenen Filter handelt es sich um ein rekursives zeitliches Filter erster Ordnung, das die Filterwirkung an die Bewegung im Bild adaptiert. Die Bewegungserkennung und Filterung erfolgt in einer Auflösungshierarchie. Im Folgenden wird das Filter als multiskalares Rauschglättungsfilter mit Bewegungsdetektion bezeichnet. Die wesentlichen Schritte der Filterung sind die Dekomposition in eine Laplace-Auflösungshierarchie [4] und eine kantenerhaltende Rauschglättung auf variablen Stufen der Laplace-Pyramide.

3.1 Laplace-Auflösungshierarchie

Die Laplace-Pyramide ist ein wesentliches Konzept in der Bildverarbeitung [4] und wird im beschriebenen Algorithmus zur Dekomposition verwendet. Die anschließende Ortsfilterung dient einerseits als Vorverarbeitungsschritt für die Bewegunsdetektion und andererseits als Ergänzung zum Temporalfilter. Bei der Verwendung von GPUs zur Beschleunigung rechenintensiver Anwendungen muss Folgendes beachtet werden: Teure Zugriffe auf den globalen Grafikspeicher, die jeweils 400 bis 600 Taktzyklen (vgl. [5], S.49) benötigen, können durch den Einsatz von Texturen (Texturcache) vermieden werden. Zugriffe auf den Texturcache erreichen dabei eine ähnliche Latenz wie auf Register. NVIDIAs Speicherverwaltungseinheit unterstützt das Lesen von 32-, 64- oder 128-bit Werten, wobei die maximale Datenrate beim Lesen von 32-bit Werten erreicht wird. In unserem Fall jedoch liefert das Akquisitionsgerät 16-bit breite Daten. Die Geschwindigkeit des Reduktions- und des Expansionsschrittes ist auf Grund der geringen Anzahl an arithmetischen Befehlen durch die Speicherbandbreite limitiert. Dies entspricht einem niedrigen Verhältnis von Rechenoperationen pro Speicherzugriff.

Beide Probleme werden durch die folgende Strategie gelöst: Durch das Zusammenfassen von zwei oder vier, in x-Richtung nebeneinanderliegenden Bildpunkten werden Speicheroperationen optimiert. Dies führt im Fall von 16-bit Werten zu Speicherzugriffen von nunmehr mindestens 32-bit, wodurch in einem Thread die optimale Speicherbandbreite ausgenutzt und das Verhältnis von Rechenoperationen pro Speicherzugriff gesteigert wird.

3.2 Varianzgesteuertes Glättungsfilter

Das varianzgesteuerte Glättungsfilter beschreibt die Tiefpassfilterung eines Bildpunktes entlang der Richtung, die bezüglich einer lokalen Nachbarschaft die minimale Varianz aufweist. Dadurch wird eine kantenerhaltende Rauschreduktion erreicht. Obwohl die Glättungsrichtung und die der minimalen Varianz übereinstimmen, muss die lokale Nachbarschaft des Glättungskerns nicht notwendigerweise der Nachbarschaft der Varianzberechnung entsprechen.

Analog zur Implementierung der Laplace-Pyramide werden hier auf Grund der lokalen Speicherzugriffe Texturen eingesetzt. Die relativ zum Mittelpunkt definierten Richtungen können aus Effizienzgründen im Constant Memory abgelegt werden, wodurch Mehrfachzugriffe pro Richtung effizient den Constant Cache nutzen.

Eine weitere Optimierung ist das Entrollen von Programmschleifen (loop unrolling). Obwohl CUDA hierfür die Compileranweisung *#pragma unroll* zur Verfügung stellt, wurden die vorkommenden verschachtelten Schleifen in unserem Fall nicht vollständig entrollt. Durch den Einsatz von (nicht offiziell unterstützter) Template-Metaprogrammierung konnten wir schleifenähnliche Strukturen nachbilden, die in jedem Fall entrollt werden.

Diese definitive Entrollung der Schleifen ermöglicht einen weiteren Optimierungsschritt: Die relativ zum Mittelpunkt definierten Richtungen der Varianzberechnung können nunmehr im Code als *switch*-Block realisiert werden, wodurch der Zugriff auf den Constant Memory für die Berechnung entfällt.

3.3 Multiskalares Rauschglättungsfilter mit Bewegungsdetektion

Ein Bewegungsdetektor kann durch den Vergleich zwischen den verschiedenen Stufen der Laplace-Hierarchie von $n-1$ bereits gefilterten Bildern ($s_{\text{filtered}}^{(n-1,2,..)}$) und dem aktuellen Bild effizient realisiert werden. Durch die Kombination einer Laplace-Pyramide, eines varianzgesteuerten Glättungsfilters und eines Bewegungsdetektors erhält man das multiskalare Rauschglättungsfilter mit Bewegungsdetektion (vgl. Abbildung 1). Dieses ermöglicht eine Rauschreduktion durch die Filterung der oberen Bandpassstufen mit dem varianzgesteuerten Filter, zusätzlich kombiniert mit der zeitlichen Änderung der Bildfolge.

Da der Registerverbrauch dem der optimierten Laplace-Pyramide ähnlich ist, können effizient mehrere Werte auf einmal verarbeitet werden.

4 Evaluierung und Ergebnisse

Aufgrund der Komplexität wurde die Optimierung des varianzgesteuerten Glättungsfilters priorisiert. Durch den Einsatz von Fließkommaarithmetik entstehen geringe Werteabweichungen zwischen der Referenz und der auf der GPU berechneten Bilder. Insgesamt entsteht dabei im Beispielbild eine durchschnittliche Abweichung aller Werte von lediglich $7.2 \cdot 10^{-6}$ für einen Wertebereich von 0 bis 4095. Die fehlerhaften Werte weichen im Schnitt um 1.27% vom Ergebnis der Referenzimplementierung ab.

Das multiskalare Filter hingegen zeigt mit einem durchschnittlichen Fehler von etwa 2.78% stärkere Abweichungen, was wiederum auf die rekursive Struktur des Filters zurückzuführen ist. Zusätzlich entsteht durch die Berechnung mit Fließkommazahlen auf der GPU ein numerischer Unterschied, der jedoch aufgrund der höheren Genauigkeit näher am theoretischen Ergebnis liegt.

Die unterschiedlichen Berechnungszeiten der einzelnen Stufen des multiskalaren Filters sind in Tabelle 1 aufgezeigt. Hierbei verdeutlicht der Vergleich zwischen einer optimierten CPU-Implementierung und der von uns vorgestellten CUDA Implementierung, gemessen auf der für unsere Tests verwendeten Grafikkarte NVIDIA GeForce 8800 GTX, die deutlich höhere Rechenleistung. Darüberhinaus liegt die Gesamtperformance mit 7.24 ms in einem Bereich, der einen Echtzeitbetrieb ermöglicht!

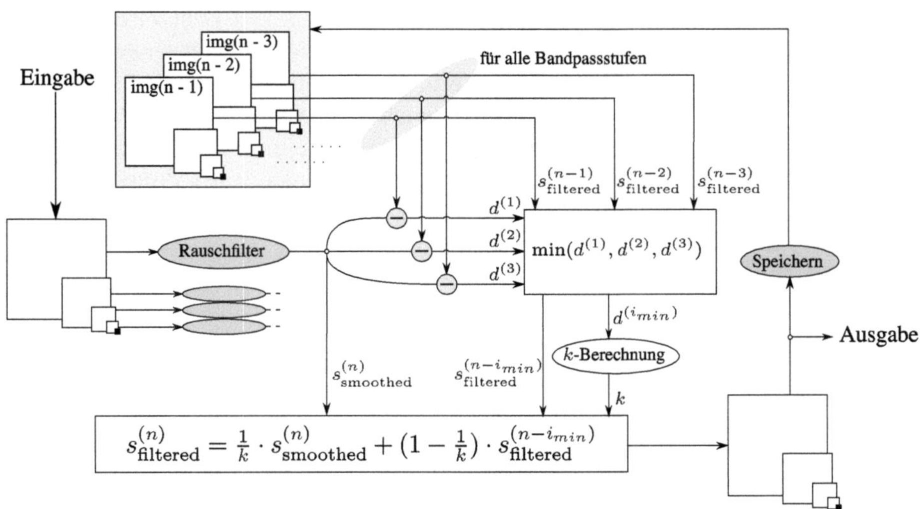

Abb. 1. Verarbeitung der Bandpassbilder mit dem multiskalaren Rauschglättungsfilter; k-Faktor steuert den temporalen Einfluss.

Tabelle 1. Gemessene Zeiten jedes Filterschrittes in ms bzw. Beschleunigungsfaktor zwischen Singlecore und GPU Implementierung.

	Glättungsfilter	Konstruktion Laplace	Rekonstruktion Laplace	Multiskalarer Filter	Kopieren CPU → GPU	Kopieren GPU → CPU	Gesamt
Xeon 2.66 1-Kern	181.59	18.38	15.99	115.35			**331.31**
Xeon 2.66 2-Kern	91.57	9.88	7.91	58.94			**168.30**
GeForce 8800 GTX	3.90	0.86	0.48	0.74	0.60	0.66	**7.24**
Speedup	×46.6	×21.4	×33.3	×155.9			×**45.8**

5 Zusammenfassung und Ausblick

Mit der Einführung von mehrkernbasierten GPUs, wie z.B. NVIDIAs G80, ist es möglich die Anforderungen für Hochleistungsfluoroskopiesysteme in Echtzeit zu erfüllen. Dabei haben wir bezüglich des implementierten Filters einen Geschwindigkeitsvorteil von Faktor 10 über den gegebenen Anforderungen erreicht. Ein weiteres wichtiges Ergebnis erzielten wir durch die Technik der Schleifenentrollung in der Optimierung. Die Verwendung des erweiterten Programmierkonzeptes für Mehrkernarchitekturen (CUDA) und deren 32-bit Gleitkommaverarbeitung kann die zukünftige Entwicklung von medizinischen Echtzeitanwendungen stark vereinfachen. Allerdings müssen interventionelle Röntgensysteme zusätzlich Netzwerkübertragungen, die Archivierung und verschiedene DICOM-Dienste parallel mit einer festen Latenz verarbeiten. Die stabile Hochleistungsverarbeitung eines Bildstroms in Kombination mit einem stark belasteten Prozessor und diesbezüglichen Betriebssystemanforderungen muss daher noch gezeigt werden.

Literaturverzeichnis

1. Mueller K, Yagel R. Rapid 3D cone-beam reconstruction with the algebraic reconstruction technique (ART) by utilizing texture mapping graphics hardware. IEEE Nuclear Science Symposium. 1998;3:1552–1559.
2. Mack M, Hornegger J, Paulus D, et al. Echtzeit-Röntgenbildverarbeitung mit Standardhardware. Proc BVM. 2004; p. 395–399.
3. Scherl H, Keck B, Kowarschik M, et al. Fast GPU-Based CT Reconstruction using the Common Unified Device Architecture (CUDA). In: Frey EC, editor. Nuclear Science Symposium, Medical Imaging Conference 2007; 2007. p. 4464–4466.
4. Burt PJ, Adelson EH. The Laplacian pyramid as a compact image code. IEEE Trans Comm. 1983;31:532–540.
5. NVIDIA. NVIDIA CUDA - Compute Unified Device Architecture - Programming Guide. 2701 San Tomas Expressway, Santa Clara, CA 95050 (USA); 2007.

Kategorisierung der Beiträge

Betrachtetes Organsystem

Primärfunktion des Verfahrens

Art des Projektes

Autorenverzeichnis

Stichwortverzeichnis

Printing: Mercedes-Druck, Berlin
Binding: Stein + Lehmann, Berlin

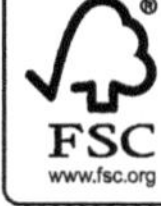

MIX
Papier aus verantwortungsvollen Quellen
Paper from responsible sources
FSC® C105338

If you have any concerns about our products,
you can contact us on
ProductSafety@springernature.com

In case Publisher is established outside the EU,
the EU authorized representative is:
Springer Nature Customer Service Center GmbH
Europaplatz 3, 69115 Heidelberg, Germany

Printed by Libri Plureos GmbH
in Hamburg, Germany